Distal Radius Fractures

Leiv M. Hove • Tommy Lindau
Per Hølmer
Editors

Distal Radius Fractures

Current Concepts

Springer

Editors
Leiv M. Hove, MD, PhD
Department of Orthopaedic Surgery
Haukeland University Hospital
Bergen
Norway

Department of Surgical Sciences
University of Bergen
Bergen
Norway

Tommy Lindau, MD, PhD
The Pulvertaft Hand Centre
Kings Treatment Centre
Royal Derby Hospital
Derby
UK

University of Derby
Derby
UK

Per Hølmer, MD
Department of Orthopedic Surgery
Hand Section
Nordsjelland Hospital
Hillerød
Denmark

Department of Hand
Surgery, Rigshospitalet
University of Copenhagen
Copenhagen
Denmark

ISBN 978-3-642-54603-7 ISBN 978-3-642-54604-4 (eBook)
DOI 10.1007/978-3-642-54604-4
Springer Heidelberg New York Dordrecht London

Library of Congress Control Number: 2014942078

Printed on acid-free paper

Springer is part of Springer Science+Business Media (www.springer.com)

Preface

The forearm represents a critical anatomical unit of the upper extremity, permitting the hand to be placed in any position, to either grasp or support an object. The distal radius and the surrounding joints and soft tissues are essential for these most vital of motions – the orientation and stabilization of the hand, wrist, and forearm. Unfortunately, this anatomical unit is one of the most injured sites of the body.

This book represents a new step in publications from Springer on fractures of the distal radius.

At the 200th anniversary for Abraham Colles' first publication in the English literature about this common fracture, we cannot conclude as he did in 1814: ....“*the limb will again enjoy perfect freedom in all its motions, and be completely free of pain*”.

After all these years, there is no international consensus on how to treat the wide variations in fracture patterns of the distal radius and their associated injuries. Why is there so much controversy in the management of distal radius fractures that the Cochrane Institute is not able to find strong evidence for anything we do in its management?

Thus, the purpose of this textbook is to discuss “all topics” of this most common of long bone fractures. We have asked an international group of 52 expert authors to write the 47 chapters about injuries to these critical “five centimetres” of the upper extremity. The majority of the authors are from the Nordic countries where the incidence of distal radius fractures is the highest in the world. The authors are all experienced and dedicated to the diagnosis, classification, treatment, and rehabilitation of distal radius fractures.

More than ten years have passed since Springer published its classic edition: *A Practical Approach to Management of Fractures of the Distal Radius*. During these ten years, half of all the papers on the topic “distal radius fracture”, listed in PubMed, have been published. Thus there is a strong need for new “current concepts” on this common injury.

This book is not intended to present an extensive review of the literature, but to discuss specific issues of these troublesome injuries.

Bergen, Norway
Derby, UK
Hillerød, Denmark
January 2014

Leiv M. Hove, MD, PhD
Tommy Lindau, MD, PhD
Per Hølmer, MD

Contents

Part III Treatment

Contributors

Antonio Abramo, MD, PhD Department of Hand Surgery, Lund University, Skane University Hospital, Malmö, Sweden

Lars Adolfsson, MD, PhD Department of Orthopaedics, Linköping University Hospital, University of Linköping, Linköping, Sweden

Rohit Arora, MD Department of Trauma Surgery, Medical University Innsbruck, Innsbruk, Austria

Per Aspenberg, MD, PhD Department of Orthopaedic Surgery, Linköping University Hospital, University of Linköping, Linköping, Sweden

Michel E.H. Boeckstyns, MD Clinic for Hand Surgery, Gentofte Hospital – University of Copenhagen, Copenhagen, Denmark

Christina Brudvik, MD, PhD Department of Surgical Sciences, University of Bergen, Bergen, Norway

Accident and Emergency Department, Bergen, Norway

Lene Buch, OT Clinic for Hand Surgery, Gentofte University Hospital, Copenhagen, Denmark

Guillem Salva-Coll, MD, PhD Consultant in Hand and Wrist Surgery, Department of Orthopaedics, Institut Balear de Cirurgia de Mà and Son Llatzer Hospital, Palma de Mallorca, Spain

Michael A.C. Craigen, MD FRCS (Tr Orth) Dipl Hand Surg The Birmingham Hand Centre, Birmingham, UK

Tim Davis, MD Department of Trauma and Orthopaedics, Nottingham University Hospitals, Nottingham University, Nottingham, UK

Karen-Lisbeth Bay Dirksen, MD Department of Radiology, University Hospital of Hillerød, Hillerød, Denmark

Andrew D. Duckworth, MSc, MRCSEd Edinburgh Orthopaedic Trauma Unit, Royal Infirmary of Edinburgh, Edinburgh, UK

Carl Ekholm, MD, PhD Department of Orthopedics, Sahlgrens' University Hospital, University of Gothenburg, Gothenburg, Sweden

Dorte Engelund, MD Hand Surgery Clinic, Department of Orthopedics, Hillerød Hospital, University of Copenhagen, Copenhagen, Denmark

Tapio Flinkkilä, MD Division of Orthopaedic and Trauma Surgery, Department of Surgery, Oulu University Hospital, Oulu, Finland

Anders Ditlev Foldager-Jensen, MD Department of Orthopedic Surgery, Section for Hand Surgery, Aarhus University Hospital, Aarhus, Denmark

Markus Gabl, MD Department of Trauma Surgery, Medical University Innsbruck, Innsbruk, Austria

Marc Garcia-Elias, MD, PhD Consultant in Hand and Upper Extremity Surgery, Institut Kaplan, Barcelona, Spain

Rakel Sif Gudmundsdottir, MD Department of Orthopaedic Surgery, Haukeland University Hospital, Bergen, Norway

Carl-Gøran Hagert, MD, PhD Department of Orthopaedic Surgery, Lund University Hospital, University of Lund, Lund, Sweden

University of Pittsburgh, Pittsburgh, PA, USA

Ola-Lars Hammer, MD Orthopaedic Department, Akershus University Hospital, University of Oslo, Oslo, Norway

Torben B. Hansen, MD, PhD Department of Orthopaedic, Regional Hospital Holstebro, University of Aarhus, Aarhus, Denmark

Jan-Ragnar Haugstvedt, MD, PhD Department of Orthopedics, Østfold Hospital Trust, Moss, Norway

Carlos Heras-Palou, MD Consultant Hand and Wrist Surgery, Pulvertaft Hand Centre, Royal Derby Hospital, Derby, UK

Per Hølmer, MD Department of Orthopedic Surgery, Hand Section, Nordsjelland Hospital, Hillerød, Denmark

Department of Hand Surgery, Rigshospitalet, University of Copenhagen, Copenhagen, Denmark

Leiv M. Hove, MD, PhD Department of Orthopaedic Surgery, Haukeland University Hospital, Bergen, Norway

Department of Surgical Sciences, University of Bergen, Bergen, Norway

Torstein Husby, MD, PhD Section for Hand and Microsurgery, Department of Orthopedic Surgery, Oslo University Hospital, Oslo, Norway

Peter Jørgsholm, MD The Hand Unit, Mølholm Private Hospital, Vejle, Denmark

Per-Olof Josefsson, MD, PhD Department of Clinical Sciences, University of Lund, Lund, Sweden

Departments of Orthopedics, Skåne University Hospital, Malmö, Sweden

Magnus K. Karlsson, MD, PhD Departments of Orthopedics and Clinical Sciences, Skåne University Hospital, Lund University, Malmö, Sweden

Yngvar Krukhaug, MD, PhD Department of Orthopedic Surgery, Haukeland University Hospital, Bergen, Norway

Department of Surgical Sciences, University of Bergen, Bergen, Norway

Hebe Désirée Kvernmo, MD, PhD, MPH Department of Orthopedic, Plastic and Hand Surgery, University Hospital of North Norway, Tromsø, Norway

Department of Clinical Medicine, University of North Norway – Arctic University of Norway, Tromsø, Norway

Benedicte Lange, MD Department of Radiology, University Hospital of Aalborg, Aalborg, Denmark

Tommy Lindau, MD, PhD The Pulvertaft Hand Centre, Kings Treatment Centre, Royal Derby Hospital, Derby, UK

University of Derby, Derby, UK

Margaret M. McQueen, MD, FRCSEd(Orth) Edinburgh Orthopaedic Trauma Unit, Royal Infirmary of Edinburgh, Edinburgh, UK

Cecilia Mellstrand-Navarro, MD Department of Orthopedics, Karolinska Institute, Södersjukhuset, Stockholm, Sweden

Adalsteinn Odinsson, MD Section of Hand Surgery, Department of Orthopaedic Surgery, St Olav's University Hospital, Trondheim, Norway

Kerstin Oestreich, MD, MSc Consultant Paediatric Plastic Surgeon, Children's Hospital, Birmingham, UK

Francisco del Piñal, MD, Dr Med Instituto de Cirugia Plastica y de la Mano, Santander, Spain

Unit of Hand-Wrist and Plastic Surgery, Hospital Mutua Montañes, Santander, Spain

Per-Henrik Randsborg, MD, PhD Health Services Research Unit, Akershus University Hospital, Oslo, Norway

Björn E. Rosengren, MD Departments of Orthopedics and Clinical Sciences, Skåne University Hospital, Lund University, Malmö, Sweden

Kerstin Runnquist, MSc (Orthopedics) Department of Orthopedics, Lunds University Hospital, Lund, Sweden

Camilla Ryge, MD, PhD Section of Hand Surgery, Department of Orthopedics, Hillerød Hospital, University of Copenhagen, Copenhagen, Denmark

Johan Scheer, MD, PhD Department of Orthopaedics, Linköping University Hospital, Linköping, Sweden

Kristbjörg Sigurdardottir, MD Orthopaedic Department, Falun Hospital, Falun, Sweden

Claire K. Simpson, MD FRCS (Tr Orth) Dipl Hand Surg The Birmingham Hand Centre, Birmingham, UK

Niels H. Søe, MD Clinic for Hand Surgery, Gentofte Hospital, University of Copenhagen, Copenhagen, Denmark

Magnus Tagil, MD Department of Hand Surgery, Lund's University Hospital, Lund, Sweden

Department of Orthopedic Surgery, University of Lund, Lund, Sweden

Niels Thomsen, MD, PhD Department of Hand Surgery, Skåne University Hospital, Lund University, Malmø, Sweden

Jarkko Vasenius, MD Hand Surgery and Therapy, Omasairaala Hospital, Helsinki, Finland

Maria Wilcke, MD, PhD Department of Hand Surgery, Karolinska Institute, Södersjukhuset, Stockhom, Sweden

John Williksen, MD Section for Hand and Microsurgery, Department of Orthopedic Surgery, Oslo University Hospital, Oslo, Norway

Part I

Introduction

Distal Radius Fractures: What Is the Problem?

1

Tommy Lindau and Carl Ekholm

Contents

T. Lindau, MD, PhD (✉)
The Pulvertaft Hand Centre, Kings Treatment Centre, Royal Derby Hospital, Uttoxeter Road, Derby, DE22 3NE, UK

University of Derby, Derby, UK
e-mail: tommylindau@hotmail.com

C. Ekholm, MD, PhD
Department of Orthopedics, Sahlgrens' University Hospital, University of Gothenburg, Gothenburg, Sweden

1.1 Summary

Why do we struggle with distal radius fractures as Abraham Colles stated 200 years ago: "… the limb will again enjoy perfect freedom in all its motions, and be completely free of pain"?

Why have half of all the publications on the topic "distal radius fracture", listed in PubMed, been published in the last ten years?

Why is there so much controversy that the Cochrane Institute (2008) cannot find any evidence for anything we do in the management of distal radius fractures?

Why could the American Association for Orthopaedic Surgeons (2009) only find one area of "moderate" evidence, namely, regarding operative treatment: "We suggest operative fixation for fractures with post-reduction radial shortening >3 mm, dorsal tilt >10°, or intra-articular displacement or step-off >2 mm as opposed to cast fixation"?

Why can't we manage this common fracture better in the twenty-first century?

1.2 Factual Background

- Fact – Since the days of Abraham Colles, we know that the number of distal radius fractures is increasing. Today, it is the commonest of all fractures with an incidence of roughly 0.3 % in industrialised countries. The burden of treatment on the orthopaedic community and society in general is obvious.

L.M. Hove et al. (eds.), *Distal Radius Fractures*,
DOI 10.1007/978-3-642-54604-4_1, © Springer-Verlag Berlin Heidelberg 2014

- Fact – Non-osteoporotic patients have more high-energy trauma and intra-articular fractures as opposed to osteoporotic patients, which have more low-energy trauma and extra-articular fractures (Lindau et al. 1999).
- Fact – Until recently few treatment options were available; different splints and casts were supplemented with the possible use of external fixation and the anatomical end result improved but was far from excellent. Fortunately, the typical patient is elderly and seems to tolerate malunion even when the deformity is visible. Today, the use of internal fixation reaches 42 % of all distal radius fractures in some centres (Chung et al. 2011), yet the overall outcome is not proven better than external fixation (Margaliot et al. 2005)!
- Fact – Our treatment goals have always been the same:
  - The patient wants a quick and safe recovery, low treatment risks, restored normal wrist function, and no complications!
  - The treating doctor wants to restore anatomy and function with a reliable method, with a low risk, and without complications or residual deformity!
  - Health-care institutions and society want a healthy population, treatments at low cost, low risk, quick recovery, and no follow-ups!

1.3 So What Is the Problem?

We have identified the following areas of concern:

- Patient-related factors
- Fracture-related factors
- Treatment-related factors
- Outcome measurements

1.4 Patient-Related Factors

- Fact – There is no "gold standard" patient (Fig. 1.1)!
- We have to differentiate whether the patient is a child; a young, active non-osteoporotic adult; an active elderly with possible osteoporosis; or a patient with low functional demands!
- Is the fracture in the dominant or non-dominant hand? Manual or sedentary worker?
- How is the patient's health, what is the socio-economic background, are there co-morbidities (Fig. 1.1a), and are there concomitant injuries?
- Will the patient's bone quality allow reduction to be maintained or implants to be fixed?
- How will the patient tolerate a possible malunion if the fracture is not completely reduced?

1.5 Fracture-Related Factors

- Fact – There is no "gold standard" fracture (Figs. 1.1 and 1.2)!
- Fact – The fracture classifications we use today:
  - Firstly, are too many (Fernandez, AO/OTA, Frykman, Older, Melone, etc.) which demonstrates that none of these fulfil the criteria of a "gold standard" classification
  - Secondly, cannot be reproduced regarding intra- and inter-observer reliability (Andersen et al. 1996)
  - Thirdly, do not correlate with outcome (Flinkkila et al. 1998)
  - Lastly, most likely do not reflect the true nature of the injury!
- Instead of classifications, ask yourself:
  - What is the type of fracture; is it extra- or intra-articular?
  - Is there comminution?
  - What is the amount and direction of displacement (Fig. 1.3)?
  - Are there signs of instability in the fracture (Lafontaine et al. 1989)?
    - Age over 60
    - Dorsal comminution
    - Dorsal displacement >20°
    - Intra-articular radiocarpal fracture
    - Associated ulnar fracture (Fig. 1.4)
  - Should I try to calculate the predictability of instability on http://www.trauma.co.uk/wristcalc (Mackenney et al. 2006)?
  - Is the ulna or DRUJ involved (Fig. 1.4)?
  - Are the fragments fixable (in terms of size and condition) (Figs. 1.2 and 1.3)?
  - Is the extent and nature of the injury visualised well enough, or do we base our fracture

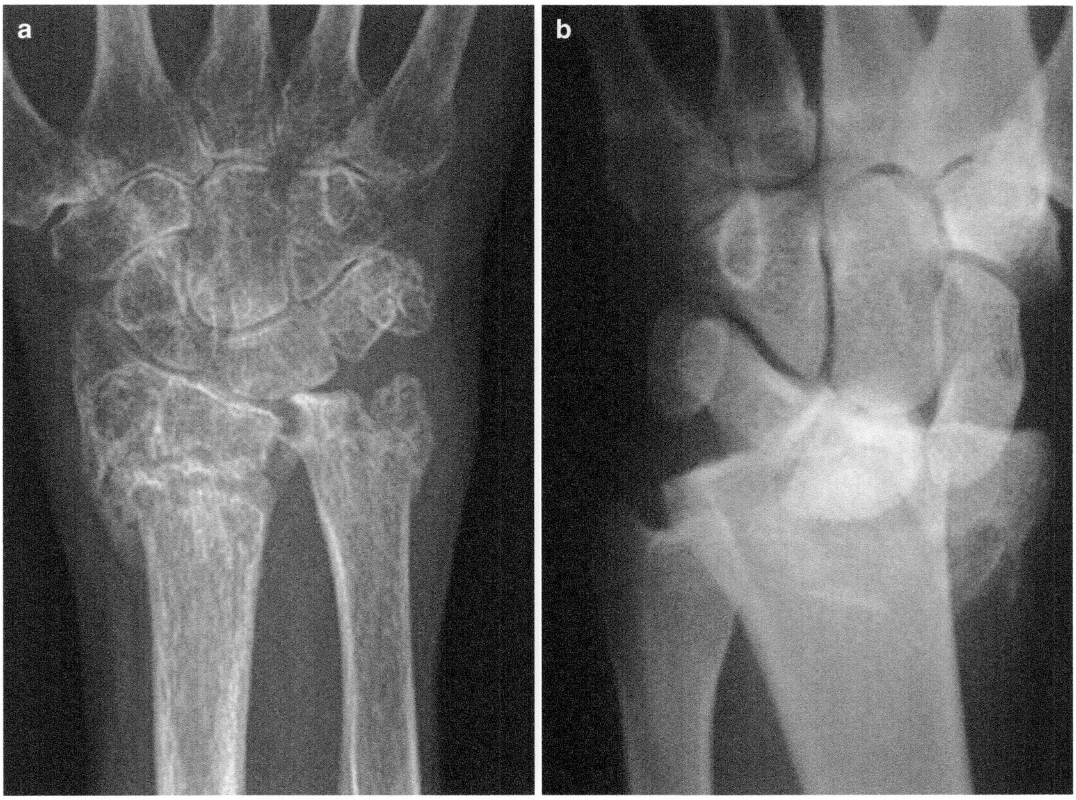

Fig. 1.1 (**a**) X-ray of an undisplaced fracture sustained by low-energy trauma in an elderly woman with rheumatoid arthritis as a significant co-morbidity. (**b**) X-ray of a fracture sustained by high-energy trauma

assessment on poor X-ray films? Do we need post-reduction films and CT (Figs. 1.3 and 1.4)? Should we use arthroscopy as an additional diagnostic tool?

- Can we assess the intermediate column, the so-called critical corner, which often involves the important lunate fossa and its strong extrinsic ligaments that are so hard to fix with standard volar locking plates? These fractures have to be identified before surgery since they require specific treatment, specific fixation methods, and possibly a dedicated wrist surgeon!?
- Can we differ "true" distal radius fractures from the extension of such difficult fractures in "the critical corner" into full-blown radiocarpal fracture dislocations with "teardrop" fragments (Figs. 1.2 and 1.3)?
- Can we understand the fracture's "personality" better by assessing the degree of secondary involvement in the carpus as a part of an incomplete greater arch mechanism injury with either carpal fractures or associated soft tissue ligament injuries (Figs. 1.2 and 1.4)?
- Although strong correlation between final anatomy and hand and wrist function is evident in patients who undergo corrective osteotomy for symptomatic malunion, the correlation is weak even in fairly large studies or meta-analyses of patients being treated for fresh fractures. This may have a number of possible explanations, but it is clear that young patients seem more sensitive to malunion than older. Whether this is due to higher demands, different ligament competence, and different (undiagnosed) soft tissue injury pattern is not known.
- *In short, do we truly understand the fracture's "personality"?*

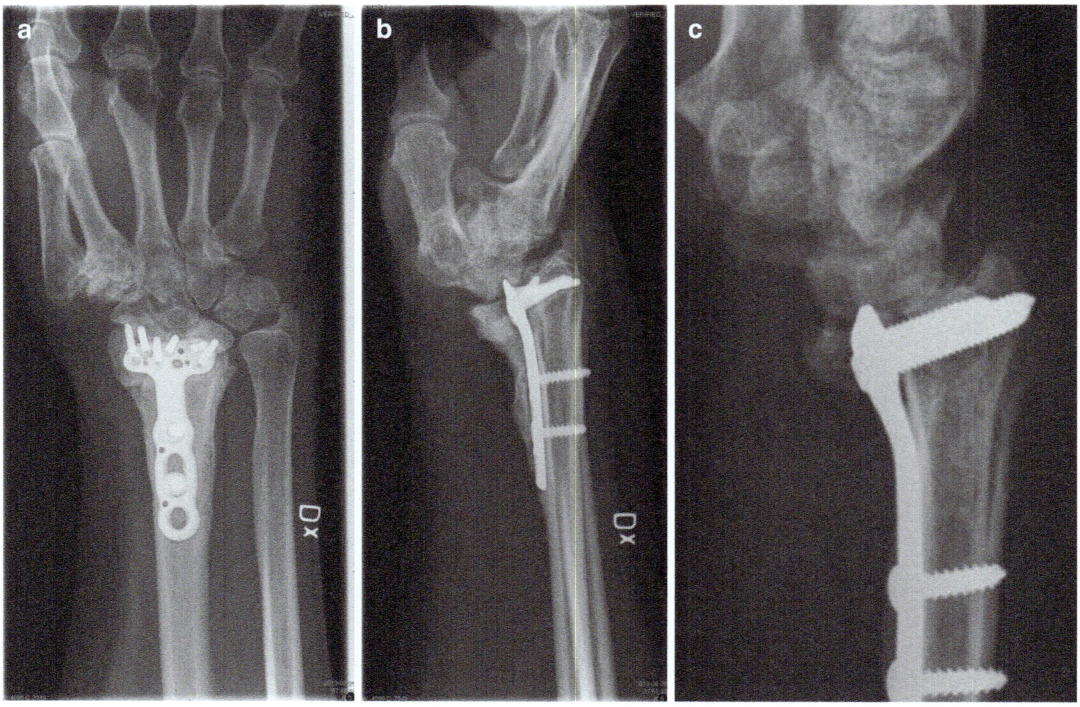

Fig. 1.2 (**a**–**c**) 61-year-old woman with known arthritis, possibly rheumatoid, sustained a dislocated distal radius fracture that was operated on with a volar locking plate. At later follow-up there she presents with radiographic volar carpal dislocation and the plate is digging into the lunate after the ORIF, where the "critical corner" was under-diagnosed and incompletely addressed with the plate. The patient is nevertheless pain-free, has good ROM, and does not want an additional procedure

1.6 Treatment-Related Factors

- Fact – There is no "gold standard" treatment!
- In a meta-analysis comparing 46 articles of 1,520 patients, there was no evidence to support internal fixation (Margaliot et al. 2005).
- A more advanced meta-analysis by the Cochrane Institute (2008) states:
  - *There is insufficient evidence regarding*:
    - *Methods of reduction*
    - *Anaesthesia – reduction*
    - *Conservative interventions*
    - *Surgical treatment*
    - *Bone graft/substitutes*
    - *Rehabilitation*
  - *There is weak support for*:
    - *Percutaneous pinning*
    - *External fixation vs conservative treatment*
  - *There is evidence regarding*:
    - *External fixation to reduce redisplacement*
- There is most likely always an "ideal" or at least "a best treatment" for a patient and his/her fracture. The decision should be "evidence-based", but adaption to the individual patient needs to be "experience-based", and thus much dependent also on the surgeon responsible for the patient.
- So, when choosing a treatment tailored for the patient, ask yourself:
  - *Is the best surgeon assessing the fracture in our fracture clinics?*
  - *What is the weakest link in the treatment chain in my unit?*
  - *Is our surgeon adequately trained for the procedure needed?*
  - *Is the rehabilitation team geared up to manage all patients' needs?*
- How can we achieve and retain reduction and fixation without complications (Figs. 1.2

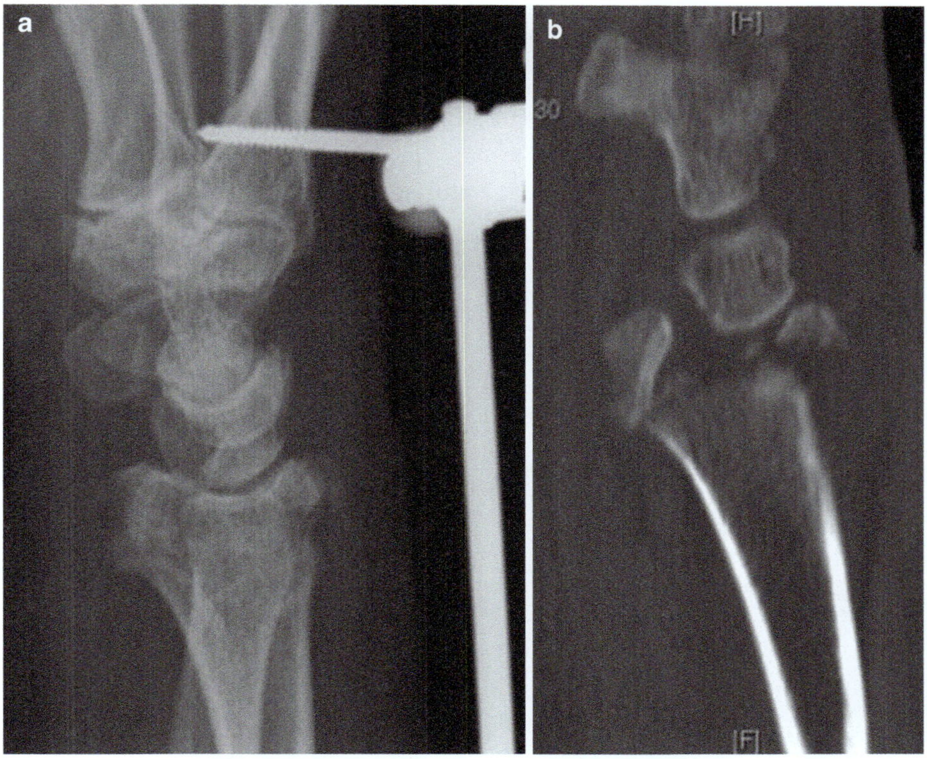

Fig. 1.3 (**a**) Fracture treated with external fixation with a reasonable postoperative X-ray. (**b**) Her X-rays were scrutinised after 10 days and the patient was called back for CT. Gross displacement and 90° rotation of a "teardrop" fragment was found despite close to normal plain film

and 1.3)? The industry has lately provided us with a large number of excellent implants – excellent in the sense that they reliably maintain adequate reduction until the fracture is healed – and volar locking plating has become the mainstay of modern treatment. Disappointingly, despite the increasing implant cost, studies have not really been able to demonstrate parallelism between radiological improvement and functional outcome. In fact, the shear number of implants makes it difficult to choose which one is the best!

1.7 Outcome Measurements

- Fact – There is no "gold standard" outcome measurement!
- What is the ideal outcome measurement?
  - Is objectively measured hand function, such as grip strength and range of motion, correlated with patient-perceived hand function?
  - Is the outcome further influenced by factors such as injury compensation and level of education?
  - Is a hybrid score better and more "objective" such as the Gartland and Werley system or the Green and O'Brien?
  - Is a patient-based questionnaire best: the Disabilities of the Arm, Shoulder, and Hand (DASH), the Patient-Related Wrist Evaluation (PRWE), the Patient-Rated Wrist/Hand Evaluation (PRWHE), or the Michigan Hand Outcomes Questionnaire (MHQ)? Do they pose the questions that best describe the perceived hand function for each patient category?
- It is virtually impossible to predict outcome in this massively diverse group of patients with distal radius fractures, where the groups are not homogenous enough in terms of age,

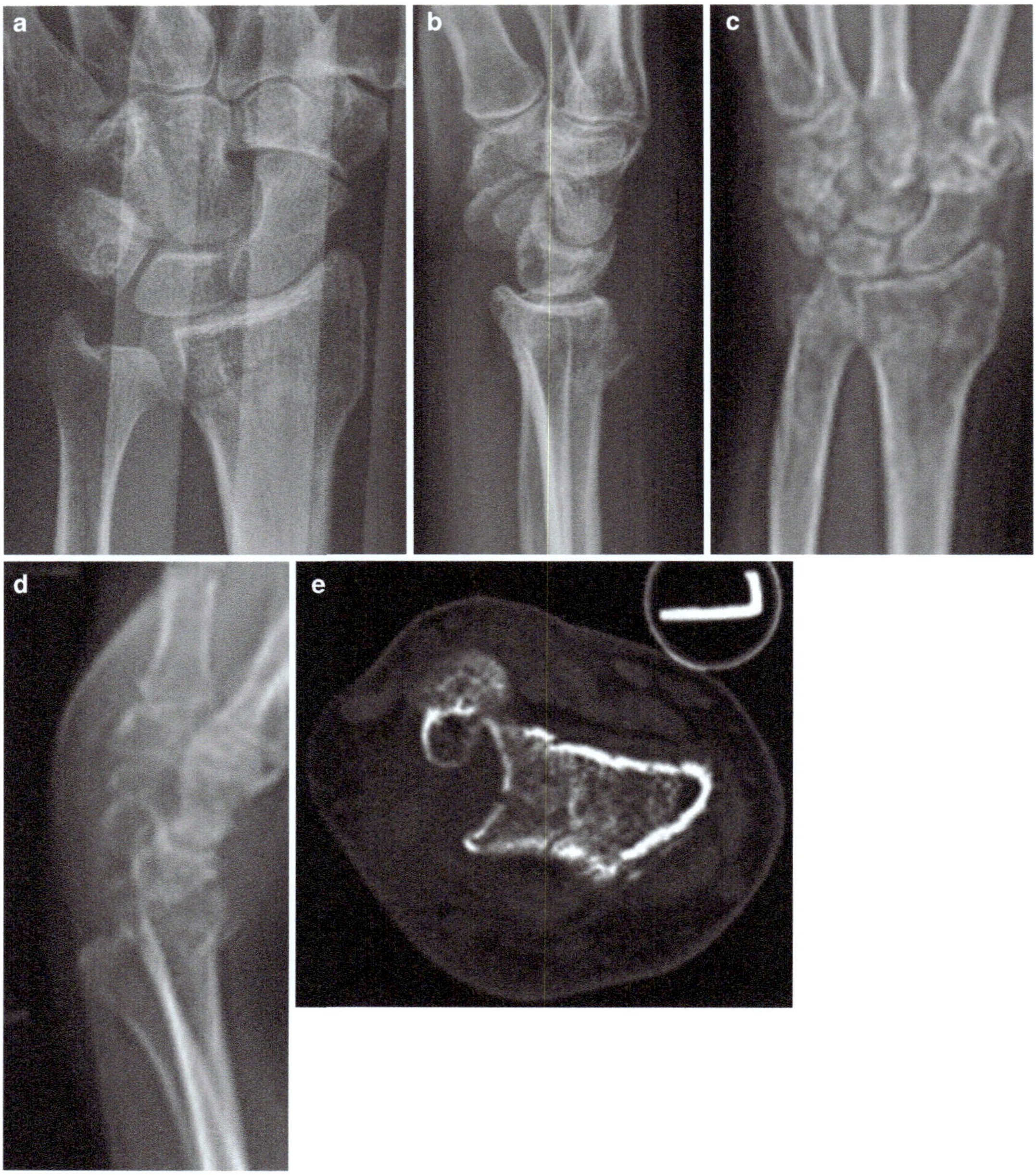

Fig. 1.4 (**a**, **b**) 52-year-old lady sustains a distal radius fracture with minimal dorsal comminution and displacement. (**c**, **d**) At follow-up consultation after 3 months, she presents with locked rotation in the distal forearm. The DRU joint was dislocated and volar corner of sigmoid notch wedged into ulnar head. (**e**) CT scan shows the severity of this supposedly simple minimally displaced distal radius fracture

gender, fracture type, soft tissue injury, demands/expectations, or other factors that we still do not know of.

- Our methods of evaluating the outcome are almost always not sensitive enough. In fact, our attempts of achieving evidence-based medicine are difficult as our sample sizes often are reasonable for a unit, but not to confirm evidence. In a randomised controlled trial of 116 patients comparing cast with external fixation, there was no difference after 2 years. A power calculation showed that 1,200 patients were needed to prove the benefit of surgery (Kreder et al. 2006). Increasing the size of the study group may not necessarily solve this dilemma, and narrowing the inclusion criteria will certainly make studies more difficult to execute. It can also be argued that if a study needs 1,200 patients to demonstrate the effect of a certain treatment, the effect may not be clinically important.

1.8 In Summary: The Future Holds the Answer!

- The future challenge will be to treat the increasing number of distal radius fractures safely, predictably, and at a reasonable cost. Ideally this means that we should operate only on patients who will benefit from the procedure and then tailor the optimal method considering costs, side effects, clinical burden, etc.
- The key to success is to identify the patient's "personality" (Fig. 1.1)!
- A further key to success is to combine the patient's personality with a full understanding of "the personality" of the fracture (Figs. 1.2 and 1.3)!
- Once these two "personalities" have been detected, then to tailor the treatment to the patients needs and the ideal way of treating the fracture ought to be easy!
- We should, however, avoid to overtreat patients. This might be difficult especially in times when volar locking plates that dominate the market may drive the surgeon into a view of "fix-them-all". Yet we should not neglect and under-treat others, who may develop long-term disability, possibly with a symptomatic malunion.
- We have to design future studies better in order to focus on solving the issues regarding patient-, fracture-, and treatment-related factors with the best outcome measurement available. Multicentre studies or studies designed by national societies must be considered rather than personal case series of outcome. Furthermore, it is equally essential to analyse the "outliers" as it is to draw conclusions based on statistical significance of the mean, mainstream patients. The outliers teach us more what to avoid, yet they skew the outcome of the study and still causes the individual and society great problems.
- We are convinced that the future holds the answer, provided we learn how to identify the right treatment for each patient!

References

American Association of Orthopaedic Surgeons (AAOS) Guideline on the treatment of distal radius fractures. 2009. http://www.aaos.org/Research/guidelines/DRFguideline.asp

Andersen DJ, Blair WF, Steyers Jr CM, Adams BD, el-Khouri GY, Brandser EA. Classification of distal radius fractures: an analysis of interobserver reliability and intraobserver reproducibility. J Hand Surg Am. 1996;21A(4):574–82.

Chung KC, Shauver MJ, Yin H, Kim HM, Baser O, Birkmeyer JD. Variations in the use of internal fixation for distal radial fracture in the United States medicare population. J Bone Joint Surg Am. 2011;93A(23):2154–62.

Flinkkilä T, Raatikainen T, Hämäläinen M. AO and Frykman's classifications of Colles' fracture. No prognostic value in 652 patients evaluated after 5 years. Acta Orthop Scand. 1998;69(1):77–81.

Handoll HHG, Huntley JS, Madhok R. External fixation versus conservative treatment for distal radial fractures in adults. Cochrane Database Syst Rev. 2007;(3):CD006194. doi:10.1002/14651858.CD006194.pub2.

Kreder HJ, Agel J, McKee MD, Schemitsch EH, Stephen D, Hanel DP. A randomized, controlled trial of distal radius fractures with metaphyseal displacement but without joint incongruity: closed reduction and casting versus closed reduction, spanning external fixation, and optional percutaneous K-wires. J Orthop Trauma. 2006;20(2):115–21.

Lafontaine M, Hardy D, Delince P. Stability assessment of distal radius fractures. Injury. 1989;20(4):208–10.

Lindau TR, Aspenberg P, Arner M, Redlundh-Johnell I, Hagberg L. Fractures in the distal forearm in young adults. An epidemiologic description of 341 patients. Acta Orthop Scand. 1999;70(2):124–8.

Mackenney PJ, McQueen, MM, Elton R. Prediction of instability in distal radial fractures. J Bone Joint Surg Am. 2006;88A(9):1944–1951. http://www.trauma.co.uk/wristcalc.

Margaliot Z, Haase SC, Kotsis SV, Kim HM, Chung KC. A meta-analysis of outcomes of external fixation versus plate osteosynthesis for unstable distal radius fractures. J Hand Surg Am. 2005;30A(6):1185–99.

A Historical Review of the Distal Radius Fracture

2

Leiv M. Hove

Contents

L.M. Hove, MD, PhD
Department of Orthopaedic Surgery,
Haukeland University Hospital,
Bergen, N-5021, Norway

Department of Surgical Sciences,
University of Bergen, Bergen, Norway
e-mail: leiv.hove@k1.uib.no

2.1 Summary

The first hint that carpal dislocations sometimes were actually fractures of the distal end of the radius came from the French surgeon Jean-Louis Petit (1673–1750). Another French surgeon, Claude Poteau (1725–1775) was the first who, without question, recognized the lesion as a fracture of the distal end of the radius. However, the Irish surgeon, Abraham Colles (1773–1843) has been given most of the credit for directing the attention of his contemporaries to the underlying nature of these injuries. His famous paper was, however, published in a provincial medical journal, and like Pouteau's paper, it received little attention. It was the famous French surgeon, Guillaume Dupuytren (1774–1835) that brought these fractures to the attention of the surgical world at large. Dupuytren based his observations on a large number of postmortem examinations and demonstrated that these injuries were fractures. He also described the morphology of the different fracture patterns.

2.2 Early History

The story must begin with Hippocrates (460–371 BC) who described different traumatic injuries of the wrist. However, he and his successors described the wrist injuries as distortions, subluxations, radiocarpal luxations, or dislocations (separation) of the distal radioulnar joint.

L.M. Hove et al. (eds.), *Distal Radius Fractures*,
DOI 10.1007/978-3-642-54604-4_2, © Springer-Verlag Berlin Heidelberg 2014

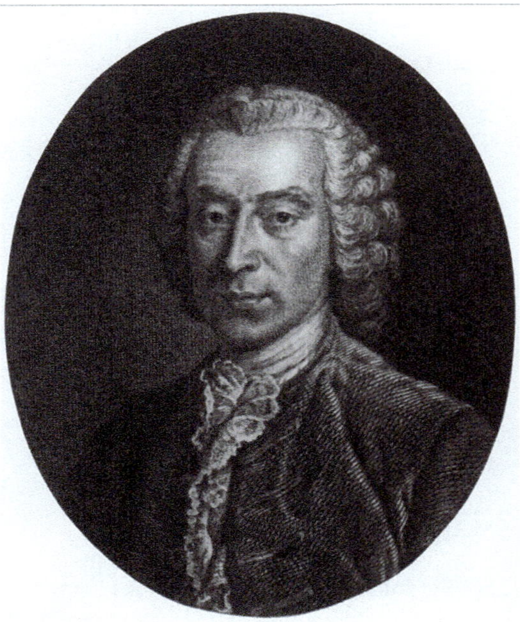

Fig. 2.1 Claude Poteau, the French surgeon who was the first to recognize a fracture of the distal end of the radius

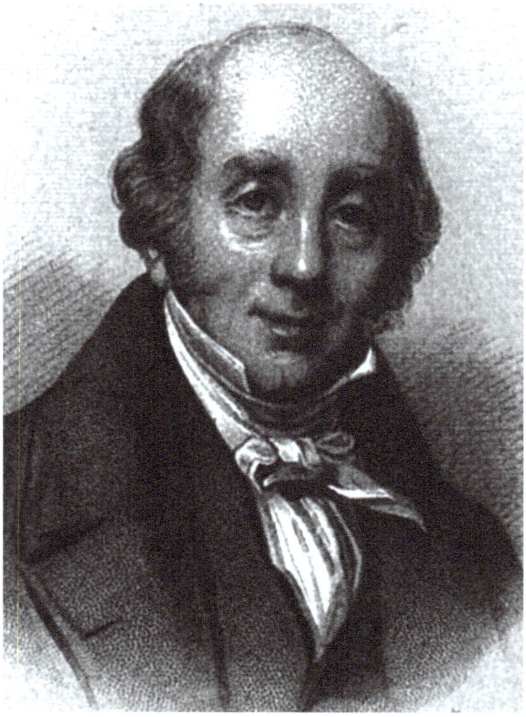

Fig. 2.2 Abraham Colles, the Irish surgeon who described Colles' fracture in 1814

The first hint that the carpal dislocations sometimes were actually fractures of the distal end of the radius came from the French surgeon *Jean-Louis Petit* (1673–1750). He was the first head of the Royal French Academy of Surgery, founded in 1731 (Petit 1705).

Another French surgeon, *Claude Poteau* (1725–1775) was the first who, without question, recognized the lesion as a fracture of the distal end of the radius (Poteau 1783, published posthumously) (Fig. 2.1)

The Irish surgeon, *Abraham Colles* (1773–1843) has been given most of the credit for directing the attention of his contemporaries to the underlying nature of these injuries (Fig. 2.2). His famous paper "On the fracture of the carpal extremity of the radius" (Colles 1814), was, however, published in a provincial medical journal and, like Pouteau's paper, received little attention (Peltier 1984).

The famous French surgeon, *Guillaume Dupuytren* (1774–1835) (Fig. 2.3), and his contemporaries brought these fractures to the attention of a host of students and surgeons, and through his published lectures, the "Lecons Orales" (1832), to the surgical world at large.

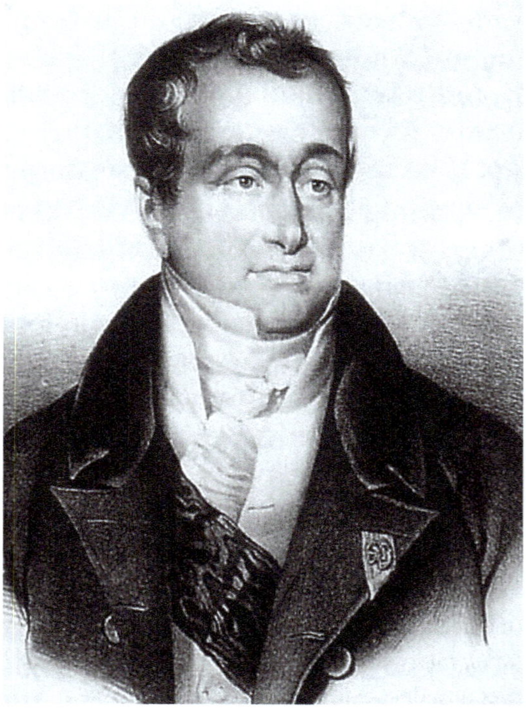

Fig. 2.3 Guillaume Dupuytren, the French surgeon who brought distal radius fracture to the attention to the surgical world at large

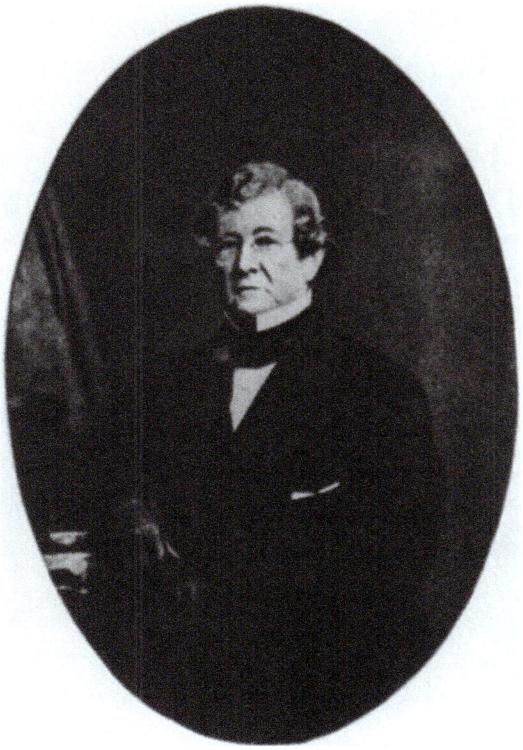

Fig. 2.4 John Lea Barton, an American surgeon described a fracture-dislocation of the radiocarpal joint, known as Barton's fracture

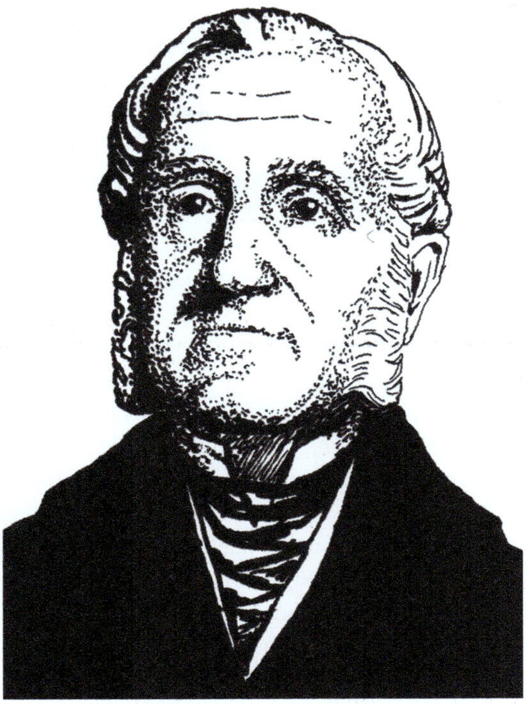

Fig. 2.5 Robert William Smith described the palmar displacement of the distal radius fracture, the Smith's fracture

Dupuytren based his observations on a large number of postmortem examinations that demonstrated to him and his colleagues that these injuries were fractures. He also described the morphology of the different fracture patterns.

Another French surgeon, one of Dupuytren's students, Jean-Gaspard-Blaise Goyrand (1803–1866), continued the anatomical studies and described several different subtypes (Goyrand 1832). Joseph-Francois Malgaigne (1806–1865) and M. Lenoir were also part of Dupuytren's study group and his successors.

In the United States, fractures of the distal end of the radius were also of interest to surgeons. The publication that has made *John Lea Barton* (1794–1871) (Fig. 2.4) most acknowledged in the medical history is his paper: *Views and treatment of an important injury of the wrist*. He described a fracture-dislocation of the radiocarpal joint, known as *Barton's fracture*. The fracture could be on either the dorsal or palmar side of the radius and, similarly, the subluxation or dislocation could displace in either direction (Barton 1838). However, Barton's paper was not based on autopsy specimens, and European surgeons, like Lenoir and Malgaigne, had already described the shearing type of fracture based on postmortem studies (Fernandez and Jupiter 2002).

Fractures featuring palmar displacement of the distal fragment have been attributed to *Robert William Smith* (1807–1873) (Fig. 2.5), the successor at the chair of Abraham Colles. In his monograph *A Treatise on Fractures in the Vicinity of Joints and on Certain Forms of Accidents and Congenital Dislocations*, he included a chapter entitled "Fractures of the Bones of the Forearm." This chapter contains a description of a fracture of the lower extremity of the radius with displacement of the lower fragment forward, i.e., *Smith's fracture* (Smith 1847).

Smith had been unable to obtain an anatomical specimen of this latter fracture, and his description was based entirely on clinical finding (Peltier 1984). Smith also firmly attached the eponym of *Colles' fracture* to the most common fracture of the distal radius.

Three rather well-defined eponymic fractures can be distinguished fractures of the distal radius: Colles', Barton's, and Smith's, although undoubtedly these fracture patterns previously had been described by Pouteau, Lenoir, Goyrand, and other French contemporaries (Peltier 1984, Fernandez and Jupiter 2002). The main reason for these historical misinterpretations may be that the latter had written their papers in the French language.

In the second part of the nineteenth century, a large number of papers were published, based on anatomical dissections and experiments to assess the different trauma types and fracture patterns. The years following *Conrad Röntgen's* (1845–1923) discovery of the x-rays (1895), a great change took place in the study of fractures. Only a few months after Röntgen presented his x-rays, Carl Beck in New York published a series of 44 fractures of the distal radius, diagnosed with the new x-rays (Beck 1898). Another early pioneer from the early days of x-rays, Frederick J. Cotton in Boston, published a series of 140 patients with fractures of the distal radius (Cotton 1900).

During the years from the introduction of the automobile in the late 1800s to the perfection of the electric starter in the 1920s, another type of fracture of the distal radius was diagnosed by x-rays, i.e., "chauffeur's fracture." It was sometimes called the "backfire fracture" as a result of a "backfire" occurring when pulling the crank while starting the car. The fracture was described the same year by F.G. Lund in Boston (1904) and by the French surgeon Just Lucas-Championniere (1904) (Fig. 2.6). The fracture was not given its own eponym, but for many years it was called "*chauffeur's fracture.*" Today, it is most often called a fracture of the radial styloid (Rang 2000).

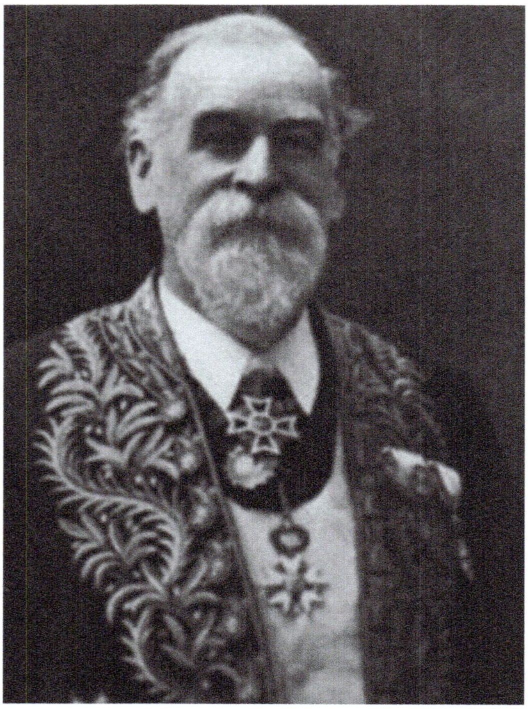

Fig. 2.6 Just Lucas-Championniere, a French surgeon was one of two that described the fracture through the radial styloid, also called "chauffeur's fracture"

2.3 Treatment

2.3.1 Splints

From the time of Hippocrates, the treatment of the "carpal dislocation" had been closed reduction and bandages with linen. Cline of London introduced a straight dorsal splint on the outside of these bandages. The arm was tied up in a sling, and the hand fell in a semiflexed and ulnar deviated position.

The tradition with the use of a splint or an "apparatus" for fractures of the forearm was continued by Colles, Dupuytren, and successors during most of the nineteenth century. Some of the splints forced the wrist into a painful and flexed position, while others kept the hand free, so it would fall on its own weight to a semiflexed and ulnar position (Fenger 1847).

2.3.2 Plaster of Paris

In the antique period of history bandages, linen wraps, or other means were used to achieve tight control over the deformity once it was reduced. The linen might be added water and corn, or wax and resin, to make the bandages stiffer. In the ninth century the Arabic surgeon, Rhazes, described how to add calk and egg

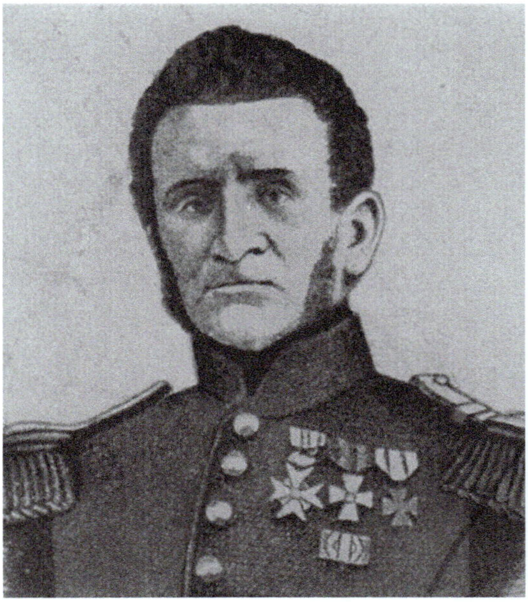

Fig. 2.7 Antonius Mathijsen, a Dutch surgeon introduced plaster treatment for fractures

white to the linen. In 970, in Persia, the surgeon Abu Mansur Muwaffak described a kind of plaster. Much later, in the nineteenth century, the English surgeon William Cheselden (1688–1752) used linen soaked in egg white and starch. Plasters from Arabia, Persia, and India were sent to Europe.

In 1814–16, Pieter Hendriks and Hubenthal were the first to use a plaster, as we know today, for fracture treatment. The man attributed as the first to introduce plaster for fracture treatment at large was the Dutch war surgeon *Antonius Mathijsen* (1805–1878) (Fig. 2.7). This was described in a short paper (1852) and in a large monograph (1854). Plaster for fracture treatment was tested in large scale during the Crimea war (1853–1856). At the same time, both the Russian surgeon, Nikolai Pirogoff, and the American surgeon, Samuel St John, introduced plasters for fracture treatment, without knowing about the papers by Mathijsen.

The treatment of distal radius fracture was non-operative until *Lorenz Böhler* (1885–1953) (Fig. 2.8), during the years after WW1, introduced "pin-and-plaster" technique which anticipated the use of more elaborate external fixators to support the fracture reduction by ligamentotaxis.

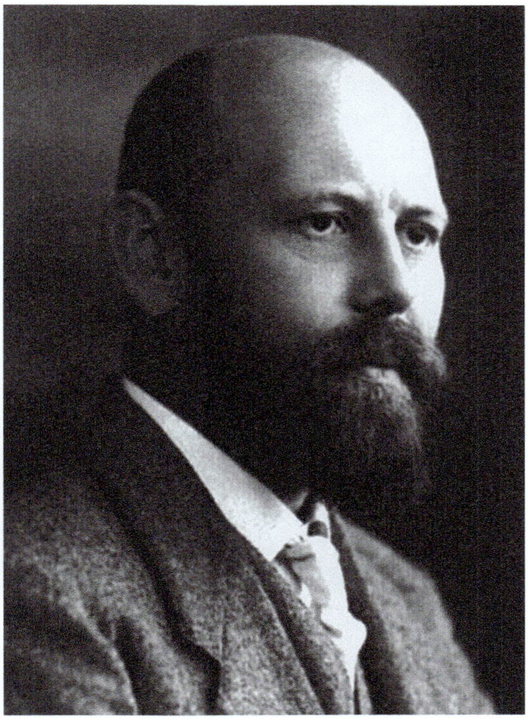

Fig. 2.8 Lorenz Böhler, a German surgeon introduced the "pin-and-plaster" technique for unstable fractures

2.3.3 External Fixation

Both Hippocrates and Paracelsus (1493–1541) made external fixators with wooden or metal bars, connected to rings around the leg. Malgaigne used a clamp to hold a patella fracture fixed. Carl Wilhelm Wutzer (1789–1863) was the first surgeon known to use external fixators with screws through the skin. Von Langenbeck (1810–1887) was a pioneer in the use of external fixation and wrote a paper about it in 1886. Clayton Parkhill (1860–1902) published his paper *A new apparatus for the fixation of bones* and reported of nine successfully treated patients (1897).

In 1900 the Belgian surgeon, *Albin Lambotte* (1866–1956) (Fig. 2.9), presented a "bone suture device." He modified the device to be used for most long bone fractures, including fractures of the distal radius (Fig. 2.10). He introduced the term "external fixation" and was the first to report on pinning of a radial styloid fracture in 1908 (Harness and Meals 2006).

Louis Ombredanne from Paris was the first to use external fixation on pediatric fractures of the distal radius (1929) (Fig. 2.11). The American *Roger Anderson* made a universal frame (Fig. 2.12) for different long bone fractures (1934) and reported on the use of external skeletal fixation to maintain fracture reduction by ligamentotaxis in a distal radius fracture (1944).

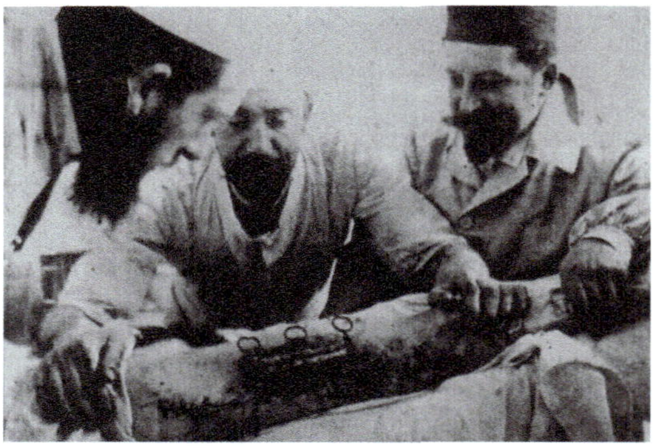

Fig. 2.9 Albin Lambotte, a Belgian surgeon, the father of fracture surgery in Europe, introduced "external fixators" and other operative techniques. The picture shows Lambotte operating in Antwerp/Belgium 1902

In 1938, the Austrian *Raul Hoffmann* (1881–1972) (Fig. 2.13) designed a universal joint for fixation of the metal frame and to adjust the position of the fracture during the treatment period. Unlike the devices designed by Lambotte and Ombredanne, which were "non-bridging," Hoffmann's forearm fixator was designed for fixation in the shaft of the radius and in the second metacarpal, thus "bridging" the wrist joint.

Terry Clyburn and Dietmar Pennig designed "ball joints" in the fixator, to allow for early movements of the wrist joint during treatment. A Norwegian dynamic frame (Dynawrist®), designed by Per Helland, was also introduced in the 1990s, based on the principle of "dynamic traction" (Hove et al. 1999). However, a new mini-fixator which was non-bridging, achieved greater success, and allowed for more "safe" motion of the wrist (McQueen et al. 1996).

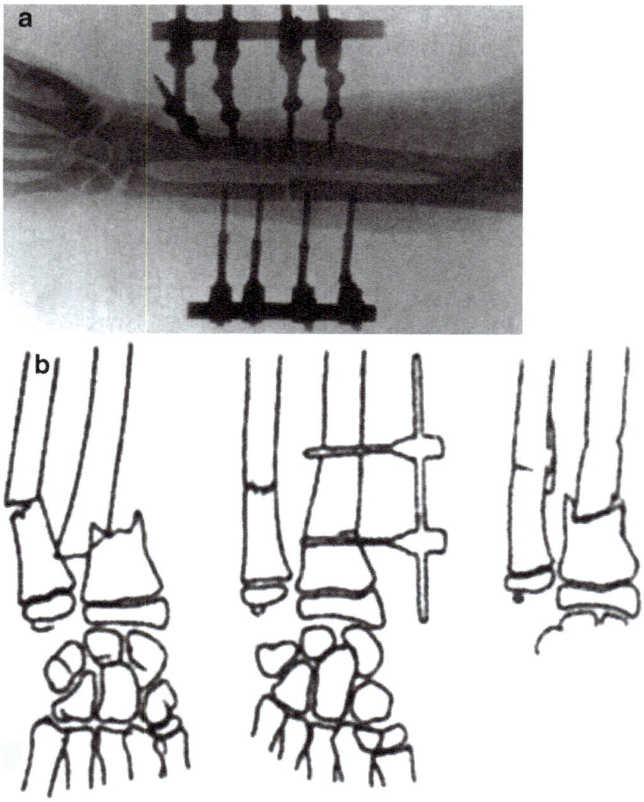

Fig. 2.10 (**a**) Forearm fracture treated with Lambotte fixator (**b**) Lambotte's own sketches of ex-fix of distal forearm fractures

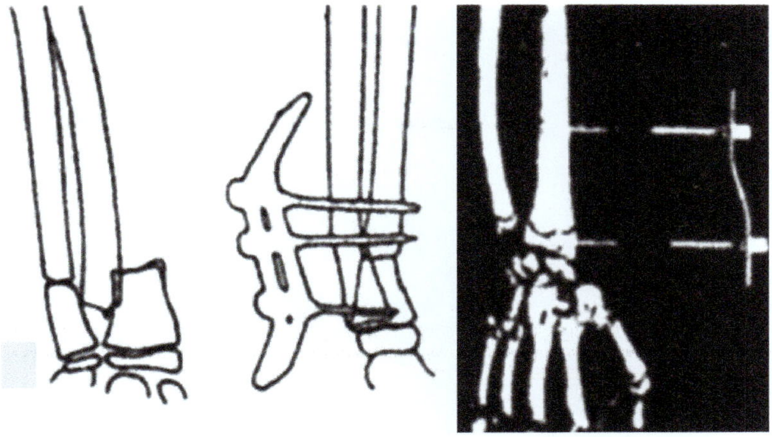

Fig. 2.11 Louis Ombredanne, a French surgeon was the first to use an external fixator on pediatric fractures of the distal radius. The figure shows his non-bridging ex-fix

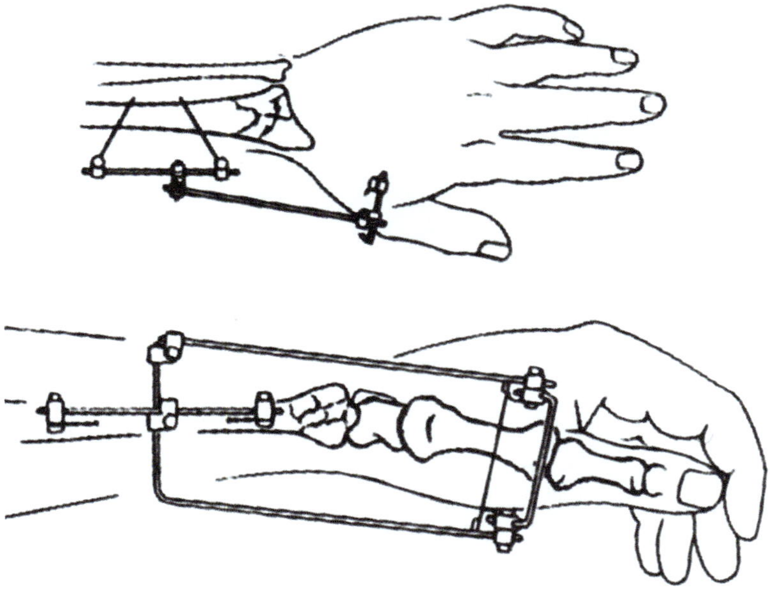

Fig. 2.12 Roger Anderson, an American surgeon, designed a universal frame for different long bone fractures and reported on the use of that device in distal radius fractures

2.3.4 ORIF

In 1861 in San Francisco, Samuel Cooper stabilized a fracture of the patella with a metal suture. He used ethyl alcohol to disinfect the wound and the suture. In 1862 Ernest Julius Gurtl (1825–1899) described the principles for fixation of a fracture with screws, nails, and cerclage. *Joseph Lister* introduced his "antiseptic principles" in 1867 and started treating comminute fractures with open reduction and internal fixation (ORIF).

Themistocles Gluck (1853–1942) made the first nickel plates for fixation of fractures. Sir William Arbuthnot Lane (1856–1938) made screws from steel and later even steel plates (1905). Lambotte introduced the term "osteosynthesis" in 1907 and made his own plates. In 1914 Henry S MacLean made the first compression plates. In 1947, Robert Danis (1880–1962) published his book on operative fracture treatment. The purpose of operative treatment of dislocated fractures was to restore normal anatomy, to create direct bone healing without visible callus formation, and to allow for early, active movements of joints and muscles.

In the early 1950s, James Ellis from England began using a specially designed T-plate to buttress the small marginal fragment in

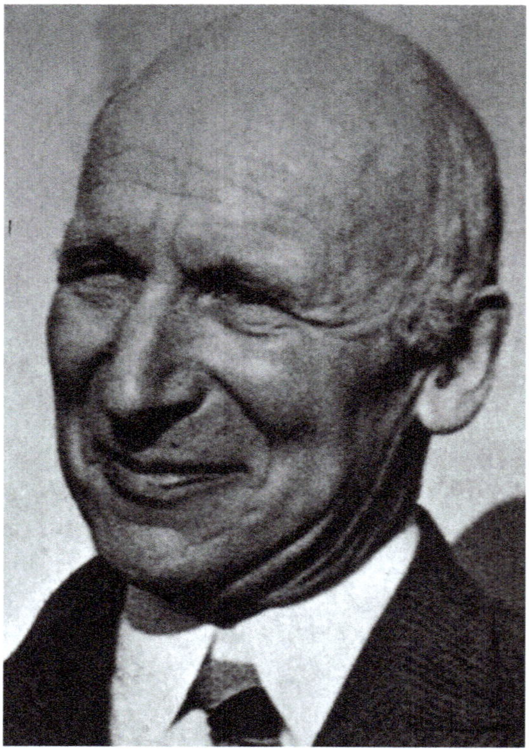

Fig. 2.13 Raul Hoffmann, an Austrian surgeon, designed a universal joint for fixation of a metal frame which could adjust the position of the fracture during treatment

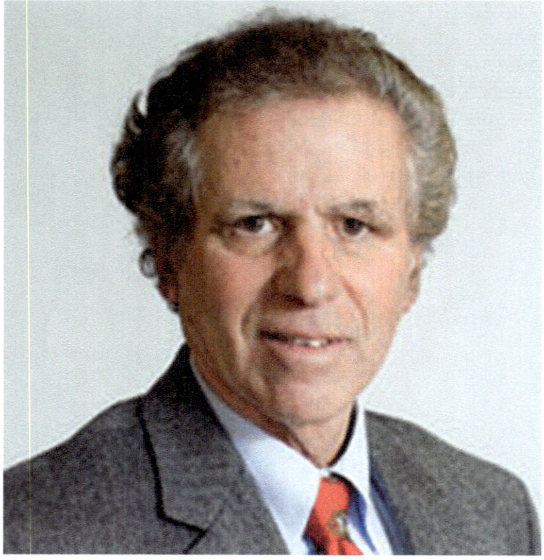

Fig. 2.14 Jesse Jupiter, professor at Harvard University, is the surgeon with the highest number of papers on this topic in the history of distal radius fractures

volar Barton's fractures. The AO-group (Die Arbeitsgemeinschaft für Osteosyntheses) was founded in 1950 by Müller, Allgöwer, and Willenegger. The first AO-fracture manual was published in 1963. The AO-group recommended dorsal plating for fractures of the distal radius. However, the technique was not in common use until the mid-1970s.

A specially designed distal radius plate, the pi plate ("π-plate"), was introduced in the 1990s (Ring et al. 1997). They recommended more fragment-specific fixation of intra-articular fractures. This multicenter study of *Jesse Jupiter* (Fig. 2.14) and co-workers popularized the use of low-profile dorsal plates for the internal fixation of distal radius fractures. The recognition that precise reduction of the distal radius is required for optimal outcome resulted in an increased interest in treating distal radius fractures with ORIF (Harness and Meals 2006).

In 1996, Rikli and Regazzoni described a new theory, "the three-column theory," as a more precise description of the biomechanics of distal radius fracture. And Medoff's fragment-specific fixation changed the way of thinking about distal radius fractures.

The biomechanical studies of Gesensway and Putnam demonstrated the superior strength of a new distal radius plate design that incorporated the concept of the fixed angel blade plate. It was the predecessor to the fixed angle plates that are widely used today (Harness and Meals 2006). The introduction of new specially designed volar fixed angle plates for fractures of the distal radius allowed more versatility in creating subchondral support and provides fixation of most distal radius fractures from a volar approach (Orbay 2000). In 2014 The Norwegian Orthopaedic Association developed guidelines based on the GRADE-system and launched these in the new MAGIC-application (MAGICapp) (Kvernmo et al. 2014).

Corrective osteotomies for mal-united fractures of the distal radius were thoroughly described by Diego Fernandez in his classic paper from 1982 (Fig. 2.15). These techniques are also part of the differentiated treatment program for fractures of the distal radius.

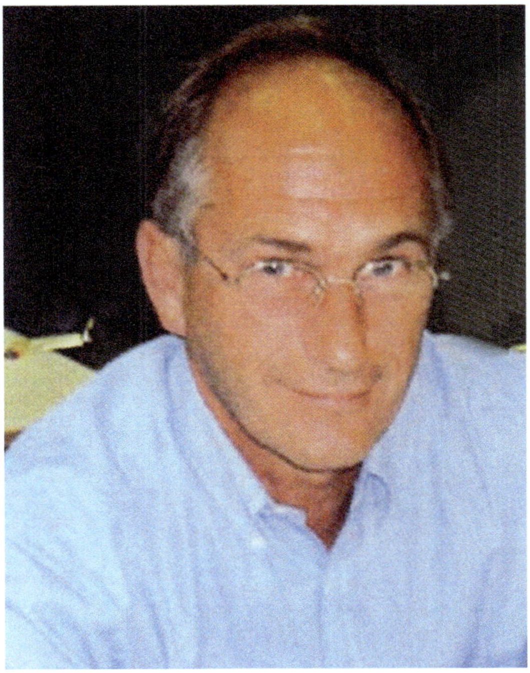

Fig. 2.15 Diego Fernandez, professor at the University of Bern, is probably most famous for his work on fractures healed with malalignment of the distal radius and his system of fracture classification

References

Barton JR. Views and treatment of an important injury of the wrist. Med Examiner. 1838;1:365–8.

Beck C. Colles' fracture and the roentgen rays. Med News. 1898;72:230–2.

Colles A. On the fracture of the carpal extremity of the radius. Edinb Med Surg J. 1814;10:182–6.

Cotton FJ. A study of the x-ray plates of one hundred and forty cases of fracture of the lower end of the radius. Boston Med Surg J. 1900;142:305.

Fenger CE. On fracture of the lower extremity of the radius. Royal medical and chirurgical society. London. Lancet. 1847;8:487–8.

Fernandez DL. Correction of posttraumatic wrist deformity in adults by osteotomy, bone-grafting, and internal fixation. J Bone Joint Surg. 1982;64A:1164–78.

Fernandez DL, Jupiter JB. Fracture of the distal end of the radius: historical perspective. In: Fernadez DL, Jupiter JB, editors. Fractures of the distal radius. A practical approach to management. 2nd ed. New York: Springer; 2002. p. 1–21.

Goyrand G. Memoires sur les fractures de l'extrémité inférieure du radius qui simulent les luxations de poignet. Gaz Med. 1832;3:664–7.

Harness NG, Meals RA. The history of fracture fixation of the hand and wrist. Clin Orthop Relat Res. 2006;445:19–29.

Hove LM, Helland P, Mølster AO. Dynamic traction for unstable fractures of the distal radius. J Hand Surg. 1999;24B:210–4.

Kvernmo HD, Krukhaug Y, Hove LM, Williksen JH, Husby T, Odinsson A, Vandvik PO, Brandt L. Guidelines for fractures of the distal radius. 2014. http://www.wristfractures.no.

Lucas-Championniere J. Fractures du radius dues au retour de manivelle d'automobile. Bull Acad Natl Med. 1904;75:209.

Lund FB. Fractures of the radius in starting automobiles. Boston Med Surg J. 1904;151:481.

Mathijsen A. Du bandage platre. Liege: Grandmont-Donders; 1854.

McQueen MM, Hajducka C, Court-Brown CM. Redisplaced unstable fractures of the distal radius: a prospective randomized comparison of four methods of treatment. J Bone Joint Surg. 1996;78:404–9.

Orbay JL. The treatment of unstable distal radius fractures with volar fixation. Hand Surg. 2000;5(2):103–12.

Peltier LF. Fractures of the distal end of the radius: an historical account. Clin Orthop. 1984;187:18–22.

Petit JL. L'Art de Guérir les Maladies de l'Os. Paris: L. d'Houry; 1705.

Pouteau C. Oeuvres posthumes de M. Pouteau: mémoire, contenant quelques réflexions sur quelques fractures de l'avant-bras sur luxations incomplétes du poignet et sur le diastasis. Paris, Ph-D Pierres 1783.

Rang M. The story of orthopaedics. Philadelphia: WB Sauders Company; 2000. p. 401–10.

Ring D, Jupiter J, Brennwald J, Büchler U, Hastings II H. Prospective multicenter trial of a plate for dorsal fixation of distal radius fractures. J Hand Surg Am. 1997;22:777–84.

Smith RW. A treatise on fractures in the vicinity of joints and on certain forms of accidental and congenital dislocations. Dublin: Hodges & Smith; 1847.

Anatomy of the Wrist

3

Tommy Lindau and Carl-Göran Hagert

Contents

T. Lindau, MD, PhD (✉)
The Pulvertaft Hand Centre,
Kings Treatment Centre, Royal Derby Hospital,
Uttoxeter Road, Derby, DE22 3NE, UK

University of Derby, Derby, UK
e-mail: tommylindau@hotmail.com

C.-G. Hagert, MD, PhD
Department of Orthopaedic Surgery, Lund University Hospital, University of Lund, Lund, Sweden

University of Pittsburgh, Pittsburgh, PA, USA

3.1 Summary

Allegedly, Gubarev (Russian anatomist, nineteenth century) stated:

> Without anatomy there is no surgery, no therapy, but only guessing and prejudices.
> A doctor who is not an anatomist is not only useless but harmful.

Let us approach anatomy bearing this in mind and let us agree that anatomy of the distal forearm, wrist and hand is exceptionally complex yet still has to be well understood!

We will in this chapter not describe anatomy in great detail, but rather focus on the important structures necessary to understand biomechanics, fracture patterns and approaches whilst managing distal radius fractures.

3.2 Osseous Anatomy

The wrist is the link between the forearm and the hand (Fig. 3.1). It is comprised of the distal radius, the distal ulna, the proximal and distal carpal rows and the five metacarpal bases.

3.2.1 The Distal Radius

- The articular surface of the radius is triangular with the apex of the triangle at the tip of the radial styloid.

L.M. Hove et al. (eds.), *Distal Radius Fractures*,
DOI 10.1007/978-3-642-54604-4_3, © Springer-Verlag Berlin Heidelberg 2014

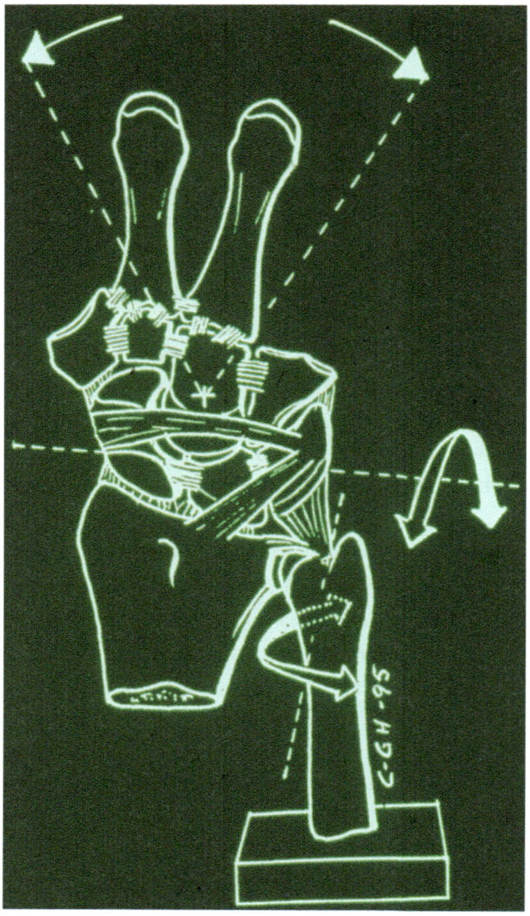

Fig. 3.1 This drawing demonstrates that the *ulna* is the stable, nonrotating and weight-bearing pillar around which the radius and carpus move in three dimensions – *the fixed point concept*

- It has a radial inclination of about 22° (13–30), which is a predisposing factor for carpal translation ulnarward in case of impaired ligamentous support as often seen in rheumatoid arthritis.
- It has a radial length of about 11 mm (8–18) and an average volar tilt of 11° (1–21). Hence, radiographic articular views have to be done to compensate for these angles to both understand the intra-articular involvement in a fracture and control that no pegs/screws will penetrate the cartilage during application of a volar locking plate.
- The dorsal cortex can be thought of as being composed of two surfaces, one radial and one ulnar to the Lister's tubercle. On a straight lateral radiogram, the ulnar part is not visualised as the Lister's tubercle forms the dorsal contour.
- Lister's tubercle acts as a fulcrum for the extensor pollicis longus (EPL).
- The dorsal cortex is thin, which leads to comminution when fractured and a high risk of dorsal tilt of the distal fragment.
- The volar side of the radius, which is covered by the pronator quadratus (PQ), is flat and makes a smooth curve that is concave from proximal to distal. The volar approach to the radius allows releasing the PQ, which is often trapped in the fracture, causing a pronation contracture and limited rotation after a distal radius fracture.
- The distal volar margin of the pronator fossa creates a line, called the "watershed line", which should not be trespassed at volar plate fixation.
- In the column theory, *the radial column* is defined as the radial styloid process and the scaphoid facet and extends to the base of Lister's tubercle. Only a small amount of load passes the radial column, which serves as a radial osseous buttress and an insertion for the radiocarpal extrinsic ligaments.
- The ulnar border of the distal radius is called *the intermediate column*. It includes the lunate facet and the sigmoid notch, or semilunar notch, which is the articulating surface to the ulnar head.
- The ulnar part of the palmar radius is the "calcar" of the wrist bearing maximal load, hence the density of the bone.
- This is further supported on the palmar surface of the lunate facet where the "teardrop" marks the insertion of the short radio-lunate (SRL) ligament, the strongest ligament in the wrist. Hence, intra-articular fractures have the key articular fragments and impaction zones at the level of *the intermediate column* due to the compressive forces. This is why this area is called *the critical corner*.

- The volar lunate facet extends more distally than expected, and an effective support of this area with a plate can be challenging.
- On a lateral x-ray view, the palmar cortex of the distal radius shaft should be collinear with the centre of the lunate and head of capitate, the so-called volar lines of Lewis.

3.2.2 The Distal Ulna and the Distal Radial-ulnar (DRU) Joint

- The distal ulna forms *the ulnar column* together with the ulnar styloid, the TFCC and the DRU joint. This area transmits a similar amount of load as the intermediate column and is therefore sensitive to radial shortening, i.e. relative ulnar lengthening.
- Stable, non-rotating and weight-bearing, the ulnar head forms a "fixed point" (Fig. 3.1) around which the radius moves on pronation-supination and the hand and wrist in extension-flexion and radial-ulnar deviation (Hagert 1996).
- The DRU joint is very complex and comes in three types (Tolat et al. 1996):
  - Type I where the apposing joint surfaces are parallel to the long axis of the radius and the ulna
  - Type II where the apposing surfaces are oblique
  - Type III where the apposing surfaces are "reverse oblique"
- In addition, the sigmoid notch most often has a flat face but may come in a C type and S type and look like a ski slope.
- All these differences may to some extent explain why certain patients develop limited ROM after gentle malunions, and others develop DRU-joint instability, while others have no symptoms at all.
- The curvature of the sigmoid notch is about 50 % larger than the one of the ulnar head, which gives a significantly larger contact area in neutral position than at the end of pronation or supination (Fig. 3.2) (af Ekenstam and Hagert 1985).
- Due to the different curvatures of the radii of the sigmoid notch and the ulnar head, the movement of the radius through the DRU joint on pronation-supination will be partly translational, partly rotational.

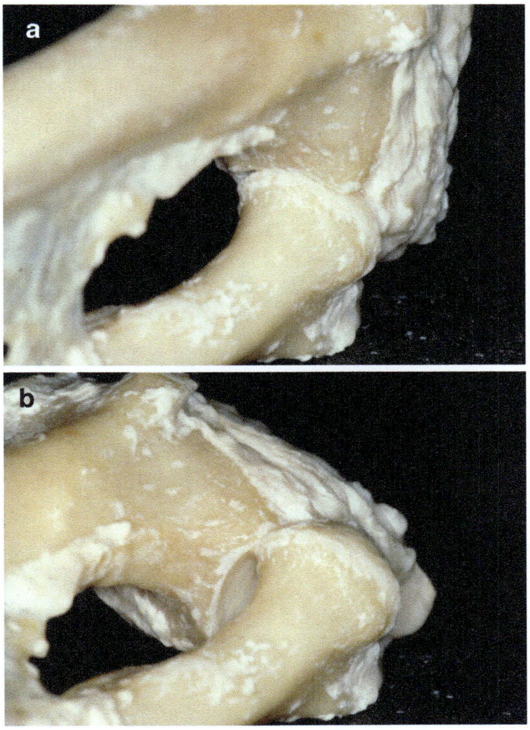

Fig. 3.2 These dissection images show a dorsal view (**a**) with the forearm in neutral position; in this projection it is clearly seen that the curvature of the semilunar notch has a larger radius than the ulnar head. At the end of pronation (**b**), the articulating surfaces are in a very marginal contact but still enough to provide full stability; with the radii of the semilunar notch and the ulnar head being of different size, the movement of the DRU joint on pronation-supination will be translational, not rotational

- From an articulation point of view, the forearm represents a bicondylar joint, the "forearm joint", with its axis of rotation in the centre of the radial and ulnar heads. With the forearm in full pronation, the radius crosses over the ulna resulting in a relative shortening in relation to the ulna.
- Stability in the DRU joint is primarily dependent on passive (ligamentous) soft tissue stabilisers; so- called stabilisers of first order but also the presence of dynamic (musculotendinous) structures; so-called stabilisers of second order (please see TFCC).

3.2.3 The Carpus

- The carpus consists of three anatomical units: the proximal and distal carpal rows and the bases of the metacarpal bones.
- *The proximal row* includes the scaphoid, lunate and triquetrum.
- The proximal row has no tendinous attachment; hence, its movements are secondary to forces distal to itself.
- The lunate is an intercalated segment within the proximal row. It flexes together with the scaphoid in radial deviation and extends together with the triquetrum in ulnar deviation.
- The scaphoid moves like a rotating triplanar pendulum, with relatively more motion at the distal palmar pole than at the proximal dorsal pole.
- *The distal row* includes the trapezium, trapezoid, capitate and hamate.
- The distal row along with the 2nd and 3rd metacarpal bones forms a unit, which has been called "the fundament of the wrist" due to its great internal stability. Wrist motion always starts here as all tendons insert distal to the proximal row.
- The carpus includes two joint systems, the radiocarpal and midcarpal joints, even if some also include the carpometacarpal (CMC) joints.
- *The radiocarpal joint* is composed of the two articular surfaces of the radius – the scaphoid and lunate facets divided by the interfossal ridge. These facets in addition to the triangular fibrocartilage complex (TFCC) form one concave articular facet towards the convex proximal part of the proximal row, "the carpal condyle".
- *The midcarpal joint* contains three articulations:
  - On the radial side is the scapho-trapezium-trapezoid (STT) joint.
  - Centrally is the scaphoid and lunate articulation with the capitate, the main mobile part of the wrist, where the capitate may be looked upon as "the femoral head of the wrist" and the concave scapholunate (SL) articulation as "the acetabulum of the wrist".
  - Ulnarly, the hamate and triquetrum form a helicoid joint.
  - The "dart-throwing motion" or the "dart-thrower's motion" runs in an oblique plane mainly in the midcarpal joint controlled by the STT joint. It runs from radial deviation and extension to ulnar deviation and flexion. This essential motion supports to consider rather radiocarpal than midcarpal fusions in situations where salvage procedures are necessary.

3.3 Paediatric Osseous Anatomy

- The growing skeleton is unique in many ways. The presence of the physis or growth plate provides longitudinal growth and a chance to remodel.
- The physis is divided into four distinct zones: germinal, proliferative, hypertrophic and provisional calcification.
- The hypertrophic and provisional calcification zones are weaker. Hence, fractures tend to go through these zones and may affect further growth with either malunion or growth arrest.

3.4 Ligamentous Anatomy

- Nearly all wrist ligaments are contained within capsular sheaths, which makes it difficult to visualise the ligaments when approaching the carpal joints surgically. The ligaments are best visualised arthroscopically.
- There are two general categories of ligaments: *intrinsic* and *extrinsic* (Fig. 3.3).
- *The intrinsic ligaments* have their origin and insertions within the carpus. They insert onto the cartilage rather than the bone and have much less elastic fibres compared with extrinsic ligaments. The intrinsic ligaments tend to avulse from insertion or origin rather than rupture midsubstance.
- The intrinsic ligaments in the distal row are very firm and hardly allow any mobility at all. Hence, the distal row should be looked upon as one functional unit cf. the previously described "the fundament of the wrist".
- Intrinsic ligaments in the proximal row comprises of the scapholunate (SL) and

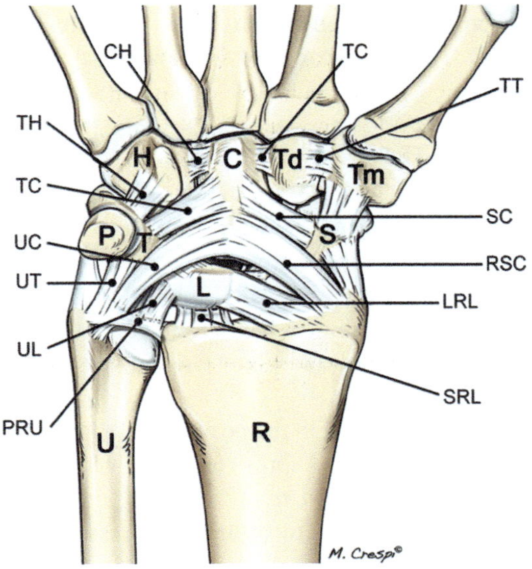

Fig. 3.3 The palmar intrinsic and extrinsic ligaments. *U* ulna, *R* radius, *L* lunate, *S* scaphoid, *Tm* trapezium, *Td* trapezoid, *C* capitate, *H* hamate, *P* pisiform, *T* triquetrum, *SRL* short radiolunate lig, *LRL* long radiolunate lig, *RSC* radio-scapho-capitate lig, *SC* scapho-capitate lig, *TT* trapezium-trapezoid lig, *TC* trapezoid-captiate lig, *CH* capito-hamate lig, *TH* triquetro-hamate lig, *TC* Triquetro-capitate lig, *UC* ulno-capitate lig, *UT* ulno-triquetral lig, *UL* ulno-lunate lig, *PRU* palmar radioulnar lig

luno-triquetral (LT) ligaments. They have dorsal, membranous and volar components.
  - The SL ligament is thickest and strongest in its dorsal part. The palmar part is fibrocartilage with no collagen fibres.
  - The LT ligament is thickest volarly and merges with fibres from the ulno-capitate (UC) ligament. The dorsal component is thinner with fibrocartilage fibres and no collagen.
- The palmar midcarpal ligaments between the proximal and distal carpal rows are functionally acting as intrinsic ligaments, but the palmar arcuate ligament forms the central third of the palmar midcarpal capsule and is composed of the blended fibres of the extrinsic radio-scapho-capitate (RSC) and UC ligaments (Fig. 3.3). They give a strong support for the head of capitate, i.e. supporting its "dart-throwing" motion in "the acetabulum of the wrist".
- The dorsal intercarpal ligament (DIC) connects the scaphoid, trapezium and trapezoid with the triquetrum. It forms a radaial (rather htan lateral) "V" shape and is indirectly stabilising the scaphoid dorsoradially. Its origin is to 100 % from the dorsal tubercle of the triquetrum, and 97 % of it inserts into the dorsoradial aspect of the waist of the scaphoid. They are important as secondary stabilisers to the SL joint, avoiding rotatory subluxation of the scaphoid.
- *The extrinsic ligaments* form connections between the forearm and the carpus. These ligaments are stiffer compared with intrinsic ligaments.
- *The palmar extrinsic* radio- and ulnocarpal ligaments have been portrayed as two inverted "V"-shaped ligament bands arising from the radius and the ulna, 'the arcuate ligaments'. The proximal "V" converges onto the palmar aspect of the lunate and the distal "V" onto the palmar aspect of the neck of the capitate (Fig. 3.3).
- These ligaments are disposed in superficial and deep layers and are best visualised arthroscopically. Non-arthroscopically, they are almost impossible to identify as they blend so intimately with the capsule.
- *Palmar radial extrinsic ligaments* (Fig. 3.3):
  - Radio-scapho-capitate (RSC) is an important second stabiliser to the scaphoid and the SL joint. It is also a key stabiliser to prevent ulnar translation of the carpus along the 22° radial inclination of the radiocarpal joint.
  - Long radio-lunate (LRL).
  - Radio-scapho-lunate (RSL) or the ligament of Testut is not a true ligament but rather a capsular tissue through which blood vessels course.
  - Short radio-lunate (SRL) ligament originates from the volar rim of the radius to insert at the volar surface of the lunate, acting as a pivot on extension of the wrist. This is the most important ligament around the wrist, well described by Mayfield (Mayfield et al, 1980) in his explanation of the biomechanics around perilunate dislocations.
- *Palmar ulnar extrinsic ligaments (please see at TFCC)* (Fig. 3.3):
  - Ulno-lunate (UL)
  - Ulno-luno-capitate (ULC)
  - Ulno-triquetro-capitate (UTC)

3.4.1 Dorsal Extrinsic Ligaments

- Dorsal radio-triquetral or dorsal radio-luno-triquetral (in spite of not having any attachment to the lunate) or dorsal radiocarpal ligament (Figs. 3.4 and 3.5). This ligament has an origin that varies from the dorsal lunate facet to areas close to the radial styloid. It is a key stabiliser to prevent ulnar translation of the carpus along the 22° radial inclination of the radiocarpal joint.

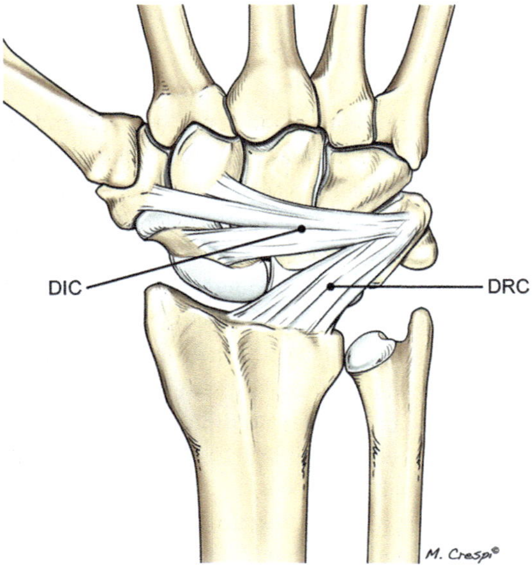

Fig. 3.4 The dorsal extrinsic radio-triquetral ligament (DRC) and the dorsal intercarpal ligaments (DIC)

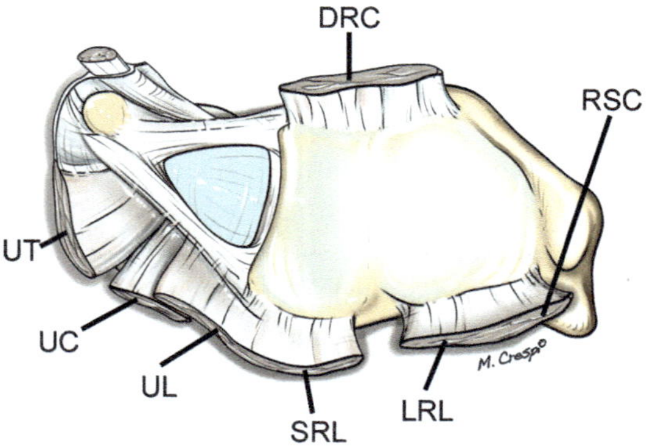

Fig. 3.5 A transverse illustration of the extrinsic ligaments: dorsal radio-triquetral or radiocarpal (*DRC*) ligament, the palmar radio-scapho-capitate (*RSC*) ligament, the long (*LRL*) and short (*SRL*) radio-lunate ligaments and the ulno-lunate (*UL*), ulnocarpal (*UC*) and ulno-triquetral (*UT*) ligaments (Adapted from Henry M. Perilunate dislocations and fracture dislocations/radiocarpal dislocations and fracture dislocations. In: del Piñal F, Mathoulin C, Luchetti R, editors. Arthroscopic management of distal radius fractures. Heidelberg: Springer; 2010, Fig. 11.2, page 128)

3.4.2 TFCC

The TFC is attached to the fovea at the base of the ulnar styloid, which represents the axis of rotation for "the forearm joint" (Figs. 3.1 and 3.6). The foveal attachment is just radial to the base of the ulnar styloid and gives rise to near-vertical fibres.

- With respect to the position of axis of rotation, the *TFC* fibres can be defined as *centric* and *eccentric.*
- With respect to arthroscopic assessment, they can be called proximal and distal (Atzei 2009).
- The centric, deep fibres represent the proximal fibres whereas the distal fibres are the superficial, exccentric ones, and they work in conjunction through the prono-supination in the following way: on supination, the dorsal, superficial (excentric) fibres become tight whereas the palmar, deep (centric) fibres become slack, and vice versa in pronation.
- The combined action of these ligaments and the limited bony contact area demonstrate the basics of joint stability: the interaction between *ligament tension* at one side of the joint and *bony compression* at the opposite side (Hagert 1994).
- Post-traumatic instability of the DRU joint is a common clinical problem that should be analysed with respect to both *tension* and *compression*, in other words, both *ligament tear* and *joint incongruity*, of which joint incongruity is the major stabiliser of the two (af Ekenstam et al. 1985).
- Stabilisers of the DRU joint "of second order" are the ECU tendon sheath, the DRU-joint capsule, the pronator quadratus (PQ) and interosseous ligament/membrane.

- The TFCC's ulnocarpal extension is a fibrous bundle that comes from the fovea of the ulnar head, adjacent to the volar bundle of the TFC, and extends distally to insert at the volar

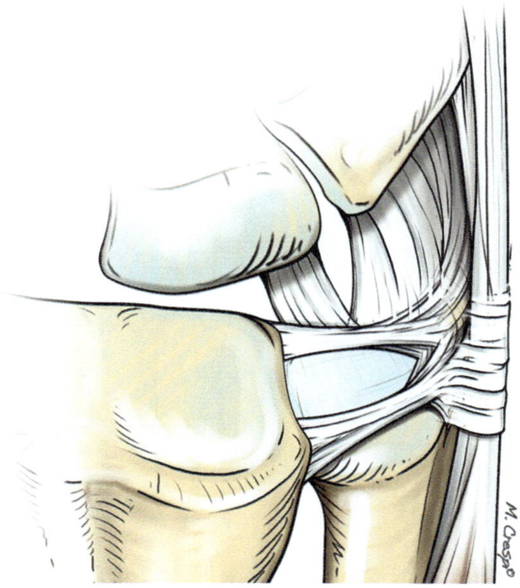

Fig. 3.6 The triangular fibrocartilage complex (*TFCC*). The ulna, radius and lunate-triquetrum are bound up by the TFCC, which extends in two perpendicular planes: the radial-ulnar portion (the radial-ulnar ligament, *TFC*) in the transverse plane and the ulnocarpal ligament in the coronal plane, enabling a three-dimensional movement, pronation-supination, wrist extension-flexion and wrist radial-ulnar deviation (Adapted from Nakamura T. Radial side tear of the triangular fibrocartilage complex. In: del Piñal F, Mathoulin C, Luchetti R, editors. Arthroscopic management of distal radius fractures. Heidelberg: Springer; 2010, Fig. 7.1, page 89)

surface of the triquetrum, the ulno-triquetral ligament (Fig. 3.6).

- The ulno-triquetral ligament is of importance to stabilise the ulnar part of the carpus and prevent the triquetrum from sagging volarly, counterbalanced by the dorsal radio-triquetral ligament.

3.4.3 The Interosseous Ligament (IOL) or Interosseous Membrane (IOM)

- The IOL/IOM has multiple biomechanical functions. It is a quadrangular sheath that extends from the radius to the ulna. Filling the interosseous space, it links both bones of the forearm and also separates the anterior and posterior compartments of the forearm.
- The IOL is loaded in tension as the forearm is loaded axially in compression.
- The IOL functions not only to transfer load from the radius to the ulna but also to pull the radius and ulna together at the proximal radial-ulnar and DRU joints.
- Fractures of the radial head may give rise to a disruption of the central third of the IOL, which in turn may give rise to a shift in the forearm load and potential injuries to the DRU joint, so-called Essex-Lopresti injuries (see Chap. 47). Such injuries contribute to loss of forearm stability and/or mobility.

3.5 Musculotendinous Anatomy

3.5.1 Dorsal Wrist

- The dorsal extrinsic muscles crossing the wrist are divided into six dorsal wrist fibro-osseous compartments at the level of the wrist. Each compartment is separated by a vertical fibrous septum that originates from the periosteum of the distal radius or ulna and extends to the extensor retinaculum. These compartments are numbered from 1 to 6 beginning at the midsagittal aspect of the radial wrist:
  1. Abductor pollicis longus (APL) is palmar and radial to the extensor pollicis brevis (EPB). The APL has 2 tendon slips in 70 %. The EPB has a separate compartment within the first compartment in 30 %.

     The brachioradialis (BR) muscle has a broad insertion to the distal radial border, proximal and deep to the APL and EPB at the wrist.
  2. Extensor carpi radialis longus and brevis (ECRL/B) cross the wrist immediately radial to Lister's tubercle.
  3. Extensor pollicis longus (EPL) is located ulnar to the Lister's tubercle and turns 45° radially distal to it where it runs dorsal to ECRL/B. It runs ulnar to the EPB further distally on the wrist/hand.
  4. Extensor digitorum communis (EDC) and extensor indicis proprius (EIP). EIP typically runs deep to the EDC. EDC is on the back of the hand interconnected with the juncturae tendinae.

5. Extensor digiti quinti (EDQ) or extensor digiti minimi (EDM) crosses the dorsal aspect of the DRU joint and is a good anatomical landmark to approach this joint.
6. Extensor carpi ulnaris (ECU) is stabilised by the extensor retinaculum, which at this level has a subcompartment, the *linea jugata*, which is a fibro-osseous tunnel as it runs in the dorsal groove on the ulnar head. This is also called the ECU subsheath.

3.5.2 Volar Wrist

- *The volar extrinsic* musculotendinous units are twofold, the superficial layer (crosses the elbow joint) and the deep layer (does not cross the elbow joint).
  - Superficial forearm flexors all arise from the medial common flexor insertion: flexor carpi ulnaris (FCU), flexor digitorum superficialis (FDS) (caput humerale), palmaris longus (PL) and flexor carpi radialis (FCR).
  - Deep forearm flexors: flexor digitorum superficialis (FDS) (caput radiale), flexor digitorum profundus (FDP), flexor pollicis longus (FPL) and pronator quadratus (PQ). Occasionally, there is a tendinous connection (Linburg-Comstock) between FPL and the index FDP
- *The volar intrinsic* musculotendinous anatomy includes:
  - Hypothenar (abductor digiti minimi (ADM), flexor digiti minimi (FDM) and opponens digiti minimi (DM))
  - Thenar muscles (abductor pollicis brevis (APB) and flexor pollicis brevis (FPB), opponens pollicis (OP) and the adductor pollicis (ADD))

3.6 Vascular Anatomy

- The distal radius and ulna receive nutrient vessels from four extraosseous vessels, namely, the radial, ulnar, anterior (AIA) and posterior (PIA) interosseous arteries (Fig. 3.7).

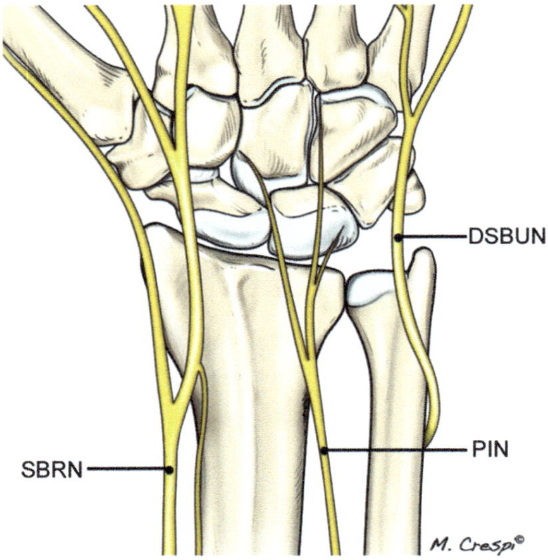

Fig. 3.7 The dorsal cutaneous nerve supply comprises the superficial branch of the radial nerve (*SRNB*) and the dorsal superficial branch of the ulnar nerve (*DSBUN*). In the floor of the 4th extensor compartment lies the posterior interosseous nerve (*PIN*)

- Most of the distal radius and the proximal carpal row are supplied via the radial artery and the AIA. In contrast, the ulna is mainly supplied via the ulnar artery and the PIA.
- The vessels supplying the dorsal radius and ulna are best described by their relationship to the extensor compartments.
- They are further divided into intercompartmental arteries if they are located within an extensor compartment or supraretinacular arteries if they are located dorsal and superficial to the retinaculum.
- On the volar aspect, the palmar carpal arch arises approximately 1.5 cm proximal to the radial styloid and courses volarly to the pronator quadratus.
- The TFCC is vascularised in its periphery where the radial-ulnar ligaments are nourished by dorsal and palmar branches of the ulnar artery. The central and the radial attachments are avascular. These vascular anatomical aspects are important when attempting to repair or debride the TFCC.

3.7 Nerve Anatomy Including Proprioception

- The distal forearm is mainly innervated by the median, ulnar and radial nerves.
- *The median nerve* gives off two branches as it courses through the forearm:
  - The anterior interosseous nerve (AIN) branch courses with the anterior interosseous artery (AIN) and innervates FPL, FDP II and part of FDP III and ends by innervating the PQ.
  - The palmar cutaneous branch of the median nerve arises at the distal part of the forearm. It supplies sensory innervation to the thenar area. This branch is at risk when approaching the distal radius from palmar.
  - The median nerve enters the hand through the carpal tunnel immediately under the flexor retinaculum together with the FDS, FDP and FPL tendons.
- *The ulnar nerve* lies under the FCU alongside the ulna. It courses with the ulnar artery.
  - The ulnar nerve enters the palm of the hand through the Guyon's canal next to the pisiform and further splits into a deep motor branch and a superficial sensory branch.
  - The dorsal cutaneous branch becomes subcutaneous 5 cm proximal to the pisiform but passes the wrist at its ulnar border around the distal part of the ulnar head.
- *The radial nerve* splits proximal in the forearm.
  - The deep branch pierces the supinator muscle, after which it is known as the posterior interosseous nerve (PIN).
  - The superficial branch of the radial nerve (SBRN) descends in the forearm under the brachioradialis (BR). The SBRN exits under the BR approximately 5 cm proximal to the radial styloid.
- The lateral antebrachial cutaneous branch can partially or completely overlap the SBRN.
- The carpus is innervated by articular branches of the AIN and PIN, the SBRN, the palmar cutaneous branch of the median nerve and the branches of the ulnar nerve.
- *Proprioception*
  - The understanding of ligament innervation and sensorimotor function has developed in the last decade. We have been made aware of the importance of Ruffini endings, Pacini corpuscles, Golgi tendon organs, free nerve endings and some unclassifiable corpuscles in the fine-tuning of neuromuscular control of the wrist (Hagert et al. 2007).
  - Most of these mechanoreceptors have been found in the dorsal ligaments. This is worth knowing in the consideration of resecting the most distal part of the PIN, also called the dorsal interosseous nerve, DIN.
  - Proprioception and neuromuscular control are also essential in the rehabilitation of post-traumatic ligament instabilities.

3.8 Summary of Anatomy in Relation to Wrist Trauma

Fall on the out-stretched hand (FOOSH) is by far the most common type of wrist trauma. With the wrist forced in extension, different injuries may occur depending on age, varying strength of the bone, the amount of trauma energy and the direction at impact. We may find:

- Sprains of unknown severity (Bergh et al. 2012)
- Isolated or combined ligament injuries (Bergh et al. 2012)
- Distal radius fractures (extra-articular, intra-articular, compound)
- Scaphoid fractures
- Combined fractures with associated ligament injuries
- Perilunate dislocation in a so-called "Mayfield's greater arc" involving fractures of the radius styloid, the scaphoid, the capitate, the triquetrum and the ulnar styloid in various forms with or without inclusion of the SL and/or LT ligaments.
- Perilunate dislocation in the so-called "Mayfields lesser arc" involving ligament injuries to the RSC, SL, LT and TFCC

In order to diagnose, understand and manage these injuries, it is essential to have sufficient knowledge of the anatomy.

References

af Ekenstam F, Hagert C-G. Anatomical studies on the geometry and stability of the distal radioulnar joint. Scand J Plast Reconstr Surg. 1985;19:17–25.

af Ekenstam F, Hagert C-G, Engkvist O, Törnvall AH, Wilbrand H. Corrective osteotomy of malunited fractures of the distal end of the radius. Scand J Plast Reconstr Surg. 1985;19:175–87.

Atzei A. New trends in arthroscopic management of type 1-B TFCC injuries with DRUJ instability. J Hand Surg Eur Vol. 2009;34(5):582–91.

Bergh TH, Lindau T, Bernardshaw SV, Behzadi M, Soldal LA, Steen K, Brudvik C. A new definition of wrist sprain necessary after findings in a prospective MRI study. Injury. 2012;43(10):1732–42. Epub 2012 Jul 21.

Hagert C-G. Distal radius fracture and the distal radioulnar joint – anatomical considerations. Handchir Mikrochir Plast Chir. 1994;26:22–6.

Hagert C-G. Current concepts of the functional anatomy of the distal radioulnar joint, including the ulnocarpal junction. In: Buchler U, editor. Wrist instability. London: Federation of European Societies for Surgery of the Hand, Martin Dunitz; 1996. p. 15–21.

Hagert E, Garcia Elias M, Forsgren S, Ljung BO. Immunohistochemical analysis of wrist ligament innervation in relation to their structural composition. J Hand Surg (Am). 2007;32(1):30–6.

Mayfield JK, Johnson RP, Kilcoyne RK. Carpal dislocations: pathomechanics and progressive perilunar instability. J Hand Surg Am. 1980;5:226–41.

Tolat AR, Stanley JK, Trail IA. A cadaveric study of the anatomy and stability of the distal radioulnar joint in the coronal and transverse planes. J Hand Surg Br. 1996;21(5):587–94.

Biomechanics and Kinematics of the Wrist

4

Yngvar Krukhaug

Contents

Y. Krukhaug, MD, PhD
Department of Orthopaedic Surgery,
Haukeland University Hospital, Bergen, Norway

Department of Surgical Sciences,
University of Bergen, Bergen, Norway
e-mail: yngvar.krukhaug@helse-bergen.no

4.1 Summary

Studies of biomechanics and kinematics are important in order to understand normal wrist function and specific pathologies of the wrist. The movement of the wrist bones is complex. Ligaments and muscle/tendons determine the position of the wrist bones during flexion/extension and radial/ulnar deviation to maintain congruency of the wrist joints. Therefore, the center of rotation shifts during the movements. As an axial force acts across the wrist, it tends to slide volarly and ulnarly. This tendency is prevented by ligaments and the bone architecture. The ulnar variance varies because of the axial movement of the radius in relation to the ulna during forearm rotation. This emphasizes the importance of taking standardized x-rays. In neutral position, an average of 18 % of the axial load applied on the metacarpus is transmitted to the ulna. The force transmitted to the ulna rises during pronation, ulnar deviation, and shortening of the radius. In the radiocarpal joint there are two different joint facets, the lunate facet and the scaphoid facet; 40 % of the load is normally borne by the lunate facet and 60 % by the scaphoid facet.

4.2 Introduction

Kinematics is important in order to understand normal wrist function. It is also important to determine the role of specific factors in the development

L.M. Hove et al. (eds.), *Distal Radius Fractures*,
DOI 10.1007/978-3-642-54604-4_4,

of specific pathologies (e.g., Kieneböck's disease and local osteoarthrosis). Kinematics helps us to understand how the balance between joint architecture, ligament tensions, and tendon forces may be altered by injury or disease, resulting in specific patterns of carpal instability.

4.3 Biomechanics

4.3.1 Tendons

- The flexor carpi ulnaris (FCU) tendon is attached to the pisiform bone.
- All other wrist tendons are attached to the base of the metacarpal bones.
- There are no tendons attached to the carpal bones in the proximal row of the wrist.
- Therefore, contraction of any forearm muscle, with a tendon crossing the wrist, generates a flexion/extension or a radial/ulnar deviation on the distal carpal row.
- The bones of the proximal row start moving after the distal row, when tightness of the ligaments crossing the midcarpal joint reaches a certain tension.
- This explains why there is no fixed point of rotation in the wrist joint. The center of rotation will change during the flexion/extension and the radial/ulnar movements of the wrist (Fig. 4.1).

4.3.2 Bones

The bones of the proximal row are less tightly bound to one another than the bones of the distal row.

- The proximal row moves in synergy as one unit during all movements of the wrist, despite differences in angular rotation of the individual bones.
- Therefore, the proximal row can be considered as one functional unit, in the same way as the distal row.
- The proximal row is acting as an intercalated segment between the distal row and the radius (Kauer 1974; Linscheid 1986).
- During flexion/extension of the wrist, the proximal row is able to keep the joint congruent even when combined with radial/ulnar deviation.
- This is achieved by the rotation between the individual bones of the proximal carpal row (Kauer 1974; Linscheid 1986; Garcia-Elias et al. 1989).

4.3.3 Forces

During normal load-bearing conditions, there are two opposite moments of force interacting in the proximal row.

- One is induced by the scaphoid, which tends to rotate the proximal row into flexion.
- The other moment is initiated by the distal row and is transmitted by the midcarpal ligaments to the triquetrum, tending to produce extension of the proximal row.
- As a result substantial torques are generated at the scapholunate and lunotriquetral joint. Under normal conditions these torques are likely to result in a cooptation that would further enhance their stability.
- Loss of this mechanism may result in articular incongruency, osteoarthrosis, and intercarpal and radiocarpal ligament disruptions.
- This may then lead to secondary instability and abnormal kinematics of the wrist. In the normal mechanics of the wrist joint, the scaphoid and the lunate share the load. For example, in cases of significant scaphoid-lunate dissociation, the lunate tends to dislocate, resulting in a significantly increased load on the scaphoid.

4.4 Kinematics

As an axial force acts across the wrist, the carpus tends to slide in the volar direction on the articular surface of the distal radius, which is inclined in the palmar/ulnar direction. The tendency to slide in the ulnar direction is resisted mainly by the palmar radiolunate and dorsal radiotriquetral ligaments. The volar arc of the radial concavity

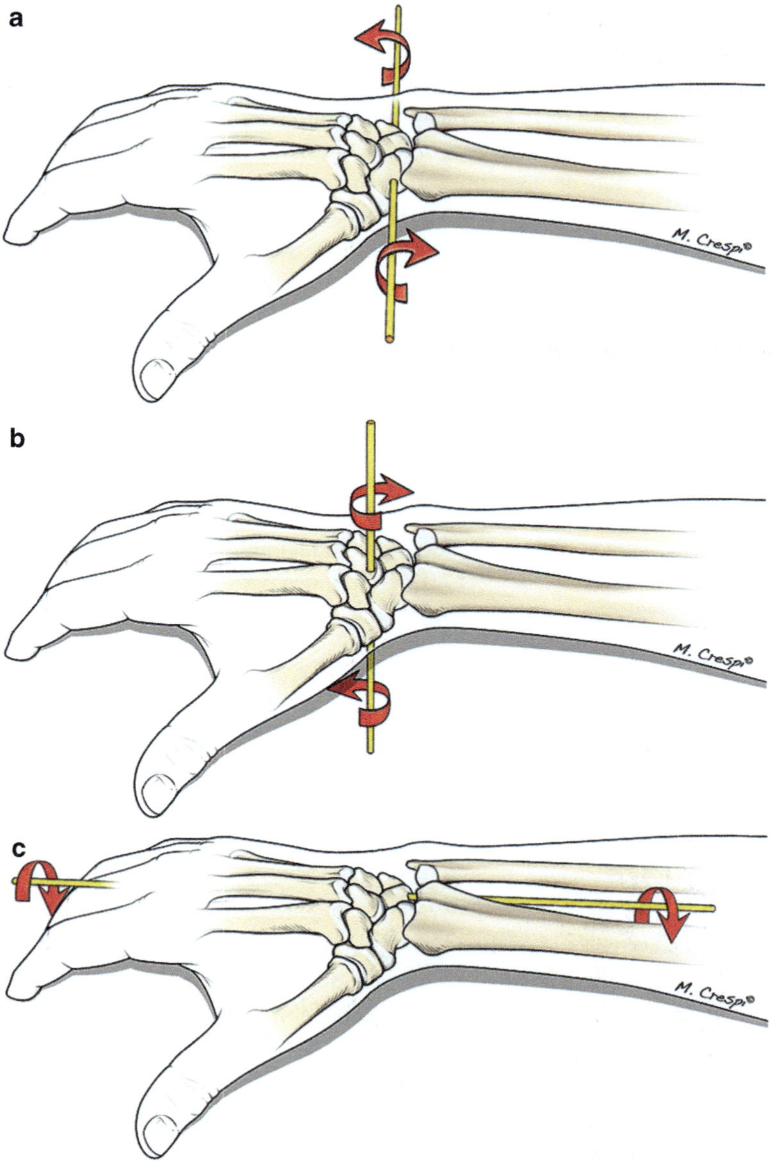

Fig. 4.1 (**a–c**) The figures show the reference axes for wrist motions

and the ulnocarpal ligament complex prevent the tendency for the carpus to slide in the volar direction on the palmar slope. These anatomical features explain why the unconstrained carpus subluxates or dislocates in a volar and ulnar direction, when the extrinsic radiocarpal ligaments are torn (Rayhack et al. 1987).

4.4.1 Ulnar Variance

The median ulnar variance is −0.8 mm (CI 95 %: −4.5 mm – +2.3 mm). Axial movement of the radius in relation to the ulna is found during forearm rotation. The ulnar variance is measured to be 1 mm more positive in pronation compared to supination (Palmer 1998). This emphasizes the importance of taking standardized x-rays (e.g., neutral rotation) (Epner et al. 1982).

In persons that have a negative ulnar variance, the radial joint gives less coverage of the lunate. This feature may create more forces to the lunate bone than is found in individuals with better coverage of the radiolunate joint and may be an explanation for the observation that people with a significant ulna minus are more likely to develop Kienebock's disease.

4.4.2 Grip Strength

When grasping an object, the total force transmitted to the distal row can reach values 10 times the applied force at the tip of the fingers (Schuind et al. 1995). The average maximum grip strength for men is 52 kPa and 31 kPa for women (Harkonen et al. 1993). Therefore, one can anticipate that the wrist may experience compressive forces as high as 520 kPa for men and 310 kPa for women.

4.4.3 Load

Fifty to sixty percent of the load experienced by the distal row is transmitted through the capitate to the scaphoid and lunate; the other joints are of less importance in this context (Fig. 4.2). A consequence of this observation is to consider that a stable osteosynthesis of the wrist must withstand considerable force to allow exercises of the hand before the fracture has healed (Krukhaug et al. 2009).

In neutral position an average of 18 % of the axial load applied on the metacarpus is transmitted to the ulna (Palmer and Werner 1984). Radial deviation of the carpal bones, shortening of the ulna, and excision of the triangular fibrocartilage complex (TFCC) decrease the load on the ulna. However, ulnar deviation of the carpal bones, lengthening of the ulna, and pronation of the forearm increase the load on the ulna (Werner et al. 1986) (Table 4.1).

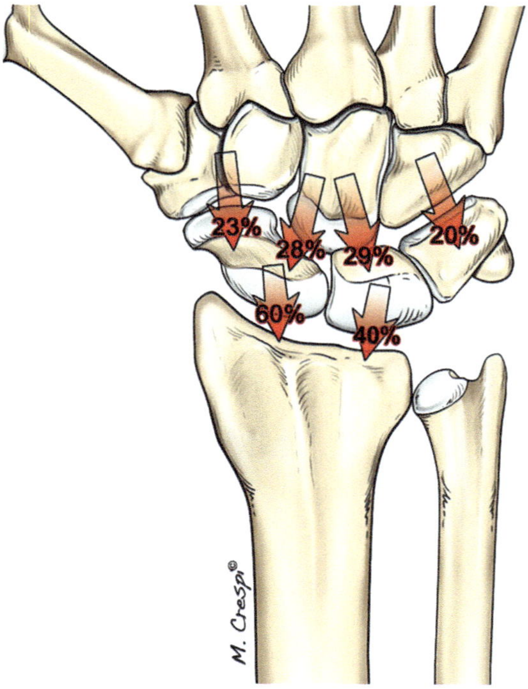

Fig. 4.2 The figure shows the force transmission in the wrist

Table 4.1 This shows the effect of wrist position on force distribution in the intact wrist (Werner et al. 1986)

	Force distribution (%)	
Wrist position	Radius	Ulna
Neutral	81.6	18.4
Radial deviation	87.2	12.8
Ulnar deviation	71.6	28.4
Supination	86.0	14.0
Pronation	63.0	37.0

In the radiocarpal joint there are two different joint facets: the lunate facet and the scaphoid facet. In normal people, approximately 40 % of the total load on the radius is borne by the lunate facet and 60 % by the scaphoid facet (Table 4.2). If the ligament between the lunate and the scaphoid is torn, a shift of load from the scaphoid fossa to the lunate fossa will occur (Viegas 2001) (Table 4.3).

Table 4.2 This shows the pressure changes on the lunate fossa and scaphoid fossa in different wrist positions (Hara et al. 1992)

	Pressure changes (MPa) and force distribution (%)	
Wrist position	Scaphoid fossa	Lunate fossa
Neutral	2.4 (62 %)	1.5 (38 %)
Radial deviation	2.6 (70 %)	1.1 (30 %)
Ulnar deviation	2.1 (42 %)	2.9 (58 %)

Table 4.3 Distribution of the axial load between the radius and ulna in an intact wrist after simulated ulnar shortening and lengthening Palmer and Werner 1984)

	Axial load (%)		
Site of measurement	−2.5 mm	0	+2.5 mm
Radius	95.7	81.6	58.1
Ulna	4.3	18.4	41.9

References

Epner RA, Bowers WH, Guilford WB. Ulnar variance–the effect of wrist positioning and roentgen filming technique. J Hand Surg Am. 1982;7(3):298–305.

Garcia-Elias M, Cooney WP, An KN, Linscheid RL, Chao EY. Wrist kinematics after limited intercarpal arthrodesis. J Hand Surg Am. 1989;14(5):791–9.

Hara T, Horii E, An KN, Cooney WP, Linscheid RL, Chao EY. Force distribution across wrist joint: application of pressure-sensitive conductive rubber. J Hand Surg Am. 1992;17(2):339–47.

Harkonen R, Piirtomaa M, Alaranta H. Grip strength and hand position of the dynamometer in 204 Finnish adults. J Hand Surg Br. 1993;18(1):129–32.

Kauer JM. The interdependence of carpal articulation chains. Acta Anat. 1974;88(4):481–501.

Krukhaug Y, Gjerdet NR, Lundberg OJ, Lilleng PK, Hove LM. Different osteosyntheses for Colles' fracture: a mechanical study in 42 cadaver bones. Acta Orthop. 2009;80(2):239–44.

Linscheid RL. Kinematic considerations of the wrist. Clin Orthop Relat Res. 1986;202:27–39.

Palmer AK, Werner FW. Biomechanics of the distal radio-ulnar joint. Clin Orthop Relat Res. 1984;187:26–35.

Palmer AK. The distal radioulnar joint. In: Lichtman DM, editor. The Wrist and its disorders. Philadelphia: Saunders; 1998. p. 220–31.

Rayhack JM, Linscheid RL, Dobyns JH, Smith JH. Posttraumatic ulnar translation of the carpus. J Hand Surg Am. 1987;12(2):180–9.

Schuind F, Cooney WP, Linscheid RL, An KN, Chao EY. Force and pressure transmission through the normal wrist. A theoretical two-dimensional study in the posteroanterior plane. J Biomech. 1995;28(5):587–601.

Viegas SF. The dorsal ligaments of the wrist. Hand Clin. 2001;17(1):65–75.

Werner FW, Glisson RR, Murphy DJ, Palmer AK. Force transmission through the distal radioulnar carpal joint: effect of ulnar lengthening and shortening. Handchir Mikrochir Plast Chir. 1986;18(5):304–8.

Epidemiology

5

Kristbjörg Sigurdardottir

Contents

K. Sigurdardottir, MD
Orthopaedic Department, Falun Hospital,
Falun, SE-791 82, Sweden
e-mail: kristbjorg.sigurdardottir@ltdalarna.se

5.1 Introduction

- Epidemiology of most fractures has been changing quickly in modern times. Improved living standards and medical treatment in the developed world have led to an increasingly aged but active population with more frequent osteoporotic fractures in both men and women.
- In the 1970s and 1980s, the most emphasis was on studying and treating younger patients with severe trauma. In recent years, osteoporotic elderly patients with low-energy trauma have become of interest because they are many and often require an expensive and complicated treatment.
- Until recently very few epidemiological studies on distal radius fractures had been carried out, but in the last 15 years, numerous studies have been published in this area.
- Understanding the epidemiology of distal radius fractures is important for identifying the health and economic burden of them. It also helps in choosing the right treatment and in the prevention of future fractures by, for example, treating at-risk patients for osteoporosis, clearing snow off pavements and securing building sites and children's playgrounds.
- Although sometimes harmless, especially in children, distal radius fractures often lead to prolonged symptoms, functional disability

L.M. Hove et al. (eds.), *Distal Radius Fractures*,
DOI 10.1007/978-3-642-54604-4_5, © Springer-Verlag Berlin Heidelberg 2014

and considerable disfigurement. Adults who present with this fracture are also at increased risk of further osteoporosis-related fractures.
- Increasing treatment costs, loss of work hours and decreased school attendance make distal radius fractures a major health issue (Brogren et al. 2007; Court-Brown and Caesar 2006; O'Neill et al. 2001; Tsai et al. 2011).

5.2 Overall Incidence

- The distal radius fracture is one of the most common fractures in humans. It is the leading cause of attendance to the orthopaedic emergency departments in the world, where it stands for 17–20 % of all diagnosed orthopaedic fractures (Court-Brown and Caesar 2006; Wilcke et al. 2013).
- The overall incidence of distal radius fractures varies in different studies around the world. In Scandinavia it is around 30 per 10,000 person-years, and almost 40 % of the fractures occur in children under the age of 18 years (Wilcke et al. 2013).

5.3 Age and Gender Distribution

- There is a bimodal distribution of distal radius fractures in young males and older females, as seen in other common fractures, such as those of femoral and tibial diaphysis and the ankle (Court-Brown and Caesar 2006).
- Eight different distribution curves can describe age and gender distribution for all fractures according to Court-Brown and Caesar. Type A curve defines distal radius fractures (Fig. 5.1) (Court-Brown and Caesar 2006).
- An example of Scandinavian age and gender distribution curve for distal radius fractures is shown in Fig. 5.2.

5.4 Paediatric Incidence

- Children and adolescents up to about 16–17 years of age have particularly high risk for distal radius fractures partly because of their fast developing immature skeletal structure and partly because of their active lifestyle (Hedström et al. 2010).
- Distal radius fractures account for 25–30 % of all fractures in children (Brudvik and Hove 2003; Hedström et al. 2010; de Putter et al. 2011).
- Around 60 % of the paediatric fractures occur in boys. This probably reflects a combination of biological and social differences with boys perhaps being more active and prone to risk taking (Brudvik and Hove 2003; Hedström et al. 2010; de Putter et al. 2011).
- The peak age for boys is 13–14, while the peak age for girls is 10–11. This may be explained by girls going earlier through puberty when there is a large dissociation between skeletal growth and mineralisation with weak points at the physis (Hedström et al. 2010; de Putter et al. 2011; Wilcke et al. 2013).
- The overall incidence of distal radius fractures in children varies considerably in different parts of the world, from 35 to 100 per 10^4 person-years, even though mechanisms of injury are similar worldwide. Differences in climate, ethnicity, activity levels and nutrition are probably responsible (Hedström et al. 2010).

5.4.1 Trends Over Time

- Some recent studies have shown a huge increase in the incidence of distal radius fractures in children in the last decade. There are two theories that are likely explanations:

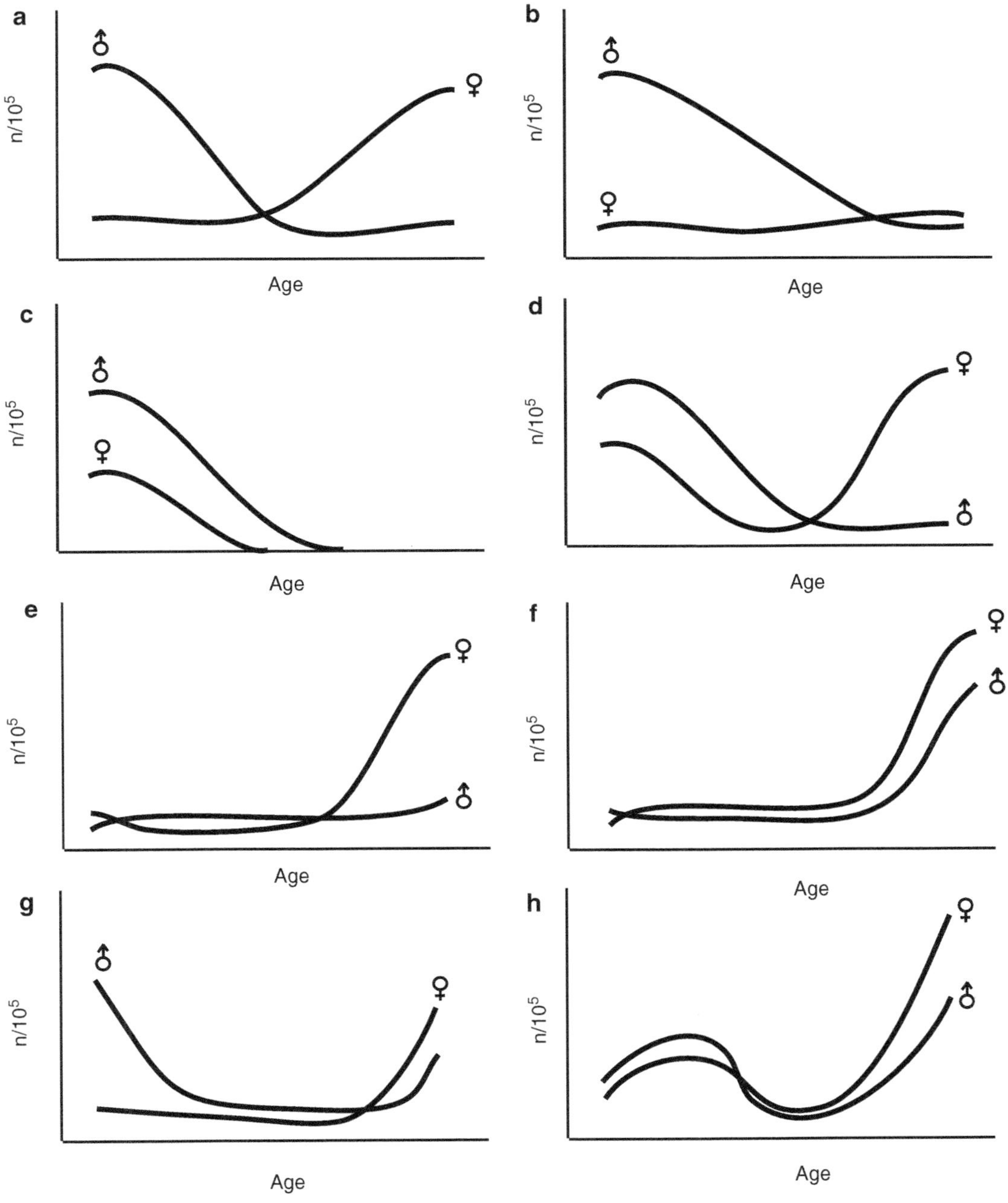

Fig. 5.1 The eight fracture distribution curves can describe age and gender distribution for all fractures. Type A curve defines distal radius fractures. Type A curve also may describe fractures of the scapula, carpus, thoracolumbar spine, metatarsus and femoral diaphysis. Type B curve shows the distribution of fractures of the scaphoid, metacarpus and fingers. Type C curve describes fractures of the talus and toe phalanges. Type D curve describes fractures of the proximal forearm, forearm diaphysis and distal tibia. Type E curve describes fractures of the distal humerus, pelvis and distal femur. Type F curve describes fractures of the proximal humerus, proximal femur and patella. Type G curve describes fractures of the clavicle, acetabulum and calcaneus. Type H curve describes fractures of the humerus diaphysis, cervical spine and proximal tibia (Published with permission from CM Court-Brown)

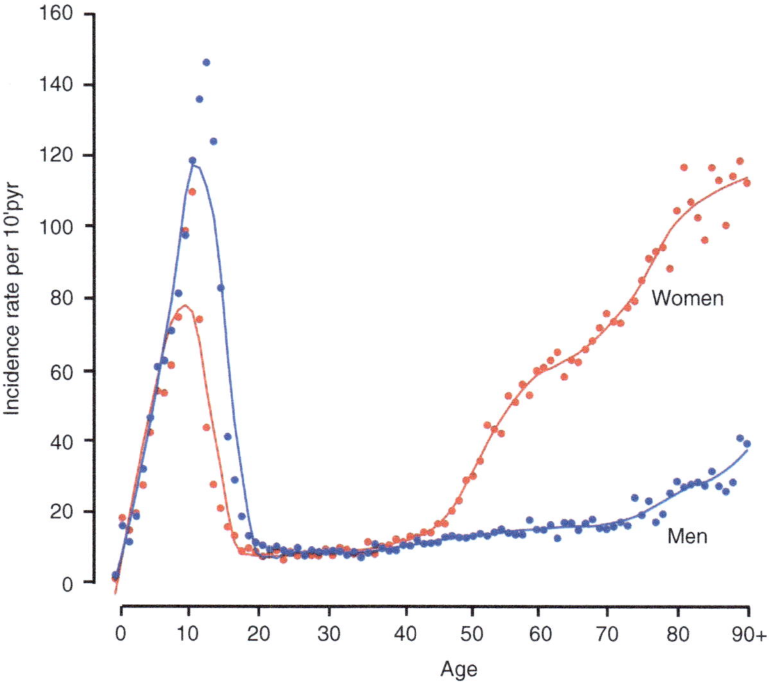

Fig. 5.2 Incidence of reported fractures of the distal radius in Stockholm, Sweden, 2004–2010. Scatter plot with a loess curve inserted. *pyr* person-years (Published with permission from the authors (Wilcke et al. 2013))

– Increased participation in sports as a result of increased awareness of the importance of physical activity
– An increase in overweight and inactivity with increased fracture risk in children with high body mass index (Hedström et al. 2010; de Putter et al. 2011)

5.5 Adult Incidence

- Distal radius fractures account for around 18 % of all adult fractures (Hove et al. 1995; Court-Brown and Caesar 2006).
- The left wrist is slightly more often broken than the right (Hove et al. 1995; Hagino et al. 1999; O'Neill et al. 2001; Lofthus et al. 2008).
- Around 70 % of the adult fractures occur in women, and they have three to five times higher incidence than men after the age of 60 (Melton et al. 1998; O'Neill et al. 2001; Jaglal et al. 2005; Brogren et al. 2007; Lofthus et al. 2008; Sigurdardottir et al. 2011; Flinkkilä et al. 2011; de Putter et al. 2013; Wilcke et al. 2013).
- The age-specific annual incidence rates of adult distal radius fractures in different recent studies are shown in Table 5.1.

5.5.1 Women's Incidence

- The lifetime risk of a distal radius fracture in white women has been reported to be around 15 % (Melton et al. 1998).
- Women's mean age for presenting with a distal radius fracture is 61–69 years (Melton et al. 1998; Brogren et al. 2007; Sigurdardottir et al. 2011; Flinkkilä et al. 2011).
- In adult women, the incidence starts to rise shortly after menopause, partly as a result of demineralisation of their bones due to lack of oestrogen and partly because of decreased neuromuscular control resulting in increased falling tendency (Melton et al. 1998; O'Neill et al. 2001; Jaglal et al. 2005; Brogren et al. 2007; Lofthus et al. 2008; Sigurdardottir et al. 2011; Flinkkilä et al. 2011; de Putter et al. 2013; Wilcke et al. 2013).

Table 5.1 The annual incidence of adult distal radius fractures in different recent studies (The rates of Jaglal et al. are estimated from a figure in the article (Jaglal et al. 2005))

First author	Study period	Country	Studied age	Women's incidence/10⁴ pyr	Men's incidence/10⁴ pyr
Scandinavia					
Wilcke et al. (2013)	2004–2010	Sweden	≥18	36	14
Flinkkilä et al. (2011)	2008	Finland	≥16	36	15
Sigurdardottir et al. (2011)	2004	Iceland	≥16	37	17
Lofthus et al. (2008)	1998–1999	Norway	≥20	56	17
Brogren et al. (2007)	2001	Sweden	≥19	39	12
UK/USA					
O'Neill et al. (2001)	1997–1998	UK	≥35	37	9
Melton et al. (1998)	1985–1994	USA	≥35	42	10
Asia					
Tsai et al. (2011)	2000–2007	Taiwan	≥20	15	10
Hagino et al. (1999)	1995	Japan	≥35	21	6
Studied age over 50 years					
Diamantopoulos et al. (2012)	2004–2005	Norway	≥50	75	19
de Putter et al. (2013)	1997–2009	Holland	≥50	46	10
Jaglal et al. (2005)	1992–2000	Canada	≥50	49	14

- In most recent studies women's incidence increases steadily with age and comes to a peak in the highest age groups, at over 80 years (Fig. 5.2), but in some older studies and studies from Asia, the incidence levels off or decreases in the oldest population (Hove et al. 1995; Melton et al. 1998; Hagino et al. 1999; O'Neill et al. 2001; Jaglal et al. 2005; Brogren et al. 2007; Lofthus et al. 2008; Sigurdardottir et al. 2011; Flinkkilä et al. 2011; Tsai et al. 2011; Diamantopoulos et al. 2012; de Putter 2013; Wilcke et al. 2013).

5.5.2 Men's Incidence

- Men's mean age for presenting with a distal radius fracture is 50–55 years (Brogren et al. 2007; Sigurdardottir et al. 2011; Flinkkilä et al. 2011; Wilcke et al. 2013).
- In adult men, the incidence is highest in the youngest and the oldest ones but otherwise fairly low throughout life. In old age it starts to rise after 70 and gets up to a rate similar to that of women in their fifties in the eighth decade of their lives (Fig. 5.2) (Melton et al. 1998; O'Neill et al. 2001; Jaglal et al. 2005; Brogren et al. 2007; Lofthus et al. 2008; Sigurdardottir et al. 2011; Flinkkilä et al. 2011; Diamantopoulos et al. 2012; de Putter 2013; Wilcke et al. 2013).

5.5.3 Trends Over Time

- The overall annual incidence of distal radius fractures has increased in many parts of the world during the twentieth century together with many other primarily osteoporotic fractures (Court-Brown and Caesar 2006).
- In Sweden the incidence almost doubled between the 1950s and 1980s, and a similar but less dramatic trend was shown in other developed countries for the same period. This trend of increase is also shown in recent Asian studies (Hagino et al. 1999; Brogren et al. 2007; Tsai et al. 2011).
- However, in recent Western world publications, the trend has been broken, with a stable or declining overall adult incidence over the last

two decades in spite of continuous aging of the population (Jaglal et al. 2005; Brogren et al. 2007; Lofthus et al. 2008; Sigurdardottir et al. 2011; Flinkkilä et al. 2011; Diamantopoulos et al. 2012, de Putter 2013).

- Furthermore, a decrease has been observed in the incidence of younger postmenopausal women (50–70 years of age) in Scandinavia in the last 15–20 years. This is perhaps a result of widespread osteoporosis prevention programmes in the 1980s and 1990s, with increased hormone replacement therapy and vitamin D/calcium intake as well as increased awareness on the importance of physical activity (Brogren et al. 2007; Lofthus et al. 2008; Sigurdardottir et al. 2011; Flinkkilä et al. 2011; Diamantopoulos et al. 2012; Wilcke et al. 2013).

5.6 Ethnicity

- The incidence of distal radius fractures varies widely in different parts of the world. The reason is probably multifactorial with possible contributing factors such as different biology of the bones, different weight/height, different living standards and activities and difference in longevity and/or environmental factors (Hagino et al. 1999; Lofthus et al. 2008; Tsai et al. 2011).
  - The highest overall adult incidence has been reported in Norway, but the other Scandinavian countries follow closely (Table 4.1). Possible explanations are that the Scandinavian population is genetically predisposed to osteoporosis and that icy ground conditions are very common in this part of the world. This however only partly explains the high incidence rate in Scandinavia, since their summer incidence is also higher than reported in other parts of the world (Brogren et al. 2007; Lofthus et al. 2008; Sigurdardottir et al. 2011; Flinkkilä et al. 2011; Hagino et al. 1999; Tsai et al. 2011; Wilcke et al. 2013).
- Distal radius fractures seem to be less frequent in populations of African and Asian heritage than of Caucasians. Studies from Japan and Taiwan show 2–3 times lower incidence figures than that of Scandinavia (Table 5.1), but their patterns of increase in incidence with age are similar (Melton et al. 1998; Hagino et al. 1999; Tsai et al. 2011).
- Possible explanations to the low rates in Asia are the low average height/weight of the population and their low prevalence of falls, even in areas with snow in winters, due to some of their traditional lifestyle characteristics. Their longevity is however similar and their bone mineral density similar or lower than that of whites (Hagino et al. 1999; Tsai et al. 2011).
- First-generation immigrants of Asian descent in Norway have a relative fracture risk of 0.72 compared to ethnic Norwegians. They have however a considerably higher rate than that reported in Asian studies. The influence of migration on fracture rates is complex, but the cold/dark climate of Norway with frequent icy ground conditions and low vitamin D levels are possible explanations (Lofthus et al. 2008).

5.7 Urban/Rural Differences

- People who live in urban areas seem to have a higher risk of distal radius fractures than their rural counterparts. This is perhaps because the rural population is generally more physically active than the urban one, resulting in higher bone density (Diamantopoulos et al. 2012).
- However, rural young men are at higher risk of high-energy distal radius fractures than their urban counterparts, especially in the summertime. This is possibly due to their more frequent hard labour and high-risk activities during this season (Diamantopoulos et al. 2012).

5.8 Seasonal Variation

- Children's distal radius fractures occur most frequently in the spring or summer, the seasons of outdoor sports and recreational activities as well as in certain winter holiday sport weeks in Scandinavia (Brudvik and Hove 2003; Hedström et al. 2010; de Putter et al. 2011).

- In contrast, adults in the Western world experience a significantly greater number of fractures in the cold winter months (Nov–Feb) with icy ground conditions than in other seasons (Hove et al. 1995; O'Neill et al. 2001; Brogren et al. 2007; Lofthus et al. 2008; Sigurdardottir et al. 2011; Flinkkilä et al. 2011; Diamantopoulos et al. 2012).
- In Finland, a 2.5-fold risk of distal radius fractures was shown on slippery winter days compared with non-winter days (Flinkkilä et al. 2011).
- In Taiwan, the highest rate of adult distal radius fractures is in the summertime, probably due to frequent typhoons that cause people to slip and fall (Tsai et al. 2011).

5.9 Mechanism of Injury

- Falling evokes a primitive motor reflex in humans to receive the fall with an outstretched arm in order to protect the head from a blow. This causes the forearm to break at its most weak part, the distal metaphysis of radius, where also the greatest load transmission acts in the fall.
- Most distal radius fractures in children are sports related, they happen during, for example, football, skiing or school gymnastics, but among the youngest children, many result from simple home accidents (Brudvik and Hove 2003; Hedström et al. 2010; de Putter et al. 2011).
- The vast majority of adult distal radius fractures (54–77 %) result from low-energy trauma. Most patients describe falling on level ground and in cold climates a fair proportion of these patients blame the fall on icy ground conditions (Melton et al. 1998; Flinkkilä et al. 2011; Sigurdardottir et al. 2011; Tsai et al. 2011).
- In younger adults, especially men, there is a greater proportion of high-energy causes of these fractures. These include falling from heights and sports or traffic accidents (Melton et al. 1998; Flinkkilä et al. 2011).
- In Taiwan, 39 % of adult fractures are associated with traffic accidents, a considerable higher percentage than that of Europe/North America where it has been reported to be 8–12 % (Melton et al. 1998; Flinkkilä et al. 2011; Tsai et al. 2011).

5.10 Summary

- *The distal radius fracture is one of the most common fractures in humans. It is the leading cause of attendance to the orthopaedic emergency departments in the world.*
- *Distal radius fractures account for 25–30 % of fractures in children and around 18 % of all adult fractures.*
- *The two major risk groups are the skeletally immature children/adolescents and the osteoporotic elderly.*
- *Around 60 % of the paediatric fractures occur in boys, while around 70 % of the adult fractures occur in women, depicting a bimodal distribution in young males and older females, as seen in other common fractures, such as those of femoral and tibial diaphysis and the ankle.*
- *Most fractures result from low-energy trauma, like falling on level ground, but sports and leisure activities account for the vast majority of the paediatric and young adult fractures.*
- *In Scandinavia and other cold climates, there is an apparent seasonal variation with the highest incidence of fractures during the winter months, largely due to icy ground conditions.*
- *The overall incidence of distal radius fractures in the developed world seems to have come to a plateau in the last two decades after a steep rise between the 1950s and 1980s. The reason for this recent plateau is unknown and probably multifactorial.*
- *The incidence in younger postmenopausal women in Scandinavia seems to be declining of recent, perhaps due to prevention and treatment of osteoporosis.*

References

Brogren E, Petranek M, Atroshi I. Incidence and characteristics of distal radius fractures in a southern Swedish region. BMC Musculoskelet Disord. 2007;8:48.

Brudvik C, Hove LM. Childhood fractures in Bergen, Norway. Identifying high-risk groups and activities. J Pediatr Orthop. 2003;23:629–834.

Court-Brown CM, Caesar B. Epidemiology of adult fractures: a review. Injury. 2006;37:691–7.

de Putter CE, Selles RW, Polinder S, et al. Epidemiology and health-care utilisation of wrist fractures in older adults in The Netherlands, 1997–2009. Injury. 2013; 44(4):421–6.

de Putter CE, van Beeck EF, Looman CWN, et al. Trends in wrist fractures in children and adolescents, 1997–2009. J Hand Surg. 2011;36A:1810–5.

Diamantopoulos AP, Rohde G, Johnsrud I, et al. The epidemiology of low- and high-energy distal radius fracture in middle-aged and elderly men and women in Southern Norway. PLoS One. 2012;7(8):e43367.

Flinkkilä T, Sirniö K, Hippi M, et al. Epidemiology and seasonal variation of distal radius fractures in Oulu, Finland. Osteoporos Int. 2011;22(8):2307–12.

Hagino H, Yamamoto K, Ohshiro H, et al. Changing incidence of hip, distal radius, and proximal humerus fractures in Tottori Prefecture, Japan. Bone. 1999;24(3):265–70.

Hedström EM, Svensson O, Bergström U, et al. Epidemiology of fractures in children and adolescents. Increased incidence over the past decade: a population-based study from northern Sweden. Acta Orthop. 2010;81(1):148–53.

Hove LM, Fjeldsgaard K, Reitan R, et al. Fractures of the distal radius in a Norwegian city. Scand J Plast Reconstr Hand Surg. 1995;29:263–7.

Jaglal SB, Weller I, Mamdani M, et al. Population trends in BMD testing, treatment, and hip and wrist fracture rates: are the hip fracture projections wrong? J Bone Miner Res. 2005;20:898–905.

Lofthus CM, Frihagen F, Meyer HE, et al. Epidemiology of distal forearm fractures in Oslo, Norway. Osteoporos Int. 2008;19:781–6.

Melton LJ, Amadio PC, Crowson CS, et al. Long-term trends in the incidence of distal forearm fractures. Osteoporos Int. 1998;8:341–8.

O'Neill TW, Cooper C, Finn JD, et al. Incidence of distal forearm fracture in British men and women. Osteoporos Int. 2001;12(7):555–8.

Sigurdardottir K, Halldorsson S, Robertsson J. Epidemiology treatment of distal radius fractures in Reykjavik, Iceland, in, 2004. Comparison with an Icelandic study from 1985. Acta Orthop. 2011;82(4):494–8.

Tsai CH, Muo CH, Fong YC, Lo WY, Chen YJ, Hsu HC, Sung FC. A population-based study on trend in incidence of distal radial fractures in adults in Taiwan in 2000–2007. Osteoporos Int. 2011;22(11):2809–15.

Wilcke MK, Hammarberg H, Adolphson PY. Epidemiology and changed surgical treatment methods for fractures of the distal radius. Acta Orthop. 2013;83(3):292–6. Epub 2013 Apr 17.

Distal Radius Fractures and Osteoporosis

6

Magnus K. Karlsson, Per-Olof Josefsson, and Björn E. Rosengren

Contents

M.K. Karlsson, MD, PhD (✉) • P.-O. Josefsson, MD, PhD
B.E. Rosengren, MD
Department of Orthopedics and Clinical Sciences, Skåne University Hospital, Lund University, Malmo SE-205 20, Sweden
e-mail: magnus.karlsson@med.lu.se

6.1 Summary

Risk factors for falls and distal radius or other fragility fractures should be evaluated in a structured way in patients with high risk for osteoporosis. This is especially true for patients with a previous distal radius or other fragility fractures since one indicates more to come. Modifiable risk factors should be addressed, and prophylactic treatment should be considered as there are a number of pharmacological and non-pharmacological regimens that reduce the risk of fragility fractures. It can no longer be acceptable clinical practice to neglect investigation or treatment of patients with osteoporosis who present with a distal radius or other fragility fractures. A bone mass scan should therefore be considered in these patients as pharmacological treatment in those with osteoporosis or with low bone mass and additional risk factors has been found to reduce fracture risk. In individuals with osteoporosis who require pharmacological treatment, bisphosphonate is usually the drug of choice, always in combination with calcium and vitamin D. Other possible treatments include selected estrogen receptor modulators (SERMs), strontium ranelate, subcutaneous parathyroid hormone (PTH), and denosumab. Physical activity should, independently of age, be recommended to all patients with a distal radius or other fragility fractures, together with a well-balanced diet. Individual risk factors should be addressed and avoided. As several interventions have been shown to reduce the fall risk in elderly, also

L.M. Hove et al. (eds.), *Distal Radius Fractures*,
DOI 10.1007/978-3-642-54604-4_6, © Springer-Verlag Berlin Heidelberg 2014

fall-preventive interventions should be initiated in elderly with a distal radius or other fragility fractures.

6.2 Introduction

- The incidence of distal radius and other fragility fractures (low-energy fractures of the proximal humerus, vertebra, pelvis, hip, and tibial condyles in individuals older than 50 years) has during the recent half-century increased in the western world (Kannus et al. 1996). The risk increases with advancing age, and half of all women and 15–30 % of all men are currently expected to sustain a fragility fracture during their lifetime. Why the number of osteoporotic fractures has increased is partially unclear, but a larger population and a higher proportion of elderly in society as well as secular changes in bone mineral density (BMD), fall frequency, and other risk factors may have influenced the fracture rate (Øyen et al. 2010, 2011a, b).
- During the recent decades, it has been shown that in individuals with osteoporosis, a BMD of 2.5 standard deviations (SD) or more below the average value in young healthy individuals of the same gender (T-score −2.5), evaluated by dual-energy X-ray (DXA) technique (WHO 1994) (Table 6.1), drug treatment could reduce the fracture risk by half (Black et al. 1996).
- Fracture reduction has however only been verified in high-risk cohorts. However, individuals with this profile only represent a small proportion in community, and even though their fracture risk is high, the absolute number of fractures in this group will be low.
- Most distal radius and other fragility fractures do instead occur in the much larger group of individuals with osteopenia.
- Pharmacological treatment should only be given to defined risk groups with osteoporosis or high fracture risk, not to patients with only osteopenia.
- The total fracture burden must instead be addressed by other general fracture-preventive strategies. These strategies must fulfill specific demands; they must reduce the fracture risk, be safe, have no or few adverse side effects, be accessible for most individuals, and be cost-effective.

Table 6.1 Definition of normal bone mass, osteopenia, osteoporosis, and established osteoporosis (WHO 1994)

Diagnostic category	Definition	BMD T-score
Normal bone mass	BMD above 1 standard deviation below the average young and adult value	> −1
Osteopenia	BMD between 1 and 2.5 standard deviations below the average young adult value	−1 to −2.5
Osteoporosis	BMD more than 2.5 standard deviations below the average young adult value	< −2.5
Severe osteoporosis or established osteoporosis	BMD more than 2.5 standard deviations below the average young adult value and at least one osteoporotic fracture	< −2.5

6.3 Risk Factors for Falls and Fractures

- Low BMD is often referred to one of the most important risk factors for distal radius fractures and other fragility fractures (Øyen et al. 2010, 2011a, b). A 1.0 standard deviation (SD) lower BMD virtually doubles the fracture risk (Cummings et al. 1995) (Fig. 6.1).
- If BMD is more than 2.5 SD lower than the mean BMD in a young healthy population, the condition is defined as osteoporosis (WHO 1994).
- Osteoporosis is classified as primary or secondary.
- Primary osteoporosis occurs at aging and is in women often related to the bone loss that follows low estrogen levels after menopause.
- Secondary osteoporosis is the result of diseases or treatments such as endocrine

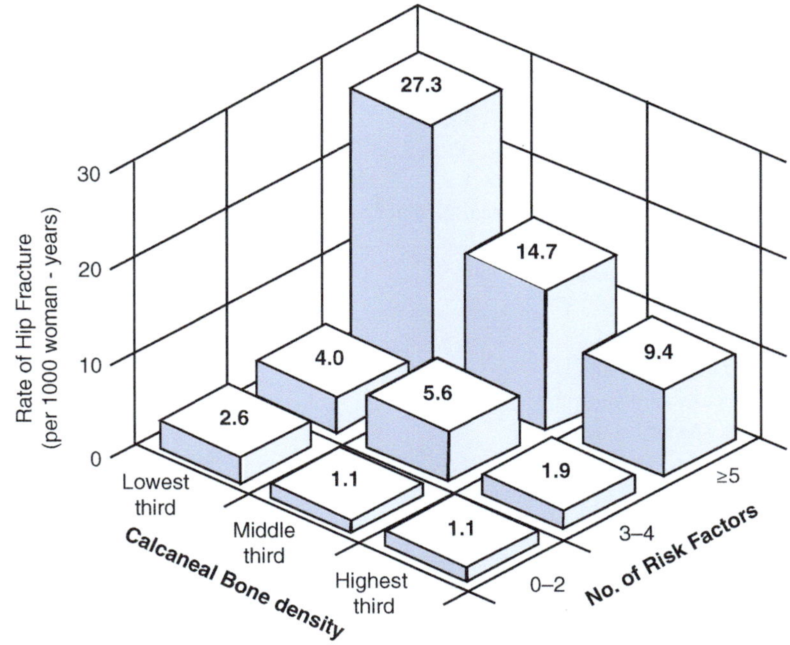

Fig. 6.1 Annual risks of hipfracture according to the number of risk factors and the age-specific calcaneal bone density (Cummingset al. 1995)

disorders, anorexia nervosa, or glucocorticoid treatment.

- Even if the risk to sustain a distal radius fracture or other fragility fractures is highest in risk cohorts, the majority of fractures arise from the much larger proportion of the population with osteopenia at low or moderate fracture risk. Pharmacological treatment in these groups is less effective.
- Other general risk factors for distal radius and other fragility fracture include female gender and high age. In fact, the same BMD value provides a much higher risk for fractures in older than younger individuals.
- Fall risk is maybe the most important independent risk factor for a distal radius or other fragility fractures, and risk factors for falls and fractures are similar (Table 6.2) (Lee et al. 2002; Cameron et al. 2010; Gillespie et al. 2012).
- Weaker risk factors are poor nutrition, low body weight, smoking, excessive alcohol consumption, excessive caffeine intake, physical inactivity, impaired vision, comorbidities, functional impairments, disabilities, and specific medication (Table 6.2).

6.4 Nutrition and Physical Activity

- For prevention of distal radius or other fragility fractures, we usually recommend a well-balanced nutritional intake with the recommended levels of energy, protein, calcium, and vitamin D.
- We also advocate an active physical lifestyle since it seems likely that there is a causal relationship between exercise, high BMD, beneficial neuromuscular function, and low fracture risk.
- During adulthood and in the postmenopausal period, physical activity should however be regarded as bone preserving more than bone building, seeing that evidence from RCTs suggests that exercise in adults at best increases BMD by a few percentage points (Heinonen et al. 1998).
- Physical activity may also induce a decrease in fracture risk through nonskeletal pathways such as higher muscle strength and better coordination and balance (Kroger et al. 1994).
- Physical activity also reduces fall risk in both community dwelling and institutionalized

Table 6.2 Risk factors for osteoporosis, fall, and fracture (Gillespie et al. 2012)

Risk factor	Osteoporosis	Fall	Fracture
Low bone mineral density			+
High age	+	+	+
Female sex	+	+	+
Primary or secondary amenorrhea	+		+
Primary or secondary hypogonadism in men	+		+
Premature menopause	+		+
Postmenopausal status	+	+	+
Tallness		+	+
Low body weight	+		+
Long hip axis length			+
Previous fragility fracture	+	+	+
Family history of fracture			+
White or Asian ethnic origin			+
Immobility/low physical activity	+	+	+
Current smoking	+	+	+
High caffeine intake			+
Alcohol abuse	+	+	+
High bone turnover	+		+
Osteomalacia/vitamin D deficiency	+	+	+
Low dietary calcium intake	+		+
Chronic illnesses	+	+	+
Glucocorticoid therapy	+		+
Sedative medications		+	+
Visual impairment		+	+
Cognitive impairment		+	+
Neurological diseases		+	+
Lower limb disability	+	+	+
Hyperthyroidism	+		+
Hyperparathyroidism	+		+
Malabsorption	+		+
Celiac disease	+		+
Gastrectomy	+		+
Chronic arthritides	+	+	+
Chronic renal/liver diseases	+		+
Cushing syndrome	+		+
Malignancies	+		+
Organ transplantations	+		+
Living in a nursing home		+	+

elderly (Cameron et al. 2010; Gillespie et al. 2012).

- Both earlier and current physical activities are associated with reduction in fracture risk by 50 % in both genders (Karlsson et al. 2001). Hence, exercise is beneficial for fracture risk at all ages and should be recommended to all patients.

6.5 Non-pharmacological Interventions for Fall and Fracture Prevention

- There has been a tradition of modifying a variety of environmental risk factors for falls and fractures in individuals with a high risk of distal radius or other fragility fractures.

- For prevention of distal radius and other fragility fractures, we usually recommend individuals at high fracture risk to modify and eliminate possible hazards for falls in the home environment. This includes removal of loose carpets and electrical cords and improved lightning and is usually a simple and cheap approach for fall and fracture risk reduction.
- Intervention strategies that reduce the risk in RCTs have also been even more cost-effective in high-risk groups than in the general population (Cameron et al. 2010; Gillespie et al. 2012).
- As a previous fall is an independent risk factor for subsequent falls and as a distal radius or other fragility fracture predicts future fractures, it is especially important to evaluate each elderly person with a fall or fragility fracture to elucidate if the patient is a high-risk individual suitable for specific intervention.
- Fall-preventive interventions that have been shown to reduce the number of falls and/or the number of fallers in RCTs are listed below:
  - Regular exercise that includes multicomponent training modalities
  - Reduction of home hazards
  - Vitamin D supplement in individuals with low levels of vitamin D
  - Adjustment of psychotropic medication
  - Structured modification of multi-pharmacy
  - Anti-slip shoe devices in old individuals walking outdoors during icy conditions
  - Multifaceted podiatry to patients with specific foot disability
  - First eye cataract surgery in patients with visual impairment
  - Pacemakers in patients with cardioinhibitory carotid sinus hypersensitivity
  - Generalized multifactorial fall prevention programs
  - Individually designed multifactorial fall prevention programs

6.6 Pharmacological Intervention for Fracture Prevention

- For prevention of distal radius or other fragility fractures, we usually recommend individuals with osteoporosis to start prophylactic drug treatment, as the fracture reductive effect is supported by high level of evidence.
- These drugs should always be given together with calcium and vitamin D.
- The following pharmacological treatments in high-risk groups for osteoporosis and/or distal radius or other fragility fractures have been shown to reduce the number of fractures in RCTs:
  - Bisphosphonates.
  - Parathyroid hormone (PTH).
  - Selective estrogen receptor modulator (SERM).
  - Calcium and vitamin D – at least in institutionalized individuals.
  - Hormone replacement therapy (HRT) – adverse effects such as breast cancer and ischemic heart disease outweigh the fracture risk reduction, and HRT is not recommended for fracture prevention in most countries.
  - Strontium ranelate.
  - Denosumab.

6.7 Who Should We Treat with Pharmacological Interventions?

- When identifying a patient with osteoporosis or with several risk factors for distal radius or other fragility fractures, it is often difficult to decide if pharmacological treatment should be initiated or not. To support decision, a free country-specific web-based tool – FRAX (*fracture index* (*http://www.shef.ac.uk/FRAX/*)) – *could be used.* By filling out information on 12 known risk factors and if also the results from a bone mass scan are available, FRAX can be used to estimate the patient's 10-year probability of fragility fractures.

- In many countries, the national health services recommend the use of FRAX in patients who have sustained a distal radius or other fragility fracture or in patients where a DXA scan has shown a BMD value below 2 SD compared to the mean value in young individuals (T-score −2.0).
- FRAX provides the probability in percent for the individual to sustain major or minor fragility fractures within a 10-year frame. With the estimate, it is easier for both the doctor and the patient to agree on pharmacological treatment or not. For example, in Sweden, the current recommendation for pharmacological treatment is a previous hip or vertebral fracture, a FRAX 10-year probability of fractures of more than 30 %, or a BMD T-score <−2 with a previous fracture.
- Recommendations for pharmacological treatment are generally country specific.
- There are now studies inferring that fracture liaison services that provide the necessary assessment and treatment of osteoporosis and evaluation and interventions for fall risk for all patients with distal radius or other fragility fracture are a cost-effective method to reduce the fracture risk. This also accounts for distal radius fractures where patients who are addressed in this way after a distal radius fracture have a significantly reduced risk to sustain a second distal radius fracture (Harness et al. 2012).

6.8 Orthopedic Surgeons and Prevention of Fractures

- The orthopedic surgeon has a central role in the prevention of distal radius or other fragility fractures.
- Osteoporosis is a silent disease until a distal radius or other low-energy-related fractures occur. The patient is then often treated by an orthopedic surgeon, and there are few medical doctors that see as many patients with osteoporosis and established osteoporosis as an orthopedic surgeon.
- However, there is an obvious risk that orthopedic surgeons concentrate on the distal radius fracture treatment itself. It cannot be considered acceptable today to neglect investigation or treatment of osteoporosis in patients presenting with a low-energy fracture.
- The evaluation of patients with a prevalent distal radius or other fragility fractures must therefore also include history of falls and assessment of other risk factors and may in many cases also include BMD scan, to identify patients at high risk of sustaining future fractures.
- We are therefore of the firm opinion that distal radius or other fragility fracture treatments must be accompanied by properly initiated investigations for osteoporosis and suitable interventions. This is the responsibility of the orthopedic surgeon. He or she does not necessarily have to conduct the investigation and/or initiate treatment but at least has to refer the patient to a clinic suitable for this.
- It is also essential to initiate pharmacological treatment only in group with proven fracture reductive effect (Table 6.3).

Table 6.3 Tricks and tips in osteoporosis

Fracture-preventive strategies must reduce the fracture risk, be safe, have no or few adverse side effects, be accessible for most individuals, and be cost-effective
Fractures and falls share common risk factors and are highly linked
There is strong evidence that a variety of intervention programs may reduce the fall risk
Physical activity has been identified as the most effective intervention for fall risk reduction
Meta-analyses of RCTs have shown that exercise-induced fall-preventive interventions do reduce not only the number of falls but also the number of injurious falls, including those that result in factures
Virtually all exercise trials are concordant and report that lifetime physical activity is associated with a low fracture risk
The evidence that improvement in nutritional intake prevents fragility fractures is only supported by trials with a lower level of evidence
The evidence that both anti-resorptive and bone-forming pharmacological treatments prevent fragility fractures is high

References

Black DM, et al. Randomised trial of effect of alendronate on risk of fracture in women with existing vertebral fractures. Fracture Intervention Trial Research Group. Lancet. 1996;348(9041):1535–41.

Cameron ID, et al. Interventions for preventing falls in older people in nursing care facilities and hospitals. Cochrane Database Syst Rev. 2010;(1):CD005465.

Cummings SR, Nevitt MC, Browner WS, et al. Risk factors for hip fracture in white women. Study of Osteoporotic Fractures Research Group. N Engl J Med. 1995;332(12):767–73.

Gillespie LD, et al. Interventions for preventing falls in older people living in the community. Cochrane Database Syst Rev. 2012;(9):CD007146.

Harness NG, et al. Distal radius fracture risk reduction with a comprehensive osteoporosis management program. J Hand Surg Am. 2012;37(8):1543–9.

Heinonen A, et al. Effect of two training regimens on bone mineral density in healthy perimenopausal women: a randomized controlled trial. J Bone Miner Res. 1998; 13(3):483–90.

Kannus P, et al. Epidemiology of hip fractures. Bone. 1996;18 Suppl 1:57S–63.

Karlsson M, Bass S, Seeman E. The evidence that exercise during growth or adulthood reduces the risk of fragility fractures is weak. Best Pract Res Clin Rheumatol. 2001;15(3):429–50.

Kroger H, et al. Bone mineral density and risk factors for osteoporosis–a population-based study of 1600 perimenopausal women. Calcif Tissue Int. 1994;55(1):1–7.

Lee SH, Dargent-Molina P, Breart G. Risk factors for fractures of the proximal humerus: results from the EPIDOS prospective study. J Bone Miner Res. 2002;17(5):817–25.

Øyen J, Gjesdal CG, Brudvik C, Hove LM, Apalseth EM, Gulseth HC, et al. Low-energy distal radius fractures in middle-aged and elderly men and women–the burden of osteoporosis and fracture risk: a study of 1794 consecutive patients. Osteoporos Int. 2010;21(7): 1257–67.

Øyen J, Apalseth EM, Gjesdal CG, Brudvik C, Lie SA, Hove LM. Vitamin D inadequacy is associated with low-energy distal radius fractures: a case–control study. Bone. 2011a;48:1140–5.

Øyen J, Brudvik C, Gjesdal CG, Tell GS, Lie SA, Hove LM. Osteoporosis as a risk factor for distal radial fractures: a case–control study. J Bone Joint Surg Am. 2011b;93(4):348–56.

WHO. Assessment of fracture risk and its application to screening for postmenopausal osteoporosis. Report of a WHO Study Group. World Health Organ Tech Rep Ser. 1994;843:1–129.

Outcome Assessment After Distal Radius Fractures

7

Markus Gabl and Rohit Arora

Contents

M. Gabl, MD (✉) • R. Arora, MD
Department of Trauma Surgery,
Medical University Innsbruck,
Anichstrasse 35, A-6020 Innsbruck, Austria
e-mail: markus.gabl@uki.at;
www.unfallchirurgie-innsbruck.at

7.1 Summary

Subjective and objective measurements after operative or nonoperative treatment of distal radius fractures (DRFs) are a fundamental key of scientific work, clinical research, and to evaluate objective and subjective parameters. For a long time, distal radius fractures were a typical injury in the older population, considered to be harmless and best treated by conservative means, as radiologically bad results did not correlate with patients' satisfaction. With a constantly increasing number of severe fractures especially in younger patients due to high-velocity trauma, work related or in sports, pain and functional impairment was not well tolerated in this more demanding population. By the change of our lifestyle during the years, the patients' individual expectations to the final outcome have changed. Range of motion, strength, pain and good radiological results can be seen, as prerequisites, but are no guarantee for patients' satisfaction.

7.2 Introduction

- The WHO included in the International Classification of Function and Health (ICF) 3 parts: body structure/function, activity and participation. A questionnaire should address items of highest priority in daily life activity.
- Measurement of treatment of DRF of either operative or nonoperative intervention does not just depend on the type of treatment

L.M. Hove et al. (eds.), *Distal Radius Fractures*,
DOI 10.1007/978-3-642-54604-4_7, © Springer-Verlag Berlin Heidelberg 2014

performed but also depends on the way it is measured (Pechlaner et al. 2007).

- There may be as much as 30 % difference in good and excellent results comparing the outcome of DRF assessed using the Gartland and Werley system and Green and O'Brien score in the same patients (Beaton et al. 2002).
- To be useful, measurement instruments should be reliable, valid and responsive.
- If the measurement instrument cannot measure the acute status in a reproducible manner, it has a poor reliability. But also the highest reliability is nothing worth if the instrument does not measure the results with accuracy, which means without validity. High responsiveness reflects the sensitivity of the instrument to assess any changes of the measured parameters during the assessment.
- There is unanimity which measurement should be used to evaluate outcome of DRF. Various different outcome measures are available to evaluate clinical and radiological outcome of DRFs. These measures include general and anatomy-specific patient-reported subjective outcomes, objective measurements and radiographic measurements. As there is not only one instrument that is optimal for all needs during a study, those instruments should be used, which are best suited to the goal of the investigation.
- Various different disease-specific instruments assessing hand-related parameters, for instance the Boston Carpal Tunnel Questionnaire, the Health Assessment Questionnaire (HAQ), the Arthritis Impact Measurement Scale (AIMS) and the Australian/Canadian Hand Osteoarthritis Index, are in use.
- Widely used measurement instruments for outcomes related to the DRF are the Disabilities of the Arm, Shoulder and Hand (DASH) (Hudak et al. 1996), the Michigan Hand Outcomes Questionnaire (MHQ) (Chung et al. 1998) and the Patient-Related Wrist Evaluation (PRWE) (MacDermid 1996), which focuses specifically on wrist function.
- This chapter provides an overview of the most currently used outcome measures for treatment of DRFs.

7.3 Patient-Reported Subjective Outcome Questionnaires

7.3.1 Disabilities of the Arm, Shoulder and Hand (DASH) and Hand/Upper Extremity Function Scale

- This instrument evaluates the disability and the function of the entire upper extremity, taking into account that the wrist and hand are part of the upper extremity (Hudak et al. 1996).
- The difference between the domains of "disability" and "function" is important.
- *Disability* is the lack of ability to perform activities (daily life, work and leisure) due to the impairment (such as not being able to use knife and fork due to the loss of flexion). *Disability* is reported by patients and can vary substantially for a given amount of clinician-measured impairment in domains such as strength or movement. There are some reports proving that patient-perceived disability depends on psychosocial factors and level of education leading to the fact that disability correlates poorly with impairment and with function. For a given degree of physically measureable impairment, patient-reported disability can vary widely.
- *Function* is a term that includes dimensions of movement, strength, joint stability, pain and cosmetic appearance. As most of these domains are not measured accurately, assessment of function as a result has limited use. Disability and function might be related but are not equal with one another.
- The DASH Questionnaire should only be used to measure results in patient-reported disability relating the upper extremity as a whole. Changes that are not correlated with much disability for patients cannot be assessed using this instrument.
- The biggest drawback using DASH for assessing results of DRF is that this questionnaire summarises the overall status of the entire upper limb as a unit. For instance, pain and movement are improved 3 months after volar plating of DRF, but the ability to perform the

evaluated activities is not changed because of poor shoulder/elbow function. In this case the impact of wrist treatment as measured by the instrument might not be as specific as expected.
- The DASH has been widely used in reports of DRFs to measure subjective patient outcomes. For instance, better short-term DASH scores have been found for patients operated on with a volar plate compared to external fixator after 3 and 6 months, with no differences at 12 months. Furthermore, the DASH score has high reliability to assess specifically outcomes of DRFs (MacDermid 1996).

Scoring

- The DASH is scored in two components: the disability/symptom questions (30 items, scored 1–5) and the optional high-performance sport/music or work section (4 items, scored 1–5).
- At least 27 of the 30 items must be completed for a score to be calculated. The assigned values for all completed responses are simply summed and averaged, producing a score out of five.
- This value is then transformed to a score out of 100 by subtracting one and multiplying by 25. This transformation is done to make the score easier to compare to other measures scaled on a 0–100 scale. A higher score indicates increased disability.

Optional Modules (Sport/Music or Work)

- Each optional module consists of four items, which may or may not be used by patients. The goal of the optional modules is to identify the specific difficulties that professional athletes/performing artists or other groups of workers might experience but which may not affect their activities of daily living and consequently may go "undetected" in the 30-item portion of the DASH.

Missing Items

- If more than 10 % of the items (i.e. more than three items) are left blank by the respondent, you will not be able to calculate neither a DASH disability/symptom score nor the high-performance sports/performing arts or work module.
- A shorter form of the DASH, the *Quick*DASH, has also been developed to be more appropriate in some clinical research settings.

7.3.2 The Michigan Hand Outcomes Questionnaire (MHQ)

- The MHQ was developed to assess overall health status and function in patients with hand disorders (Chung et al. 1998). It has excellent reliability and has been shown to be valid and responsive for a wide spectrum of conditions affecting the hand including hand injuries, rheumatoid arthritis and other inflammatory pathologies. It contains 6 scales: overall hand function, activities of daily living, pain, work performance, hand appearance and patient satisfaction.
- Better MHQ scores for volar locking plating compared to fragment-specific fixation were only found at 3 months, whereas at 12 months there were better MHQ scores for aesthetic and work (Chung et al. 1999).

Scoring

- In the pain scale, high scores indicate greater pain, while in the other five scales high scores denote better hand performance. The raw scale score for each of the six scales is the sum of the responses of each scale item. The raw score is converted to a score ranging from 0 to 100. The response categories for one of the questions are reversed and recoded. The score for the affected hand is obtained by selecting either the right or the left hand score. If both hands are affected (e.g. rheumatoid arthritis patients), the right and left hand scores are averaged to get the score.
- An overall MHQ score can be obtained by summing the scores for all six scales after reversing the pain scale (pain = 100-pain score) and then dividing by six.
- An abbreviated version of the MHQ, the Brief MHQ has been developed primarily for clinical use.

Missing Items

- Missing values in each scale may affect the validity of the scores. If 50 % or more of the items in a scale are missing, then that particular scale cannot be scored. For scales with less than 50 % missing, the average of the existing scale items may be imputed for the missing items.

7.3.3 Patient-Related Wrist Evaluation (PRWE) or Patient-Rated Wrist/Hand Evaluation (PRWHE)

- The aim of the PRWE questionnaire is to provide a reliable and valid tool for quantifying patient-rated wrist pain and disability in order to assess outcome in patients with distal radius fractures (MacDermid 1996).
- Objective clinical parameters compared with patient-related disability after DRFs show that although grip strength is a good predictor of the PRWE score, active range or wrist motions are not predictive for this score.
- However, since its introduction, validity, reliability and responsiveness have been tested, and the instrument has gained widespread use and was used in more than 70 published wrist/hand studies.

Scoring

- It is constructed in 15 domains. There are five items in the pain domain and ten items in the function domain.
- The response to each item is scored on a scale of 0–10. The pain score is the sum of five items, a worse score of 50; the disability (function) score is the sum of ten items, divided by 2. Thus, the total function on the PRWE scale ranges from 0 (normal wrist) to 150 (worst possible score).

Missing Items

- If there is an item missing, you can replace the item with the mean score of the subscale.
- The Patient-Rated Wrist/Hand Evaluation (PRWHE) is identical to the PRWE except that "wrist" is replaced with "wrist/hand".

7.4 Objective Measures of Outcome

7.4.1 Physical Examination

- Clinical examination of the wrist should assess range of motion (ROM), grip strength and pain. Normal and functional wrist range of motion is presented in Table 7.1.
- The benchmark for satisfaction regarding wrist arc of motion following DRF is achieving 95 % of the uninjured contralateral side.
- Grip strength as an objective outcome parameter is assessed in most recent studies due to its good predictive value for patient satisfaction (Fujii et al. 2002).
- Grip strength can be measured quantitatively using a hand dynamometer. The Jamar hand dynamometer (Lafayette Instrument Company, USA) is the most widely cited in the literature and accepted as the gold standard by which other dynamometers are evaluated. The Jamar is a variable hand span dynamometer with five handle positions. Most studies have used the second position for all participants. This has been assumed to be the most reliable and consistent position and is the position advocated for routine use (Fess 1992).
- The American Society of Hand Therapists (ASHT) recommends standardised positioning: subject seated, shoulders adducted and neutrally rotated, elbow flexed at 90°, forearm in neutral and wrist between 0 and 30° of dorsiflexion (Fess 1992). The need for a standard protocol to improve the validity of assessment is illustrated by Spijkerman et al. (1991),

Table 7.1 Normal and functional wrist range of motion (ROM)

	Normal ROM	Functional ROM
Extension (deg)	64	35
Flexion (deg)	74	10
Pronation (deg)	90	40
Supination (deg)	90	45

who found that allowing subjects to assume a comfortable position produced significantly different readings from the ASHT protocol.

- The ASHT protocol uses the mean of three trials of grip strength in each hand, which had higher test–retest reliability among female students than either one trial alone or the maximum of three trials.
- Normal values of grip strength depend on gender and age exhaustion, and the use of measuring instrument can vary from 5 kg (women aged above 75 years, nondominant hand) to 73 kg (men, aged between 24 and 43 years, dominant hand). The 10 % rule used by therapists treating patients with injured hands states that the dominant hand has a 10 % stronger grip than the nondominant hand.
- The benchmark for satisfaction regarding grip strength following DRF is achieving 65 % of the uninjured contralateral side.
- Patient satisfaction after DRFs correlates highly with the final range of motion and grip strength. In our experience (Arora et al. 2009), treating unstable dorsally displaced DRF using volar locking plate fixation in an elderly population, the ROM reaches about half for flexion and extension and about 80 % regarding pronation and supination of the uninjured contralateral side. The grip strength could be restored to 75 % of the normal side.
- Assessment of pain is always a self-report by patients. The experience and recognition of pain are highly influenced by a multitude of factors. This fact should always be kept in mind when interpreting the results of pain evaluation. Visual analogue scale (VAS) is the widely used method of semi-quantifying pain (VAS 0 = no pain, VAS 10 = severe pain).
- The pain level decreases during the postoperative course. The majority of patients experience mild pain at rest (average VAS 2) and high levels of pain (average VAS 6) with active wrist motion during the first 2 months following DRF. The majority of pain recovery occurs within 6 months (average VAS 1). High levels of pain persist only for a small minority of patients at 1 year following fracture.

7.4.2 Radiographic Evaluation

- Radiographic parameters are commonly used for evaluation of the outcome after DRFs. All are based on the quantitative assessment of plain x-rays in 2 planes. Specific radiographic parameters with biomechanical and clinical implications have been developed to assess the radiocarpal joint (see Chaps. 9 and 10).
- It is general agreement that there is a close relationship between the restoration of radiographic anatomy and function in young, non-osteoporotic and functional active patients (McQueen and Caspers 1988).
- There is evidence that the relationship between radiological alignment and outcome may not be reflected in self-reported function, particularly in the elderly (>70 years) and low-demanding patients.
- In our experience (Arora et al. 2011), we evaluated and compared nonoperative treatment and locked volar plating for DRFs. At 3, 6 and 12 months postoperatively, final results showed that dorsal radial tilt, radial inclination and radial shortening were significantly better in the operatively treated group, whereas the nonoperative group had a 100 % malunion rate (defined as greater than 10° dorsal tilt, greater than 2 mm of radial shortening and greater than 1 mm of articular incongruity). Despite these findings, the operative group had lower DASH and PRWE scores only at 3 months but not at any other time. At the 12-month follow-up examination, the range of motion, the level of pain and the PRWE and DASH scores were not different between the operative and nonoperative treatment groups. Achieving anatomical reconstruction did not convey any improvement in terms of the range of motion or the ability to perform daily living activities in our cohort.

Conclusion

- There are several different methods of evaluating patient recovery after distal radius fracture, including strictly subjective measures, objective examination measurements or a combination of both and radiographic outcomes. Only reliable and valid outcome measures should be used to assess functional recovery after DRFs.
- There are few studies that directly compare outcome measures in a single population to identify the best outcome measures to evaluate the treatment of DRFs.
- The Gartland and Werley score is one of the most widely used outcome measures because it takes into consideration objective measurements to predict overall recovery, but it has never been validated.
- The Disabilities of the Arm, Shoulder and Hand (DASH) questionnaire is a validated outcome measure of the upper extremity, and although it is frequently used to assess DRF outcomes, it can be skewed by ipsilateral injury to the upper extremity and neck. The DASH score after 1 year sustaining a DRF averages 6 points.
- The Patient-Rated Wrist Evaluation (PRWE) and the Michigan Hand Outcomes Questionnaire (MHQ) are the most frequently used outcome measures to assess DRF outcomes, as they are more specific to wrist function. The PRWE score after 1 year sustaining a DRF averages 12 points.
- We reviewed the consistency of the PRWE with only the wrist-specific items of the DASH (Gabl et al. 2007). It identified a high correlation between both of these scores and found that all of the questions that were used were specific for wrist function and subjective comfort after a distal radius fracture when compared with a pathologic condition without wrist involvement. Of the 25 questions, however, only 14 of these correlated well with radiographic features of malunion, which one could consider to be a high determinant of overall functional outcome.
- If there is no substantial improvement for the used scores between the baseline and 2-month follow-up, more intensive therapy may be indicated, and further investigation to look for undetected associated injuries or complications might be appropriate. The role of nonmedical issues that could be contributing to the patient's disability should be questioned.
- Physical examination is one of the most important predictors of overall functional outcomes. However, the contralateral extremity may be an unreliable control. In addition, average values are highly dependent on sex, age, comorbidity and hand dominance. The benchmark for satisfaction following DRF is achieving 95 % of wrist arc range of motion and 65 % of grip strength of the uninjured contralateral side (Ritting and Wolf 2012).
- Pain level should start decreasing after 6 weeks. If patients are reporting abnormally high scores for pain at rest at a 6-week visit, the treating surgeon may become concerned that this patient is presenting with early signs of complex regional pain syndrome (CRPS) and look for other signs/evidence suggestive of this problem (MacDermid et al. 2003).
- If pain level remains high after 6 weeks during activities of daily life without any evidence of CRPS, signs of flexor tendon irritations due to volar plate protrusion or extensor tendon irritations caused by too long screws penetrating the extensor compartments should be checked.
- Radiographic parameters have been created to establish normal anatomy, although they may not be predictive of functional recovery, specifically in the elderly population.

References

Arora R, et al. A comparative study of clinical and radiologic outcomes of unstable colles type distal radius fractures in patients older than 70 years: nonoperative treatment versus volar locking plating. J Orthop Trauma. 2009;23(4):237–42.

Arora R, Lutz M, Deml C, et al. A prospective randomized trial comparing nonoperative treatment with volar locked plate fixation for displaced and unstable distal radius fractures in patients sixty-five years of age and older. J Bone Joint Surg Am. 2011;93(23):2146–53.

Beaton DE, Boers M, Wells GA. Many faces of the minimal clinically important difference (MCID): a literature review and directions for future research. Curr Opin Rheumatol. 2002;14(2):109–14.

Chung KC, Pillsbury MS, Walters MR, et al. Reliability and validity testing of the Michigan Hand Outcomes Questionnaire. J Hand Surg Am. 1998;23(4):575–87.

Chung KC, Hamill JB, Walters MR, et al. The Michigan Hand Outcomes Questionnaire (MHQ): assessment of responsiveness to clinical change. Ann Plast Surg. 1999;42(6):619–22.

Fess EE. Grip strength. 2nd ed. Chicago: American Society of Hand Therapists; 1992.

Fujii K, Henmi T, Kanematsu Y, et al. Fractures of the distal end of radius in elderly patients: a comparative study of anatomical and functional results. J Orthop Surg (Hong Kong). 2002;10:9–15.

Gabl M, Krappinger D, Arora R, et al. Acceptance of patient-related evaluation of wrist function following distal radius fracture. Handchir Mikrochir Plast Chir. 2007;39(1):68–72.

Hudak PL, Amadio PC, Bombardier C. Development of an upper extremity outcome measure: the DASH (disabilities of the arm, shoulder and hand). The Upper Extremity Collaborative Group (UECG). Am J Ind Med. 1996;29(6):602–8.

MacDermid JC. Development of a scale for patient rating of wrist pain and disability. J Hand Ther. 1996;9(2):178–83.

MacDermid JC, Roth JH, Richards RS. Pain and disability reported in the year following a distal radius fracture: a cohort study. BMC Musculoskelet Disord. 2003;4:24.

McQueen MM, Caspers J. Colles fracture: does the anatomical result affect the final function? J Bone Joint Surg Br. 1988;70:649–51.

Pechlaner S, Gabl M, Lutz M, Arbeitsgruppe AMUDIRA, et al. Distal radius fractures—aetiology, treatment and outcome. Handchir Mikrochir Plast Chir. 2007;39:19–28.

Ritting AW, Wolf JM. How to measure outcomes of distal radius fracture treatment. Hand Clin. 2012;28:165–75.

Spijkerman DC, Snijders CJ, Stijnen T, Lankhorst GJ. Standardization of grip strength measurements. Effects on repeatability and peak force. Scand J Rehabil Med. 1991;23:203–6.

Medicolegal Aspects of Distal Radius Fractures

8

Tim Davis

Contents

T. Davis, MD
Department of Trauma and Orthopaedics,
Nottingham University Hospitals,
Nottingham University, Nottingham, UK
e-mail: tim.davis@nuh.nhs.uk

8.1 Summary

Most surgeons will at some time be sued for negligent treatment by a patient. A successful claim requires the patient to demonstrate that his/her surgeon made a mistake, which no competent surgeon should have made. It is not good enough for the patient to demonstrate that an expert surgeon could have achieved a better result. In my experience, most successful negligence claims against surgeons are due to very simple errors and mistakes, as well as a failure to communicate with the patient and involve him/her in treatment decisions.

8.2 Introduction

- It is difficult to generalise between different countries and different health care systems, with different cultural and national climates for complaints. This chapter will basically refer to the United Kingdom (UK) and experiences from this country, but with general application to most parts of the world.
- All doctors have patients who are dissatisfied with their treatment, usually as a result of an unsatisfactory functional or cosmetic outcome. Some will make a financial claim on the basis that their treatment was negligent, and most surgeons will be sued for damages due to claimed negligence on at least one occasion during their careers.

L.M. Hove et al. (eds.), *Distal Radius Fractures*,
DOI 10.1007/978-3-642-54604-4_8, © Springer-Verlag Berlin Heidelberg 2014

- In the UK a patient can only gain financial compensation through the courts for "negligent" treatment if "Breach of Duty" and "Causation" are proven.
- "Breach of Duty" indicates that the treatment provided to the patient was of an unacceptably poor quality, lower than that which would have been provided by an average surgeon. With this definition of "Breach of Duty" the quality of treatment must have been of lower than the standard quality you would expect to receive throughout UK.
  - A claim for negligent treatment cannot be made on the basis that the outcome of treatment would have been better if the most modern sophisticated treatment had been provided instead of the standard treatment, which is provided throughout the UK.
  - Thus, surgeons, particularly those with a particular interest in fractures of the distal radius, should be cautious not to criticise standard treatment when considering the outcomes of treatments of fractures of the distal radius by colleagues. This is even if they believe that a better outcome could have been provided with the more sophisticated treatment, which they personally would have offered.
- "Causation" indicates that the patient has suffered a "loss" as a result of the "Breach of Duty". The loss is a worse outcome from the injury/surgery than would have occurred if treatment of adequate quality had been provided. This might result in:
  - A longer recovery from injury/surgery than would have occurred if treatment of a satisfactory standard had been provided
  - Permanent loss of function, which is greater than would normally have been expected
  - The requirement for additional treatment, such as a corrective osteotomy, which would otherwise have been unnecessary
- In many cases, lawyers and medical experts acting for both the patient and the surgeon are uncertain if they can prove to the court that the treatment was, or was not, negligent and has, or has not, worsened the outcome. As a result many cases are settled "out of court" for a compromise payment agreeable to both parties.

8.3 Choice of Treatment Modality

- Most fractures of the distal radius can be managed adequately and safely with a variety of treatments ranging from nonoperative treatment in a below elbow plaster to open reduction and internal fixation (ORIF) with a volar locking plate.
- This is highlighted by the chapters in this book, which describe a wide variety of different treatment options.
- Each treatment option has a number of unique benefits, as well as a number of unique disadvantages. Whichever way one treats a fracture of the distal radius, one will always encounter some unsatisfactory outcomes, but the type of unsatisfactory outcome is often determined by the treatment modality selected. For example, fracture malunion causing cosmetic deformity is common after nonoperative treatment of displaced fractures of the distal radius by closed reduction and immobilisation in plaster. In contrast, rupture of the flexor pollicis longus (FPL) tendon is a complication, which is almost unique to the use of volar locking plates.
- Cochrane reviews, which have looked at the generality of distal radius fractures, have concluded that there is no firm evidence to demonstrate benefit of one form of treatment (whether nonoperative in plaster or external fixation, EF) over any other mode of treatment (e.g. volar locking plates or closed reduction and percutaneous wiring). To quote the conclusion of one Cochrane review (Handoll and Madhok 2003):
  - The 48 randomised trials do not provide robust evidence for most of the decisions necessary in the management of these fractures. Although, in particular, there is some evidence to support the use of external fixation or percutaneous pinning, their precise role and methods are not established. It is also unclear whether surgical intervention of most fracture types will produce consistently better long-term outcomes.
- Further systematic reviews of randomised controlled studies have also failed to show definite superiority of one treatment over

others (Handoll et al. 2007). It is thus my belief that, for most distal radius fractures, it is difficult to claim that the choice of treatment modality was negligent, though the manner in which it was administered might be.

8.4 Effect of Malunion

- It has been suggested that acceptable alignment for isolated closed distal radius fractures is:
  - Dorsal tilt (angulation) <15° but with a palmar tilt <20°
  - Radial inclination >15°
  - Radial shortening ≤5 mm
  - Intra-articular step-off <2 mm (Ilyas and Jupiter 2010).
- The American Academy of Orthopaedic Surgeons (AAOS) has created guidelines for the treatment of fractures of the distal radius using systematic evidence-based processes designed to combat bias, enhance transparency, and promote reproducibility. They suggest operative fixation as opposed to cast fixation for fractures with post-reduction radial shortening >3 mm, dorsal tilt >10°, or intra-articular displacement or step-off >2 mm. However, they only found "moderate" (i.e. not conclusive) evidence to support operative fixation for fractures with greater persistent displacement (Lichtman et al. 2011).
- Thus, there is great debate on the significance of the most common complication of fractures of the distal radius, extra-articular malunion, on the outcome. For example, one recent study concluded that fracture malunion only had a minor influence on the functional outcome of fractures of the distal radius (Finsen et al. 2013), whereas another (Brogren et al. 2013) found malunion had a greater impact on function. Some studies have reported that some, but not other, parameters of malunion (shortening, dorsal tilt, and loss of radial angle) influence the functional outcome, whereas other papers have found no influence of the same parameter of malunion, but detected significant effects of others on function (Table 8.1). Few studies have quantified the influence of "small" compared to "large" amounts of malunion on the functional outcome and most have set a boundary between malunion and no malunion for each parameter. Thus, although large malunions may cause poor functional outcomes in a significant number of patients, one cannot assume that smaller malunions will affect function.
- What is often forgotten is that the greater any malunion, the more likely there will be a significant, and permanent, cosmetic deformity. The patients' perception of the cosmetic appearance of their fracture is often of great importance, but it is not assessed in many outcome studies. For example, the DASH score does not consider the appearance of the wrist, only symptoms and function.

Table 8.1 Conclusions of papers published during 2008–2013 on the effects of three parameters of extra-articular malunion on the clinical outcome of fractures of the distal radius. There is no or little consistency in their findings

Authors	Dorsal tilt	Radial Inclination	Radial Length
Abramo et al. (2008)	–	–	–
Forward et al. (2008)	–	–	+
Kumar et al. (2008)	–	+(<15°)	+
Ng and McQueen (2011)	–	–	+(≥2 mm)*
Brogren et al. (2013)	+(>10°)	–	+(≥1 mm)#

–, no effect; +, effect but not quantified; *, radial height; #, ulnar positive variance

8.5 Minimising the Risk of Litigation Against Yourself and Others

I believe that patients pursue negligence claims due to:

- Lack of communication between the surgeon and the patient
- The provision of misinformation, often well intentioned, to the patient

  For example:
- The patient is initially seen by one surgeon, who emphatically advises that one particular

form of treatment is necessary for his/her fracture. The patient is then transferred to the care of another surgeon who disagrees that this treatment is "best", or does not use this form of treatment. This surgeon advises and undertakes a different form of treatment. If the cosmetic or functional outcome of the fracture is poor, or complications occur, then these may be blamed on the second surgeon's choice of treatment as the patient assumes no problems would have occurred if the first surgeon's treatment had been provided. The first surgeon had "set the second surgeon up for failure" by emphatically stating how the fracture should be treated. Such dissatisfaction is readily avoided by explaining to patients that there are several entirely acceptable ways of treating most fractures of the distal radius, rather than strongly over-stating the need for his/her favoured form of treatment. This problem typically occurs when a patient fractures his/her wrist when away from home, such that he/she is first seen in the town where the injury occurred but is then transferred back to his/her home town (in a temporary plaster) for definitive treatment of his/her fracture. The first surgeon is often a keen young trainee, who wishes to demonstrate his knowledge and competence, but lacks wisdom.

- Failure of the surgeon to communicate to the patient that, however their fracture is treated, there is a risk of developing a poor outcome due to an unavoidable complication of the fracture or its treatment.
- Poor note-keeping. Clinic consultation records should not just record what treatment is to be provided. They should also record what treatment options were discussed with the patient and whether the potential benefits and drawbacks of the selected treatment were described to the patient.
- Operation notes should not just describe the operative technique and record screw lengths. They should also record whether particular difficulties were encountered during the operation and, if the preoperative plan is abandoned and a different method of fixation is used, explain why this decision was made (e.g. ORIF abandoned as fracture too comminuted, or implant kit unavailable as accidently de-sterilised or components missing).
- In my opinion, poor communication between the surgeon and his/her patient is the most potent cause of negligence claims. The basic premise is that the patient must feel involved in his/her treatment and understand what is happening and why it is happening.
- Also, I think patients are far more likely to sue if they feel that something went wrong during their treatment and an attempt has been made to cover this up.
- The risk of litigation is minimised by explaining to the patient frankly and honestly
  - What is being, and has been, done
  - What has gone wrong

8.6 Common Causes of Negligence Claims

In my view, the following are common causes of claims for negligent treatment against surgeons:

1. *Treating the X-ray rather than the patient.*
   - No fracture can be considered in isolation, without assessing the patient who is "attached" to the fracture.
   - The X-ray is not the fracture, but an image of the fracture and the outcome of the "true" fracture cannot be accurately predicted from the "X-ray" image of the fracture.
   - Much will depend on the patients' perception of his/her injury and the quality of his/her treatment. It will also probably depend on the character of the patient.
   - Demographic data, such as age and sex, should not be used to categorise patients and assign them to treatment pathways; it is imperative that the treating surgeon talks to the patient and assesses his/her level of activity, as well as his/her ambitions, both functional and cosmetic, and requirements of treatment.
   - At the initial assessment of the patient, before any treatment is instituted, all patients should be warned that, however

the fracture is treated, there is always a risk of a poor outcome due to:
  - Complications of the fracture itself, such as complex regional pain syndrome
  - Specific complications of the preferred treatment option
- Failure to explain to patients that they may obtain a poor result however expertly their fracture is treated or whichever treatment option is advised is likely to cause dissatisfaction afterwards.
- It is imperative that the patient feels that he/she is being treated, rather than the X-ray image of his/her fracture.

2. *Failure to consider the likely cosmetic outcome of the injury.*
   - Orthopaedic surgeons are taught that the absolute aim of treatment is to restore function, but they may fail to consider the cosmetic outcome.
   - However, the cosmetic outcome is of utmost importance to some patients and important to many.
   - Fractures, which unite with loss of radial height and dorsal angulation, can produce very unsightly wrists, and the greater the degree of malunion, the worse the cosmetic outcome.
   - If it is decided that the best form of treatment of a displaced fracture is nonoperative, by closed reduction and immobilisation in a plaster cast, then the patient should be warned at the beginning of treatment that this may result in the fracture uniting with sufficient malunion to cause a significant cosmetic deformity.
   - As a general rule displaced fractures treated nonoperatively in a plaster, at worst, may unite in the position in which they presented to the A&E Department. This will give an indication of the severity of the cosmetic deformity, which could occur.
   - Additionally, when discussing cosmesis, it should be explained that other techniques such as percutaneous K-wiring or ORIF are likely to produce a better cosmetic outcome, but both treatments carry risks of other complications.
   - Also, although treatment with a volar locking plate most reliably results in union in near anatomical alignment, and thus achieves a good cosmetic result, it leaves a scar, which is normally accepted. Scars on the dorsum of the distal radius will have a greater impact, as this is the side of the forearm which is visible to others for most of the time.

3. *Failure to provide appropriate follow-up treatment after nonoperative treatment by closed reduction and plaster immobilisation.*
   - Nonoperative treatment of displaced distal radius fractures by closed reduction and plaster immobilisation requires careful follow-up during the first few weeks. This is to ensure that the fracture remains in "acceptable" alignment, but what is "acceptable" will vary from surgeon to surgeon and patient to patient.
   - If follow-up appointments and check X-rays are not made at appropriate times, then the fracture may displace unnoticed into an "unacceptable position" resulting in a poor outcome.
   - Problems develop when clinics are cancelled and in these situations alternative clinic appointments within a day or two of the required follow-up time should be made. Unfortunately, patients are sometimes not given an alternative appointment during the week when the clinic is cancelled and instead may be instructed (sometimes without the surgeon's knowledge) to attend in the following week. If the fracture displaces into "unacceptable alignment" during this period, the chance to perform a "simple" procedure to realign the fracture (e.g. remanipulation and percutaneous Kirschner wiring) may be missed, as the fracture can no longer be reduced with a closed manipulation. Instead either:
     - The position of the fracture has to be accepted and nonoperative treatment in plaster continued with the intention of performing a corrective osteotomy after fracture consolidation, or

    - If indicated, the fracture is realigned immediately by ORIF.
  - A similar problem occurs with patients who fracture their wrist just before going away on a planned holiday. Many wish to continue with their holiday, particularly if they have not purchased travel cancellation insurance. The temptation to be kind to the patient and tell him/her "that's fine – go on your holiday and we'll see you when you're back" should be resisted. This is, as you are taking a risk on his/her behalf by arranging follow-up which is inadequate and reduces the chances of a good result. Instead it should be made quite clear to such patients that their treatment requires them to attend clinic for check X-rays during the period that they are on holiday, and if they are away and cannot attend, then they (and not you) are increasing the risk of the fracture uniting with malunion and producing a poor cosmetic, and possibly functional, outcome. Such advice should be clearly recorded in the notes so there is no doubt that this warning/advice was given.

4. *Tunnel vision*
   (a) Nonoperative treatment of displaced fractures by closed reduction and immobilisation in plaster.
   - If this treatment is not working because:
     - There are repeated plaster problems
     - The fracture displaces into unacceptable alignment and obviously has an unstable configuration (dorsal cortical comminution or step-off of the palmar surface), or
     - The fracture re-displaces after a remanipulation.
     - Then it is time to reflect!

   Rather than continuing with nonoperative treatment in plaster as this is "how I always treat these fractures", it is better to stand back and consider whether this is the best form of treatment for this particular patient, or whether it would be best to abandon nonoperative treatment in plaster and change to an alternative form of treatment.
   - The earlier alternative options are considered, the easier it is to salvage the situation.
   - Prevarication beyond 2 weeks post-fracture will only make matters worse by reducing the range of salvage options available. As always the patient must be involved in the management of his/her fracture and, after an explanation of the dilemma, be allowed to consider the benefits and risks (both functional and cosmetic) of
     - Continuing with nonoperative treatment in plaster
     - Abandoning this treatment and continuing treatment with an alternative modality
   - In essence, the final decision rests with the patient, but it is the surgeon's duty to explain the situation to the patient so that he/she understands the logic behind your advice and can make an informed decision. A record of these discussions needs to be in the notes.

   (b) ORIF
   - If an adequate reduction and fixation of the fracture is not readily achieved by percutaneous K-wire fixation or ORIF, then, rather than continuing to try and achieve an adequate reduction and satisfactory fixation with the chosen technique (which may be impossible), it is better to stand back and think whether an alternative treatment method might produce a better outcome and be safer for the patient.
   - For example, a fracture, which is found to be "unfixable", may be best managed by application of an EF, however great the surgeon's dislike of this treatment option.
   - When such problems are encountered with the fixation of a fracture which are due to the nature of the fracture, the limitations of the selected fixation device, or the unexpected unavailability of the chosen fixation device (perhaps used earlier in the day and not yet cleaned and sterilised), then these should be carefully recorded in the notes and explained to the patient after they have fully recovered from the anaesthetic. This is so that he/she is aware of the difficulties,

that their fracture has been difficult to treat, and that there is an increased risk of an unsatisfactory outcome. This is particularly the case if the method of fracture fixation is changed during the surgery. Again the basic premise is that the patient must be involved in his/her treatment and understand what is happening and why it has happened.
  - Sometimes I wonder if there has been particular determination to continue to fix a fracture with a new fixation device, when the surgeon may have little, if any, past experience of the device and may not have read the instruction manual.

5. *Locking plates and their distal pegs and screws.*
   - It is not always easy to be certain that the screws and pegs for a volar locking plate are the correct length and that none of their tips penetrate into the radiocarpal joint. This is because the depth gauge may be difficult to use if there is dorsal cortical comminution and also because it is not always possible to obtain good quality image intensifier images of the fracture during the operation. However, the images which are obtained, particularly the stored images which are retained as a record of the procedure, must be carefully scrutinised to check if:
     – The wrist is correctly positioned for the X-rays
     – No screw or peg is obviously standing proud of the dorsal cortex of the distal radius
     – No peg/screw tip is obviously lying within the radiocarpal joint
     – The distal end of the locking plate is not standing proud of the volar cortex, thus allowing it to abrade the flexor tendons
     – Any the temporary distal rod/screw guides (fixed angle targeting devices), which come attached to some locking plates, have been removed
   - It sounds simple, but concentration levels sometimes fall allowing stupid errors to be made at the end of a stressful procedure.

6. *The damning second opinion.*
   - Inevitably some fractures of the distal radius have poor outcomes and some patients then seek the advice of another surgeon on what further can be done to improve their outcome.
   - The surgeon who sees the patient for a second opinion may review the previous treatment of the fracture and disagree with the initial management and firmly feel that an alternative treatment should have been given.
   - Sometimes he/she strongly expresses his opinion to the patient, and the patient has a right to know if his/her original treatment was of an unacceptably low quality.
   - However, the surgeon providing the second opinion, whatever his view on how the fracture was treated, should ensure that his criticism of the original treatment does not suggest negligence unless he/she feels that surgeons of average standard throughout the same country would have provided significantly better treatment.
   - Unjustified criticism of treatment by a surgeon whose personal belief is that the original treatment was negligent can lead a patient into a time-consuming and costly legal case, which is likely to be unsuccessful (Table 8.2).

Table 8.2 Tips and tricks to avoid medicolegal problems in managing distal radius fractures

Treat the patient, not the X-ray
Assess each patient's long-term functional requirements
Consider and discuss with the patient the likely cosmetic, as well as, functional, outcome
Warn the patient before starting treatment that there is a risk of a bad outcome, however his/her fracture is treated
Do not be dogmatic as to how the patient's fracture "must be treated". This is especially if another surgeon will be providing the treatment
If problems occur, explain them frankly and honestly to the patient
If nonoperative treatment is not working well, then discuss with the patient whether to change to a different treatment
If a fracture fixation is proving difficult, consider alternative options
Patients are more likely to sue if they feel that something went wrong during their treatment and an attempt was made to cover this up

References

Abramo A, Kopylov P, Tagil M. Evaluation of a treatment protocol in distal radius fractures: a prospective study in 581 patients using DASH as outcome. Acta Orthop. 2008;79:376–85.

Brogren E, Wagner P, Petranek M, Atroshi I. Distal radius malunion increases risk of persistent disability 2 years after fracture: a prospective cohort study. Clin Orthop Relat Res. 2013;471:1691–7.

Finsen V, Rod O, Rod K, Rajabi B, Alm-Paulsen PS, Russwurm H. The relationship between displacement and clinical outcome after distal radius (Colles') fracture. J Hand Surg Eur Vol. 2013;38:116–26.

Forward DP, Davis TR, Sithole JS. Do young patients with malunited fractures of the distal radius inevitably develop symptomatic post-traumatic osteoarthritis? J Bone Joint Surg Br. 2008;90:629–37.

Handoll HH, Madhok R. Surgical interventions for treating distal radial fractures in adults. Cochrane Database Syst Rev. 2003;CD003209.

Handoll HH, Vaghela MV, Madhok R. Percutaneous pinning for treating distal radial fractures in adults. Cochrane Database Syst Rev. 2007;CD006080.

Ilyas AM, Jupiter JB. Distal radius fractures–classification of treatment and indications for surgery. Hand Clin. 2010;26:37–42.

Kumar S, Penematsa S, Sadri M, Deshmukh SC. Can radiological results be surrogate markers of functional outcome in distal radial extra-articular fractures? Int Orthop. 2008;32:505–9.

Lichtman DM, Bindra RR, Boyer MI, et al. American Academy of Orthopaedic Surgeons clinical practice guideline on: the treatment of distal radius fractures. J Bone Joint Surg Am. 2011;93:775–8.

Ng CY, McQueen MM. What are the radiological predictors of functional outcome following fractures of the distal radius? J Bone Joint Surg Br. 2011;93:145–50.

Part II

Diagnosis

Imaging

9

Benedicte Lange and Karen-Lisbeth Bay Dirksen

Contents

B. Lange, MD (✉)
Department of Radiology,
University Hospitals of Aalborg, Aalborg, Denmark
e-mail: bl@benedictelange.dk

K.-L.B. Dirksen, MD
Department of Radiology,
University Hospital of Hillerød, Hillerød, Denmark

9.1 Summary

Imaging plays a central role in the diagnosis and treatment of distal radius fractures. Conventional radiography in 2 planes is still considered first choice imaging for wrist injuries. Image quality and a systematic diagnostic approach are however essential. Computer tomography (CT) is indicated in cases of uncertain radiograph findings and in comminuted, complex or intra-articular fractures and occasionally for presurgery assessment. Magnetic resonance imaging (MRI) is useful in assessment of tissue lesions and suspicion of fracture despite normal radiograph. Ultrasound is not considered routine modality in radius fracture diagnosis.

9.2 Introduction

Wrist traumas are amongst the most common injuries in the emergency department with fracture of the distal radius reported to be the most common upper extremity fracture (Larsen and Lauritsen 1993). There are few prospective, randomized trials to support different diagnostic strategies. Since wrist injuries are often complex comprising not only fractures but also a continuum of soft-tissue damages, great demands are put on a judicious imaging

L.M. Hove et al. (eds.), *Distal Radius Fractures*,
DOI 10.1007/978-3-642-54604-4_9, © Springer-Verlag Berlin Heidelberg 2014

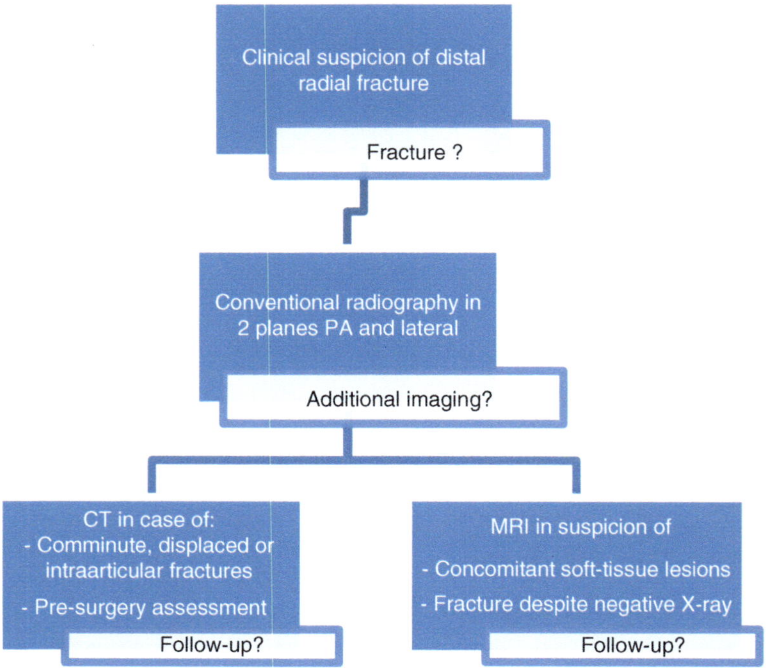

Fig. 9.1 Imaging strategy

strategy, ensuring they are developed in close cooperation between the clinician and the radiologist (Fig. 9.1). This strategy should include immediate as well as possible follow-up imaging. Conventional radiography in at least 2 planes is still considered first choice imaging. In cases of uncertain radiograph findings, comminuted, displaced or intra-articular fractures or for presurgery assessment, computer tomography (CT) is the modality of choice (Trumble et al. 1999; Arora et al. 2010; Harness et al. 2006). Magnetic resonance imaging (MRI) is useful in the assessment of soft-tissue lesions and fracture suspicion despite negative radiograph (Goldfarb et al. 2011; Metz and Gilula 1993; Larsen et al. 1993). Ultrasound is not routine modality; however, it can be considered in an austere environment (McNeil et al. 2009) (Fig. 9.1).

9.3 Conventional Radiography

Wrist radiographs, which include the distal radius, distal ulna, carpal bones and metacarpal bases, can be a challenge. The 15 bones have subtle relationships that change with wrist positioning, which is why the adequacy of the radiograph is of utmost importance. The standard wrist series includes a posterior-anterior (PA – with shoulder in 90° abduction and elbow in 90° flexion) (Fig. 9.2) and lateral view (Fig. 9.3); more views can be added (Goldfarb et al. 2011).

First: Check the adequacy of the radiograph, the alignment and angles of the bones and the bone shapes (Table 9.1).

Second: Carefully evaluate and describe the radiograph systematically. Distal radial fractures are normally not difficult to identify but since they often are accompanied by soft

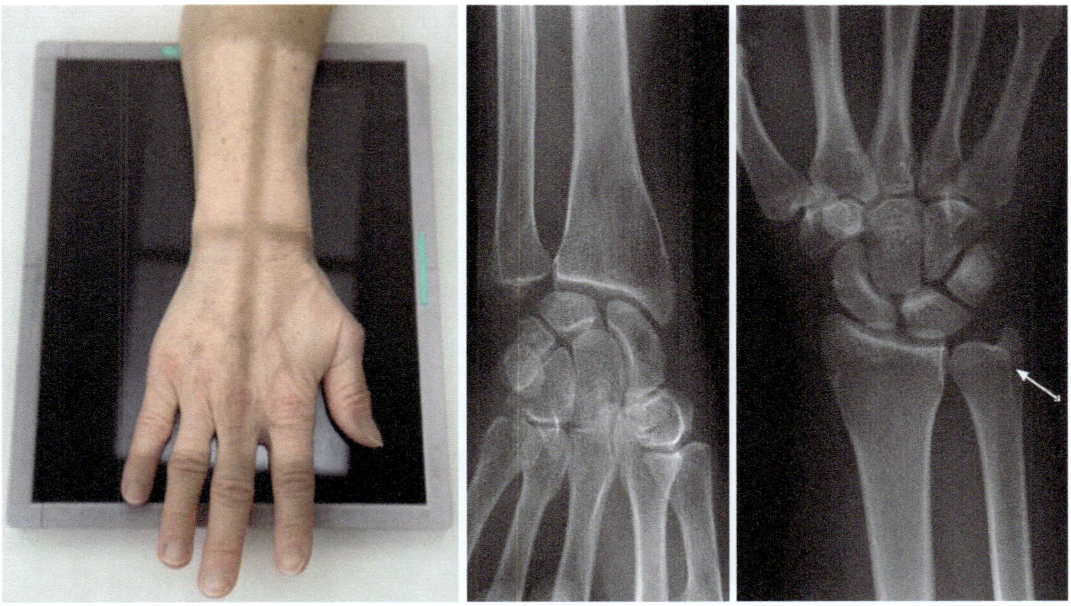

Fig. 9.2 PA view; should profile the extensor carpi ulnaris tendon groove, which should be at the level of or radial to the base of the ulnar styloid (*arrow*)

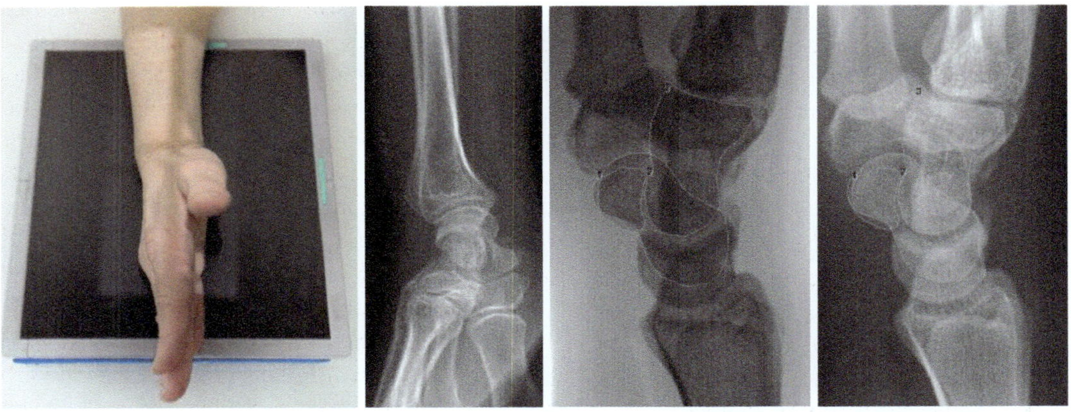

Fig. 9.3 Lateral view; the volar cortex of the pisiform bone (*1*) should overlie the central third of the interval between the volar cortices of the distal scaphoid pole (*2*) and the head of the capitate bone (*3*)

A meticulous 3-step approach to radiograph interpretation can be taken.

Tips and tricks –3-step approach for reading the radiograph

1. *Check adequacy, alignment and angles – see table 9.1*
2. *Evaluate and describe systematically – see table 9.2*
3. *Diagnose and decide treatment – see table 9.3*

tissue injuries resulting in dislocations of carpal bones, careful examination of all the structures in the wrist is necessary (Spence et al. 1998; Geissler et al. 1996) (see Table 9.2). Examples of fractures are displayed in Fig. 9.7.

Third: Diagnose and decide treatment. The classification of fractures is described elsewhere in this book. Table 9.3 displays how injuries are best viewed and Fig. 9.7 displays examples.

Table 9.1 Systematic assessment of the wrist radiograph

Adequacy of the radiograph	Alignment and angles of bones	Bony shapes
Distal 5 cm of radius to carpal-metacarpal junction is included	The three smooth articulating lines of the carpals are visible in PA view (Fig. 9.4)	*PA view* (Fig. 9.4)
Hand neutral in both the PA and lateral views. The axis of the middle metacarpal lines up with the middle of the radius (Figs. 9.2 and 9.3)	No more than 2–3 mm between individual carpal bones (Fig. 9.4)	The scaphoid should be "boat" shaped (scaphos is Greek for boat); a cortical ring implies displacement (signet-ring sign)
PA view	The radius articulates with at least half the lunate (Fig. 9.4)	The lunate should be quadrangular; a triangular shape implies rotation or displacement
Should profile the extensor carpi ulnaris tendon groove, which should be at the level of or radial to the base of the ulnar styloid (Fig. 9.2)	Articular surface of ulna at the same height or slightly shorter as the articular surface of radius (shorter ulna, ulna minus; longer ulna, ulna plus)	The pisiform is the last carpal to ossify up to age 12 years
Lateral view	*PA view* (Fig. 9.5)	
The palmar cortex of the pisiform bone should overlie the central third of the interval between the palmar cortices of the distal scaphoid pole and the capitate head (Fig. 9.3)	Radial inclination 21–25° Radial height 10–13 mm *Lateral view* (Figs. 9.4 and 9.5) Radial volar tilt 0–22° (average 11°) Scapholunate (SL) angle 30–60° Capitolunate (CL) angle < 30°	

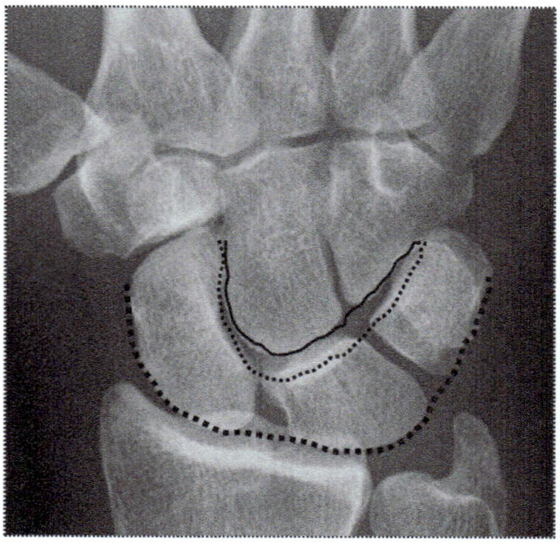

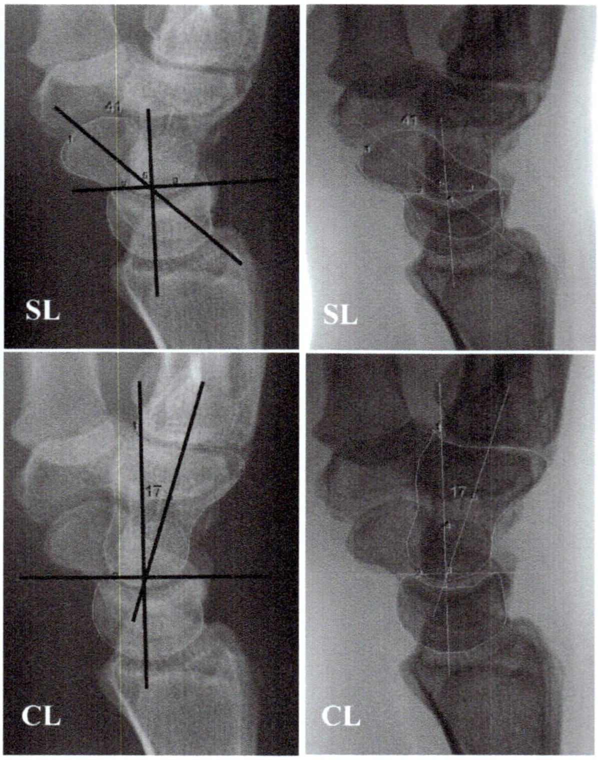

Table 9.2 Evaluation and description of findings on the radiograph

Evaluation and description of pathological findings on the radiograph
Check both PA and lateral views!
Look for:
Soft tissue swelling – observe underlying cortices
Bone cortices discontinuity: PA: cortices of scaphoid, lunate and distal radius Lateral: all cortical structures (distal radius, ulna, carpal bones, metacarpal cortices)
Articular surface discontinuity
Distance between carpals – carpal instability Scapholunate instability: Distance between scaphoid and lunate > 3 mm (Terry-Thomas sign) PA view: abnormal angle of the scaphoid (signet-ring sign) Lateral view (Fig. 9.6): scapholunate angle can be increased (dorsal scapholunate instability, DISI) or decreased (volar scapholunate instability, VISI) Perilunate dislocation (severe, seldom, requires forced injury to the wrist) – distal carpal row dislocates dorsal together with the capitate in relation to the lunate
Describe the fracture: Simple or compound Transverse, oblique or spiral Comminute Complex Impacted Dislocation Avulsion Fissure Greenstick
Measure: Radial height Radial angle
Note other findings: Osteoporosis Osteoarthritis Arthritis Other abnormal findings

Fig. 9.4 Normal wrist radiograph: three smooth articulating lines of the carpals are visible, there is no more than 2–3 mm between individual carpal bones and the radius articulates with at least half the lunate. The scaholunate angle (*SL*) is measured by drawing a line through or parallel to the long axis of the scaphoid bone (*5*), then a helping line parallel to the articular surface of the lunate (*3*) and then a line perpendicular to the articular distal surface of the lunate (*4*). The SL angle is measured between line 4 and 5 and should normally be 30–60° (in this example it is 41°). 1 and 2 represents the outlines of the scaphoid and the lunate. The capitolunate angle (*CL*) is measured by drawing a line through the longitudinal axis of the capitate (*5*), then a helping line parallel to the articular surface of the lunate (*3*) and then a line perpendicular to the articular distal surface of the lunate (*4*). The CL angle is measured between line 4 and 5 and is normally <30° (in this example 17 °). 1 and 2 represents the outline of the capitate and the lunate

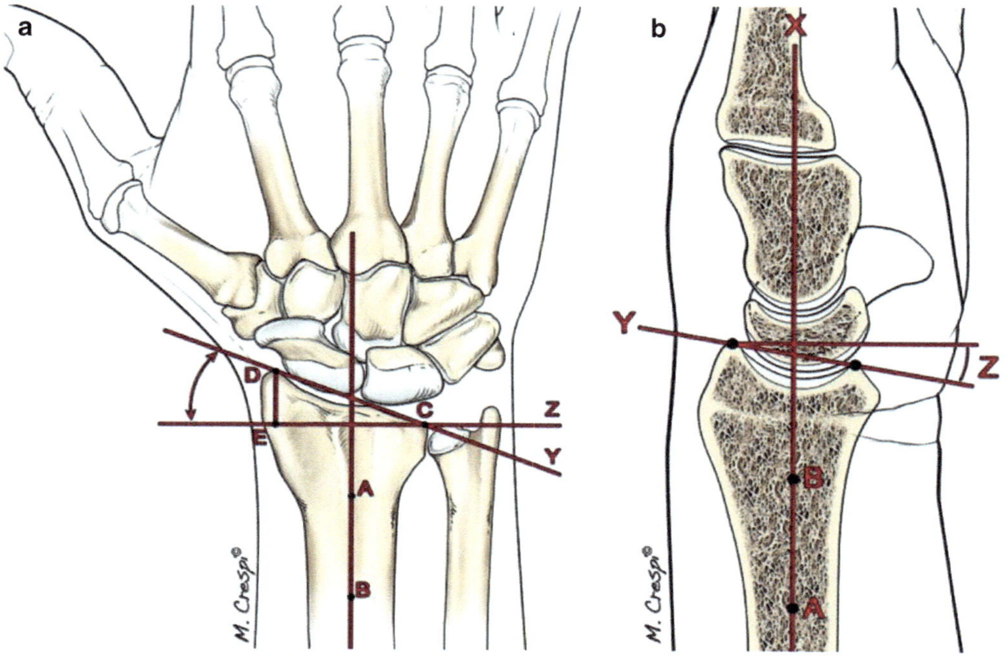

Fig. 9.5 Measurement of radial inclination and radial volar tilt. (**a**) Radial inclination angle (*arrow*) is measured by drawing a perpendicular line (line *EC*) to the radial axis (*AB*) through the ulnar edge of the lunate fossa and another line (line *DC*) joining the distal tip of the radial styloid and the ulnar edge of the lunate fossa. These two lines form the radial inclination angle (normal angle, 21–25°). Radial height is the measured distance between points *D* and *E*, where *D* represents the distal-most tip of the radial styloid and *E* is a point on line *EC*. Line *DE* is the shortest distance between point *D* and line *EC*. Normal radial height is 10–13 mm. (**b**) The palmar (volar) tilt is the angle created between the line (*Y*) joining the most distal points of the dorsal and ventral rims of the distal articular surface of the radius and the line (*Z*) drawn perpendicular to the long axis (line *XBA*) of the radius. The average tilt is 11°, with a range of 0–20°

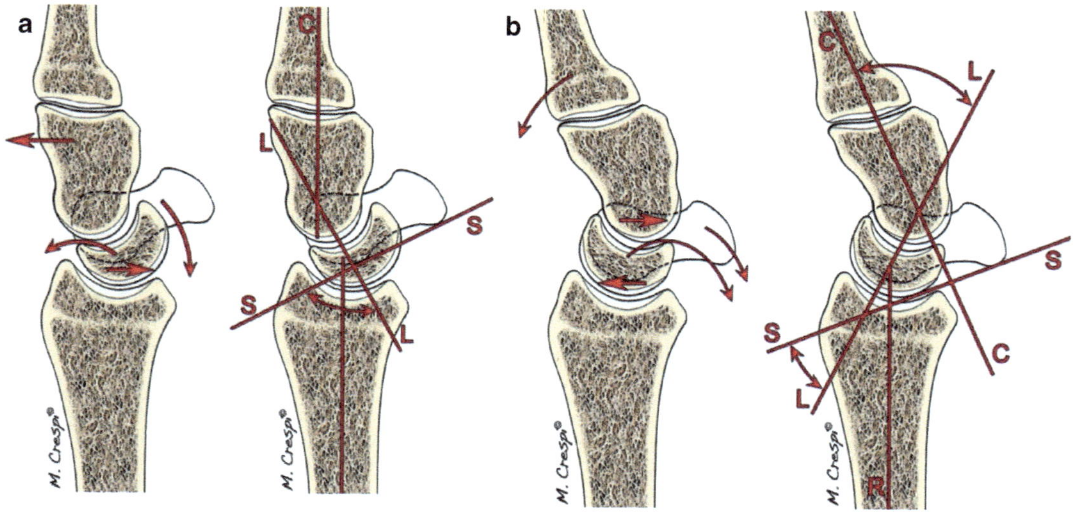

Fig. 9.6 (**a**) Dorsal scapholunate instability – (DISI). *SL* angle is increased. (**b**) Volar scapholunate instability – (VISI). *SL* angle is decreased. *S* line along the base or center of the scaphoid, *L* line perpendicular to the lunate, *C* line along the long axis of the capitate, *R* line along the long axis of the radius, *S–L* lines form the scapholunate angle (SL), *C-L* lines form the capitolunate angle (CL)

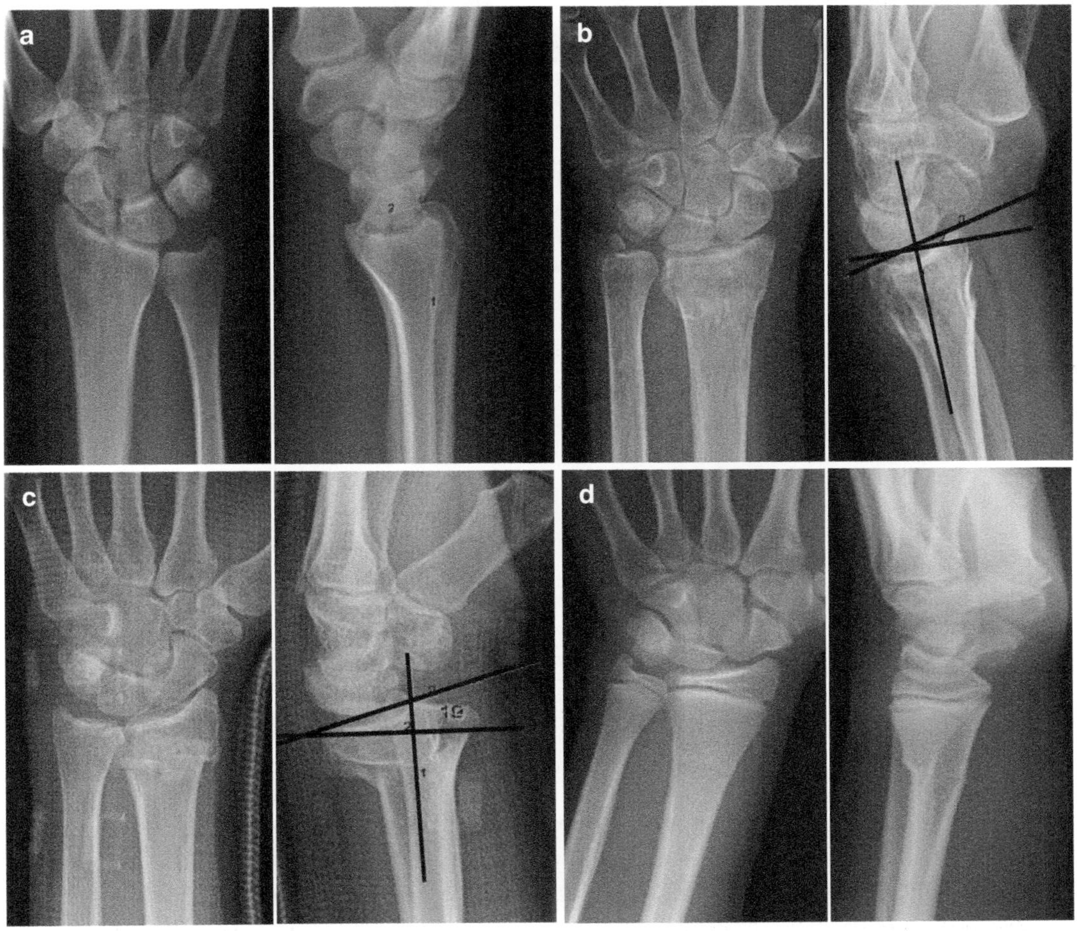

Fig. 9.7 Examples of common fractures and injuries. (**a**) Intra-articular fracture of the radial styloid. (**b**) Smith's fracture with a volar tilt. (**c**) Colles fracture with dorsal tilt of distal fragment. (**d**) Greenstick fracture of distal radius. The lines (1, 2, 3 and 19) drawn at the lateral radiographs show how to measure the tilt of the articular surface of the radius according to Fig. 9.5

9.4 Computer Tomography (CT) Scanning

As mentioned, conventional radiography is usually sufficient for correct diagnosis and adequate treatment of distal radius fractures. CT scans provide more accurate information regarding the anatomy of intra-articular fractures than radiography, and 70–81 % distal radius fractures have been reported to have intra-articular extension. Healing with residual incongruity of 2 mm or more carry a risk of almost 100 % of developing secondary radiographic visible osteoarthritis. The addition of CT to plain films frequently changes the therapeutic recommendations for such cases, and CT is also valuable in case of comminute fractures and before surgery (Trumble et al. 1999; Arora et al. 2010; Harness et al. 2006; Slutsky 2013).

A CT scanner emits a series of narrow beams through an arc moving spirally 360° around the body. A 64-slice CT scanner has 64 rows of 0.625 mm slices giving a 40 mm detector width, which transmits the collected data to a computer, from which 2D and 3D images in high resolution are reconstructed. The patient is placed supine with the arm stretched over the head and the wrist angled a little to the central beam to avoid artefacts (Fig. 9.8). CT scan examples are displayed in Figs. 9.9 and 9.10.

Promising results regarding demonstration of instability between the carpal bones have been shown using dynamic CT scans; however,

Table 9.3 Views best suitable for diagnoses

Views	Diagnoses
PA	Colles or Smith's fracture (transverse fracture of distal radius with dorsal or volar tilt of distal fragment associated with avulsion of ulnar styloid)
	Radial styloid/Chauffeur/Hutchinson fracture (oblique, intra-articular fracture of the radial styloid which may be associated with intercarpal ligamentous injuries, especially of the scapholunate ligament)
	Galeazzi fracture (distal 1/3 of the diaphysis of the radius associated with luxation of the distal radioulnar joint)
	Essex-Lopresti fracture (fracture of radial head and/or luxation of the proximal radioulnar joint associated with rupture of interosseous membrane with dislocation of distal radioulnar joint)
	Ulnar variance (plus/minus)
	Distal radial ulnar joint (DRUJ) injury
	Perilunate dislocation
	Scapholunate or other ligament lesions
Lateral	Colles fracture (transverse fracture of the distal radius with dorsal tilt of distal fragment associated with avulsion of ulnar styloid)
	Smith's fracture (a reversed Colles fracture with volar tilt of the distal fracture fragment)
	Barton's fracture (comminuted fracture of the distal articular surface + volar or dorsal subluxation of fragment and carpus)
	Galeazzi fracture (distal 1/3 of the diaphysis of the radius associated with luxation of the distal radioulnar joint)
	Essex-Lopresti fracture (fracture of radial head and/or luxation of the proximal radioulnar joint associated with rupture of interosseous membrane with dislocation of distal radioulnar joint)
	(Radio-)carpal subluxations
	Ligament lesions between the carpals

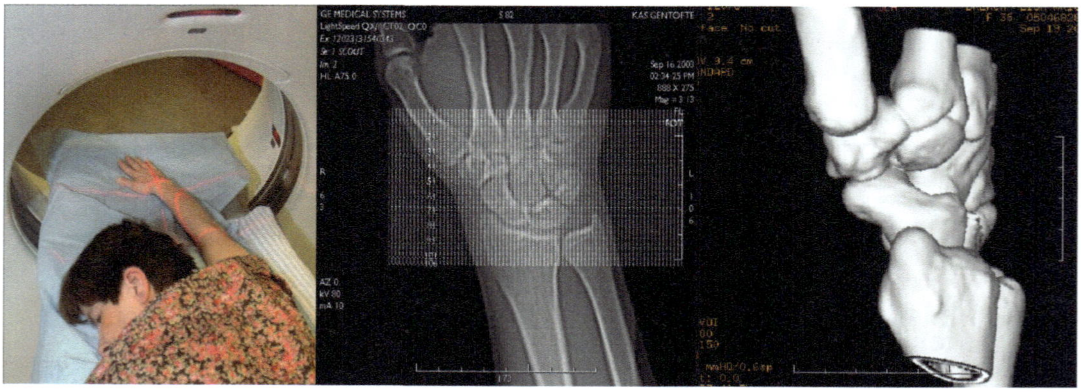

Fig. 9.8 CT scan in 3 planes with reconstruction

more studies are needed (Kalia et al. 2009; Leng et al. 2011).

9.5 Magnetic Resonance Imaging (MRI)

MRI is the modality of choice for visualization of soft-tissue injuries and hidden fractures of the wrist (Fotiadou et al. 2011). The MRI technique is entirely different from conventional radiography and CT scanning, not creating images based upon high-energy electromagnetic waves (X-rays), but upon magnetic and radio waves. The patient lies inside a large, cylinder-shaped magnet, the strength of which is measured in tesla, which is 10,000–30,000 times stronger than the magnetic field of the earth. This strong magnetic field causes alignment of the positively charged body hydrogen protons, themselves acting like small

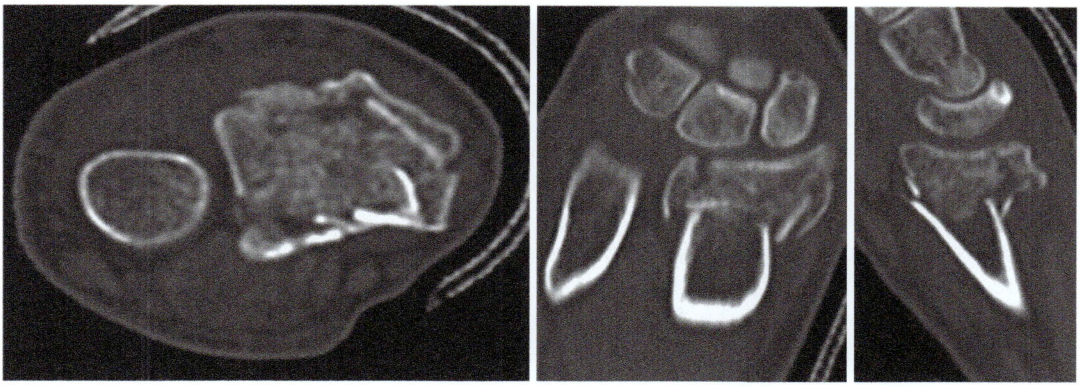

Fig. 9.9 CT scan in axial, coronal and sagittal plane

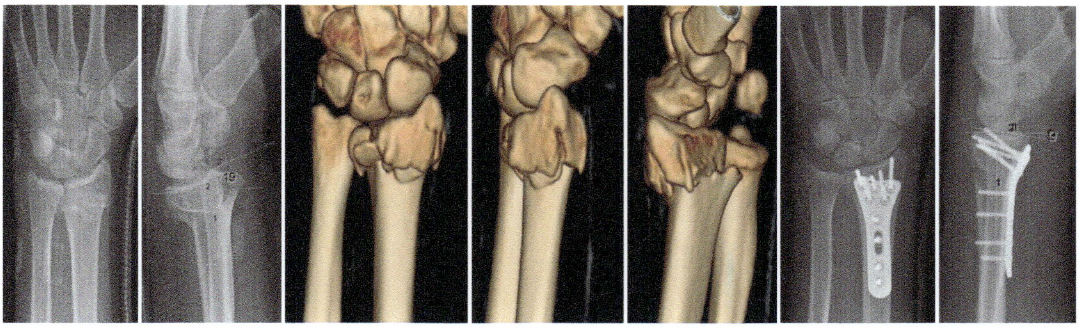

Fig. 9.10 Comminuted distal intra-articular radial fracture with dorsal tilt: conventional radiograph, preoperative 3D CT scan and postoperative control radiograph. The lines (1, 2, 3, 9, and 19) at the lateral radiograhps shows the tilt of the articular surface before and after operation according to Fig. 9.5

magnets. Radio waves are then sent through the body causing disturbance of this alignment. When the waves are switched off again, the hydrogen protons spin back to their original aligned position, projecting radio waves of their own. The scanner receives these signals, and a computer turns them into pictures in axial, coronal and sagittal planes. Since the signals are tiny, the wrist is placed in a coil (antenna). By changing the timing of the radio wave pulses, it is possible to gain information about the different types of tissue. Since movable hydrogen protons are mainly found in fat, water and soft tissue, these structures will project the strongest signals, which appear white on the MRI picture. Low signals, such as calcified bones, appear dark. Depending on when the radio waves are turned off, different signals, the so-called sequences, are developed.

It can now be understood why MRI is of benefit in cases of suspected concomitant ligamentous injuries or fractures not demonstrated on routine radiographs, since the MRI will visualize soft tissue and oedema. The ligamentous elements are important for the stabilization of the wrist. They dictate much of the injury pattern and account for many missed wrist injuries seen in association with distal radius fractures (Larsen et al. 1993). It has been reported that 68 % of patients requiring operative repair of a radius fracture had injuries to the soft tissues, including the triangular fibrocartilage complex and the scapholunate or the lunate-triquetral ligaments (Geissler et al. 1996). Arthrography is valuable when looking for such defects (Goldfarb et al. 2011). MRI is also valuable for follow-up in case of persistent discomfort after injury (Fotiadou et al. 2011).

The MRI is considered harmless to the patient as opposed to conventional radiographs and CT scans; however, they are costly, time consuming and challenging for patients suffering from claustrophobia. The cost-benefit of additional MRI is still under debate (Nikken et al. 2005).

The sequences used for imaging of the wrist are called T1, T2, STIR (short tau inversion recovery) and T2 with fat suppression, and opposed to CT, reconstruction is not possible; the sequences have to be chosen before the examination. Table 9.4 illustrates which types of tissue give high and low signals in the different sequences. For strengths and weaknesses of the different sequences, see Table 9.5. Examples of soft-tissue injuries are displayed in Fig. 9.11.

Table 9.5 Strengths and weaknesses of MRI sequences

Sequence	Strengths	Weaknesses
T1	Anatomy Fat tissue Meniscus Contrast enhancement	Oedema
T2	Oedema Pathological processes	Movement sensitive
STIR or T2 fat suppressed	Oedema Pathological processes	Not as good as T2 for details

Tips and tricks – difficult to remember in which sequences water is white?

STIR WHITE WATER IN THE TEA TOO!!
(Water is white in STIR and T2)

Table 9.4 Water and fat signals in different MRI sequences – insufficient healing of radial styloid fracture

	T1	T2	STIR or T2 fat suppressed
Water signal	Black	White	White
Fat signal	White	Grey/white	Black
	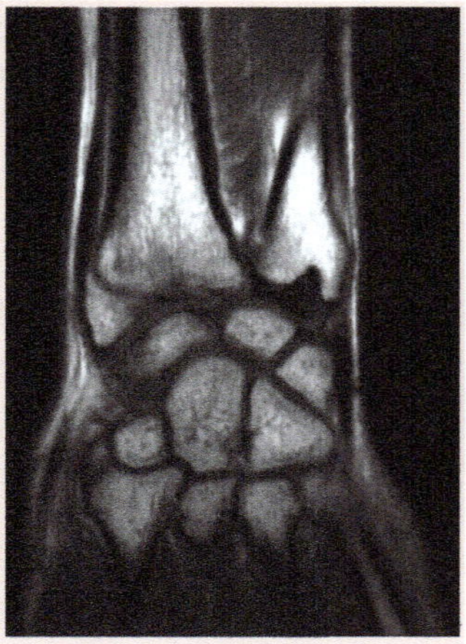	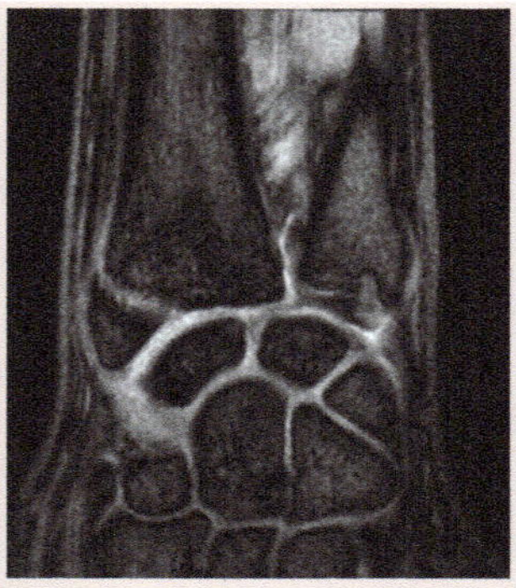	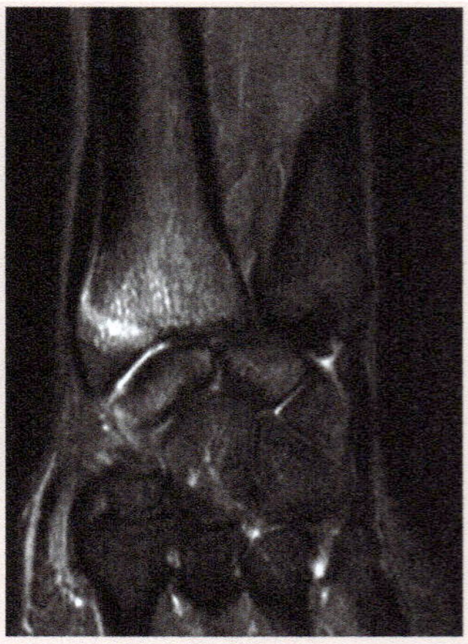

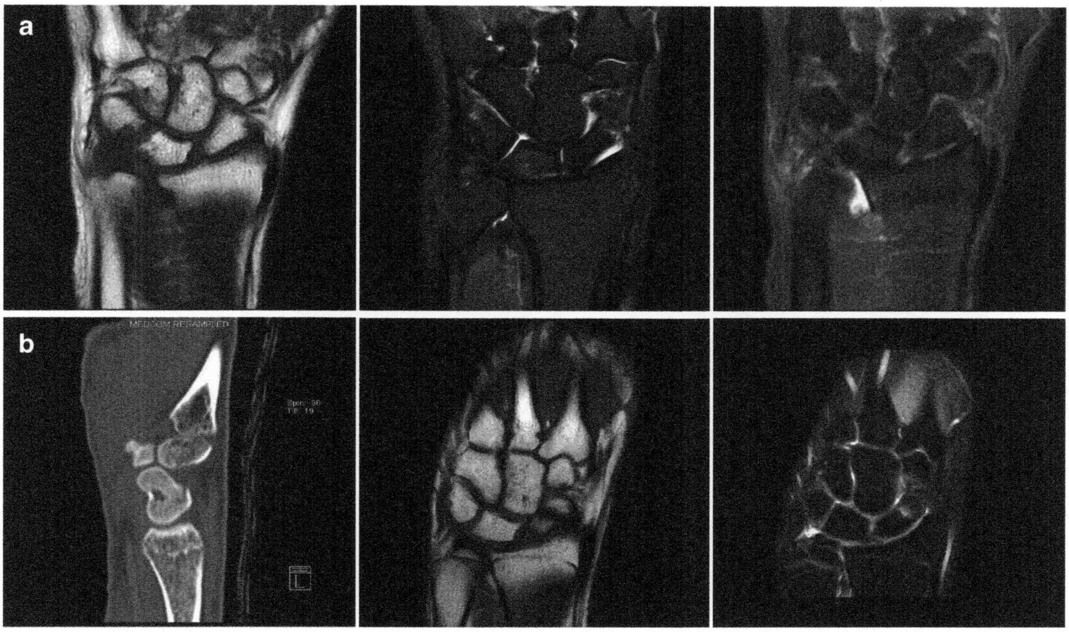

Fig. 9.11 Examples of soft tissue and bone injuries on MRI. (**a**) Lesion of the triangular fibrocartilage discus with water signal in the distal radioulnar joint. (**b**) Scaphoid fracture: sagittal CT and MRI T1 and STIR

9.6 Ultrasound

Ultrasound is not considered to be routine modality in the diagnosis of wrist injuries. It has been shown that the use of ultrasound by an experienced clinician in an austere environment can be performed accurately and may possibly prevent unnecessary evacuations for suspected fractures requiring radiographic verification (McNeil et al. 2009).

References

Arora S, Grover SB, Batra S, Sharma VK. Comparative evaluation of postreduction intra-articular distal radial fractures by radiographs and multidetector computed tomography. J Bone Joint Surg Am. 2010; 92(15):2523–32.

Fotiadou A, Patel A, Morgan T, Karantanas AH. Wrist injuries in young adults: the diagnostic impact of CT and MRI. Eur J Radiol. 2011;77(2):235–9.

Geissler WB, Freeland AE, Savoie FH, McIntyre LW, Whipple TL. Intracarpal soft-tissue lesions associated with an intra-articular fracture of the distal end of the radius. J Bone Joint Surg Am. 1996;78(3):357–65.

Goldfarb CA, Yin Y, Louis AG, Fisher AJ, Boyer MI. Wrist fractures: what the clinician wants to know. Radiology. 2011;219:11–28.

Harness NG, Ring D, Zurakowski D, Harris GJ, Jupiter JB. The influence of three-dimensional computed tomography reconstructions on the characterization and treatment of distal radial fractures. J Bone Joint Surg Am. 2006;88(6):1315–23.

Kalia V, Obray RW, Filice R, Fayad LM, Murphy K, Carrino JA. Functional joint imaging using 256-MDCT: technical feasibility. Am J Radiol. 2009;192(6):w295–9.

Larsen CF, Lauritsen J. Epidemiology of acute wrist trauma. Int J Epidemiol. 1993;22(5):911–6.

Larsen CF, Brondum V, Wienholtz G. An algorithm for acute wrist trauma. A systematic approach to diagnosis. J Hand Surg Br. 1993;18(2):207–12.

Leng S, Zhao K, Qu M, An K, Berger RA, McCollough CH. Dynamic CT technique for assessment of wrist joint instabilities. Med Phys. 2011;38(7):50–6.

McNeil CR, McManus J, Mehta S. The accuracy of portable ultrasonography to diagnose fractures in austere environment. Prehosp Emerg Care. 2009;13: 50–2.

Metz VM, Gilula LA. Imaging techniques for distal radius fractures and related injuries. Orthop Clin North Am. 1993;24(2):217–28.

Nikken JJ, Oei EH, Ginai AZ, Krestin GP, Verhaar JA, van Vugt AB, et al. Acute peripheral joint injury: cost and effectiveness of low-field-strength MR imaging–

results of randomized controlled trial. Radiology. 2005;236(3):958–67.

Slutsky D. Predicting the outcome of distal radius fractures. Hand Clin. 2013;21(2005):289–94.

Spence LD, Savenor A, Nwachuku I, Tilsley J, Eustace S. MRI of fractures of the distal radius: comparison with conventional radiographs. Skeletal Radiol. 1998; 27(5):244–9.

Trumble TE, Culp RW, Hanel DP, Geissler WB, Berger RA. Intra-articular fractures of the distal aspect of the radius. Instr Course Lect. 1999;48:465–80.

Classification Distal Radius Fractures

10

Tapio Flinkkilä

Contents

T. Flinkkilä, MD
Division of Orthopaedic and Trauma Surgery,
Department of surgery, Oulu University Hospital,
Oulu, Finland
e-mail: tapio.flinkkila@ppshp.fi

10.1 Summary

Distal radius fractures result in typical fracture patterns and it is important to recognize these. Some fractures behave differently and may have great influence on the treatment method. Careful analysis of good quality radiographs should allow recognition of fracture lines and fragments, to classify the injury and make a treatment plan. Ideal fracture classification should be reliable (inter-observer and intra-observer reliability), should describe severity of the injury, should help in choosing the appropriate method of treatment, and should have prognostic value. An ideal classification of distal radius fractures should take into account fracture pattern, articular involvement, comminution, and lunate load fragment; degree of displacement; articular step-off; stability; ulnar-sided lesions; and soft tissue involvement.

10.2 Introduction

Distal radius fractures result in typical fracture patterns and it is important to recognize these. Some fractures behave differently and may have great influence on the treatment method. Careful analysis of good quality radiographs should allow recognition of fracture lines and fragments, to classify the injury and make a treatment plan.

Ideal fracture classification should be reliable (inter-observer and intra-observer reliability), should describe severity of the injury, should help

L.M. Hove et al. (eds.), *Distal Radius Fractures*,
DOI 10.1007/978-3-642-54604-4_10, © Springer-Verlag Berlin Heidelberg 2014

Table 10.1 Classifications of distal radius fractures

Classification	Use
Destot (1923)	No (historical)
Taylor and Parsons (1938)	No (historical)
Nissen-Lie (1939)	No (historical)
Gartland and Werley (1951)	Sometimes (mainly historical)
Lidström (1959)	No (historical)
Older (1965)	Seldom, best reproducibility
Frykman (1967)	Seldom, widely studied
Melone (1984)	Seldom
Sennwald and Segmuller (1984)	Seldom
Castaing (1964)	No (historical)
Sarmiento (1975)	No (historical)
Jenkins (1989)	No (historical)
AO (1990)	Yes, poor reproducibility
Rayhack (1990)	Seldom
Cooney (Universal) 1990	Yes
McMurtry and Jupiter (1992)	Sometimes
Mayo Clinic (1992)	Sometimes
Fernandez (1993)	Yes
Saffar (1995)	Seldom
Column (Rikli and Regazzoni 1996)	Yes, treatment oriented
Fragment specific (Medoff 2009)	Yes, treatment oriented
Buttazzoni (2009)	New, not in routine use

in choosing appropriate method of treatment, and should have prognostic value (Burstein 1993).

An ideal classification of distal radius fractures should take into account:

1. Fracture pattern. Articular involvement, comminution (metaphyseal, articular), and lunate load (die punch) fragment
2. Degree of displacement
3. Articular step-off. Incongruence of the articular surface
4. Stability. The tendency of reduced fracture fragments to collapse and cause late displacement
5. Ulnar-sided lesions. Ulnar styloid fractures, fracture of distal ulna, and distal radioulnar (DRU) joint involvement including instability
6. Soft tissue involvement

More than 20 classifications of distal radius fractures (Table 10.1) have been presented in the literature and no single classification so far has fulfilled these requirements. Some early classifications are purely descriptive and describe number of fracture fragments or fracture lines. Some classifications take metaphyseal comminution and direction and degree of displacement into account and try to assess stability of the fracture. New classifications have added important features like involvement of the DRU joint, fracture stability, and even osteoporosis.

10.3 Classifications

Eponyms are the oldest classifications and still in clinical use:

- Colles' fracture (Fig. 10.1a, b)
- Smiths's fracture (Fig. 10.2)
- Barton's fracture (Figs. 10.3 and 10.4)
- Chauffeur's fracture (Fig. 10.5)
- "Die punch fracture" (depression of dorsal (or central) aspect of the lunate fossa) (Fig. 10.6)

Many classifications (Table 10.1) have only historical relevance, but each classification has increased our understanding of the pathoanatomy of distal radius fractures. The most common contemporary classifications are:

- AO classification (Fig. 10.7)
- Fernandez' classification (Fig. 10.8)
- Fragment-specific classification (Fig. 10.9)
- Column classification (Fig. 10.10)

Both fragment-specific and column classifications are treatment oriented and specific implants can be used to fix fragments.

The *AO classification* is based on sequential recognition of fracture pattern. The AO classification divides fractures into:

- Extra-articular (type A)
- Partially articular (type B)
- Completely articular (type C)

These basic types are further divided to 27 subtypes according to fracture pattern (Muller et al. 1990). Although the AO classification is very comprehensive in classifying the radius component, it only classifies ulnar involvement as isolated extra-articular fractures (A1).

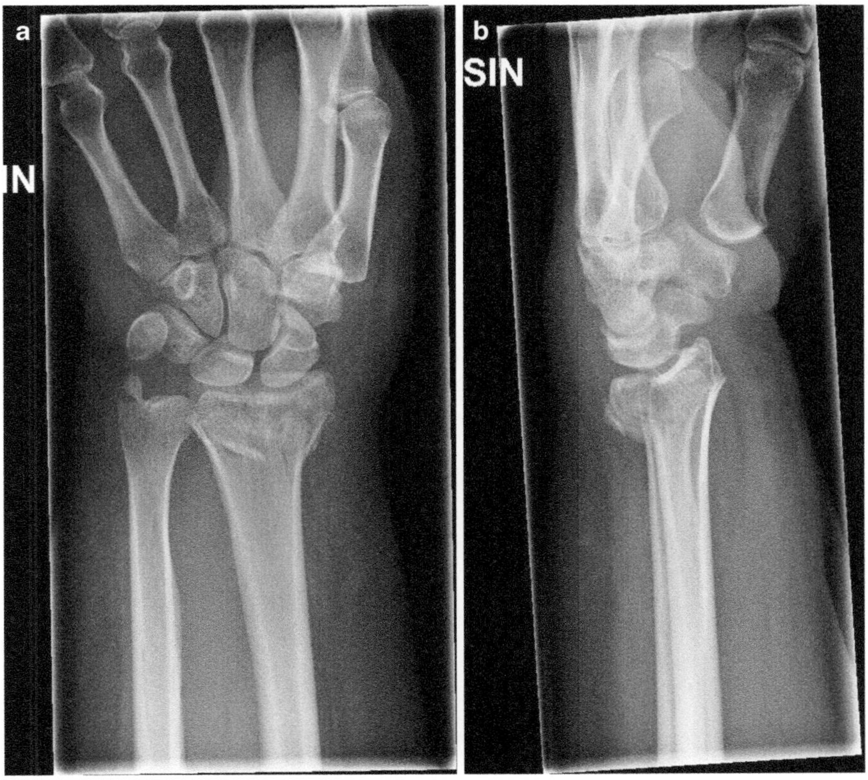

Fig. 10.1 (**a**) Colles' fracture (ap view). (**b**) Colles' fracture (lateral view)

Some authors have added a classification of distal ulnar lesions to AO classification:

1. Ulnar styloid fracture
2. Stable ulnar neck fracture
3. Comminuted ulnar neck fracture
4. Ulnar head and neck fracture
5. Fracture of the ulna proximal to the neck

Fernandez' classification (Fig. 10.8) is based on the mechanism of injury. In addition to the radius fracture, it takes distal ulnar lesions into account. It divides radial fractures into:

- Extra-articular bending fractures (type I)
- Shearing fractures (type II)
- Compression fractures of the joint surface (type III)
- Avulsion fractures of ligament attachments (type IV)
- Combined fractures (type V) involving bending, shearing, compression, and possible bone loss and metaphyseal extension of the fracture

  Associated ulnar injuries include:

- Type I stable lesions (avulsion of the tip of ulnar styloid or stable fracture of ulnar neck)
- Type II unstable (tear of TFCC and capsular ligaments or avulsion of the base of the ulnar styloid)
- Type III potentially unstable (intra-articular fracture of the sigmoid notch or intra-articular fracture of the ulnar head)

The *fragment-specific classification* (Fig. 10.9) is a simple classification of intra-articular fractures based on five main fragments (CT is often needed to identify all fragments) (Medoff 2009):

- Radial styloid
- Volar rim
- Dorsal ulnar corner

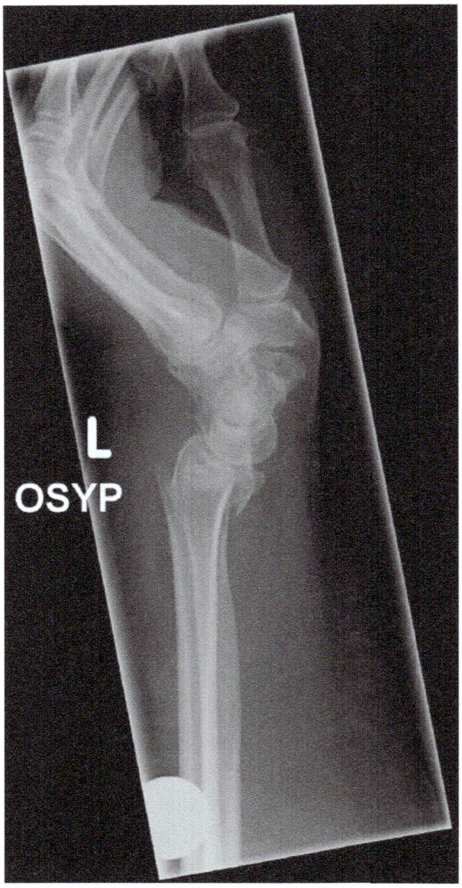

Fig. 10.2 Smith's fracture

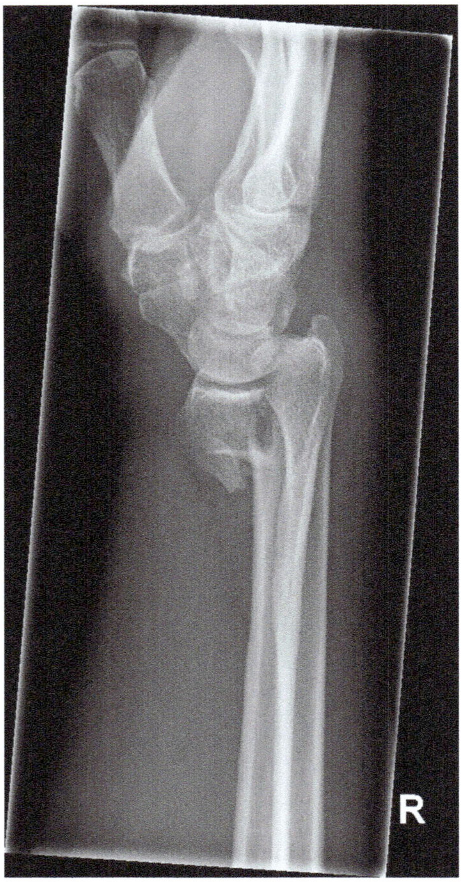

Fig. 10.3 Volar Barton's fracture

- Dorsal wall
- Impacted articular fragments

Column classification (Fig. 10.10) identifies three columns of the distal forearm (Rikli and Regazzoni 1996):

- Lateral column (radial styloid, scaphoid facet of the radius)
- Intermediate column (lunate facet including dorsal and volar ulnar corners)
- Medial column representing the distal ulna

10.4 Studies on Classifications

- Most studies of distal radius fracture classifications have focused on their inter-observer and intra-observer reliability.
- Their prognostic value or ability to choose appropriate treatment method has received little attention.
- Nearly all classifications (AO, Frykman, Melone, Mayo, Fernandez, Cooney, Universal, Older) have only fair to moderate inter-observer or intra-observer reliability (Anderson et al. 1996; Navqi et al. 2009).
- Simplified AO classification (A, B, C) has shown acceptable inter-observer reliability (Kreder et al. 1996; Flinkkilä et al. 1998a).
- The AO and Melone classifications may correlate with functional outcome (Trumble et al. 1994). However, other studies have shown no prognostic value of AO, Frykman, or Mayo classifications to functional or subjective result (Flinkkilä et al. 1998b).

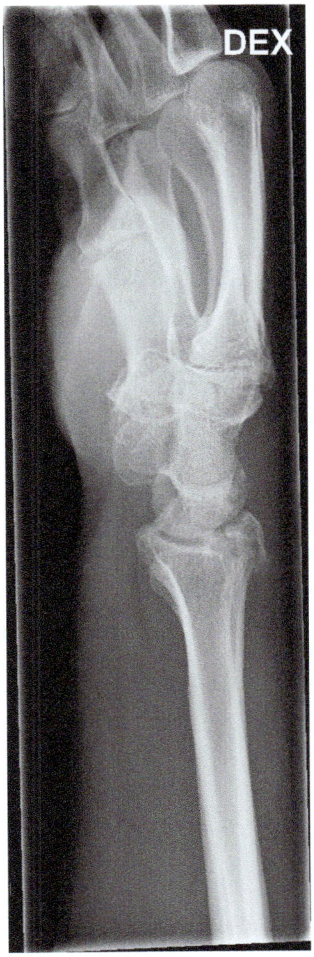

Fig. 10.4 Dorsal Barton's fracture

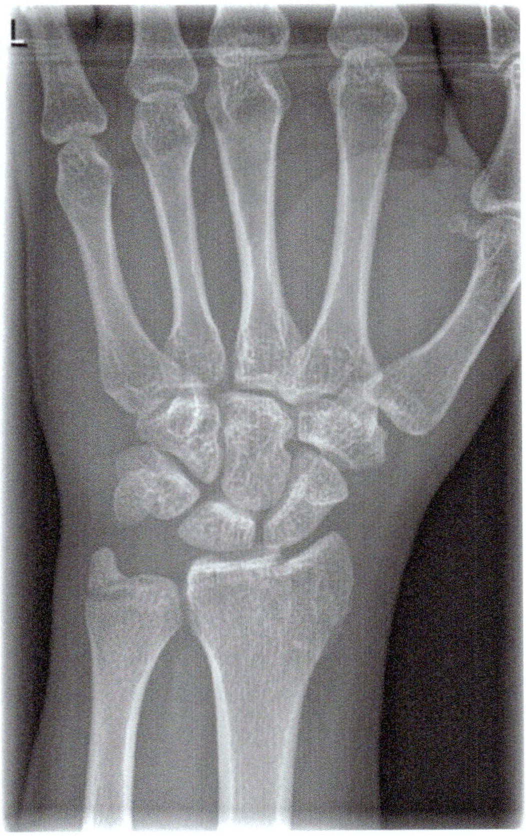

Fig. 10.5 Chauffeur's fracture

- Intra-articular fractures in general have worse prognosis than extra-articular fractures, even if articular congruity has been restored operatively. However, correlation of classifications and treatment outcome is yet again controversial.
- CT is normally useful for the surgeon (Fig. 10.11), but seems controversial and with mixed messages in the literature (Flinkkilä et al. 1998a; Katz et al. 2001; Doornberg et al. 2006). CT seems to increase intra-observer reliability of number of fragments, intra-articular fracture lines, and articular step-off, but its role in improving inter-observer reliability especially classifications is controversial (Flinkkilä et al. 1998a; Katz et al. 2001; Doornberg et al. 2006).
- Decreased bone density, not surprisingly, increases risk of comminuted fractures. It has been suggested that osteoporosis should be included in fracture classifications (Kettler et al. 2008).
- Traction radiographs may increase reliability of fracture characterization.

10.5 Clinical Use

- Most classifications unquestionably describe fracture severity. However, no classification has been proven universally accepted for clinical use.
- Some classifications are too complex to be used in normal clinical practice, and poor reliability limits their scientific value, while other classifications are too simple to describe fracture severity accurately enough.

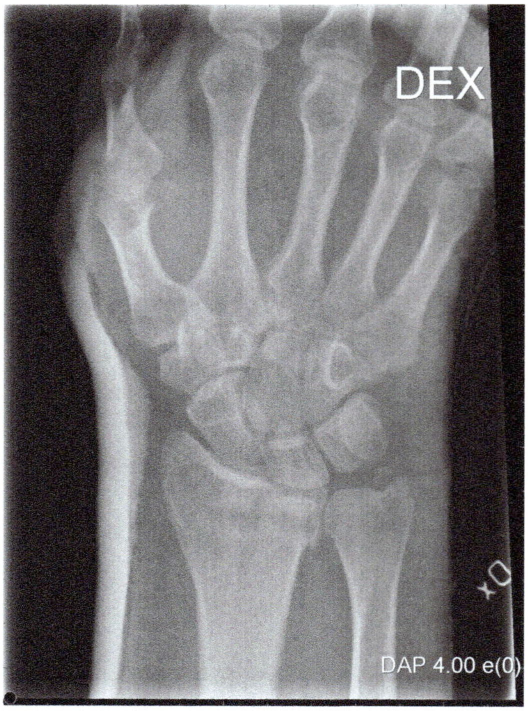

Fig. 10.6 Die punch fracture

- Simple radiological parameters and articular step-off are more often used as a guide to choose the appropriate treatment method.
- CT improves detection of articular step-off, gapping, and distal radioulnar joint involvement and influences treatment recommendations more than fracture classifications (Harness et al. 2006; Katz et al. 2001).
- Despite severe problems, classifications have some role in communication between surgeons, perhaps less in the clinical setting than in scientific papers.
- The AO classification's main types A, B, and C describe progressive articular involvement and help to assess fracture severity.
- Eponyms also have some use, since Smith's fractures as well as volar Barton's fractures often need operative treatment.
- Poor inter-observer reliability of detailed classifications is the main problem of classifications and limits their clinical or scientific use.

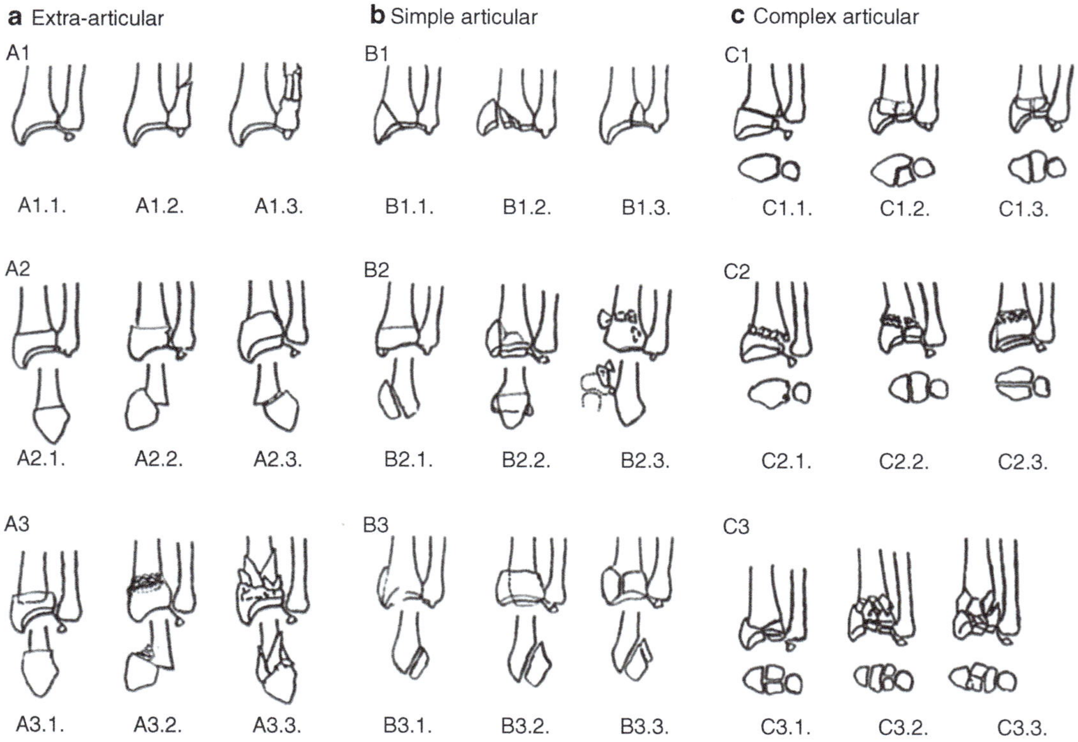

Fig. 10.7 AO classification of distal radius fractures. (a) Extra-articular. (b) Partial articular. (c) Complex articular (Flinkkilä et al. 1998a)

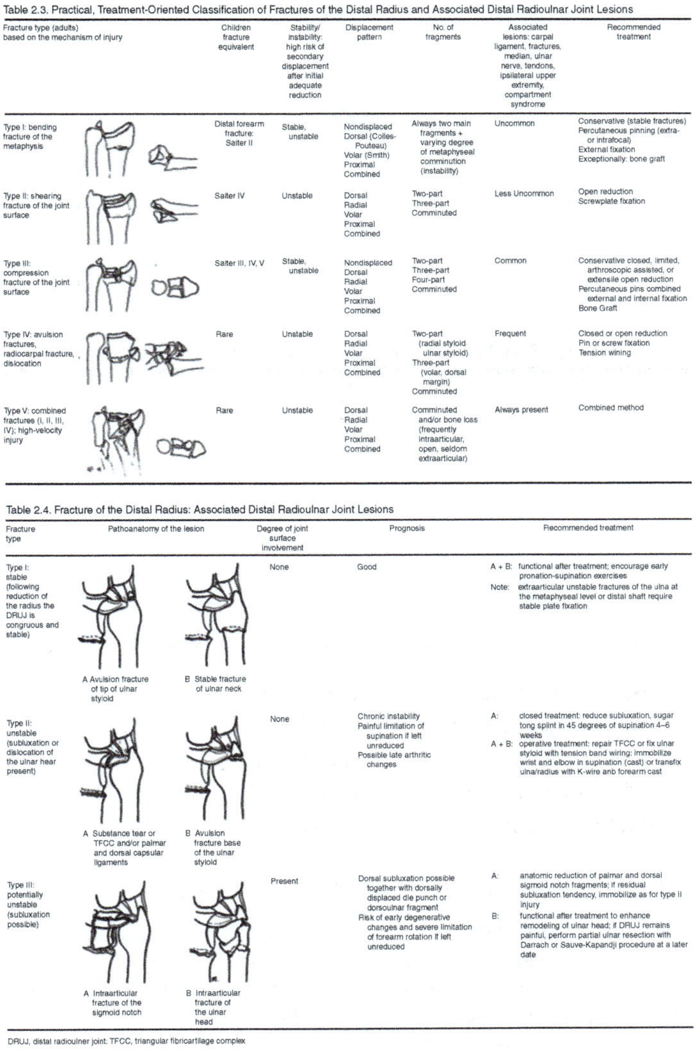

Table 2.3. Practical, Treatment-Oriented Classification of Fractures of the Distal Radius and Associated Distal Radioulnar Joint Lesions

Fracture type (adults) based on the mechanism of injury	Children fracture equivalent	Stability/ instability: high risk of secondary displacement after initial adequate reduction	Displacement pattern	No. of fragments	Associated lesions: carpal ligament, fractures, median, ulnar nerve, tendons, ipsilateral upper extremity, compartment syndrome	Recommended treatment
Type I: bending fracture of the metaphysis	Distal forearm fracture: Salter II	Stable, unstable	Nondisplaced Dorsal (Colles-Pouteau) Volar (Smith) Proximal Combined	Always two main fragments + varying degree of metaphyseal comminution (instability)	Uncommon	Conservative (stable fractures) Percutaneous pinning (extra- or intrafocal) External fixation Exceptionally: bone graft
Type II: shearing fracture of the joint surface	Salter IV	Unstable	Dorsal Radial Volar Proximal Combined	Two-part Three-part Comminuted	Less Uncommon	Open reduction Screwplate fixation
Type III: compression fracture of the joint surface	Salter III, IV, V	Stable, unstable	Nondisplaced Dorsal Radial Volar Proximal Combined	Two-part Three-part Four-part Comminuted	Common	Conservative closed, limited, arthroscopic assisted, or extensile open reduction Percutaneous pins combined external and internal fixation Bone Graft
Type IV: avulsion fractures, radiocarpal fracture, dislocation	Rare	Unstable	Dorsal Radial Volar Proximal Combined	Two-part (radial styloid ulnar styloid) Three-part (volar, dorsal margin) Comminuted	Frequent	Closed or open reduction Pin or screw fixation Tension wining
Type V: combined fractures (I, II, III, IV); high-velocity injury	Rare	Unstable	Dorsal Radial Volar Proximal Combined	Comminuted and/or bone loss (frequently intraarticular, open, seldom extraarticular)	Always present	Combined method

Table 2.4. Fracture of the Distal Radius: Associated Distal Radioulnar Joint Lesions

Fracture type	Pathoanatomy of the lesion	Degree of joint surface involvement	Prognosis	Recommended treatment
Type I: stable (following reduction of the radius the DRUJ is congruous and stable)	A Avulsion fracture of tip of ulnar styloid B Stable fracture of ulnar neck	None	Good	A + B: functional after treatment; encourage early pronation-supination exercises Note: extraarticular unstable fractures of the ulna at the metaphyseal level or distal shaft require stable plate fixation
Type II: unstable (subluxation or dislocation of the ulnar hear present)	A Substance tear or TFCC and/or palmar and dorsal capsular ligaments B Avulsion fracture base of the ulnar styloid	None	Chronic instability Painful limitation of supination if left unreduced Possible late arthritic changes	A: closed treatment: reduce subluxation, sugar tong splint in 45 degrees of supination 4–6 weeks A + B: operative treatment: repair TFCC or fix ulnar styloid with tension band wiring: immobilize wrist and elbow in supination (cast) or transfix ulna/radius with K-wire anb forearm cast
Type III: potentially unstable (subluxation possible)	A Intraarticular fracture of the sigmoid notch B Intraarticular fracture of the ulnar head	Present	Dorsal subluxation possible together with dorsally displaced die punch or dorsoulnar fragment Risk of early degenerative changes and severe limitation of forearm rotation if left unreduced	A: anatomic reduction of palmar and dorsal sigmoid notch fragments; if residual subluxation tendency, immobilize as for type II injury B: functional after treatment to enhance remodeling of ulnar head; if DRUJ remains painful, perform partial ulnar resection with Darrach or Sauve-Kapandji procedure at a later date

DRUJ, distal radioulner joint: TFCC, triangular fibricartilage complex

Fig. 10.8 Fernandez' classification (Fernandez and Jupiter 2002)

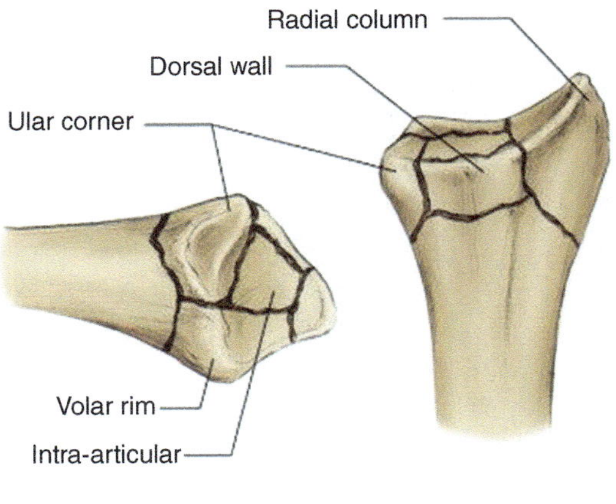

Fig. 10.9 Fragment-specific classification (Medoff 2009)

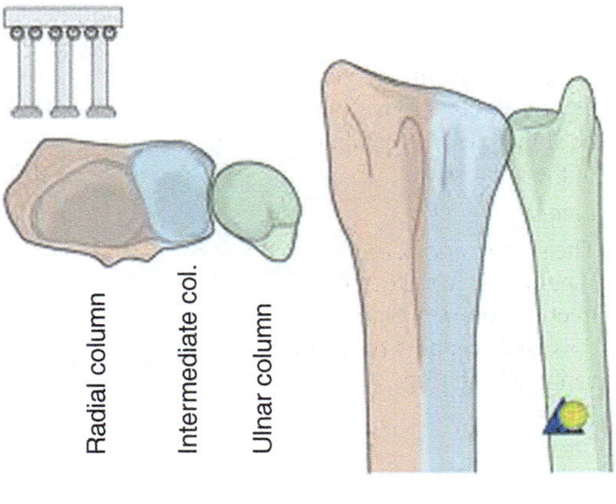

Fig. 10.10 Column classification

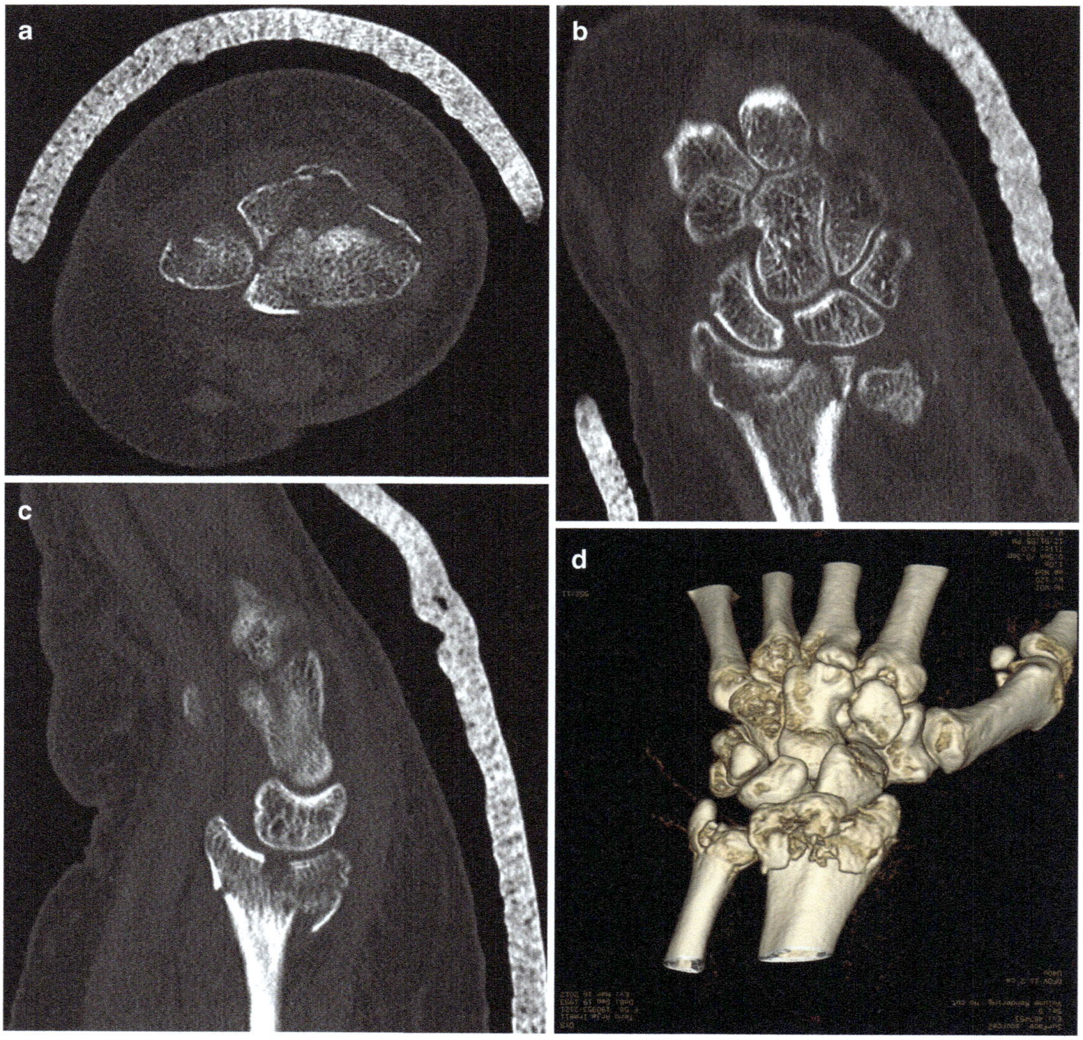

Fig. 10.11 (**a**–**d**) Computed tomography (CT)

Key Points

- There are >20 classification systems of distal radius fractures. No classification is universally accepted for clinical use.
- All classifications have only fair to moderate inter- and intraobserver reliability and this limits their clinical or scientific value.
- Classifications may help in choosing the treatment method. In general they do not have prognostic value.
- Simple radiological parameters, articular step-off, and fracture stability are more important in choosing the appropriate treatment method than classifications.

References

Anderson DJ, Blair WR, Steyers CM, Adams BD, El-Khouri GY, Brandser EA. Classification of distal radius fractures: an analysis of intraobserver and interobserver reproducibility. J Hand Surg Am. 1996; 21:574–82.

Burstein AH. Fracture classification systems: do they work and are they useful? J Bone Joint Surg. 1993; 75:1743–4.

Doornberg J, Lindenhovius A, Kloen P, Van Dijk N, Zurakowski D, Ring D. Two and three-dimensional computed tomography for the classification and management of distal humeral fractures. Evaluation of reliability and diagnostic accuracy. J Bone joint Surg. 2006;88-A:1795–801.

Fernandez DL. Fractures of the distal radius: operative treatment. Instr Course Lect. 1993;42:73–88.

Fernandez D, Jupiter J. Fractures of the distal radius. A practical approach to management. 2nd ed. 2002. Springer.

Flinkkilä T, Nikkola-Sihto A, Kaarela O, Pääkkö E, Raatikainen T. Poor interobserver reliability of the AO classification of fracture of the distal radius: additional computed tomography is of minor value. J Bone Joint Surg Br. 1998a;80:670–2.

Flinkkilä T, Raatikainen T, Hämäläinen M. AO and Frykman's classifications of Colles' fracture. no prognostic value in 652 patients evaluated after 5 years. Acta Orthop Scand. 1998b;69:77–81.

Harness N, Ring D, Zurakowski D, Harris GJ, Jupiter JB. The influence of three-dimensional computed tomography reconstructions on the characterization and treatment of distal radial fractures. J Bone Joint Surg. 2006;88A:1313–22.

Katz MA, Beredjiklian PK, Bozentka DJ, Steinberg DR. Computed tomography scanning of intra-articular distal radius fractures: does it influence treatment? J Hand Surg. 2001;26A:415–21.

Kettler M, Kuhn V, Scieker M, Melone CP. Do we need to include osteoporosis in today's classification of distal radius fractures? J Orthop Trauma. 2008;22: 79–82.

Kreder HJ, Hanel D, McKee M, Jupiter J, McGillivary G, Swiontkowski MF. Consistency of AO fracture classification for the distal radius. J Bone Joint Surg Br. 1996;78:726–31.

Medoff R. Radiographic evaluation and classification of distal radius fractures. In: Slutsky DJ, Osterman AL, editors. Fractures and injuries of the distal radius and carpus. Philadelphia: Saunders; 2009. p. 19–31.

Muller ME, Nazarian S, Koch P, et al. The comprehensive classification of long bones. New York: Springer; 1990. p. 54–63.

Navqi SG, Reynolds T, Kitsis C. Interobserver reliability and intraobserver reproducibility of the Fernandez classification for distal radius fractures. J Hand Surg. 2009;34-B:483–5.

Rikli D, Regazzoni P. Fractures of the distal end of the radius treated by internal fixation and early function. A preliminary report of 20 cases. J Bone Joint Surg. 1996;78-B:588–92.

Trumble TE, Schmitt SR, Vedder NB. Factors affecting functional outcome of displaced intra-articular distal radius fractures. J Hand Surg. 1994;19:325–40.

How to Assess Fracture Instability

11

Yngvar Krukhaug

Contents

Y. Krukhaug, MD, PhD
Department of Orthopaedic Surgery,
Haukeland University Hospital, Bergen, Norway

Department of Surgical Sciences,
University of Bergen, Bergen, Norway
e-mail: yngvar.krukhaug@helse-bergen.no

11.1 Summary

Malunion is the most common complication following conservative treatment. There is a general agreement that there is a close relationship between anatomy and function. Patients with malunited fractures of the distal radius often complain of weakness, pain and reduced motion of the wrist and forearm. Even after anatomical correction of a malunited fracture, function is not restored fully in all patients. Therefore, every effort should be made to prevent malunion in the primary treatment of distal fractures of the radius. It appears to be more common to see loss of reduction in patients suffering from high-energy injuries and in patients suffering from osteoporosis. With that in mind, the type of injury should be taken into account when trying to predict instability. The most important factors to predict loss of reduction and malunion is old age, any type of fracture comminution, high-energy injuries, positive ulnar variance (shortening of the radius) and dorsal angulation of the distal fragment

11.2 Introduction

Malunion is the most common complication following conservative treatment (Fernandez 1982, 1993). Patients with malunited fractures of the

L.M. Hove et al. (eds.), *Distal Radius Fractures*,
DOI 10.1007/978-3-642-54604-4_11, © Springer-Verlag Berlin Heidelberg 2014

distal radius often complain of weakness, pain and reduced motion of the wrist and forearm.

- Corrective osteotomy may improve the alignment of the distal radius in relation to the carpus and to the distal part of the ulna.
- Restoration of the anatomical variables improves the biomechanics of the wrist, resulting in improved grip strength, wrist and forearm motion and reduced pain (af Ekenstam et al. 1985; Fernandez 1982; Prommersberger et al. 1999; Shea et al. 1997).
- But the ROM is still found to be significantly better for all directions on the uninjured side, except radial deviation even after corrective osteotomy of the injured wrist.
- Therefore, every effort should be made to prevent malunion in the primary treatment of distal radius fractures. Even after surgical correction to normal skeletal anatomy, function is not restored fully in all patients (Krukhaug and Hove 2007).

11.3 Loss of Reduction

Previously standard initial management of all displaced fractures was closed manipulation followed by application of a cast. Instability was diagnosed by fragment dislocation on the radiographic examination between 1 and 2 weeks later. At this stage, definitive surgical treatment was instituted, if appropriate, for fractures showing early instability. However, fractures that exhibited instability after 2 weeks were not detected by this management protocol and might heal with malunion that could reduce function or produce unacceptable pain. So far, a system that can predict all kind of instability has not yet been developed. Still we know neither all details about how to assess fracture instability nor the residual degree of fracture malunion.

The measures used on radiographs to describe dislocation of the distal radius fragment are shown in Fig. 11.1.

- It is more common to see loss of reduction in patients suffering from high-energy injuries and in patients suffering from osteoporosis.
- With that in mind, the type of injury and patient age should be taken into account when trying to predict instability.

There is a general agreement that there is a close relationship between anatomy and function (Cooney 1989; Fernandez 1982; McQueen and Caspers 1988; McQueen et al. 1992). Therefore, anatomical reduction should be the goal in the primary treatment. Until this day, the degree of non-perfect reduction or secondary dislocation that can be tolerated is not known. However, malunion seems to be better tolerated by the elderly.

Different factors have been found to correlate with secondary displacement:

- Dorsal comminution (Cooney et al. 1979).
- Dorsal angulation.
- Radial shortening (Vaughan et al. 1985; Hove et al. 1994).
- Advanced age (Solgaard 1986).
- Severe primary displacement (Dias et al. 1987).
- Distal radius fractures with an initial shortening of more than 4 mm are more likely to dislocate.
- Shortening of the distal radius of more than 4 mm has been found to be the most important factor when addressing loss of reduction (Abbaszadegan and Jonsson 1989).
- The degree of shortening and volar tilt has been found to be the most important factors (Leone et al. 2004).
- One-third of the patients older than 65 years with non-displaced fractures will lose the reduction of the fracture (Leone et al. 2004).
- Initial dorsal angulation, loss of radial length and the patients' age were the most important factors to predict loss of reduction (Hove et al. 1994).

11.4 Instability

Lafontaine and his group (1989) defined an unstable distal radius fracture according to the following anatomical criteria based on the radiological study on admission:

Fractures with three or more of the following criteria are likely to fail in a cast:

- Dorsal comminution
- Associated ulnar fracture
- Dorsal angulation more than 20°
- Intra-articular radiocarpal fracture
- Age over 60 years (Lafontaine et al. 1989)

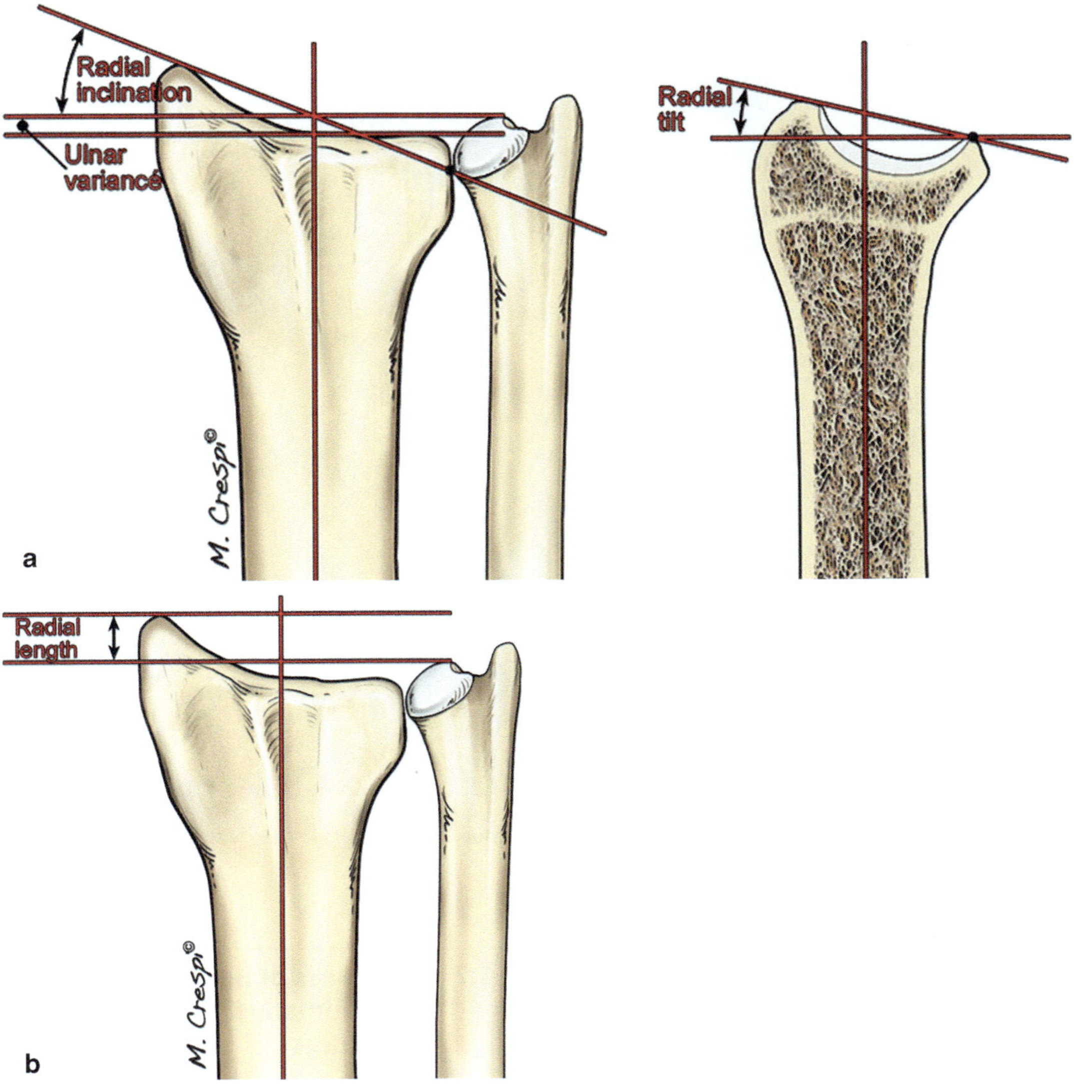

Fig. 11.1 The most common radiological parametres. (**a**) Radial inclination, ulnar variance and radial tilt. (**b**) Radial length

11.5 Early Loss of Reduction in Minimally Displaced Fractures

Fractures with minimal displacement at presentation (i.e. dorsal angulation less than 10° and ulnar variance less than 3 mm):

If treated with plaster cast, early loss (i.e. within 2 weeks) of reduction is:

- Ten times more common in old patients compared to young patients.
- Loss of reduction is six times more common in patients with fractures with any form of comminution (Fig. 11.2).
- If the patient presents with a fracture with a dorsal tilt of 5–10°, it is five times more likely to dislocate, compared to a fracture that maintains only one degree of dorsal tilt.
- If a positive ulnar variance is present at admission, the risk for loss of reduction is twice as large as if the ulnar variance is 0 mm or less (Mackenney et al. 2006).

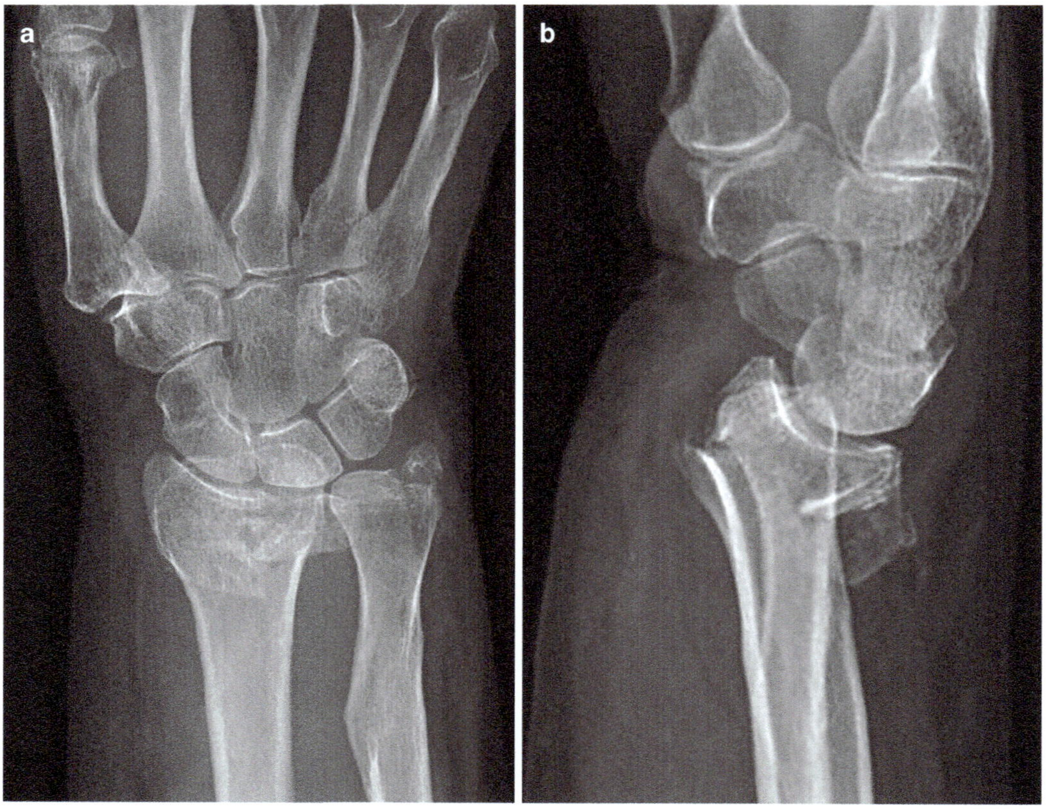

Fig. 11.2 An unstable fracture of the distal radius. (**a**) Distal radius fracture; A-P view. (**b**) Distal radius fracture; lateral view

11.6 Early Loss of Reduction in Displaced Fractures

When it comes to fractures that are displaced at presentation (dorsal tilt >10°, ulnar variance >3 mm), the most important factors to predict early loss (i.e. within 2 weeks) of reduction are:

- Old age
- Positive ulnar variance
- Any type of fracture comminution

Early loss of reduction when treated with plaster cast occurs three times more frequently in old patients, compared to young patients (Mackenney et al. 2006).

11.7 Late Loss of Reduction in Minimally Displaced Fractures

To predict late loss of reduction (later than 2 weeks after reduction) in minimally displaced fractures, we have to assess the angulation and ulnar variance at the 1-week follow-up (Mackenney et al. 2006). The most important factors are:

- Fracture comminution
- Old age
- Dorsal angulation
- Positive ulnar variance

Table 11.1 The most important factors to predict the loss of reduction in distal radius fractures treated with plaster cast

Old age
Any type of fracture comminution
High-energy injuries
Positive ulnar variance (shortening of the radius)
Dorsal angulation
Osteoporosis

11.8 Late Loss of Reduction in Displaced Fractures

Old age, dorsal angulation (dorsal tilt) of the distal fragment and a positive ulnar variance measured at 1 week are factors found to be of significance to predict late loss of reduction. As in minimally displaced fractures, the radiographic measurements at presentation are of no significance in predicting late instability (Mackenney et al. 2006) (Table 11.1).

References

Abbaszadegan H, Jonsson U. Prediction of instability of Colles' fractures. Acta Orthop Scand. 1989;60(6): 646–50.

af Ekenstam F, Hagert CG, Engkvist O, Tornvall AH, Wilbrand H. Corrective osteotomy of malunited fractures of the distal end of the radius. Scand J Plast Reconstr Surg. 1985;19(2):175–87.

Cooney WP. Management of Colles' fractures. J Hand Surg Br. 1989;14(2):137–9.

Cooney III WP, Linscheid RL, Dobyns JH. External pin fixation for unstable Colles' fractures. J Bone Joint Surg Am. 1979;61(6A):840–5.

Dias JJ, Wray CC, Jones JM. The radiological deformity of Colles' fractures. Injury. 1987;18(5):304–8.

Fernandez DL. Correction of post-traumatic wrist deformity in adults by osteotomy, bone-grafting, and internal fixation. J Bone Joint Surg Am. 1982;64(8): 1164–78.

Fernandez DL. Malunion of the distal radius: current approach to management. Instr Course Lect. 1993;42: 99–113.

Hove LM, Solheim E, Skjeie R, Sorensen FK. Prediction of secondary displacement in Colles' fracture. J Hand Surg Br. 1994;19(6):731–6.

Krukhaug Y, Hove LM. Corrective osteotomy for malunited extra-articular fractures of the distal radius: a follow-up study of 33 patients. Scand J Plast Reconstr Surg Hand Surg. 2007;41(6):303–9.

Lafontaine M, Hardy D, Delince P. Stability assessment of distal radius fractures. Injury. 1989;20(4):208–10.

Leone J, Bhandari M, Adili A, McKenzie S, Moro JK, Dunlop RB. Predictors of early and late instability following conservative treatment of extra-articular distal radius fractures. Arch Orthop Trauma Surg. 2004;124(1):38–41.

Mackenney PJ, McQueen MM, Elton R. Prediction of instability in distal radial fractures. J Bone Joint Surg Am. 2006;88(9):1944–51.

McQueen MM, Caspers J. Colles fracture: does the anatomical result affect the final function? J Bone Joint Surg Br. 1988;70(4):649–51.

McQueen MM, Michie M, Court-Brown CM. Hand and wrist function after external fixation of unstable distal radial fractures. Clin Orthop Relat Res. 1992; 285:200–4.

Prommersberger KJ, Moossavi S, Lanz U. Results of corrective osteotomy of malunited extension fractures of the radius at the usual site. Handchir Mikrochir Plast Chir. 1999;31(4):234–40.

Shea K, Fernandez DL, Jupiter JB, Martin C. Corrective osteotomy for malunited, volarly displaced fractures of the distal end of the radius. J Bone Joint Surg Am. 1997;79(12):1816–26.

Solgaard S. Early displacement of distal radius fracture. Acta Orthop Scand. 1986;57(3):229–31.

Vaughan PA, Lui SM, Harrington IJ, Maistrelli GL. Treatment of unstable fractures of the distal radius by external fixation. J Bone Joint Surg Br. 1985;67(3): 385–9.

Part III

Treatment

Pharmacologic Treatment of Distal Radial Fractures

12

Per Aspenberg

Contents

P. Aspenberg, MD, PhD
Department of Orthopaedic Surgery, Linköping University Hospital, University of Linköping, Linköping, Sweden
e-mail: per.aspenberg@liu.se

12.1 Summary

There is consensus that selective cox inhibitors inhibit fracture healing in animal experiments. There is also very good evidence that 1 week of cox-inhibitor treatment greatly reduces the risk of ectopic bone formation after hip surgery in humans. Still, cox inhibitors are commonly used for postoperative pain relief. This is obviously because clinical experience tells us that it works well, with few problems. This is a paradox. Are the animal fracture data irrelevant for humans?

So far, there is no evidence that any drug treatment aiming at accelerating fracture healing can make a difference for the patients. It is however possible that in the future, bisphosphonates or PTH might shorten the time till full loading.

12.2 Drugs Can Have Potent Effects on Fracture Healing in Animals, but Effects in Humans Are Difficult to Measure

Biopsies from distal radial fractures show that they heal almost entirely through membranous ossification, which occurs in the marrow space between injured trabeculae (Aspenberg and Sandberg 2013). This is quite different from conventional textbook descriptions of fracture healing.

L.M. Hove et al. (eds.), *Distal Radius Fractures*,
DOI 10.1007/978-3-642-54604-4_12, © Springer-Verlag Berlin Heidelberg 2014

Almost all our knowledge about the biology of fracture healing comes from animal experiments. However, animal models have two main weaknesses that preclude a safe translation to distal radial fractures in humans. Firstly, almost all animal data is derived from cortical, mid-shaft fractures of long bones, whereas the distal radius is to a large extent cancellous. Mid-shaft fractures do not, in contrast to fractured trabeculae in cancellous bone, have surrounding bone marrow with abundant mesenchymal stem cells. Therefore, most available animal data may be largely irrelevant for metaphyseal fractures.

Secondly, a most important difference between animals and humans is size. The micro-perspective is similar regarding repairing cells. The macro-perspective is hugely different: a 1 mm wide hole in the mouse tibia engages the whole bone, whereas in humans it is neglectable, so it is unclear what the hole in the mouse represents.

Large clinical fracture trials are difficult to perform, in comparison to trials on elective procedures. Patients are difficult to recruit, it is unclear exactly what to measure, and clinical variation requires studies to be inaccessibly large in order to provide statistical power. No wonder then that we know that several drugs are likely to influence healing, but are so uncertain about it.

12.3 NSAIDs Inhibit the Fracture Healing Response: How Much Does It Matter?

There is consensus that NSAIDS, or rather unspecific or selective cox inhibitors, inhibit fracture healing in animal experiments. There is also very good evidence that 1 week of cox-inhibitor treatment greatly reduces the risk of ectopic bone formation after hip surgery in humans. Still, cox inhibitors are commonly used for postoperative pain relief. This is obviously because clinical experience tells us that it works well, with few problems. This is a paradox. Are the animal fracture data irrelevant for humans?

In a large randomized trial on high-energy fractures of long bone shafts, patients who received indomethacin for 6 weeks had more than 3 times more non-unions than controls (Burd et al. 2003). So humans are no exception. However, non-unions of distal radial fractures are extremely rare, and because cox inhibitors produce such good pain relief, an increase in this very small risk could be worth taking. On the other hand, we don't know if healing of distal radial fracture is delayed by this treatment.

12.4 No Proven Effect of BMPs: What About Side Effects?

Bone morphogenic proteins (BMPs) were once the wonder drug of the future, but those prophecies appear not to have been fulfilled. No superiority over autogenous bone grafting had been demonstrated in fractures.

BMP-2 has shown a clear acceleration of healing and reduction in complication rate in patients operated without reamed marrow nailing in the treatment of open tibial fractures (Govender et al. 2002). In contrast, no positive effect and an increased rate of infections were seen in patients with reamed marrow nailing in open tibial fractures (Aro et al. 2011). These trials used no extra treatment as a comparator. A number of fracture trials with BMP-2 have been terminated prematurely after interim analyses showed no positive effect.

BMP-7 (OP-1) compared with autograft, in correction osteotomies of the distal radius with malunited fractures, showed a dramatic delay in healing and increased rate of complications (Ekrol et al. 2008).

These mainly negative effects of BMPs in metaphyseal fractures should not have been unexpected, as it has been known for more than a decade that BMPs cause increased resorption and often complete loss of bone locally, after insertion in cancellous bone. BMPs also cause local inflammation which can be dramatic and painful.

12.5 Bisphosphonates Increase Bone Density in the Fracture Region: Why So Few Studies?

Bisphosphonates are relatively safe, cheap and common. They have potent anti-catabolic effects on the bone. They improve the fixation of knee and hip replacements in randomized trials, and also the fixation of external fixator pins and dental implants is improved (Aspenberg 2009; Abtahi et al. 2012).

No effects on clinical variables and conventional radiography were seen in a randomized trial on volarly plated distal radial fractures (Gong et al. 2012). This is in contrast to a randomized trial, where a dramatic increase in mineral density in the distal radius fracture region was seen with DEXA (Adolphson et al. 2000). Therefore, there are no current recommendations for such treatment.

12.6 Parathyroid Hormone Increases Callus Density: Does It Matter?

Parathyroid hormone (PTH; or a related molecule, teriparatide) has a potent anabolic effect on bone. It stimulates fracture healing in animals. There are only two randomized trials on PTH and fracture healing (Aspenberg 2013). One of them concerns conservatively treated distal radial fractures and shows a moderate shortening of the time to cortical bridging on radiographs (Aspenberg et al. 2010). However, there are uncertainties, as a higher than normal dose did not show this effect. In a post-hoc analysis, it appeared that PTH had a strong, dose-dependent stimulatory effect on early callus formation (Aspenberg and Johansson 2010). This is what could be expected: PTH stimulates osteoblasts and prolongs their survival; therefore, the most obvious effects will appear where there are a lot of osteoblasts, i.e. in an early fracture callus. At later stages, when the bony contours are restored and the healing process is dominated by remodelling, the effects of PTH are probably more unpredictable.

The other randomized trial concerns pelvic fractures and appears to show a dramatic shortening of the time to clinical and radiographic healing (Peichl et al. 2011). However, the study design is not really randomized and opens for the risk of bias.

Even though these results appear compelling, they should not be taken as proof of accelerated healing. There is a need for a confirmatory study. Furthermore, it remains to demonstrate that earlier visible callus formation leads to clinical benefit for the patients (Aspenberg 2013).

Conclusion

So far, there is no evidence that any drug treatment aiming at accelerating fracture healing can make a difference for the patients. It is however possible that in the future, bisphosphonates or PTH might shorten the time till full loading.

References

Abtahi J, Tengvall P, Aspenberg P. A bisphosphonate-coating improves the fixation of metal implants in human bone. A randomized trial of dental implants. Bone. 2012;50(5):1148–51.

Adolphson P, Abbaszadegan H, Boden H, Salemyr M, Henriques T. Clodronate increases mineralization of callus after Colles' fracture: a randomized, double-blind, placebo-controlled, prospective trial in 32 patients. Acta Orthop Scand. 2000;71(2):195–200.

Aro HT, Govender S, Patel AD, Hernigou P, Perera de Gregorio A, Popescu GI, et al. Recombinant human bone morphogenetic protein-2: a randomized trial in open tibial fractures treated with reamed nail fixation. J Bone Joint Surg Am. 2011;93(9):801–8.

Aspenberg P. Bisphosphonates and implants: an overview. Acta Orthop. 2009;80(1):119–23.

Aspenberg P. Annotation: parathyroid hormone and fracture healing. Acta Orthop. 2013;84(1):4–6.

Aspenberg P, Johansson T. Teriparatide improves early callus formation in distal radial fractures. Acta Orthop. 2010;81(2):234–6.

Aspenberg P, Genant HK, Johansson T, Nino AJ, See K, Krohn K, et al. Teriparatide for acceleration of fracture repair in humans: a prospective, randomized, double-blind study of 102 postmenopausal women with distal radial fractures. J Bone Miner Res. 2010;25(2):404–14.

Aspenberg P, Sandberg O. Distal radial fractures heal by direct woven bone formation. Acta Orthop. 2013;84(3): 297–300.

Burd TA, Hughes MS, Anglen JO. Heterotopic ossification prophylaxis with indomethacin increases the risk of long-bone nonunion. J Bone Joint Surg Br. 2003; 85(5):700–5.

Ekrol I, Hajducka C, Court-Brown C, McQueen MM. A comparison of RhBMP-7 (OP-1) and autogenous graft for metaphyseal defects after osteotomy of the distal radius. Injury. 2008;39 Suppl 2:73–82.

Gong HS, Song CH, Lee YH, Rhee SH, Lee HJ, Baek GH. Early initiation of bisphosphonate does not affect healing and outcomes of volar plate fixation of osteoporotic distal radial fractures. J Bone Joint Surg Am. 2012;94(19):1729–36.

Govender S, Csimma C, Genant HK, Valentin-Opran A, Amit Y, Arbel R, et al. Recombinant human bone morphogenetic protein-2 for treatment of open tibial fractures: a prospective, controlled, randomized study of four hundred and fifty patients. J Bone Joint Surg Am. 2002;84A(12):2123–34.

Peichl P, Holzer LA, Maier R, Holzer G. Parathyroid hormone 1–84 accelerates fracture-healing in pubic bones of elderly osteoporotic women. J Bone Joint Surg Am. 2011;93(17):1583–7.

Flow Chart for Treatment: A Standardized Treatment Program as an Aid in Primary Treatment of Distal Radius Fractures

13

Antonio Abramo

Contents

A. Abramo, MD, PhD
Department of Hand Surgery,
Lund University, Skane University Hospital,
Malmö, Sweden
e-mail: tony.abramo@med.lu.se

13.1 Summary

Distal radius fractures are most often treated non-operatively, but sometimes they are treated surgically when deemed unstable. Based on the literature, a consensus protocol for treatment has been developed in the mid-1990s in southern Sweden to aid clinicians in their decision-making. It has been in use in several hospitals since then and the effect of the treatment program has been evaluated showing that the patients reach similar final outcome regardless of fracture type when the protocol has been used.

Distal radius fractures are a heterogeneous group of fractures, and to describe a specific treatment for each fracture would be hardly impossible due to the diversity of the fractures. Therefore, a flow chart including general rules in the treatment of distal radius fractures is of value for the emergency room doctors as well as the orthopedic surgeons (Abramo et al. 2008). Younger patients may have more fractures of multi-trauma type and may also have greater demands for a better wrist and hand function than elderly patients, and a treatment protocol has to consider that. On the other hand also patients in the older groups may have high demands to their wrists, needing a good hand function while gardening, playing golf, or other activities.

The current classifications of distal radius fractures do not in general consider the final outcome and seldom give any indication of how to treat the fractures. Usually classifications are based upon radiologic or macro-anatomic

L.M. Hove et al. (eds.), *Distal Radius Fractures*,
DOI 10.1007/978-3-642-54604-4_13, © Springer-Verlag Berlin Heidelberg 2014

appearance of the fracture. The widely used AO classification divides fracture types into extra and intra-articular fractures and also considers the comminution of the fracture suggesting that more complex fractures are in need of more aggressive treatment. The AO foundation website may give the surgeon help in decision-making as well (https://www2.aofoundation.org/wps/portal/surgery?showPage=diagnosis&bone=Radius&segment=Distal).

Numerous other classifications exist, mainly due to the complexity and diversity of the distal radius fractures, but it is difficult to draw any conclusions from the classifications on how to treat and to predict the outcome.

We suggest a simple flow chart for decision-making and treatment of the distal radius fractures.

Based on current literature, there are some predictors involving the initial fracture appearance telling us about the final outcome.

- Studies suggest that a shortening of the distal radius of 2 mm can impair the final outcome (Aro and Koivunen 1991).
- An intra-articular incongruency of more than 1 mm is a predictor for evolvement of radiocarpal osteoarthritis (Kopylov et al. 1993)
- A dorsal angulation of more than 15° is correlated to worse outcome for the patient (Leung et al. 2000; Wilcke et al. 2007), often with poor range of motion in the forearm rotation. This applies for a volar angulation of 20–30° (Finsen and Aasheim 2000).
- Fractures tend to dislocate during the treatment in the cast, with radial length being the strongest predictor for secondary dislocation (Hove et al. 1994).
- Most of the secondary dislocation after conservative treatment happens early, before the fracture starts to heal; therefore, it is important to radiologically reevaluate the fracture after 7–10 days. If the fracture then is dislocated, surgery should be considered. If the fracture shows sign of dislocation but still keeps an acceptable position, a second reevaluation is advised.

The treatment program (Fig. 13.1) has been in use at the Lund university hospital since 1998 and has been evaluated looking at the subjective outcome measured with DASH score (Abramo et al. 2008). Since 2001 all distal radius fractures have been followed with the DASH questionnaire mailed to the patients 3 and 12 months after the first visit to the ER. The response rate was 70 %. An evaluation of the treatment protocol was done looking at the patient data during 2 years (September 2001 to August 2003). To evaluate the program the patients were divided in three groups in the treatment protocol:

1. Undisplaced fractures treated in cast
2. Displaced fractures treated in cast after reposition
3. Surgically treated fractures

Patients were treated according to the flow chart, and the final outcome was similar regardless of the severity of the fracture at 3 and 12 months follow-up indicating that the flow chart is usable for selecting the proper treatment for each patient.

Dislocations subject to further treatment (reposition or surgery if reposition fails)

- Dorsal angulation of more than 10° or volar angulation of more than 25°
- Ulna plus of more than 2 mm in younger patients and more than 5 mm in older low demand patients
- Articular incongruence of more than 1 mm
- Radial inclination of less than 10°

- Distal radius fractures are a heterogenic group and a standardized and simplified treatment program is of great value.
- Simple guidelines can result in acceptable results for all types of fractures.
- For fractures with dislocations after attempted reposition surgery should be considered.
- A routine check with x-rays and clinical reevaluation within the first 10 days can catch most of the re-dislocating fractures.
- Unstable fractures such as highly comminuted fractures, high energy trauma, or volar Barton fractures are subject to surgical intervention.

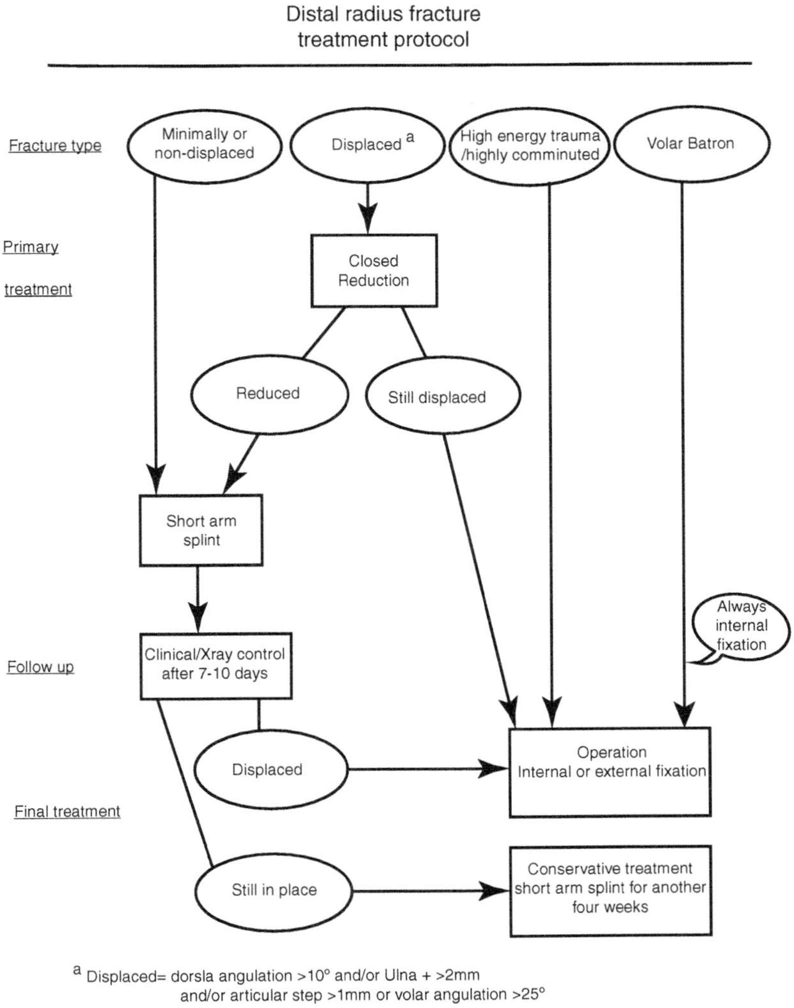

Fig. 13.1 A standard treatment protocol for distal radius fractures. Fractures are considered displaced when any of the criteria for dislocation is met. However in patients with low demands, elderly with osteoporotic fractures, or generally disabled younger persons with low demands, the cutoff for treatment is higher

References

Abramo A, Kopylov P, Tagil M. Evaluation of a treatment protocol in distal radius fractures: a prospective study in 581 patients using DASH as outcome. Acta Orthop. 2008;79(3):376–85.

Aro HT, Koivunen T. Minor axial shortening of the radius affects outcome of Colles' fracture treatment. J Hand Surg Am. 1991;16(3):392–8.

Finsen V, Aasheim T. Initial experience with the Forte plate for dorsally displaced distal radius fractures. Injury. 2000;31(6):445–8.

Hove LM, Solheim E, Skjeie R, Sorensen FK. Prediction of secondary displacement in Colles' fracture. J Hand Surg Br. 1994;19(6):731–6.

Kopylov P, Johnell O, Redlund-Johnell I, Bengner U. Fractures of the distal end of the radius in young adults: a 30-year follow-up. J Hand Surg Br. 1993; 18(1):45–9.

Leung F, Ozkan M, Chow SP. Conservative treatment of intra-articular fractures of the distal radius–factors affecting functional outcome. Hand Surg. 2000;5(2): 145–53.

Wilcke MK, Abbaszadegan H, Adolphson PY. Patient-perceived outcome after displaced distal radius fractures. A comparison between radiological parameters, objective physical variables, and the DASH score. J Hand Ther. 2007;20(4):290–8.

The Clinical Dilemma: Nonoperative or Operative Treatment

14

Anders Ditlev Foldager-Jensen

Contents

A.D. Foldager-Jensen, MD
Department of Orthopaedic Surgery,
Section for Hand Surgery, Aarhus University
Hospital, Aarhus, Denmark
e-mail: anders.ditlev@aarhus.rm.dk

14.1 Summary

Deciding whether to operate or not might be the most difficult decision to make in the process of treating distal radius fractures. A multitude of variables must be taken in consideration before one can present a treatment plan for the patient. The patient should be an active part of the decision-making, based on the surgeon's recommendations for treatment.

In this chapter, we will take a deeper look at the different factors to consider, when you are planning to treat a distal radius fracture.

Though most distal radius fractures are managed nonoperatively, in the last decade we have seen a shift towards stable internal fixation along with the development of new fixation devices (Wilcke et al. 2013). In spite of this change, no strong evidence has been published to support this increase in operative treatment. At present, the number of publications regarding treatment of distal radius fractures is increasing rapidly, and we hope in the near future to have better evidence to support our decision-making. Until then, the treatment and information given to the patient must be based on the current best evidence (Lichtman 2010; Bales and Stern 2012).

As we have seen in the rest of the chapters, we have extensive knowledge about distal radius fractures. We know the anatomy in detail and know how to classify the fractures, evaluate stability, and make flow charts for the treatment. We know different kinds of treatment, either nonoperative or operative, and in principle this

L.M. Hove et al. (eds.), *Distal Radius Fractures*
DOI 10.1007/978-3-642-54604-4_14, © Springer-Verlag Berlin Heidelberg 2014

is pretty straightforward, but the moment the patient enters the scene, things get a lot more complicated.

The patient presents multiple variables to consider: age, gender, occupation, dominant hand, hobbies/sports, bone quality, co-morbidity, medication, functional and mental level, etc. Each of these variables might influence the choice of treatment, and a normal flow chart cannot integrate all possible factors. This combined with the heterogeneous group of fractures spanning from undisplaced, stable fractures to intra-articular comminuted fractures and different mechanisms of injury renders the decision-making quite complex.

This complex mix of variables may also explain why it is difficult to reach consensus regarding the treatment strategy; the multitude of variables make studies difficult to compare in search for evidence.

- Handoll and Madhok made five systematic reviews, published in the Cochrane Library in 2003, regarding treatment of distal radius fractures. Even though they made some very thorough studies, they could not provide robust evidence regarding the decision-making of the treatment. Surgical treatment typically gave better anatomical reduction after fracture healing compared to nonoperative treatment, but there was no evidence to support a better functional and clinical outcome for the patients. These reviews were made just before the operative boom using fixed-angle devices, and the question is whether the new operative methods will make a difference in future reviews (Handoll and Madhok 2003).
- In a paper from 2012, Ng and McQueen reviewed the radiological parameters measured in distal radius fractures, in an attempt to identify potential predictors of functional outcome among patients with high functional demands. They concluded that in order to have the best possibility to gain a pain-free, mobile wrist joint without functional limitations, there should be less than 2-mm gap or step-off in the joint surface, the radius should be restored to within 2 mm of its normal length, and carpal alignment should be restored.
- Carpal alignment is measured drawing two lines in the lateral view along the long axis of the capitate and the radius. These lines should cross within the carpus, and if not so, the carpus is malaligned (Ng and McQueen 2011).
- In an earlier study, McQueen and Caspers (1988) found that dorsal tilt ≥12° from neutral and >2 mm of radial shift was clearly associated with significant functional limitation. In their most recent review, they include carpal alignment in the evaluation of dorsal tilt: the most important indication for correction is the presence of carpal malalignment, with the measured dorsal/palmar tilt being of secondary importance. Thus, some dorsal tilt can be accepted if the carpus remains aligned. In contrary, correction should be made, if the carpus is not aligned and the dorsal tilt is above neutral (McQueen and Caspers 1988).
- In 2009, the American Academy of Orthopaedic Surgeons (AAOS) made a clinical practice guideline based on a systematic review of published studies. They made 29 recommendations but none were graded "strong". With grade strength, moderate, they recommended operative treatment for fractures with postreductional radial shortening >3 mm, dorsal tilt >10° from neutral or intra-articular displacement, or step-off >2 mm (Lichtman 2010).

These recommendations are in line with the practice in most orthopaedic departments today. However, these recommendations are based on physiological young and active patients, and the question is whether the same principles apply to elderly patients.

The shift towards more operations combined with an aging population makes the treatment of distal radius fractures a potential economic challenge. Operative treatment with internal fixation is quite expensive compared with reposition and cast and increases the risk of complications; thus, there should be a clinical advantage in choosing the expensive, operative treatment. Reviewing recent literature does not support the use of operative treatment for the elderly population (Diaz-Garcia 2011).

Arora compared nonoperative treatment with volar locking plate fixation for patients aged 65 years or older and found no difference in range of motion, level of pain, nor functional scores at follow-up, 12 months later. Patients in the operative treatment group had better grip strength through the entire period of time. Achieving anatomical reconstruction in the operative group did not improve the range of motion or the ability to perform daily living activities (Arora et al. 2011). Similar results were found in a study by Ergol et al. (2010). These studies suggest that patients aged 65 years and older might not benefit from operative treatment, when looking at the subjective outcome after 1 year.

Operations with stable internal fixation often allow the patient to mobilize earlier, and the cast can typically be replaced with a removable splint after 2 weeks. Three months after surgery, the wrist motion, and DASH scores are better than when treating nonoperatively, but this difference seems to disappear after 1 year when treating the elderly. Some patients are willing to wait for the positive effect after 1 year, whereas others would like to have the fastest recovery possible.

The choice of treatment must also include an evaluation of the available implants and whether the surgeon is skilled in using it or not. In some departments, only a few expert surgeons operate distal radius fractures, whereas in other departments the surgeons are generalists and might have only little experience with the chosen type of operation (Karantana and Davis 2012). Many complications to surgery are seen because the surgeon does not master the technique. When using volar locking plates, a common fault is screws penetrating into the radiocarpal joint, or dorsal into the extensor tendons, or placing the plate volar to the volar rim of the radius with increased risk of flexor tendons injuries.

Our primary goal for treatment is to gain bone union without symptomatic malunion. Some degree of displacement is usually tolerated, but only to a certain extent. For the physiologically young and active patient these measurements should indicate an acceptable range of values:

- Radial shortening <2 mm
- Intra-articular gap or displacement <2 mm
- Dorsal tilt $\leq 10^{\circ}$ and carpus aligned

14.2 Treatment Strategy

- Unless the fracture is undisplaced, closed reduction and immobilization in a forearm cast is almost always indicated in an attempt to gain the best possible anatomical restoration (Steward et al. 1985). If the patient is senile, or otherwise severely mentally impaired, reduction might not be indicated.
- If the reduction is acceptable, and there are no other operative demanding injuries, nonoperative treatment is chosen.
- If the reduction is acceptable, but the fracture is unstable, operation should be considered, e.g. volar angulated fractures (Smiths fractures), shear fractures (volar or dorsal Barton's fractures), etc. If nonoperative treatment is chosen, the patient must be followed closely with radiographs until union is complete.
- If the fracture position is not acceptable, the surgeon must evaluate the situation with all the variables in mind.
- In the frail elderly patient who is dependent on help to perform daily living activities, a nonoperative treatment will typically suffice.
- If the patient for other reasons is not suitable for surgery, the patient should be informed about the situation and what could be expected in the future in terms of function, and nonoperative regimen is chosen.
- If the physician considers the patient suitable for surgery, he should inform that he assesses that the situation is not ideal and that surgery might be indicated.
- The patient should be involved in the clinical decision-making, so-called shared decision-making Slover et al. (2012). The surgeon informs the patient about the advantages and disadvantages regarding nonoperative versus operative care and what treatment options are available. The patient indicates how their preferences and values relate to these options. Subsequently, the surgeon and the patient reach a consensus regarding which treatment to choose (Wilcke et al. 2013).

Authors Method

- When I examine my patient I ensure that I have all the details available. If there is any doubt about the nature of the fracture, I consider performing supplementary radiographs of the contra lateral wrist for comparison and/or do a CT-scan, especially in the young patients with high energy involved in the accident.
- Next, I talk to the patient to get a full medical history. Learn about their needs for daily activities, occupation and hobbies. I examine the arm including the shoulder and elbow, and look for associated injuries like soft tissue damages, nerve compression and carpal injuries.
- At this point I have a good idea about the nature of the fracture and possible associated injuries, and have an idea about how to address the fracture either, nonoperatively or with some kind of operation, and I know if the patient is medically suitable for operation.
- I present my assessment to the patient, but do not offer a recommendation for treatment yet. I try to explain what to expect if we operate or not, and try to inform about advantages and disadvantages with the possible options, including possible complications. It is important to note, that you can direct the patient towards any treatment in the way you weight your words, and you must be aware of this.
- I explain, that we want to avoid a symptomatic malunion, but also that not all malunions are symptomatic, and that if the patient ends up with a symptomatic malunion, there are often ways of dealing with this.
- I ask the patient about their expectations and preferences, and only then do we try to reach consensus regarding the treatment.
- For the young and active, I typically recommend operative treatment as it gives the best chance for a quick return to normal function with good mobility and strength of the wrist.
- For the elderly, I explain that we expect that function will be good after one year, regardless of which treatment we choose, although there might be better strength to some degree after stable internal fixation, and if they end up with a symptomatic malunion after nonoperative treatment, it is often possible to address this later. Often the patients choose nonoperative treatment, and it is very rare, that these patients return with problems.

In 1980 Gregory Benford stated the Benford's law of controversy:

> Passion is inversely proportional to the amount of real information available.

In other words, the fewer facts are known to and agreed on by the participants, the more controversy there is, while the more is known, the less controversy there is.

For the treatment of distal radius fractures, there are numerous scientific papers, but in spite of this there is no strong evidence suggesting a certain treatment. The treatment of distal radius fractures has changed along with the development of new treatment methods and material. With the new trend, angular stable locking plates, a new era has begun, and we look forward to see whether the increasing preference for operative treatment on behalf of nonoperative treatment is based on evidence.

References

Arora R, et al. A prospective randomized trial comparing nonoperative treatment with volar locking plate fixation for displaced and unstable distal radial fractures in patients sixty-five years of age and older. J Bone Joint Surg Am. 2011;93:2146–53.

Bales JG, Stern PJ. Treatment strategies of distal radius fractures. Hand Clin. 2012;28:177–84.

Diaz-Garcia RJ, et al. A systematic review of outcomes and complications of treating unstable distal radius fractures in the elderly. J Hand Surg. 2011;36A:824–35.

Ergol KA, Walsh M, Romo-Cardoso S, et al. Distal radial fractures in the elderly: operative compared with non-operative treatment. J Bone Joint Surg Am. 2010; 92(9):1851–7.

Handoll HHG, Madhok R. Conservative interventions for treating distal radial fractures in adults. Cochrane Database Syst Rev. 2003:CD000314.

Karantana A, Davis TRC. Extra-articular fractures of the distal radius – a European view point. Hand Clin. 2012;28:145–50.

Lichtman DM, et al. Treatment of distal radius fractures. J Am Acad Orthop Surg. 2010;18:180–9.

McQueen M, Caspers J. Colles fracture: does the anatomical result affect the final function? J Bone Joint Surg Br. 1988;70-B:649–51.

Ng CY, McQueen MM. What are the radiological predictors of functional outcome following fractures of the distal radius? J Bone Joint Surg Br. 2011;93-B:145–50.

Slover J, Shue J, Koenig K. Shared decision-making in orthopaedic surgery. Clin Orthop Relat Res. 2012;470: 1046–53.

Steward HD, Innes AR, Burke FD. Factors affecting the outcome of Colles' fracture: an anatomical and functional study. Injury. 1985;16:289–95.

Wilcke MKT, et al. Epidemiology and changed surgical treatment methods for fractures of the distal radius. Acta Orthop. 2013;84(3):292–6.

Clinical Diagnosis, Closed Reduction, and Plaster

15

Carl Ekholm

Contents

C. Ekholm, MD, PhD
Department of Orthopaedics, Sahlgrens' University Hospital, University of Gothenburg, Göteborg, Sweden
e-mail: carl.ekholm@vgregion.se

L.M. Hove et al. (eds.), *Distal Radius Fractures*,
DOI 10.1007/978-3-642-54604-4_15,

15.1 Summary

Almost 2/3 of all fractures will have an acceptable outcome with plaster treatment if used properly. A prerequisite for a good radiological outcome is the absence of volar comminution, since radial length can be maintained only with contact between the opposing volar cortices of the main fragments. Closed reduction usually employs ligamentotaxis, but distraction alone will not fully reduce the fracture; the concept of multiplanar ligamentotaxis has to be used. The wrist should be immobilised in neutral or slight extension as this preserves finger function and diminishes the risk for redisplacement. Secondary displacement may occur after >2 weeks into treatment and the fracture may need to be monitored for 2–3 weeks. If redisplacement occurs, operative fixation is needed to maintain reduction of the fracture.

15.2 Introduction: Clinical Diagnosis

- Little has changed since the days of Abraham Colles and Claude Pouteau; patients still present with complaints of local tenderness and pain.
- Clinical examination of the wrist is done as in any sprained wrist in order to diagnose fractures and displacement and to assess neurovascular status of the hand.

- On inspection the wrist may demonstrate a so-called dinner-fork deformity if the fracture is displaced. Sometimes the distal end of the ulna may be prominent.
- X-ray and other imaging modalities are used to diagnose type of fracture, displacement, and possible associated fractures or ligament injuries.

15.3 Plaster Treatment: General Aspects

- Plaster is the "workhorse" for treating fractures of the distal radius. Almost 2/3 of all fractures will have an acceptable final outcome with this treatment if properly used.
- In addition, it is used for temporary fixation in fractures awaiting surgery and to supplement a semi-stable internal fixation or simply for comfort for patients with operated fractures.
- The fracture is always shortened or compressed by the trauma itself, worsened by the compressive forces from the extrinsic, long tendons across the wrist.
- The fracture is reduced mainly by distraction and the idea of plaster immobilisation is to maintain the reduced position, i.e. to counteract the compressive and displacing forces. Since plaster immobilisation itself cannot maintain distraction, preservation of length relies solely on bone contact between the fracture fragments and therefore proper reduction of the main fragments.
- Extra-articular bending fractures (Fernandez type 1) are therefore the ones best suited for this form of treatment.
- If some compression with shortening is acceptable (in the low-demand patient or the medically unfit patient), more complex fractures (Fernandez 3 and 4) may also be treated with a cast.
- Shearing fractures (Fernandez type 2 – partially intra-articular fractures) are rarely suited since displacement of the partial joint fragment will inevitably lead to an intra-articular step-off and radio-carpal dislocation.
- High-energy comminuted fractures (Fernandez type 5) are never suitable for cast treatment, but require at least fixation with a spanning external fixator for reasonable preservation of length and alignment.
- A prerequisite for a good outcome is restoration of radial length. Fractures to be treated with a cast therefore need an intact volar cortex, i.e. no volar comminution (Fig. 15.1). After perfect reduction, the distal fragment will be supported by volar cortical contact, the cortical hinge, and the purpose of the plaster is to prevent dorsal angulation or dorsal displacement of the distal fragment (Fig. 15.1). It therefore needs to exert a volarly directed pressure on the distal fragment, which requires a counterforce generated more proximally on the volar surface of the forearm (Fig. 15.1). This requires a well-moulded full cast or well-designed prefabricated brace that can be adjusted to the patient.
- By tradition (or by fear for cast induced compartment syndrome), a full cast is not routinely used in Scandinavian countries. Instead a dorsal plaster slab is wrapped to the forearm with a crepe bandage. The mechanical function of a dorsal slab has not been demonstrated. However, it supports the hand and thereby promotes the normal use of the fingers.

15.4 Closed Reduction

- Closed reduction is normally done in the A&E department with either a hematoma block or a Bier block.
- Closed reduction is performed through *direct manipulation* of the fracture or indirectly via *ligamentotaxis*.
- *Direct manipulation* typically involves a bi-digital grip across the distal fragment by which it can be manoeuvred into a reduced position. Often this starts with exaggeration of the initial displacement to disengage the distal fragment from the shaft, whereafter the volar cortices can be brought into contact and distal fragment be pivoted into reduction. Once

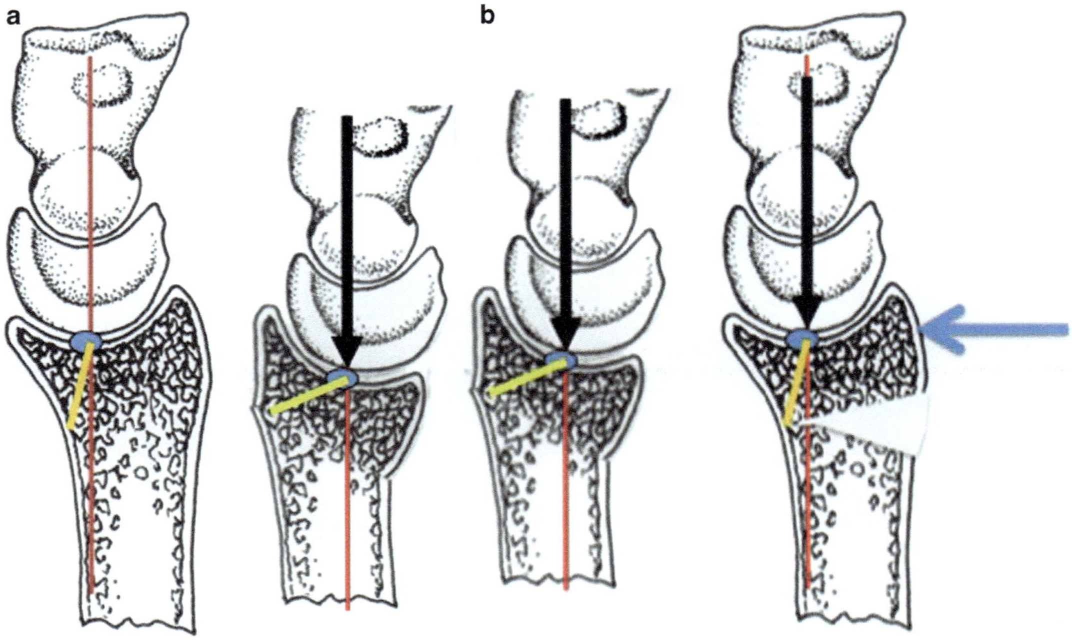

Fig. 15.1 (**a**) An extra-articular Colles type of fracture has the distal fragment dorsally tilted, but volar cortical contact may be maintained. The distal fragment is thus pivoted on the volar cortex hinge. This dorsally displaced fragment causes radial shortening and further dorsal displacement as the centre axis for load through the radio-carpal joint is transferred dorsally. This will also cause a dorsal shift of the carpus relative to the radius. The capito-lunate axis will be malaligned dorsally rather than centred in the radio-carpal joint. Once this displacement is established, continuous load through the carpus will further displace the distal fragment. (**b**) Nonoperative treatment is only successful if the volar cortical contact is realigned, which will retain reduction and preserve the length of radius. Hereby, the compression forces across the joint will return to its slightly palmar location, in order for the load to be transmitted in its normal direction. This reduction is maintained with a moderate dorsal pressure and a dorsal slab

reduced, further traction is not necessary to maintain reduction (which of course is a prerequisite for successful plaster treatment) – a moderate dorsal pressure on the distal fragment is sufficient.

- *Direct manipulation* can also be done towards individual fragments, e.g. dorsally displaced fragments could be possible to push into place with a moderate pressure.
- *Ligamentotaxis* is the process of applying traction forces to the distal radius fragment through the surrounding soft tissues. Longitudinal traction alone will not completely reduce the fracture. When the fingers are pulled distally (e.g. by using "Chinese" finger traps) traction of the distal fragment is exerted mainly via the volar ligaments since the dorsal ligaments are weak (Agee 1994) and the technique of "multiplanar" ligamentotaxis has to be employed..
- Normally, closed reduction is a combination of both techniques.
- Open or percutaneous reduction also uses all the techniques of closed reduction, now of course aided by improved visibility, access instruments, and implants.

15.5 Immobilisation: Position

- The comfortable and safe position to immobilise the wrist is in neutral radial-ulnar deviation and neutral or slight extension.
- Moderate ulnar deviation is accepted to preserve radial length with the support from the intact ulna.
- This is the natural position for undisplaced, or minimally displaced, fractures.
- In displaced fractures, reduction with manipulation is done before immobilisation is done.

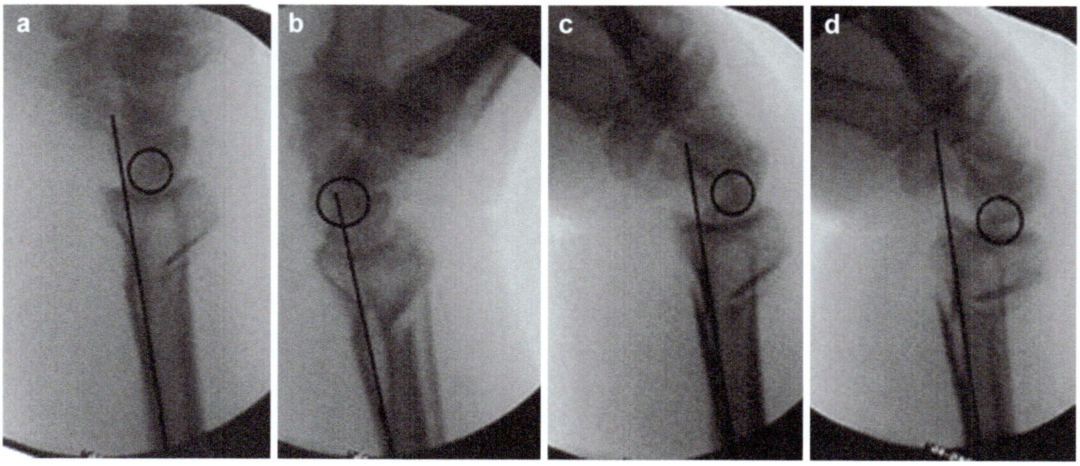

Fig. 15.2 The effect of compressive forces over the fracture is mimicked by manual compression on the knuckles along the metacarpal axes. (**a**) Shows the reduced fracture, wrist neutral. (**b**) Shows that the extension of the wrist shifts the lunate in a volar direction and that pure compression may increase the volar tilt when the wrist is extended. (**c**) Shows the wrist in flexion where the lunate shifts dorsally. (**d**) Shows that compression combined with wrist flexion will displace the fracture. *Circles* show the position of the tip of the radial styloid

- Intuitively, the wrist is often placed in flexion in order to achieve an acceptable reduction and good post-reduction X-ray. This is based on the assumption that ligamentotaxis via dorsal ligaments can prevent dorsal displacement. However, since plaster cannot maintain traction, and dorsal ligaments are flaccid, ligamentotaxis will not work.
- Flexion of the wrist will move the loading forces dorsally in the radio-carpal joint and thereby cause dorsal redisplacement of the fracture (Fig. 15.2). This has been shown in a prospective randomised study, which compared circular plaster immobilisation in moderate extension with immobilisation in flexion (Gupta 1991).
- Immobilisation in extreme flexion and ulnar deviation was historically the only option (Lidstrom 1959; Frykman 1967) as internal fixation was not available. However, the advice at the time was to not use this position for the entire immobilisation period due to the detrimental effects on hand function as finger flexion is difficult, stresses the median nerve, and prevents oedema drainage.
- The goal with plaster treatment is to maintain the reduced position of the fracture without compromising finger function. The cast should be well moulded, without obstructing full motion of the MCP-joints or the elbow.
- A well-moulded cast minimises fracture movement, which will decrease pain.
- The use of a dorsal slab will obviously decrease the risk of plaster-induced compartment syndrome; on the other hand, instability of the fracture with associated pain might make using the fingers difficult and aggravate oedema.
- For minimally displaced fractures, an adjustable brace gave better patient satisfaction than a plaster cast with equal hand function (O'Conner et al. 2003).
- Above elbow plaster, for instance, "sugar-tong plaster", may occasionally be used when there is a concomitant distal ulna fracture and still conservative management is the treatment of choice

15.6 Immobilisation: Time

- Treatment period should be long enough to allow consolidation of the fracture before mobilisation. With a functional cast or brace this period would normally be 4–6 weeks depending on fracture type.
- With immobilisation is in an extreme position, as outlined above, a treatment period of 6 weeks is not recommended, but rather a

change after 3–4 weeks into a cast or a splint for the remaining 2–3 weeks to optimise finger mobility.

- Some further settling of the fracture may take place after 6 weeks; this can be expected to be more pronounced in fractures with poor contact between fragments.

15.7 Prognostic Factors

- Minimally displaced, simple fractures that do not require manipulation have a good prognosis for healing in an anatomically acceptable position.
- The risk for secondary displacement increases with increasing initial displacement and comminution.
- Five factors have been suggested to predict instability (Lafontaine et al. 1989):
  - Dorsal angulation >20°
  - Dorsal comminution
  - Intra-articular fracture
  - Concomitant ulnar fracture
  - Age >60 years
- If three of these factors are involved, and the fracture is well reduced after manipulation, there is a further age- and time-correlated risk for redisplacement (Nesbitt et al. 2004). The risk for redisplacement was less if reduction could be maintained for 2 weeks, yet the redisplacement risk was still 50 % in patients >80 years (Table 15.1).
- Radial shortening (as decided by ulnar variance) has been suggested to be equally important (Mackenney et al. 2006). There is also a formula, using these factors, to predict the instability (Mackenney et al. 2006); however, it is not extensively used.
- Volar comminution has recently been suggested as yet another important factor for instability (Wadsten et al. 2009), as >90 % of fractures with volar comminution had radiologically unacceptable results with nonoperative treatment (Wadsten MA, 2013; unpublished data).
- AAOS has recommended radiological follow-ups for up to 3 weeks in nonoperatively treated fractures.
- If redisplacement occurs, closed re-reduction and continued plaster treatment cannot improve radiological outcome (McQueen et al. 1996), rather some type of fixation is needed.
- If redisplacement occurs late, after the third week, no general recommendation can be made. The problem is whether to consider the condition as a "nascent malunion" where the redisplaced fracture with certainty will lead to long-term bad outcome or whether the patient may do well without intervention.
- Secondary pain, or neuropathy, is a symptom in favour for an early "nascent" osteotomy. However, there has not been any difference demonstrated between early and late correction osteotomies (Pillukat et al. 2013) as some patients adapt and manage well without correction. Consequently, there is insufficient evidence how to manage late redisplacement

Table 15.1 Probability for unsatisfactory radiological outcome at 4 weeks for fractures having three of the Lafontaine instability factors with initial acceptable reduction. Three different age groups are shown (Nesbitt et al. 2004)

Reduction still acceptable at:	0 week	1 week	2 weeks
58 years	50 %	25 %	5 %
76 years	70 %	50 %	25 %
82 years	80 %	60 %	50 %

"Top tricks"

- Select the patient
  - The volar cortex should not be comminuted
  - Closed reduction should be possible
  - Assess the patient's demands of hand function
- Try to reduce opposing volar cortices to "carry" the distal fragment and preserve length. Remember that the plaster itself will not prevent fracture shortening
- Do not use awkward hand positions to hold the fracture

- The plaster, preferably a circular cast, should be well moulded and not obstruct free finger or elbow motion
- If redislocation occurs, plaster treatment alone is insufficient. After re-reduction use a different method of fixation/immobilisation
- Remember that redislocation may take place even after two successful weeks in plaster

References

Agee JM. Application of multiplanar ligamentotaxis to external fixation of distal radius fractures. Iowa Orthop J. 1994;14:31–7. Epub 1994/01/01.

Frykman G. Fracture of the distal radius including sequelae—shoulder-hand-finger syndrome, disturbance in the distal radio-ulnar joint and impairment of nerve function. A clinical and experimental study. Acta Orthop Scand. 1967;(Suppl 108):3+. Epub 1967/01/01.

Gupta A. The treatment of Colles' fracture. Immobilisation with the wrist dorsiflexed. J Bone Joint Surg Br. 1991;73(2):312–5. Epub 1991/03/01.

Lafontaine M, Hardy D, Delince P. Stability assessment of distal radius fractures. Injury. 1989;20(4):208–10. Epub 1989/07/01.

Lidstrom A. Fractures of the distal end of the radius. A clinical and statistical study of end results. Acta Orthop Scand. 1959;41:1–118. Epub 1959/01/01.

Mackenney PJ, McQueen MM, Elton R. Prediction of instability in distal radial fractures. J Bone Joint Surg Am. 2006;88(9):1944–51. Epub 2006/09/05.

McQueen MM, Hajducka C, Court-Brown CM. Redisplaced unstable fractures of the distal radius: a prospective randomised comparison of four methods of treatment. J Bone Joint Surg Br. 1996;78(3):404–9. Epub 1996/05/01.

Nesbitt KS, Failla JM, Les C. Assessment of instability factors in adult distal radius fractures. J Hand Surg. 2004;29(6):1128–38. Epub 2004/12/04.

O'Connor D, Mullett H, Doyle M, Mofidi A, Kutty S, O'Sullivan M. Minimally displaced Colles' fractures: a prospective randomized trial of treatment with a wrist splint or a plaster cast. J Hand Surg Br. 2003;28(1):50–3. Epub 2003/01/18.

Pillukat T, Schadel-Hopfner M, Windolf J, Prommersberger KJ. The malunited distal radius fracture – early or late correction? Handchir Mikrochir Plast Chir. 2013;45(1):6–12. Epub 2013/03/23.

Wadsten MA, Sayed-Noor AS, Sjoden GO, Svensson O, Buttazzoni GG. The Buttazzoni classification of distal radial fractures in adults: interobserver and intraobserver reliability. Hand. 2009;4(3):283–8. Epub 2009/01/28.

Closed Re-reduction: Is It an Alternative

16

Margaret M. McQueen and Andrew D. Duckworth

Contents

16.1 Summary

Fractures of the distal radius are commonly low-energy osteoporotic fractures, with an increasing number of elderly women affected. The functional demands of the patient along with the risk factors for instability and malunion are essential when considering the role of re-reduction for displaced distal radius fractures. The literature would suggest that there are few indications for re-reduction of a distal radius fracture that loses position following primary manipulation and casting. For patients requiring the best anatomical and functional result, internal or external fixation is superior to re-reduction. The only possible exception to this is the patient who has undergone an inadequate primary reduction, likely due to poor anesthesia, and has a low probability of losing position following an adequate reduction. For older patients with a lower functional demand in whom a malunion will likely provide a satisfactory outcome, re-reduction and even primary reduction are not routinely indicated.

16.2 Introduction

- On first reading of the chapter title, one could quite simply consider the answer to be "there is no role" and turn to the next chapter. However, the topic of re-reduction highlights many of the key considerations related to the assessment and management of displaced distal radius fractures.

M.M. McQueen, MD, FRCSEd(Orth) (✉)
A.D. Duckworth, MSc, MRCSEd
Edinburgh Orthopaedic Trauma Unit, Royal Infirmary of Edinburgh, 51 Little France Crescent, Edinburgh, EH16 4SU, UK
e-mail: mmcqueen@staffmail.ed.ac.uk

L.M. Hove et al. (eds.), *Distal Radius Fractures*,
DOI 10.1007/978-3-642-54604-4_16, © Springer-Verlag Berlin Heidelberg 2014

- The two clinical scenarios where re-reduction will be most frequently considered are:
  1. The patient who has undergone a successful initial reduction but the fracture re-displaces on subsequent review.
  2. The patient who has undergone an unsuccessful primary reduction, because of either inadequate anesthesia or severe fracture instability. If the former, the patient may be a candidate for attempted re-reduction and casting.
- There is limited data in the literature that analyzes the role of re-manipulation for fractures of the distal radius. The primary reasons for this are better-defined indications for surgery, increasing use of operative fixation at an earlier stage following injury, and an improved understanding of the consequences of malunion in relation to the physical demands of the patient.

16.3 Clinical Scenario

- For undisplaced or minimally displaced fractures of the distal radius, early instability occurs in 10 % of patients, with late instability in approximately 20 % (although figures are wide ranging) (Mackenney et al. 2006).
  - The rate of malunion for minimally displaced fractures managed with a single primary closed reduction only is almost 30 %.
- For displaced fractures of the distal radius early instability occurs in just over 40 % of patients, with late instability in almost 50 % (Roumen et al. 1991; Mackenney et al. 2006).
  - The rate of malunion for displaced fractures managed with a single primary closed reduction only is 60 %.

16.4 Clinical Assessment: Risk Factors for Instability

- After primary manipulation, patients are routinely reviewed at 1 and 2 weeks following injury. This should include:
  - A full clinical assessment including neurovascular status
  - Standard PA and lateral radiographs of the affected wrist
  - Reinforcement or change of cast as required
- Recommended criteria for defining displacement and re-displacement that would warrant intervention are found in Table 16.1.
- These are only applicable to the younger, fit, and active patient.
- Knowledge of risk factors for instability, malunion, and carpal malalignment can help guide the management and follow-up of distal radius fractures (Table 16.2) (Hove et al. 1994; Mackenney et al. 2006).
- Increasing age, metaphyseal comminution, ulnar variance, and patient independence are important predictors of fracture stability (Mackenney et al. 2006).
  - If these factors are present, the patient is more likely to lose position from the primary reduction and develop a malunion.
- Age, patient independence, fracture comminution, AO/OTA subgroup classification, and dorsal angulation at presentation are predictors of carpal malalignment (Mackenney et al. 2006).
- Primary reduction of displaced distal radius fractures is of minimal value in the very old and frail, dependent, or demented patient where almost 90 % develop a malunion (Beumer and McQueen 2003; Mackenney et al. 2006).

Table 16.1 Recommended criteria for displacement when assessing fractures of the distal radius in young, fit, and active patients

Radiographic measurement	Criteria
Lateral view	
Carpal alignment	No malalignment allowed
Gap or step in joint	2 mm
Palmar tilt	Neutral if carpus malaligned
Dorsal tilt	Neutral if carpus malaligned (<10° if carpus aligned)
PA view	
Positive ulnar variance	2–3 mm
Gap or step in joint	2 mm

Adapted from Ng and McQueen (2011)

Table 16.2 Risk factors for early instability, late instability, and malunion for minimally displaced and displaced fractures of the distal radius

Fracture type	Predictors of early instability	Predictors of late instability	Predictors of malunion
Undisplaced/minimally displaced fracture (dorsal angulation ≤10°, ulnar variance <3 mm)	Age, comminution, dorsal angle (presentation), ulnar variance (presentation)	Age, comminution, dorsal angle (1 week), ulnar variance (1 week)	Age, comminution, dorsal angle (presentation), ulnar variance (presentation), radial shift (presentation), independence, AO/OTA classification, Frykman classification
Displaced fracture	Age, comminution, ulnar variance (presentation)	Age, dorsal angle (1 week), ulnar variance (1 week)	Age, comminution, ulnar variance (presentation), independence

- A Cochrane analysis of various anesthetic techniques for the primary reduction of a displaced distal radius fracture found that a hematoma block resulted in poorer analgesia and a compromised reduction when compared with intravenous regional anesthesia (Handoll et al. 2002).

16.5 Re-reduction: Current Evidence

- When considering the various treatment options for a fracture of the distal radius including the role of re-reduction, the primary aim is to regain adequate wrist/hand strength, mobility, and function for the patient.
  - It is essential to have a clear understanding of the functional demands of the patient, which are often associated with their age and physiological state, e.g., preexisting comorbidities.
  - However, an agreed gold standard on how to accurately define the demands of any patient is yet to be determined.
  - The use of objective measures such as the Physical Activity Scale of the Elderly (PASE) score may be the future (Washburn et al. 1993).
- Age, fracture characteristics, and the timing of re-manipulation are important factors in determining the efficacy of maintaining position post re-reduction and casting of a re-displaced fracture of the distal radius.
- Older patients (Figs. 16.1, 16.2, and 16.3) have been found to be significantly more likely to lose fracture position following re-reduction of a re-displaced fracture of the distal radius, with a superior outcome in patients under 60 years of age (McQueen et al. 1986).
- The rate of maintained reduction may be influenced by the timing of re-reduction with a better result if performed in the second week after primary reduction (Collert and Isacson 1978). However, fractures that present as "late slippers" in week 2 are likely to be more stable and therefore will maintain reduction.
- There is data to support that for re-displacement following primary reduction and casting, re-reduction and immobilization results in an inferior anatomical result when compared to surgical treatment options for unstable distal radius fracture (Noordeen et al. 1992; McQueen et al. 1996).
- There is one prospective randomized trial of external fixation versus continued conservative management for re-displaced Colles' fractures in patients over 55 years of age, which found no functional benefit to external fixation and no correlation between function and anatomical outcome as measured on radiographs (Roumen et al. 1991) (Box 16.1).

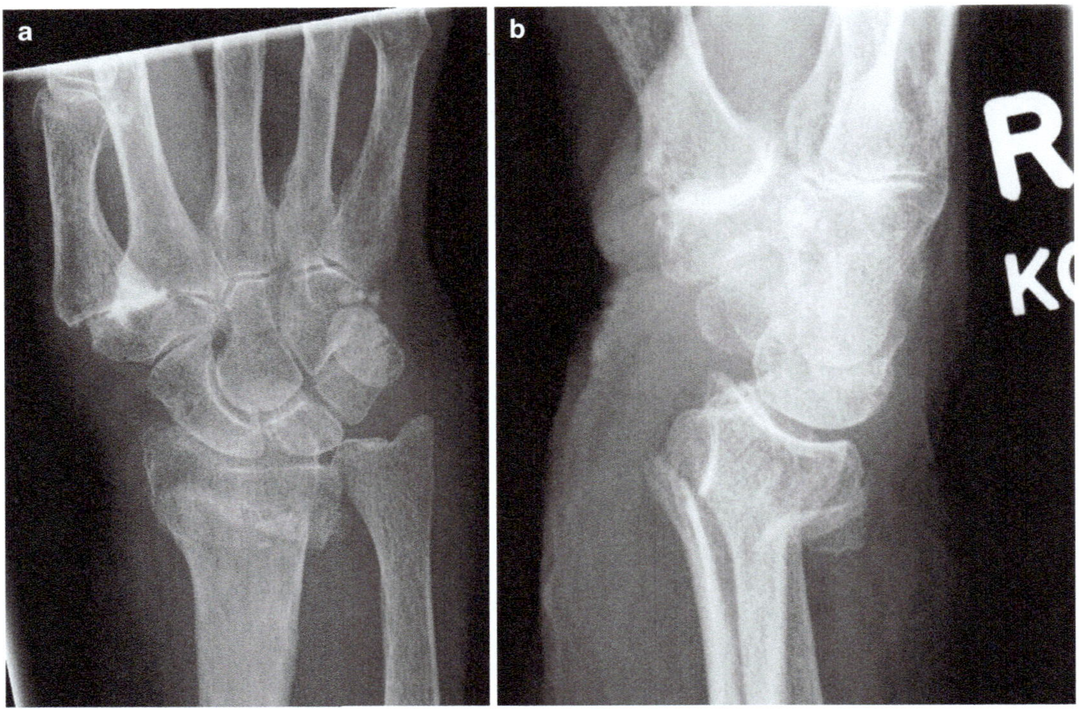

Fig. 16.1 AP (**a**) and lateral (**b**) radiographs of a dorsally displaced distal radius fracture in a 92-year-old woman

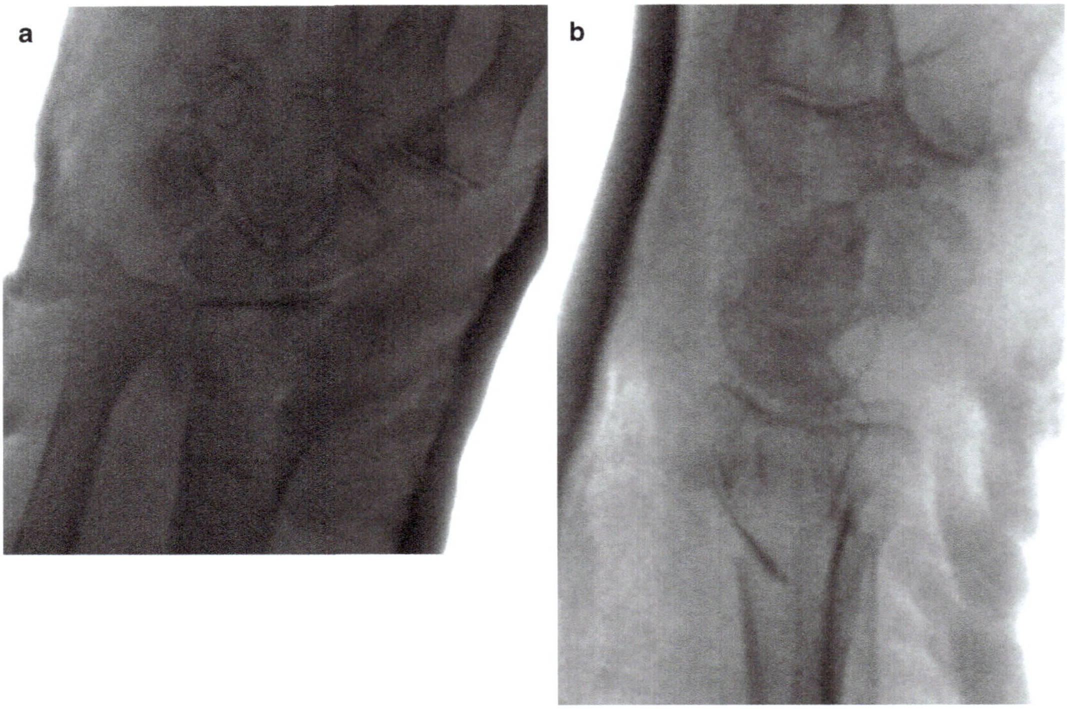

Fig. 16.2 AP (**a**) and lateral (**b**) image intensifier views demonstrating a satisfactory reduction performed 2 days following injury

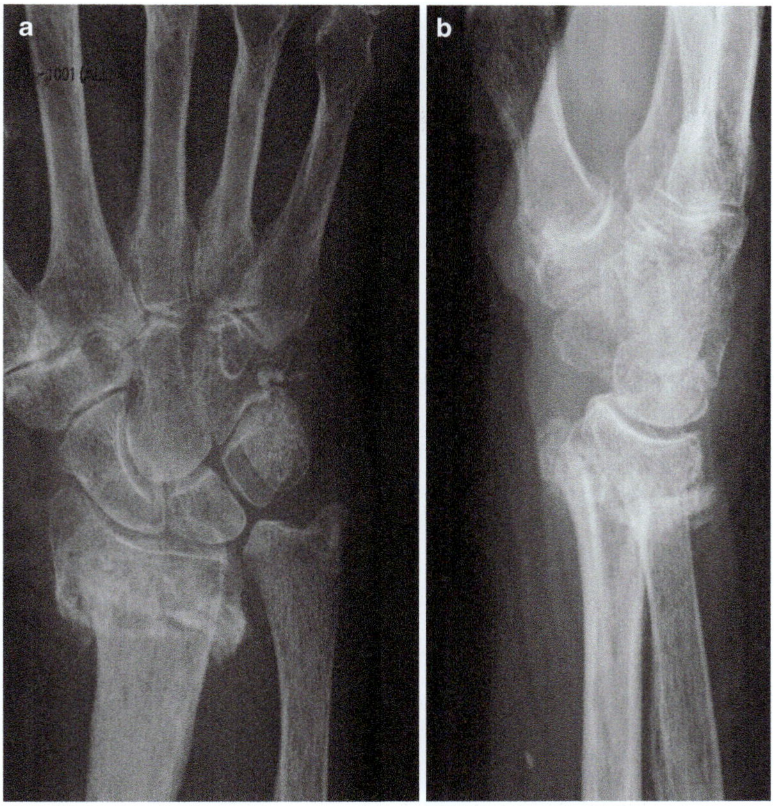

Fig. 16.3 AP (**a**) and lateral (**b**) radiographs demonstrating the fracture has lost position and malunited in the original position 7 weeks following injury

Box 16.1 Top Tips in Considering Re-reduction

- For elderly low demand patients, we would not recommend primary reduction or re-reduction and would simply treat the patient in a cast for 4–6 weeks until they progress to a malunion
  - The only exception to this is the patient with neurological compromise or an open fracture
- For the patient who has undergone an inadequate primary reduction, e.g., under a hematoma block:
  - Risk of instability >70 %: operative intervention without attempting closed re-reduction
  - Risk of instability <70 %: second closed re-reduction under a regional or general anesthesia
- For displaced fractures, we assess both the risk of instability and articular alignment
  - Gap or articular displacement >2 mm and/or risk of instability >70 %: operative reduction and fixation
  - Gap or articular displacement ≤2 mm and/or risk of instability ≤70 %: primary reduction under regional anesthesia

    Acceptable reduction: neutral position in a forearm back slab; review 1 and 2 weeks with repeat radiographs of the wrist and if there is any loss of position we recommend surgery; total time in cast 6 weeks

    Unacceptable reduction: fixation
- Undisplaced or minimally displaced distal fractures in younger patients
  - Undisplaced fractures are routinely managed with a below elbow cast for a period of 4 weeks
  - For minimally displaced fractures, we would review the patient at 1 and 2 weeks to check for evidence of instability. If there is no further displacement, we would treat in a below elbow cast for 6 weeks

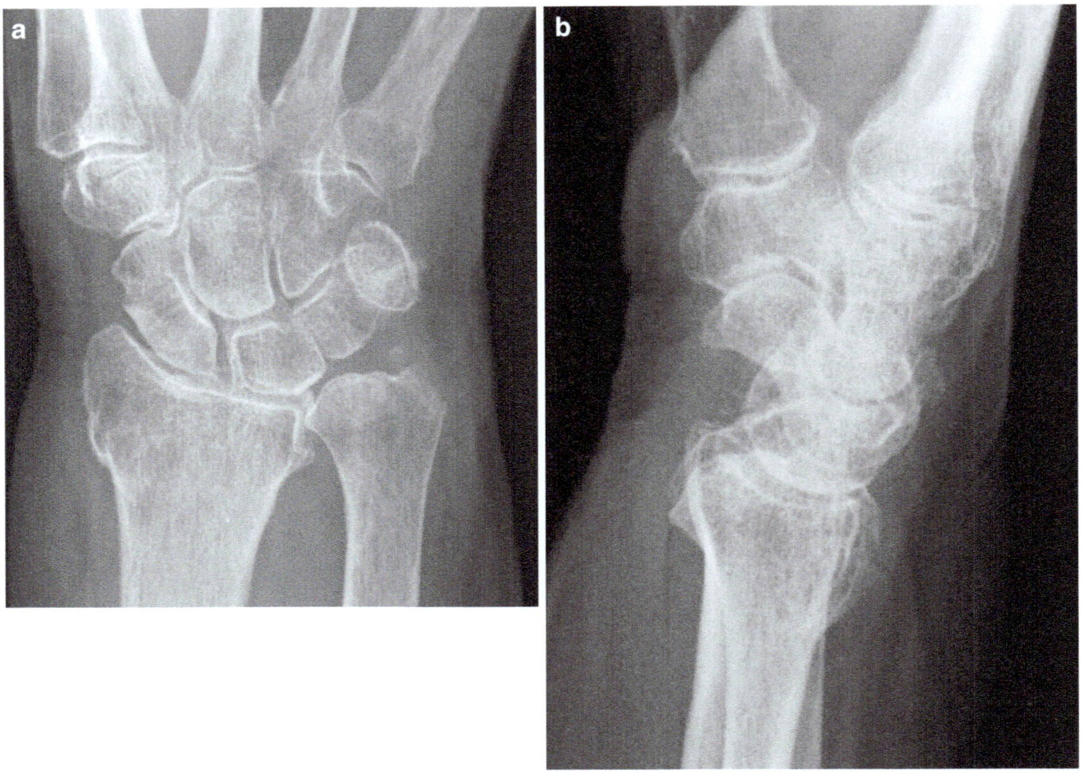

Fig. 16.4 AP (**a**) and lateral (**b**) radiographs of a malunited fracture in an 89-year-old woman 3 months following injury. The patient had no significant complaints and was managing her day-to-day activities

16.6 Re-displacement and Malunion: Does It Matter?

- The consequences of a distal radius fracture malunion, i.e., doing nothing following loss of position, are inherently related to the functional demands of the patient. Therefore, the patient must be involved in your decision-making process, not only when re-reduction is considered, but also when attempting a primary reduction.
  - The relative risk of a poorer outcome following a distal radial malunion decreases with increasing age (Fig. 16.4) (Grewal and MacDermid 2007).
- There is increasing evidence that older lower demand patients with displaced distal radius fracture gain a satisfactory outcome with nonoperative management and subsequent malunion.
  - Several studies have demonstrated that in elderly patients (>60 years of age) with a fracture of the distal radius conservative management is associated with a poorer radiographic outcome. However, functional outcomes are similar when compared to other surgical treatment options (volar plate, non-bridging EF, bridging EF, percutaneous K wire fixation) (Diaz-Garcia et al. 2011).
  - Radiographic results and grip strength may be superior in operatively treated patients compared to conservative management, but without any difference in function or pain (Egol et al. 2010).

16.7 Current Recommendations

- Two clinical scenarios are likely when considering re-reduction.
- The most common is a displaced fracture of the distal radius that is manipulated into a satisfactory position following a primary

closed reduction, which is then found to lose position on follow-up radiographs performed within the first 2 weeks following injury.
  - Patients at high risk of instability and malunion at presentation and/or following primary reduction should be identified using the risk factors defined above (www.wristcalc.org).
  - For younger higher functional demand patients, operative fixation is superior to a closed re-reduction.
  - For older lower functional demand patients, re-reduction (and even a primary reduction) is not required as a malunion will provide a satisfactory outcome in this patient group.
- The less frequent second scenario is the patient who undergoes an inadequate primary reduction, likely secondary to inadequate anesthesia.
  - Patients at high risk of instability and malunion should be considered for operative intervention without attempting closed re-reduction.
  - Patients at low risk of instability and malunion can be considered for a second closed re-reduction under improved anesthesia.
- Any patient with a persistent neurovascular deficit following attempted primary reduction warrants surgical exploration and fracture fixation.

Box 16.2 Pearls and Pitfalls
- Fractures of the distal radius are increasing in elderly women
- It is essential to consider the functional demands of the patient when determining the optimal treatment for displaced distal radius fractures
- The only possible indication for attempted re-reduction is the patient, who has undergone an inadequate primary reduction due to poor anesthesia for a fracture that has no articular malalignment and a low risk of instability
- For older patients with a lower functional demand in whom a malunion will likely provide a satisfactory functional outcome, primary reduction and re-reduction are not routinely indicated
- Young, fit, and active patients with a low risk of instability and good articular alignment can be treated with primary reduction and close regular follow-ups
- Young, fit, and active patients with a high risk of instability and/or articular malalignment warrant early surgical intervention

16.8 Technique for Re-reduction

- Adequate anesthesia should be used, e.g., regional or general anesthesia, which permits surgery to be used if a closed re-reduction is not achieved.
- The reduction method is similar to that for primary reduction:
  - Longitudinal traction to the forearm/wrist with another person providing counter traction just proximal to the elbow.
  - Direct pressure applied to the distal radial fragment from dorsal to volar can aid reduction.
  - Flexion of the wrist can aid in restoring volar tilt, but avoid extreme positions that can lead to nerve injury or stiffness.
  - Agee's maneuver (Agee 1993).
    Palmar translation of the hand in relation to the forearm, i.e., translation of the lunate on to the distal radius
- Casting
  - Randomized trials have demonstrated no advantage to either above or below elbow casting for maintaining fracture reduction, with some problems associated with rotational contracture following the use of above elbow casts (Stewart et al. 1984).
  - Position: slight flexion and ulnar deviation with free finger movement (distal extent of cast is proximal to the MCPJs).
  - Length of time: there is no definitive evidence; however, the generally accepted length of time in a cast is 5–6 weeks (Box 16.2).

References

Agee JM. Distal radius fractures. Multiplanar ligamentotaxis. Hand Clin. 1993;9(4):577–85.

Beumer A, McQueen MM. Fractures of the distal radius in low-demand elderly patients: closed reduction of no value in 53 of 60 wrists. Acta Orthop Scand. 2003;74(1):98–100.

Collert S, Isacson J. Management of redislocated Colles' fractures. Clin Orthop Relat Res. 1978;135:183–6.

Diaz-Garcia RJ, Oda T, Shauver MJ, Chung KC. A systematic review of outcomes and complications of treating unstable distal radius fractures in the elderly. J Hand Surg Am. 2011;36(5):824–35.

Egol KA, Walsh M, Romo-Cardoso S, Dorsky S, Paksima N. Distal radial fractures in the elderly: operative compared with nonoperative treatment. J Bone Joint Surg Am. 2010;92(9):1851–7.

Grewal R, MacDermid JC. The risk of adverse outcomes in extra-articular distal radius fractures is increased with malalignment in patients of all ages but mitigated in older patients. J Hand Surg Am. 2007;32(7): 962–70.

Handoll HH, Madhok R, Dodds C. Anaesthesia for treating distal radial fracture in adults. Cochrane Database Syst Rev. 2002;(3):CD003320.

Hove LM, Solheim E, Skjeie R, Sorensen FK. Prediction of secondary displacement in Colles' fracture. J Hand Surg Br. 1994;19(6):731–6.

Mackenney PJ, McQueen MM, Elton R. Prediction of instability in distal radial fractures. J Bone Joint Surg Am. 2006;88(9):1944–51.

McQueen MM, MacLaren A, Chalmers J. The value of remanipulating Colles' fractures. J Bone Joint Surg Br. 1986;68(2):232–3.

McQueen MM, Hajducka C, Court-Brown CM. Redisplaced unstable fractures of the distal radius: a prospective randomised comparison of four methods of treatment. J Bone Joint Surg Br. 1996;78(3): 404–9.

Ng CY, McQueen MM. What are the radiological predictors of functional outcome following fractures of the distal radius? J Bone Joint Surg Br. 2011;93(2): 145–50.

Noordeen MH, Lavy CB, Woodwards RT. Remanipulation or external fixation after slipped Colles' fractures? An anatomical study. Injury. 1992;23(5):303–4.

Roumen RM, Hesp WL, Bruggink ED. Unstable Colles' fractures in elderly patients. A randomised trial of external fixation for redisplacement. J Bone Joint Surg Br. 1991;73(2):307–11.

Stewart HD, Innes AR, Burke FD. Functional cast-bracing for Colles' fractures. A comparison between cast-bracing and conventional plaster casts. J Bone Joint Surg Br. 1984;66(5):749–53.

Washburn RA, Smith KW, Jette AM, Janney CA. The Physical Activity Scale for the Elderly (PASE): development and evaluation. J Clin Epidemiol. 1993;46(2): 153–62.

Closed Reduction and External Fixation of Unstable Distal Radius Fractures

17

John H. Williksen

Contents

J.H. Williksen, MD
Section for Hand and Microsurgery,
Department of Orthopaedic Surgery,
Oslo University Hospital, Oslo, Norway
e-mail: john.williksen@hotmail.no

17.1 Summary

Until some years ago external fixation was a more popular method for operative treatment of unstable fractures of the distal radius fractures, but now volar locking plates are the most commonly used operative treatment in many hospitals. There is still, however, a place for external fixation in unstable distal radius fractures, in multi-trauma management, and in severe comminuted fractures. It is therefore necessary to have this method in the surgical toolbox. It is important to use adjuvant pin fixation in order to secure the volar tilt, and it is also important to avoid overdistraction of the radiocarpal joint. The main complication of external fixation is pin site infection which is treated with pin care and antibiotics.

17.2 Introduction

External fixation with or without adjuvant pin fixation has been used for many years in the treatment of unstable distal radius fractures and is a reliable and relatively easy way of treating these fractures. In the last decade, there has been a large increase in the use of volar locking plates and not so many surgeons now use external fixation on a regular basis (Downing and Karantana 2008), but it is still important to have this method in the surgical tool box.

L.M. Hove et al. (eds.), *Distal Radius Fractures*,
DOI 10.1007/978-3-642-54604-4_17, © Springer-Verlag Berlin Heidelberg 2014

17.3 The Principles of External Fixation

17.3.1 Ligamentotaxis

External fixation relies on closed reduction and ligamentotaxis. According to Agee (1993) ligamentotaxis is "the principle of molding fracture fragments into alignment as a result of tension applied across a fracture by the surrounding intact soft tissues."

17.3.2 Suction Effect

Trans-articular wrist distraction causes a decrease in intra-articular pressure, and this might have a suction effect on small intra-articular fragments (Schuind et al. 1997).

17.3.3 Indications

- Unstable fractures of the distal radius
- Acute multi-trauma situations in order to stabilize the extremity as a temporary measure both in carpal dislocations and distal radius fractures
- Damage control surgery
- Severe comminuted fractures or bone loss when it is impossible to reconstruct the articular surface, but important to reestablish the radial length
- Open fractures with soft tissue injuries and contamination
- To stabilize the wrist after infections
- In unstable fractures of the distal radius where volar plating is not an option, or pin or plate fixation will be too weak and need additional fixation

17.3.4 Contraindications

- Patients that do not want an external fixator
- Noncompliant patients (and patient selection is therefore important)
- Barton's fractures (AO type B fractures) (these fractures need pin or screw fixation (B1), or dorsal or volar plating (B2/B3)

17.4 Problems of External Fixation in Unstable Fractures

17.4.1 Intra-articular Fragments

It is difficult to reduce impacted intra-articular fracture fragments. Therefore, these fragments have to be reduced by closed means with the "joystick technique" or open reduction and internal fixation.

17.4.2 Displacement

- *Radial length* and *radial inclination* are usually relatively easy restored.
- To retain the *volar tilt* is important.
- To augment the fixation, it is therefore recommended to use adjuvant pin fixation (Seitz et al. 1991; Braun and Gellman 1994; Wolfe et al. 1998).
- The problem with the volar tilt in external fixation might be due to the fact that the dorsal ligaments are weaker than the volar ligaments.
- A cadaveric study showed that only after transecting the volar ligaments it was possible to restore the volar tilt (Bartosh and Saldana 1990).
- This might explain that the volar ligaments pull out to the maximal length before the weaker dorsal ligaments are able to exert any traction.

17.4.3 Distraction

- Overdistraction across the wrist joint in bridging external fixation might lead to reduced motion of the fingers.
- Increasing distraction increased the load required for the finger flexors to generate flexion at the MCP joint.

- In the middle, ring, and little finger, more than 5 mm significantly increased the load.
- For the index finger only 2 mm of distraction significantly increased the load for flexion of the MCP joint (Papadonikolaikis et al. 2005).
- When the flexion of the fingers is reduced, this might lead to increased pain and edema, the precursors of complex regional pain syndrome (CRPS), and finger stiffness.

17.5 Surgical Technique

17.5.1 Bridging External Fixation (Figs. 17.1 and 17.3a–g)

- General anesthesia or a brachial nerve block.
- Manual traction and reduction under fluoroscopic control to align the fracture fragments into position.
- 4-cm incision 7–10 cm proximal to the fracture site and on the dorsoradial side of the radius.
- Protect the superficial branch of the radial nerve that emerges between the brachioradialis (BR) and the extensor carpi radialis longus (ECRL) (Fig. 17.2).
- Two half-pins are screwed into the bone between ECRL and ECRB with the aid of the pin clamp in a dorsoradial position in order to ensure bicortical purchase.
- The type of pins is important. Thicker pins are stronger, but occupy more space in the bone and might lead to secondary pinhole fractures. Cylindrical pins (Schanz screws) are preferred to tapered pins because the latter ones cannot be backed out.
- Two half-pins into the second metacarp. Either both in the diaphysis or one in the proximal metaphysis and the other one in the diaphysis.
- The screws should be in the center of the bone since an eccentric position might lead to a fracture, especially in fragile patients.
- When the pins are in position, always prestress them before fixation to the external fixator.
- Apply the fixation devices and then do the final reduction under fluoroscopic control by distraction and molding.
- Temporary overdistraction may be used intraoperatively, but final distraction should be checked with fluoroscopy and should not exceed 2 mm in the radiocarpal joint.
- Always passively flex the patient's fingers at the end of the operation. If you without tension can fold the patient's fingers into the

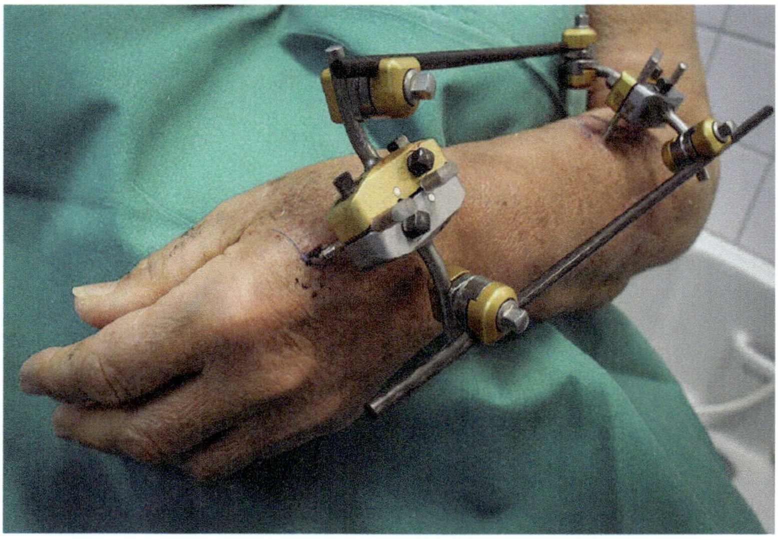

Fig. 17.1 External fixation (Hoffmann® II) with two connecting rods. Photo: Børge Olsen

palm at the level of the proximal crease, the tension and distraction is acceptable.

- The fixator clamps should be 2 cm away from the skin in order to allow for postoperative swelling and pin care.
- 2 connecting rods are stronger than 1 especially in large patients.
- 2 or 3 adjuvant pins across the fracture site 1.6–1.8 mm in order to secure the volar tilt.
- When transfixing the radial styloid, care must be taken not to injure the sensory branches of the radial nerve.
- The incisions are closed without tension and proper dressing applied.

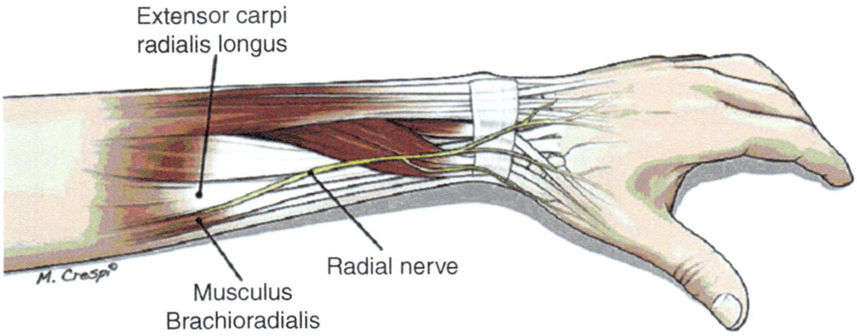

Fig. 17.2 The sensory branch of the radial nerve

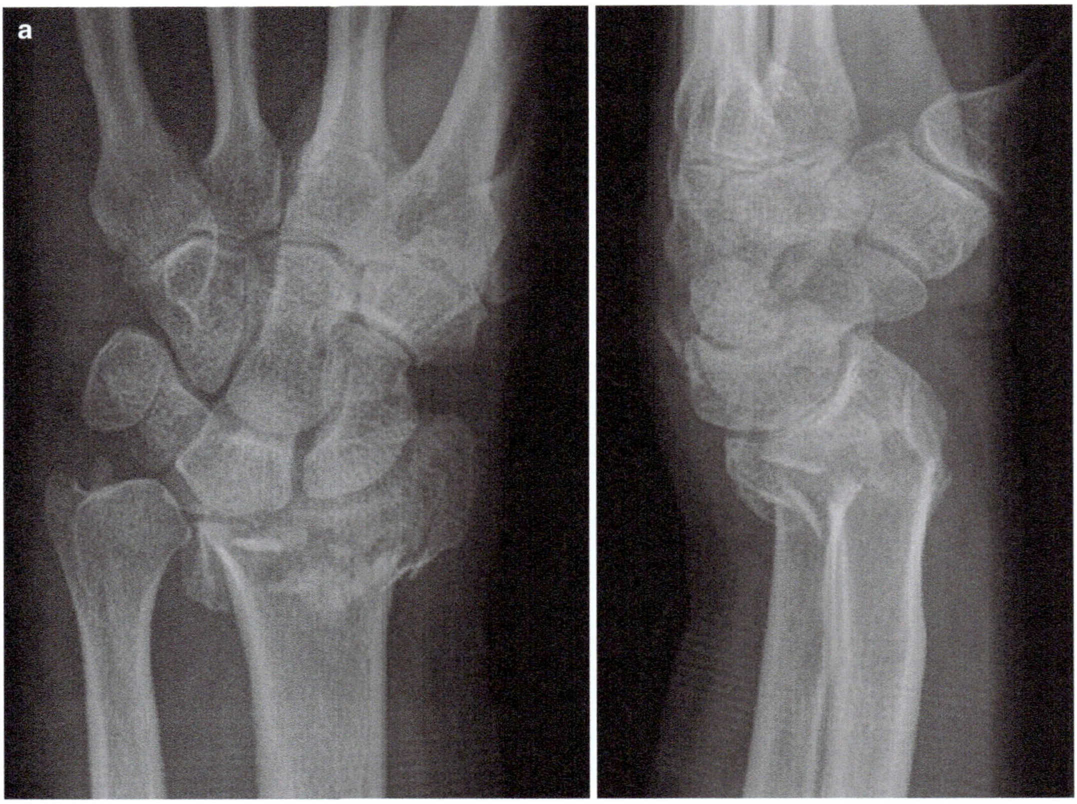

Fig. 17.3 (**a**) AO type C fracture left wrist in a 50 years old man, (**b**) External fixation (Dynawrist®) and adjuvant pin fixation. The fixator was left in place for 8 weeks and there were no dynamization or hand therapy. (**c**) Radiological results after 5 years. (**d**) Flexion after 12 years. (**e**) Extension after 12 years. (**f**) Supination after 12 years. (**g**) Pronation after 12 years. Photo: (**d–g**) Børge Olsen

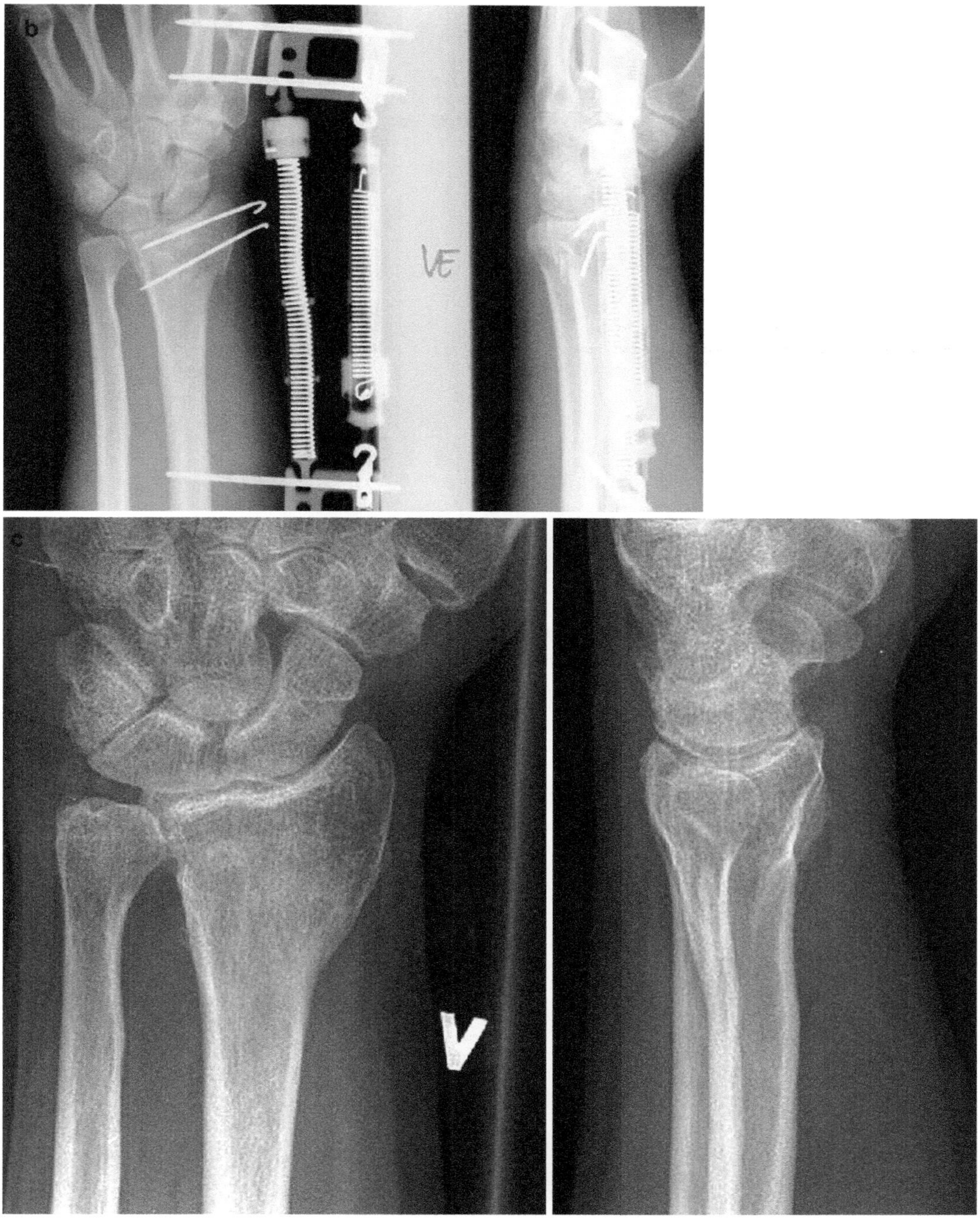

Fig. 17.3 (continued)

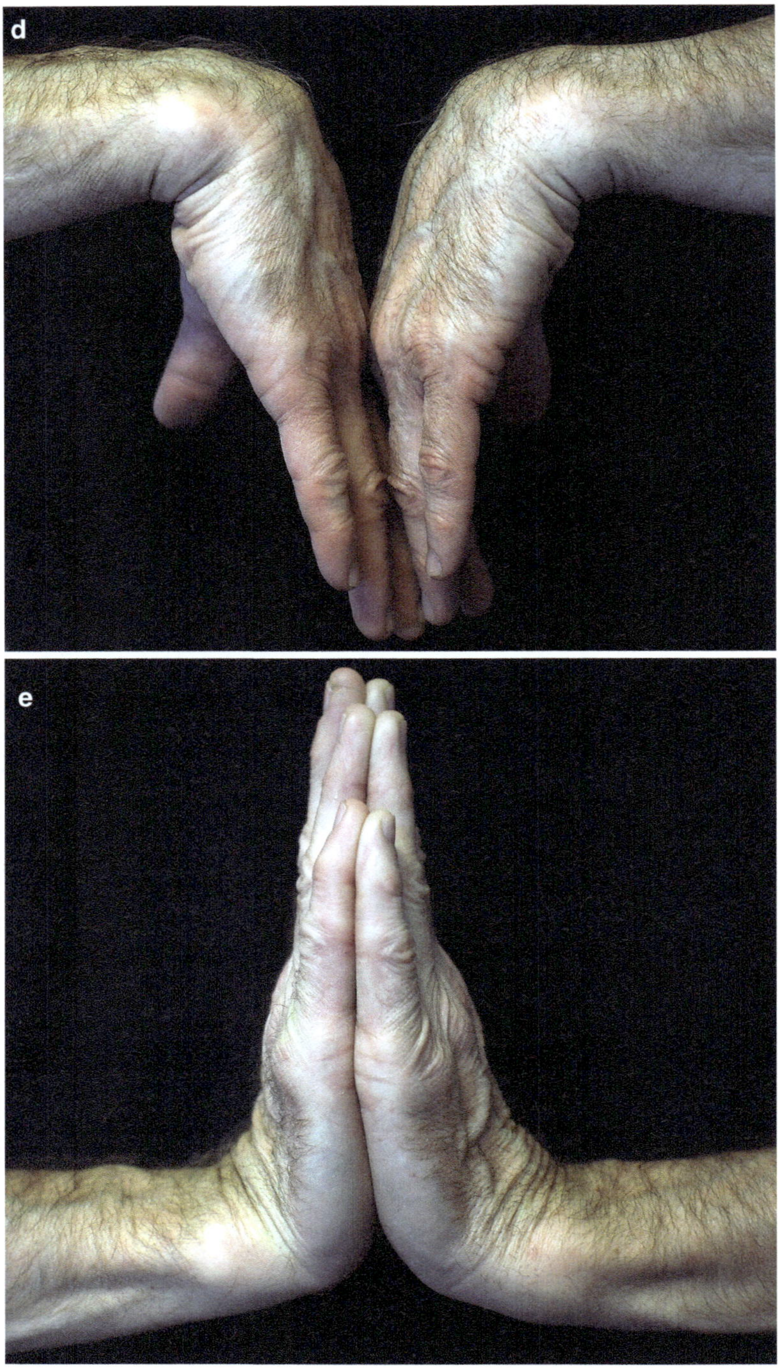

Fig. 17.3 (continued)

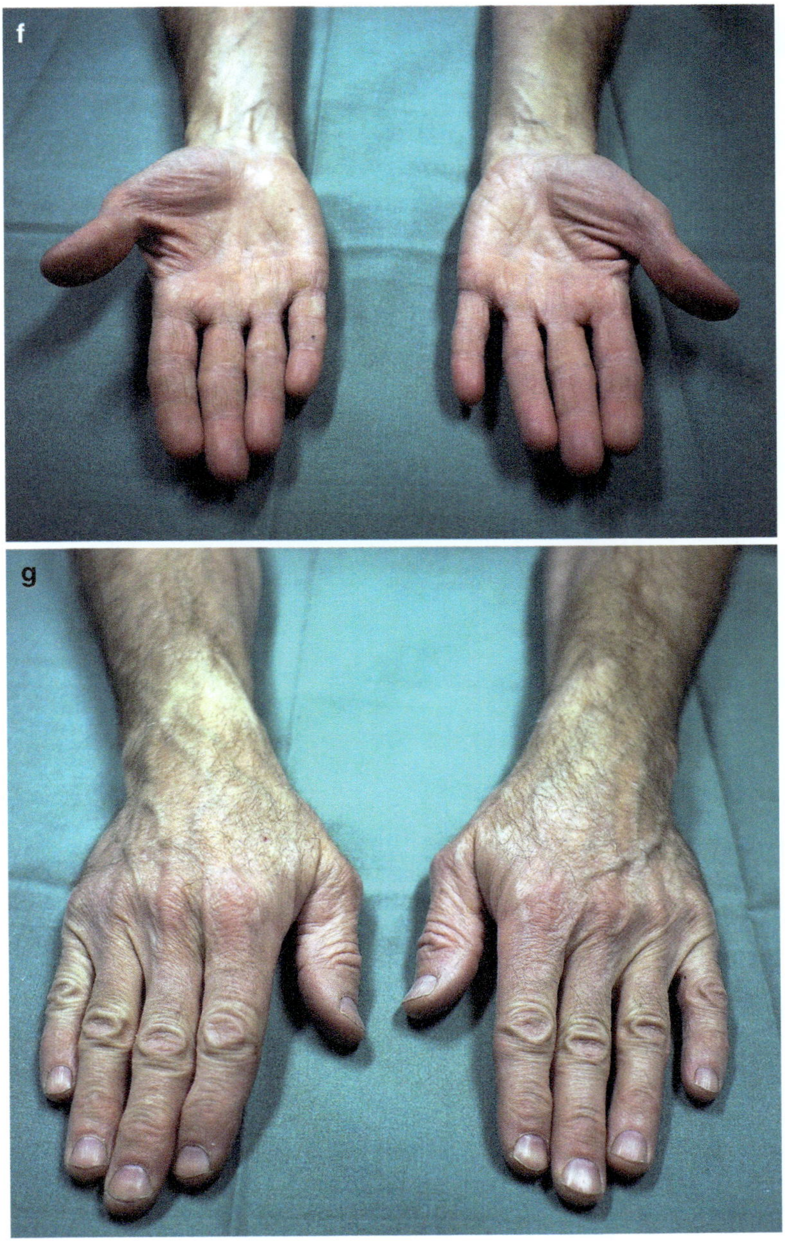

Fig. 17.3 (continued)

Complications	External fixation n = 59	Volar plates n = 52	Plate removals
CTS*	3(5%)	3(6%)	1
CRPS**	4(7%)	2(4%)	1
Fixation failure	1(2%)	0	
Incomplete reduction	2(3%)	1(2%)	
Pininfection	6(10%)	0	
Prominent plate	0	2(4%)	2
Too long screws	0	3(6%)	2
Intraarticular screw position	0	1(2%)	1
Scarproblems	2(3%)	0	
Synovitis	0	3(6%)	1
Total	18(30%)	15(29%)	8(15%)

*Carpal tunnel syndrome. **Complex regional pain syndrome.

Fig. 17.4 Complications after external fixation and volar locking plates in unstable distal radius fractures (Williksen et al. 2013)

17.5.2 Non-bridging External Fixator

Unstable extra-articular/simple intra-articular distal radius fractures:

- Proximal pin placement 7–10 cm from the fracture site.
- Two pins are placed in the distal fragment.
- The pins are placed sagittally and parallel to the joint surface engaging the volar surface.
- Good bone stock is necessary in the distal fragment, and 1 cm of intact volar cortex is required for pin purchase (McQueen 2005).

17.5.3 Dynamic or Static External Fixator

- Dynamic external fixator may facilitate wrist movement and a faster recovery (Hove et al. 2010).
- Fear of fracture collapse, especially in severe comminuted fractures.
- Long-term clinical benefits from a dynamic external fixator still lack scientific evidence (Modi et al. 2010).

17.6 Postoperative Care

- Check and tighten the fixator bolts at the follow-ups if necessary.
- Patients are instructed to start active and passive finger motion in order to reduce edema and prevent pain. If they cannot do it themselves, referral for formal hand therapy should be done.
- Fixator removal at 6–8 weeks in local anesthesia.
- No need for particular pin care if the incisions are closed without tension.

17.7 Complications (Fig. 17.4)

- Distal radius fractures lead to complications whatever the fracture treatment.
- Pin infections are the most common complication in external fixation and are best treated with pin care and antibiotics. Osteomyelitis is rare.
- Radial sensory neuropathy is avoided by a precise pin placement during an open procedure.
- Complex regional pain syndrome has previously been associated with external fixation, but current literature does not support this (Margaliot et al. 2005).
- Carpal tunnel syndrome is most commonly a result of the fracture itself, but external fixation in a flexed position might create a median nerve compression. A neutral position of the wrist is therefore recommended.

Pearls and Pitfalls

- Avoid injuring the radial nerve by placing a 4-cm long incision in the forearm to visualize the superficial branch of the radial nerve.
- Be careful when placing the distal screws and avoid eccentric position. The bone might be thin and this might lead to a fracture in the metacarpal bone.
- Overdistraction of the radiocarpal joint might lead to pain syndromes and reduced finger movements. Always check that it is possible to fold the patient's fingertips into the palm.
- The wrist should be placed in a neutral position. Extreme ulnar or flexed position may lead to pain syndromes, finger stiffness, and nerve entrapment (i.e., carpal tunnel syndrome).
- Securing the volar tilt with 2–3 adjuvant pins augments the strength of the fixation.
- It is more difficult to do a closed reduction of the fracture after 7–10 days.

References

Agee JM. Distal radius fractures. Multiplanar ligamentotaxis. Hand Clin. 1993;9(4):577–85.

Bartosh RA, Saldana MJ. Intraarticular fractures of the distal radius: a cadaveric study to determine if ligamentotaxis restores palmar tilt. J Hand Surg Am. 1990;15(1):18–21.

Braun RM, Gellman H. Dorsal pin placement and external fixation for correction of dorsal tilt in fractures of distal radius. J Hand Surg Am. 1994;19(4):653–5.

Downing ND, Karantana A. A revolution in the management of fractures of the distal radius? J Bone Joint Surg Br. 2008;90(10):1271–5.

Hove LM, Krukhaug Y, Revheim K, Helland P, Finsen V. Dynamic compared with static external fixation of unstable fractures of the distal part of the radius: a prospective, randomized, multicenter study. J Bone Joint Surg Am. 2010;92(8):1687–96.

Margaliot Z, Haase SC, Kotsis SV, Kim HM, Chung KC. A meta-analysis of outcomes of external fixation versus plate osteosynthesis for unstable distal radius fractures. J Hand Surg Am. 2005;30(6):1185–99.

McQueen MM. Non-spanning external fixation of the distal radius. Hand Clin. 2005;21:375–80.

Modi CS, Ho K, Smith CD, Boer R, Turner SM. Dynamic and static external fixation for distal radius fractures- a systematic review. Injury. 2010;41(10):1006–11.

Papadonikolaikis A, Shen J, Garret JP, Davis S, Ruch DS. The effect of increasing distraction on digital motion after external fixation of the wrist. J Hand Surg Am. 2005;30(4):773–9.

Schuind FA, Cantraine FRL, Fabeck L, Burny F. Radiocarpal articular pressures during the reduction of distal radius fractures. J Orthop Trauma. 1997;11(4):295–9.

Seitz WH, Froimson AI, Leb R, Shapiro JD. Augmented external fixation of unstable distal radius fractures. J Hand Surg Am. 1991;16(6):1010–6.

Williksen JH, Frihagen F, Hellund HD, Husby T. Volar locking plates versus external fixation and adjuvant pin fixation in unstable distal radius fractures: a randomized, controlled study. J Hand Surg Am. 2013; 38(8):1469–76.

Wolfe SW, Swigart CR, Grauer J, Slade 3rd JF, Panjabi MM. Augmented external fixation of distal radius fractures: a biomechanical analysis. J Hand Surg Am. 1998;23(1):127–34.

Closed Reduction and Percutaneous Pinning

18

Torstein Husby

Contents

T. Husby, MD, PhD
Section for Hand and Microsurgery,
Department of Orthopedic Surgery,
Oslo University Hospital, Oslo, Norway
e-mail: thusby@ous-hf.no

18.1 Summary

Percutaneous pinning supplemented with a cast is a cheap, simple, quick and still a popular treatment option for unstable distal radius fractures under given circumstances. Using the AO classification system, unstable both A-, C-1 and C-2 fractures may be suitable for percutaneous pinning. The prerequisites are acceptable reducibility under fluoroscopic view and good purchase in the bone stock. The method has versatility and is suitable for all age groups regardless of gender, but is mostly used for fractures with limited instability and comminution. The most common and recommended method used includes two pins (1.5–1.8 mm) introduced in a crossed fashion respectively through the volar and dorsal radial styloid tip and one pin from the dorsal/ulnar border of the radius. Despite the fact that there is some radial subsidence postoperatively after pinning, this method yields acceptable radiological and satisfactory long-term clinical results, especially in the elderly. Complications after pinning are few, mainly transitory pin infections.

18.2 Introduction

Using the AO classification system, unstable both A-, C-1 and C-2 fractures may be suitable for percutaneous pinning supplemented with a cast:

L.M. Hove et al. (eds.), *Distal Radius Fractures*,
DOI 10.1007/978-3-642-54604-4_18, © Springer-Verlag Berlin Heidelberg 2014

- The fractures must be reducible under traction and fluoroscopic view, and the patient must have a good purchase in the bone stock.
- *Crossed pinning* is the biomechanical most favourable pinning construct for distal radius fixations (Naidu et al. 1997). A standardised method using at least three 1.5–1.8 mm pins in a crossed fashion might prevent the fractures from significant secondary redislocations.
- Many papers confirm the findings that the dorsal angulations and radial inclinations are maintained in acceptable reduction indicating that this is a fairly stable construct, despite the fact that there is some subsidence of the radius (Glickel et al. 2008; Kennedy et al. 2010; Husby et al. 2008).
- A mean radial shortening of 1.3 mm between fracture reduction and union for fractures treated with extra-focal pinning may be expected (Barton et al. 2005).
- A prerequisite for the pinning method should be a postoperative radial shortening close to zero to allow for some loss of height.

18.3 Method

The pinning procedure is performed in the operation theatre, usually under brachial block anaesthesia. A bloodless field is not necessary. An image intensifier is mandatory. The hand and underarm is prepped sterile, and under traditional stretching and manipulation, the fracture is reduced to an acceptable position.

- An assistant in addition to the operator is obligate. Finger traps may be used if preferred, but is not mandatory. While the assistant (or the finger traps) maintain the reduction, pinning is performed.
- A great variety of pinning techniques are used: intra-focal pinning within the fracture site, trans-ulnar oblique pinning (without pinning of the DRUJ), one radial styloid pin and a second across the DRUJ, and multiple trans-ulnar to radius pins including the DRUJ (Fig. 18.1).
- Pins (1.5–1.8 mm) are preferred for a stronger osteosynthesis, and these should be introduced in a standardised fashion: we advocate two pins inserted from the volar and the dorsal prominences of the radial styloid, respectively, and one pin inserted from the dorsal/ulnar radial edge.
- It is mandatory that all the pins have a firm grip through the cortical bone proximal to the fracture line. Thus the fractures are fixed in a crossed pinned fashion (Fig. 18.2).
- When needed (intra-articular fractures) additional pin(s) parallel to the joint surface should be introduced (Fig. 18.3).
- Additional pins may be necessary when the instability is gross. When the control biplanar fluoroscopic images are acceptable, the pins are bent and cut 1 cm above the skin and protected with bandages or pin caps. All patients get a low arm plaster cast, and the cast and pins are removed 5–6 weeks postoperatively.

18.4 Tips

- In order to maintain the radial length, it is beneficial to achieve bony contact between the volar cortices of the distal radius. Even for experienced surgeons, this may be difficult.
- One possible trick is to introduce one or two percutaneous thick pin(s) from the dorsal side and under fluoroscopic viewing manipulate these into the volar fracture line. Using the pins as a lever arm, it might be possible to reduce the fracture while flexing the wrist (Fig. 18.4).

18.5 Outcome

American Academy of Orthopaedic Surgeons (2009) suggests operative fixation as opposed to cast fixation for fractures with:

- Post-reduction radial shortening >3 mm
- Dorsal tilt >10°

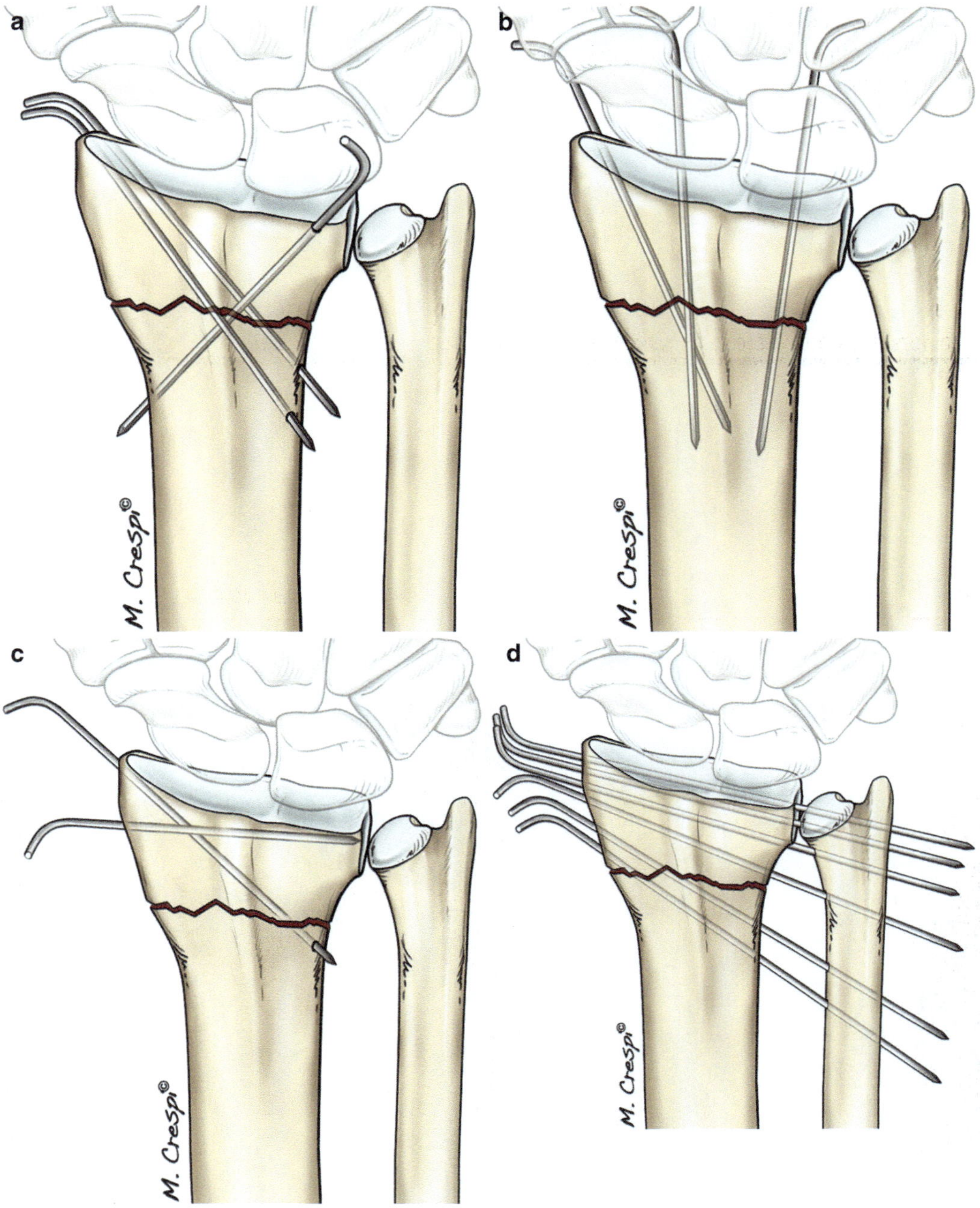

Fig. 18.1 Several different techniques of percutaneous pinning of instable distal radius fractures. (**a**) Two pins inserted from the volar and the dorsal prominences of the radial styloid, respectively, and one pin inserted from the dorsal/ulnar radial edge. (**b**) Crossing pins from the radial and ulnar sides of the distal fragment into the shaft of the radius in a more random fashion. (**c**) Two pins inserted from the radial styloid. (**d**) Multiple pins introduced through the radial styloid transfixing the fracture and the DRUJ

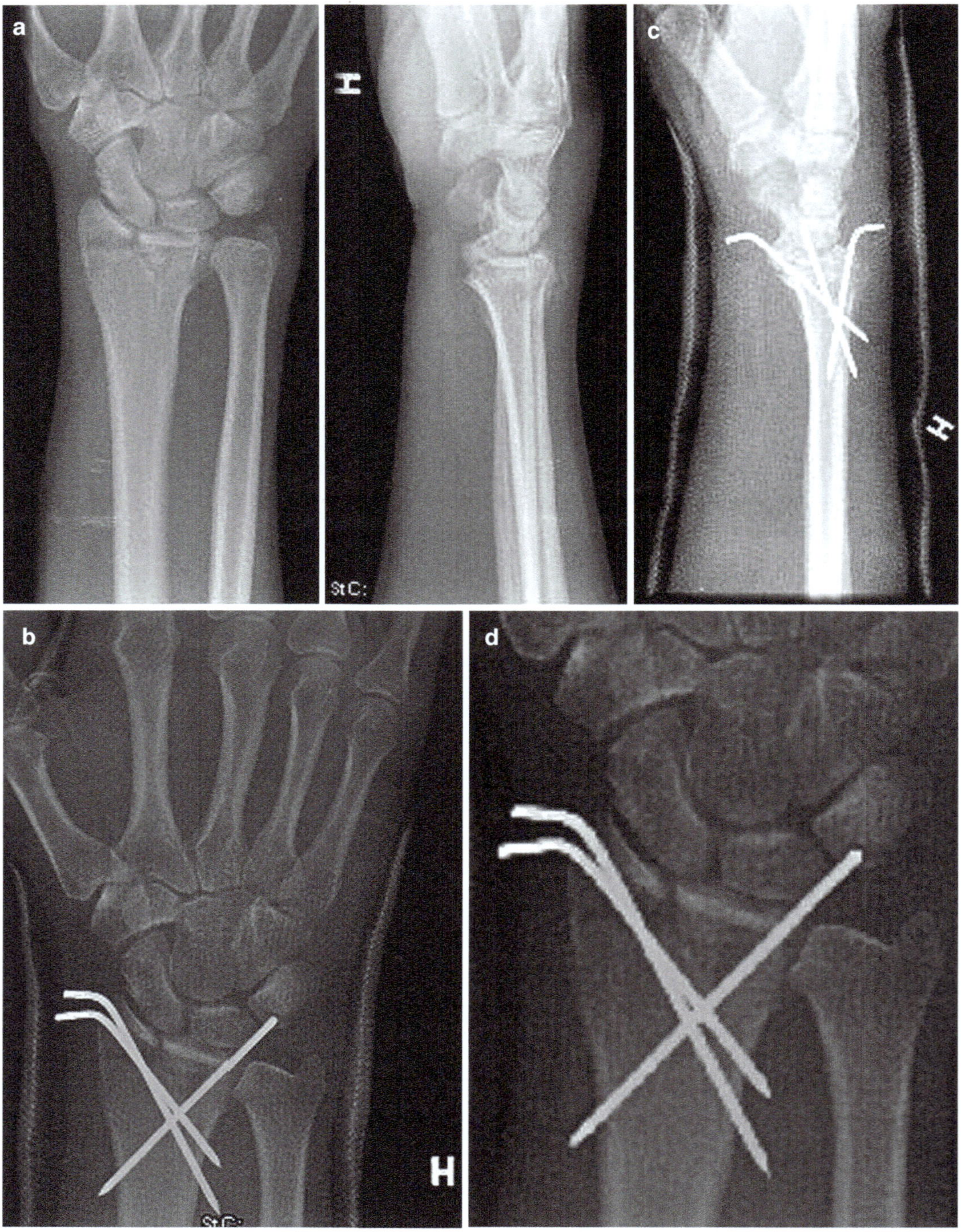

Fig. 18.2 Unstable distal radius fracture treated with standardised percutaneous pinning from the radial styloid and the dorsal/ulnar radial edge

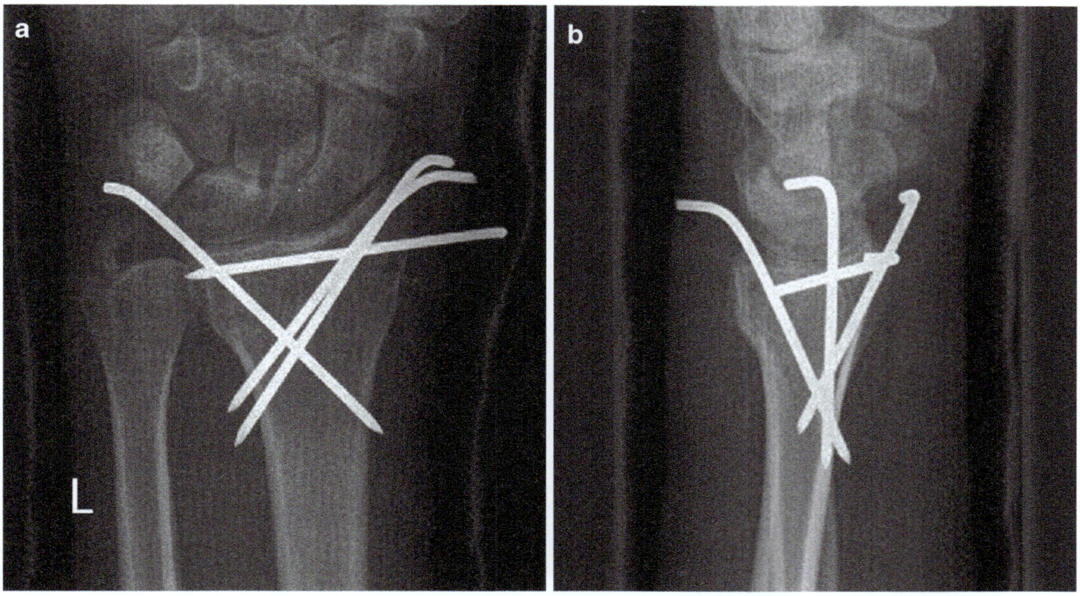

Fig. 18.3 Unstable intra-articular distal radius fracture treated with standardised pinning and one additional transfixing pin

- Intra-articular displacement (gap) >2 mm
- Intra-articular step-off >2 mm

According to these guidelines, the radiological findings at follow-ups from several studies are acceptable after the pinning procedure for distal radius fractures (Ludvigsen et al. 1997; Rozental and Blazar 2006; Rozental et al. 2009; Handoll et al. 2007; Husby et al. 2008).

- Shortening of >2 mm is related to worse functional outcome. A radial shortening ≤2 mm is probably tolerable and has negligible functional effects (Leung et al. 2008).

Other studies have as well documented that focal pinning yields improvement in anatomical reduction in unstable distal radius fractures (Ludvigsen et al. 1997; Harley et al. 2004; Rosati et al. 2006; Glickel et al. 2008).

The above studies also finds that the average ROM exceeds the *functional* ROM as described by Palmer et al. (1985), indicating well-functioning wrists after the pinning procedure.

- Interestingly the patient's subjective satisfaction rate after pinning is good and is obviously more important than the radiological results (Rosati et al. 2006; Glickel et al. 2008).
- Most of these materials are from a heterogenic elderly population with both intra- and extra-articular fractures. This might demonstrate the versatility of this simple method when comminution is not gross and the intra-articular steps are limited.
- Although there is a tendency that pinning and casting has a longer short-term rehabilitation (Rozental et al. 2009) compared to ORIF, there are reasons to believe that the long-term results are comparable to ORIF (Hauksson et al. 2008; Lozano-Calderon et al. 2008; Glickel et al. 2008).
- Most papers addressing the pinning method find that the grip strength of the injured side is insignificantly different from the uninjured

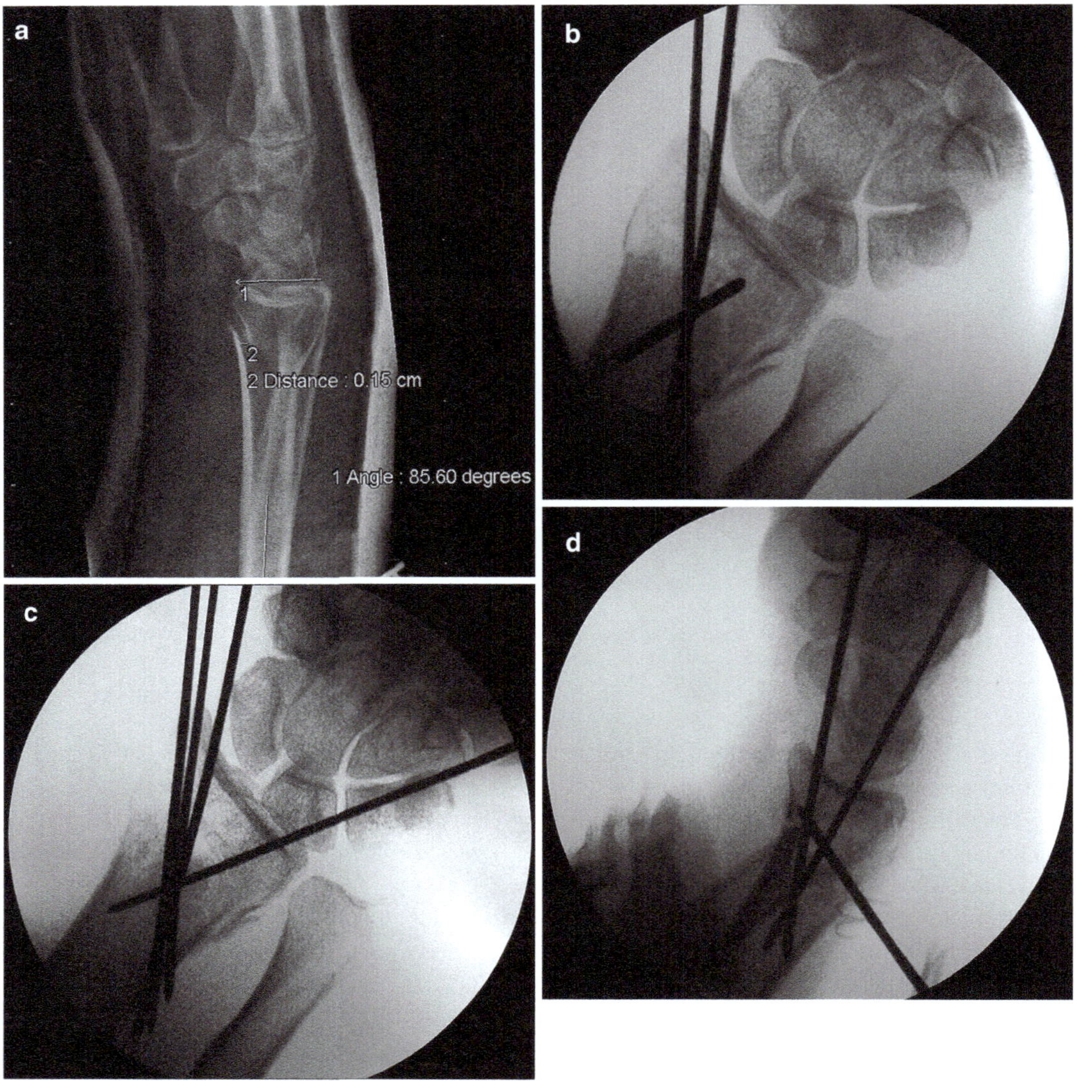

Fig. 18.4 (**a**) X-ray of elderly woman with a volar cortex difficult to reduce closed. (**b**) Introduction of a percutaneous dorsal pin as a lever arm for the volar cortex. (**c**) Transfixation of the fracture. (**d**) Postoperative control x-rays

side, indicating a re-establishing of the pre-injured wrist strength (Rosati et al. 2006; Hauksson et al. 2008).

- A rough economic calculation of distal radius fractures at our department shows that the total costs of external fixation or volar plating yields 10–15 times the total costs of percutaneous pinning and a low arm cast.

18.6 Complications

The most common complication is pin track infection (Ludvigsen et al. 1997; Rosati et al. 2006). These pin infections are superficial, transient complications that do not require secondary procedures. Other more unusual complications are CTS and CRPS (type I).

Conclusion

Despite the fact that there is some radial subsidence postoperatively after pinning of unstable distal radius A- and C-fractures, this method yields acceptable radiological and satisfactory long-term clinical results. This is especially true in the elderly population. Complications after pinning are few, mainly transitory pin infections. There are reasons to believe that closed reduction and percutaneous pinning still is a versatile and valuable tool among the treatment options of unstable distal radius fractures.

References

AAOS. The treatment of distal radius fractures. Guideline and evidence report; 2009.

Barton T, Chambers C, Lane E, Bannister G. Do Kirschner wires maintain reduction of displaced Colles fractures? Injury. 2005;36:1431–4.

Glickel SZ, Catalano LW, Raia FJ, Barron OA, Grabow R, Chia B. Long term outcomes of closed reduction and percutaneous pinning for the treatment of distal radius fractures. J Hand Surg Am. 2008;35A:1700–5.

Harley BJ, Scharfenberger A, Beaupre LA, Jomha N, Weber DW. Augmented external fixation versus percutaneous pinning and casting for unstable fractures of the distal radius – a prospective randomised trial. J Hand Surg. 2004;29A:815–24.

Handoll HHG, Vaghela MV, Madhok R. Percutaneous pinning for treating distal radius fractures in adults (Review). The Cochrane Library. 2007;(3):7–16.

Hauksson I, Husby T, Hellund J, Bjørnstad L, Maurstad L. Percutaneous pin fixation of unstable distal radius fractures. Clinical results. Proceedings Norwegian Orthopedic Society; 2008. p. 85–6.

Husby T, Hauksson I, Hellund J, Bjørnstad L, Maurstad L. Percutaneous pin fixation of unstable distal radius fractures. Radiological long term results. Proceedings Norwegian Orthopedic Society; 2008. p. 86–7.

Kennedy C, Kennedy MT, Niall D, Devitt A. Radiological outcomes of distal radius fractures treated with extra-focal kirschner wires. Injury. 2010;41:639–42.

Leung F, Tu Y, Winston Y, Chew C, Chow S-P. Comparison of external and percutaneous pin fixation with plate fixation for intra-articular distal radial fractures. A randomized study. J Bone Joint Surg Am. 2008; 90:16–22.

Lozano-Calderon SA, Souer S, Mudgal C, Jupiter JB, Ring D. Wrist mobilization following volar plate fixation of fractures of the distal part of the radius. J Bone Joint Surg Am. 2008;90:1297–304.

Ludvigsen T, Johansen S, Svenningsen S, Saetermo R. External versus percutaneous pinning for unstable colles fracture. Acta Orthop Scand. 1997;68:255–8.

Naidu SH, Capo JT, Moulton M, Ciccone W, Radin A. Percutaneous pinning of distal radius fractures: a biomechanical study. J Hand Surg. 1997;22A:252–7.

Palmer AK, Werner FW, Murphy D, Glisson R. Functional wrist motion: a biomechanical study. J Hand Surg. 1985;10A:39–46.

Rosati M, Bertagnini S, Digrandi G, Sala C. Percutaneous pinning for fractures of the distal radius. Acta Orthop Belg. 2006;72:138–46.

Rozental TD, Blazar PE. Functional outcome and complications after volar plating for dorsally displaced, unstable fractures of the distal radius. J Hand Surg. 2006;31A:359–65.

Rozental TD, Blazar PE, Orrin I, Franko BS, Aron T, Chacko BS, Earp BE, Day CS. Functional outcomes for unstable distal radius fractions treated with open reduction and internal fixation or closed reduction and percutaneous fixation. J Bone Joint Surg AM. 2009; 91:1837–46.

Closed Reduction and Intramedullary Fixation of Distal Radius Fractures

19

Torben B. Hansen

Contents

T.B. Hansen, MD, PhD
Department of Orthopaedics,
Regional Hospital Holstebro,
University of Aarhus, Aarhus, Denmark
e-mail: torben.baek.hansen@vest.rm.dk

19.1 Summary

Evolution of locking nails has led to the introduction of interlocking nails for fractures of the distal radius as a possible effective minimally invasive surgery for instable fractures. So far locked intramedullary nailing of instable extra-articular fractures AO type A has been proven as an elegant minimally invasive method with a low complication rate and a low need of hardware removal after fracture healing. However, the indications are quite narrow compared to locked volar plating, and the indications of intramedullary locked fixation of distal radius fractures should primarily be limited to dorsally displaced extra-articular fractures, and the procedure should be avoided if the fracture cannot be reduced by closed or percutaneous means. Also special attention should be taken to avoid damage to the sensory branch of the radial nerve and to avoid locking screws penetrating into the soft tissue and into the DRUJ joint.

19.2 Background

Intramedullary locking nailing has been used for years in the treatment of diaphyseal fractures providing a stable fixation of fractures and rapid joint mobilization. More refined designs of the interlocking systems have improved fragment stabilization and have widened the indications to metaphyseal fractures and fractures adjacent to joints.

L.M. Hove et al. (eds.), *Distal Radius Fractures*,
DOI 10.1007/978-3-642-54604-4_19,

This evolution of locking nails has led to the introduction of interlocking nails for fractures of the distal radius as a possible effective minimally invasive surgery for instable fractures. So far two different principles have been presented.

- An approach where the fracture is stabilized using a nail introduced in the dorsal part of the radius at Lister's tubercle and maintaining the length of the dorsal part of the radius after reduction of dorsally angulated instable fractures without volar comminution (DNP®). As this nail only has to support the distraction of the comminuted dorsal part of the radius, the DNP nail is very thin, but still has to be locked by three screws/pegs distally and three screws proximally to stabilize the fracture and form a three-dimensional scaffold for a strong and stable construct.
- Another approach is the insertion of an interlocking nail through the radial styloid after reduction of the fracture. This biomechanically different approach attacking the radius in a horizontal plane and the fracture at a right angle requires a more bulky nail (Targon®, Micronail®, Sonoma WRx®) with increased strength but similar number of interlocking screws to form a three-dimensional scaffold for a strong and stable construct.

The stability of these new devices have been tested and compared in experimental biomechanical studies. McCall et al. (2007) compared DNP® nails with volar locking plates and found that the DNV® volar plate provided a better stability compared to the DNP® nailplate in dorsally comminuted instable fractures. In radial styloid nails, Burkhart et al. (2010) found that a locking nail (Targon®) inserted through the radial styloid gave a more rigid fixation than volar plating. However, Capo et al. (2009) found the stability of volar plating and a locking nail inserted through the radial styloid to be equal.

19.3 Indications and Clinical Use

- So far the recommended indications have been adult patients with dorsally displaced instable extra-articular fractures of the AO type A (Nishiwaki et al. 2011; van Vugt et al. 2010), but nailing may also be considered in AO type C1 with a nondisplaced intra-articular fracture line.
- It is absolutely mandatory that the fracture is reduced before the insertion of the nail, as further reduction is almost impossible after introduction of the nail while placing the locking screws, contrary to open reduction and volar plating, where the plate may be used for further reduction of the fracture. If this is not possible, an alternative method of fracture fixation should be considered.
- Intramedullary locking nailing is contraindicated in patients with an open epiphysis due to the nail possibly interfering with bone growth as introduction of the nail is located in the growth zone.
- Use with care if the radius fracture is combined with a fracture of the distal ulna, because the shape of the locking nail will increase the risk of changing the rotation axis of the DRUJ (Fig. 19.1a).

19.4 Operative Technique

The operation is performed in general anaesthesia or in a regional bloc and using a tourniquet to improve visualizing the sensory nerve branches of the radial nerve and the tendons. Start by reducing the fracture by a closed technique or by introducing small elevators through stab incisions followed by a temporary fixation with K-wires. Always use a fluoroscope. Especially pay attention to restoration of volar tilt, as this may be difficult to visualize when the nail and locking screws are inserted due to hardware and instruments blocking the view on the fluoroscope. If this is not possible, an alternative method of fracture fixation should be considered. Incisions for the nail and locking screws are made with blunt dissection to avoid damage to sensory branches of the radial nerve and tendon lesions especially the EPL tendon in dorsal nailing.

Insert the distal screws first. When placing the screws in the distal part of the nail fixating the distal fragment, it is important to get a good

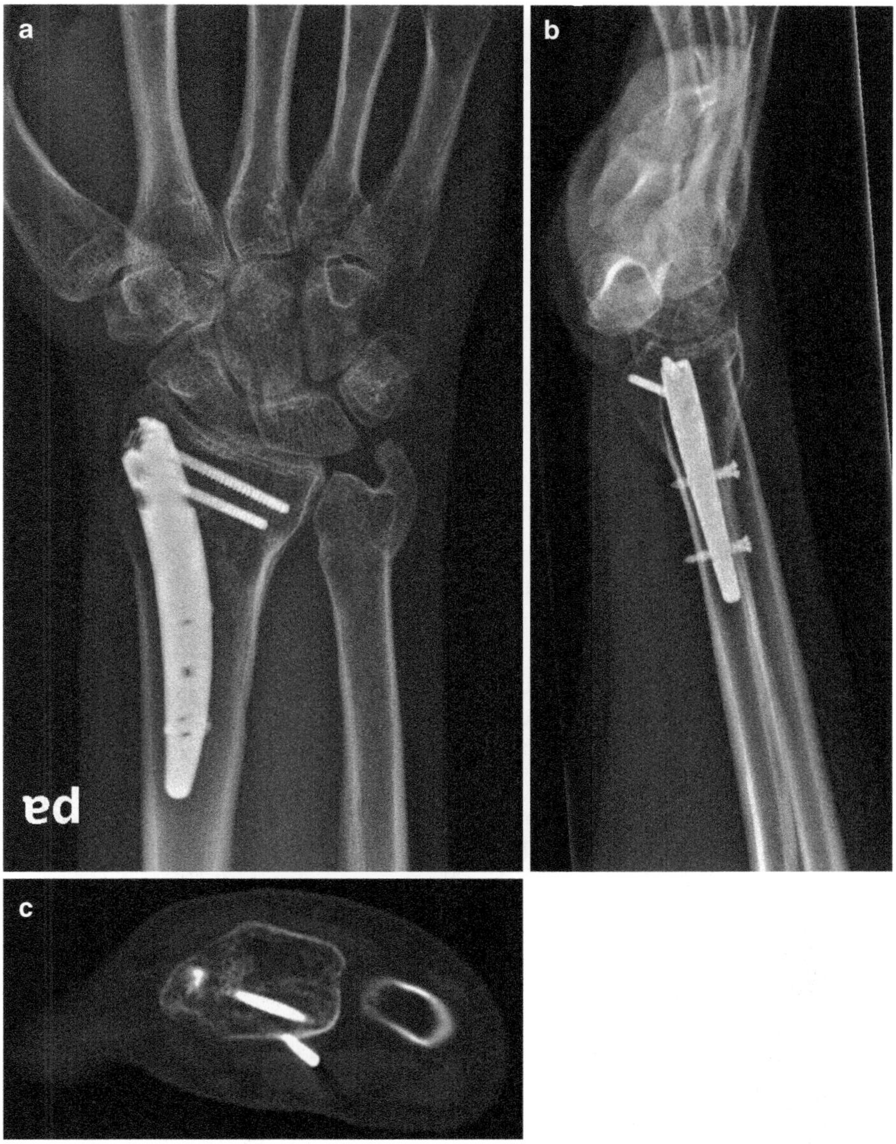

Fig. 19.1 (**a**) An example of a Micronail® used in a distal forearm fracture resulting in tilt of the DRUJ and a change in the axis of rotation in the DRUJ due to a change in the ulnar inclination of the radius. (**b**) Also the volar tilt has not been restored. (**c**) CT scan of the same case illustrating how the distal locking screws penetrates into the soft tissue

subchondral fixation of the screws to ensure a three-dimensional scaffold with a strong and stable construct. However, pay special attention to the DRUJ in placing the screws and check carefully using fluoroscopy that they do not perforate into the joint. With the proximal locking screws, it is important too to check the correct length of the screws, as screws penetrating into the soft tissue may result in discomfort and a necessity for unplanned hardware removal.

Postoperative immobilization may be reduced to a minimum after locked nailing if a stable fixation is achieved at the operation. A splint may be used for 1–2 weeks and non-loaded wrist movements allowed after removal of the splint. A removable brace may be used as protection for another 4 weeks depending on the patient and the bone quality until fracture union permits loading of the fracture.

19.5 Clinical Results

- Tan et al. (2012) compared the use of Micronail® with a simple reduction and splinting of extra-articular radius fractures and found better radiological and functional results in the initial treatment period and after 12 months when treated with Micronail® fixation.
- Comparing Micronail® with non-bridging external fixation, Schønnemann et al. (2011) found no relevant clinical difference in the results, but the Micronail® was a more cost-effective treatment option due to a reduction in the number of postoperative follow-up visits at the hospital.
- Safi et al. (2013) compared Micronail® with volar plating and found faster rehabilitation with Micronail®, but no other differences in radiological or clinical outcome.
- Lerch et al. (2009) compared another radial styloid nail (Targon®) with volar plating and found no difference in clinical or radiological outcome.
- Comparing DNP® dorsal nailing with volar plating in a randomized controlled study, Chappuis et al. (2011) found better clinical and radiological results after volar plating.

19.6 Complications

- A high risk of sensory nerve injury has been reported (Schønnemann et al. 2011; Ilyas and Thoder 2008; Safi et al. 2013; Dremstrup et al. 2013) using Micronail® with up to 30 % of the patients complaining of sensory disturbances at the radial styloid after 12 months. However, Dremstrup et al. (2013) found that after 5 years the initial observed sensory disturbances were reduced to less than 10 %.
- The closed nailing techniques also open for an increased risk of tendon damage, and especially damage to the EPL tendon in dorsal nailing should be considered (Chappuis et al. 2011; Espen et al. 2007).
- A lack of restoration of volar tilt is important before introduction and fixation of the nail. However, both in dorsal nailing (Chappuis et al. 2011) and radial styloid nailing (Schønnemann et al 2011; Dremstrup et al. 2013), this may be technically difficult leading to an insufficient restoration of volar tilt after fixation of the fracture (Fig. 19.1b). Also lack of bony support at the volar cortex due to volar comminution may lead to transforming the dorsal angulation into a Smith type configuration, and in this case another fixation method should be considered.
- Intramedullary nailing is primarily recommended in dorsally displaced instable extra-articular fractures of the AO type A, but nailing of AO type C1 with a nondisplaced intra-articular fracture line has also been described. This may introduce a risk of converting a nondisplaced intra-articular fracture into a displaced intra-articular fracture, and in this situation the intra-articular fracture should be carefully evaluated using the fluoroscope during the operation.
- Stabilizing the fracture and forming a three-dimensional scaffold for a strong and stable construct with diverging locking screws make the use of fluoroscopy mandatory in placing the locking screws, as they easily penetrate into the DRUJ or into the soft tissue (Fig. 19.1c). However, the use of an oblique view on the fluoroscope may reduce the problem, and Dremstrup et al. (2013) found that hardware removal was only needed in 2 % during the first 5 years after the operation using the Micronail®, indicating that this may not be a universal problem in intramedullary nailing of distal radius fractures.

Conclusion

Locked intramedullary nailing of instable extra-articular fractures AO type A is an elegant minimally invasive method with a low complication rate and a low need of hardware removal after fracture healing. However, there are quite narrow indications compared to volar locked plating, and the indication for intramedullary locked fixation of distal radius fractures should primarily be limited to dorsally displaced extra-articular fractures, and the procedure should be avoided if the fracture cannot be reduced by closed or percutaneous means.

Pearls and Pitfalls

- Keep indications to primarily dorsally displaced extra-articular fractures.
- Avoid intra-articular fractures apart from nondisplaced AO type C1.
- Fracture reduction has to be perfect before insertion of the nail.
- The procedure should be avoided if the fracture cannot be reduced by closed or percutaneous means.
- Use temporary K-wire fixation before insertion of the nail.
- Pay attention to the radial sensory branch of the radial nerve.
- In dorsal nailing avoid damaging the EPL tendon.
- Avoid damage to the DRUJ when introducing locking screws.
- In a stable fracture fixation, early mobilization is allowed resulting in rapid rehabilitation of hand and wrist function.
- Pay attention to the correct length of the locking screws, thereby creating a fracture fixation with a very low need for implant removal.

References

Burkhart KJ, Nowak TE, Gradl G, Klitscher D, Mehling I, Mehler D, Mueller LP, Rommens PM. Intramedullary nailing vs. palmar locked plating for unstable dorsally comminuted distal radius fractures: a biomechanical study. Clin Biomech. 2010;25(8):771–5.

Capo JT, Kinchelow T, Brooks K, Tan V, Manigrasso M, Francisco K. Biomechanical stability of four fixation constructs for distal radius fractures. Hand. 2009;4(3):272–8.

Chappuis J, Bouté P, Putz P. Dorsally displaced extra-articular distal radius fractures fixation: dorsal IM nailing versus volar plating. A randomized controlled trial. Orthop Traumatol Surg Res. 2011;97(5):471–8.

Dremstrup L, Skjærbæk SS, Olesen S, Høgh A, Hansen TB. Good radiological and functional results after intramedullary nailing of distal radius fractures. J Plast Surg Hand Surg. 2013;47:286–8.

Espen D, Lauri G, Fernandez D. Stabilisation of distal radius fractures by a novel endomedullary, fixed-angle plate: first experience. Handchir Mikrochir Plast Chir. 2007;39(1):73–7.

Ilyas AM, Thoder JJ. Intramedullary fixation of displaced distal radius fractures: a preliminary report. J Hand Surg Am. 2008;33(10):1706–15.

Lerch S, Sextro HG, Wilken F, Wittenberg CE. Clinical and radiological results after distal radius fracture: intramedullary locking nail versus volar locking plate osteosynthesis. Z Orthop Unfall. 2009; 147(5):547–52.

McCall TA, Conrad B, Badman B, Wright T. Volar versus dorsal fixed-angle fixation of dorsally unstable extra-articular distal radius fractures: a biomechanic study. J Hand Surg Am. 2007;32(6):806–12.

Nishiwaki M, Tazaki K, Shimizu H, Ilyas AM. Prospective study of distal radial fractures treated with an intramedullary nail. J Bone Joint Surg Am. 2011;93(15): 1436–41.

Safi A, Hart R, Teknedzjan B, Kozák T. Treatment of extra-articular and simple articular distal radial fractures with intramedullary nail versus volar locking plate. J Hand Surg Eur. 2013;38:774–9.

Schønnemann JO, Hansen TB, Søballe K. Randomised study of non-bridging external fixation compared with intramedullary fixation of unstable distal radial fractures. J Plast Surg Hand Surg. 2011;45(4–5): 232–7.

Tan V, Bratchenko W, Nourbakhsh A, Capo J. Comparative analysis of intramedullary nail fixation versus casting for treatment of distal radius fractures. J Hand Surg Am. 2012;37(3):460–8.

van Vugt R, Geerts RW, Werre AJ. Osteosynthesis of distal radius fractures with the Micronail. Eur J Trauma Emerg Surg. 2010;36(5):471–6.

20 Closed Reduction and External Fixation or Open Reduction and Volar Internal Fixation: The Clinical Dilemma

Maria Wilcke and Cecilia Mellstrand-Navarro

Contents

M. Wilcke, MD, PhD (✉)
Department for Hand Surgery, Karolinska Institute, Södersjukhuset, Stockholm, Sweden
e-mail: maria.wilcke@sodersjukhuset.se

C. Mellstrand-Navarro, MD
Department of Orthopedics, Karolinska Institute, Södersjukhuset, Stockholm, Sweden

20.1 Summary

This chapter presents a discussion of the choice between external fixation (EF) and open reduction and internal, mainly volar, fixation (ORIF) in the everyday clinical situation. Both methods have a place in the treatment of distal radius fractures. Many times the choice between external fixation and open reduction and internal fixation for unstable fractures of the distal radius is not obvious. Looking for guidance in the literature does not make the decision easier. Few comparison studies have been done and there is no consensus on which technique is superior. The available evidence suggests that volar plating is advantageous compared with bridging external fixation in the short term, but after 1 year, the outcome is similar. In spite of this, there has been a shift from closed reduction and external fixation to open reduction and volar plating.

20.2 Introduction

- Many times the choice between external fixation (EF) and open reduction and internal, mainly volar, fixation (ORIF) for unstable fractures of the distal radius is not obvious. Looking for guidance in the literature does not make the decision easier. Few comparison studies have been done and there is no consensus on which technique is superior.
- The available evidence suggests that volar plating is advantageous compared with

L.M. Hove et al. (eds.), *Distal Radius Fractures*,
DOI 10.1007/978-3-642-54604-4_20, © Springer-Verlag Berlin Heidelberg 2014

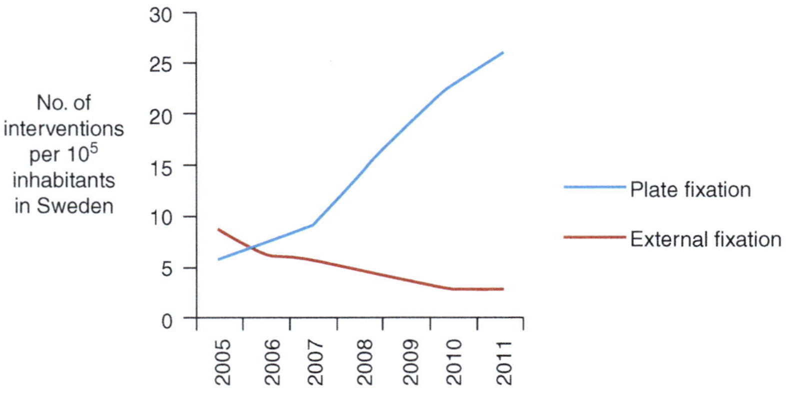

Fig. 20.1 The change in surgical methods from EF to ORIF (Data from Swedish Health Authorities www.socialstyrelsen.se)

Table 20.1 Advantages and disadvantages with external fixation (EF) and volar plating

External fixation	Volar plating
Advantages	*Advantages*
Low hardware costs	Exact reduction of the fracture possible
Short OR time	Allows early mobilization and rapid rehabilitation
Simple, minimally invasive procedure	Comfortable for the patient
No remaining hardware	Stabilizes the fracture during the entire healing process
Well established	
No late complications	
Disadvantages	*Disadvantages*
Risk for metacarpal fractures	Long OR time
Risk for damage to radial nerve branches	Invasive and technically demanding procedure
Relative stability with risk for loss of reduction	Risk for damage to or compression of median nerve or radial artery
Long fixation time (5–6 weeks)	Risk for screws or drill holes penetrating the joint surface
Slow rehabilitation	Postoperative pain
Risk for pin tract infection	Risk for tendon damage or tendinitis due to drilling, long screws or suboptimal placed plate
Inconvenient for the patient	
Requires a second procedure to remove the EF pins	

bridging EF in the short term, but after 1 year, the outcome is similar (Egol et al. 2008; Wei et al. 2009; Rozental et al. 2009; Wilcke et al. 2011). In spite of this, there has been a shift from closed reduction and EF to open reduction and volar plating (Koval et al. 2008; Mattila et al. 2011; Wilcke et al. 2013) (Fig. 20.1).

- Fractures of the distal radius that require surgical fixation occur in patients of all ages with very different demands on their wrist. There is a great variety of injury pattern and bone quality. The treatment should be tailored for the individual patient, bearing in mind the possibilities and disadvantages with each method (Tables 20.1).

20.3 When Volar Plating Is Recommended

- For an active, high-demand, working-age patient to whom a fast rehabilitation and return to normal activities is of high priority, a volar plate may be preferred. The plate fixation allows early mobilization of the wrist joint, which seems to improve short-term outcome. The wrist function returns to nearly normal within a few months and a minimum of loss of income for the patient and society is ensured. When there are concurrent injuries in the upper or lower extremities, stabile fixation with a volar plate is a good choice to facilitate the overall rehabilitation.
- Volar plating is also recommended for secondary surgery necessitated by loss of reduction during conservative treatment. Closed reduction is unable to achieve proper reduction when the healing process has reached beyond 10 or 12 days, leaving ORIF

as the reasonable option. In addition, the time of immobilization is less after plating than after bridging EF.

- In intra-articular fractures with a step or gap exceeding 1–2 mm after closed reduction, ORIF, with or without arthroscopic assistance, is necessary to restore joint congruity. We recommend open reduction and plate fixation for these cases.
- For volarly displaced fractures, a volar buttress plate is recommended (volar locked plating is not needed). EF has a very limited role for this fracture type.

20.4 When External Fixation Is Recommended

- In the majority of distal radius fractures, EF is a good and reliable treatment option, in particular for low-energy fractures that can be properly reduced with closed manipulation. EF is an easy procedure with a low risk of severe complications and with a clinical result similar to volar plating (Egol et al. 2008; Wei et al. 2009; Rozental et al. 2009; Wilcke et al. 2011).
- EF is a safe and minimally invasive method suitable for any orthopaedic trauma surgeon. It causes a minimum of hardware side effects and is, with a few exceptions (Fig. 20.2a, b), almost never wrong as a first step in complex wrist trauma and particularly open fractures.
- Additional K-wires can be used as a reduction tool or as inter-fragmentary fixation, in combination with the EF. Furthermore, this is supported by Cochrane to improve the overall outcome of these fractures (Handoll et al. 2008). Even severe displacements and reduction of several intra-articular fragments can be handled in this manner. Bear in mind the risk of injuring the radial cutaneous nerve branch when approaching the radial styloid.
- To protect the radial cutaneous nerve branches, always make a small incision and use a blunt technique to get access to the radius for your EF pins and/or for your K-wires.

20.5 When Both Techniques Are Needed

- High-energy trauma often results in severely comminuted fractures in which a combination of internal and external fixation may be necessary to restore and maintain anatomical reduction.
- EF may be the only suitable treatment modality during the first days or weeks after the injury when there is damaged soft tissues.
- At a later stage, exact reduction and fixation of the fracture fragments with a plate may be required.
- An EF device is an excellent intraoperative aid to restore and maintain length during an ORIF procedure of an unstable fracture.
- In severely comminuted fractures, the volar plate may need additional support by EF or ORIF with a combination of volar and dorsal plates. It can be advisable to keep the EF to neutralize the internal fixation during the first postoperative weeks.

20.6 Elderly "Osteoporotic" Patients

- In elderly "osteoporotic" patients, the primary clinical dilemma is not limited to the choice between external and internal fixation, but also involves the question whether the wrist should be operated on at all as the overall outcome seems independent on treatment option (Arora et al. 2011).
- Elderly, low-demand patients seem to tolerate malunion better than younger patients (Grewal and MacDermid 2007; Arora et al. 2011). Moreover, return to normal activities may not be as urgent. When surgical fixation is required, a less invasive and inexpensive EF can be suggested.
- Osteoporotic bone increases the risk for complications after both methods. Many of the failures associated with EF (e.g. pin loosening, pin tract infections and metacarpal fractures) occur more frequently in frail bone. After ORIF with volar plating, the risk of screws

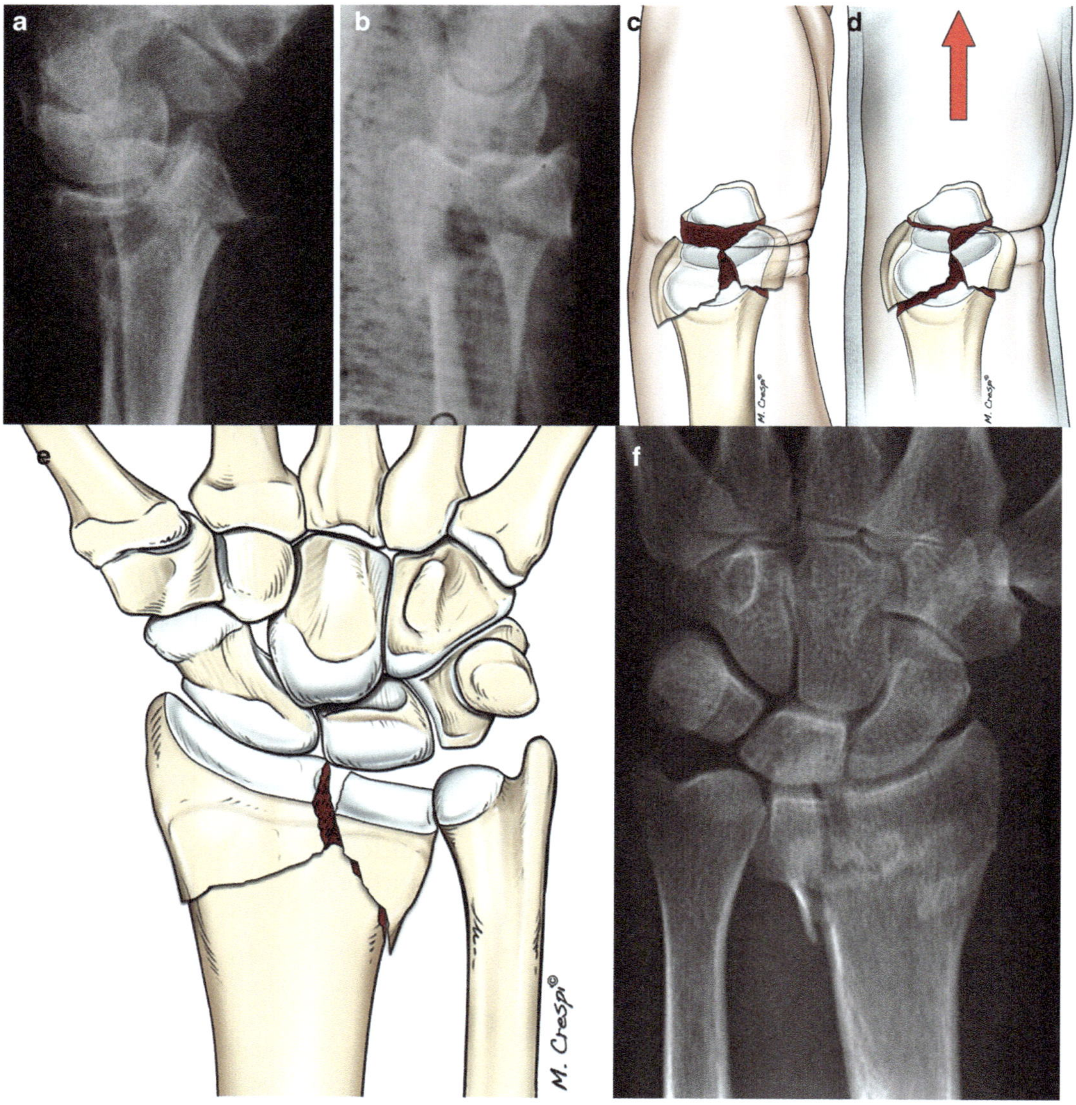

Fig. 20.2 (**a–d**) This case illustrates an example where EF is *not* a good option. Ligamentotaxis will force the volar fragment in dorsiflexion due to the volar ligaments being pulled. The reduction is most often better handled with a volar open approach. (**e–f**) Another example where external fixation alone is *not* a good option. The ulnar die punch depression will not be properly reduced by closed reduction

cutting into the joint is increased in comminuted osteoporotic bone, and even locked plates sometimes fail to maintain reduction.

20.7 General Discussion

- The EF may be looked upon as bulky and uncomfortable compared with ORIF.
- To "hide" the implant on the volar aspect of the distal radius may be subjectively preferred by many patients as a contrast to the EF "out-rigger", whilst offered the two treatment methods.
- However, EF is less invasive and leaves no remaining hardware.
- It is not uncommon that patients require plate removal due to a sense of discomfort, even though no objective signs of mechanical disturbance are present. This necessitates additional surgery with associated costs and risks. The plate removal can be challenging, and there is a risk of injuring the median nerve, in

particular the cutaneous branch, when dissecting the scarred tissue.

- Long-term patient-rated results have been reported to be similar between EF and ORIF with a volar plate. Hence, complications and costs are important outcome variables.
- Complications after EF are minor and occur early during the fixation. The risk of pin loosening and imperfect reduction associated with EF must be balanced with the risk of hardware complications associated with ORIF.
- Complications after ORIF may be tendon attrition or rupture, nerve compression or wrist stiffness due to imperfectly performed plating. The tendon ruptures may occur early or present late (Al-Rashid et al. 2006; Arora et al. 2007). These tendon injuries require reconstruction and long rehabilitation.
- Costs for the procedure may differ significantly. A volar plate with screws cost between €100 and 800, whereas the cost for the EF is about €100–120 per patient. In the absence of any superior outcome in well-designed studies, these seemingly trivial aspects ought to be brought into the decision making process whilst comparing EF or ORIF. Closed manipulation and percutaneous fixation of a wrist fracture takes approximately half the time of ORIF (Shyamalan et al. 2009).
- Indirect costs for sick leave and social services are more difficult to estimate but may hypothetically be lesser after ORIF on the assumption that patients regain wrist functions sooner. Economical aspects must be taken into consideration when dictating general recommendations regarding surgical techniques for distal radius fractures.
- Non-bridging EF may present with an advantage in the management of distal radius fractures in relation to ORIF, but requires a sizable distal fracture fragment. It is more technically demanding and it has not yet been spread to general use.

Conclusion

The choice of management of an unstable distal radius fracture is highly dependent on the surgeon's preference. Available medical evidence shows little difference between EF and ORIF. A balanced decision should be made based on the surgeon's experience, patient's need and local economic conditions.

Top 5 Tips

- In the absence of evidence, either EF or ORIF can be used for most distal radius fractures.
- Choose surgical option according to the patient's general presentation and needs in combination with the fracture pattern.
- ORIF with a volar plate is preferable in cases with concurrent musculoskeletal injuries or secondary displacement.
- EF with additional percutaneous K-wires is an excellent and cheap option for reduction in simpler cases or in open fractures.
- Never underestimate the technical skills needed for exact reduction and proper implant placement, whichever technique you favour.

References

Al-Rashid M, Theivendran K, Craigen MA. Delayed ruptures of the extensor tendon secondary to the use of volar locking compression plates for distal radial fractures. J Bone Joint Surg Br. 2006;88(12):1610–2.

Arora R, Lutz M, Hennerbichler A, Krappinger D, Espen D, Gabl M. Complications following internal fixation of unstable distal radius fracture with a palmar locking-plate. J Orthop Trauma. 2007;21(5):316–22.

Arora R, Lutz M, Deml C, Krappinger D, Haug L, Gabl M. A prospective randomized trial comparing nonoperative treatment with volar locking plate fixation for displaced and unstable distal radial fractures in patients sixty-five years of age and older. J Bone Joint Surg Am. 2011;93(23):2146–53.

Egol K, Walsh M, Tejwani N, McLaurin T, Wynn C, Paksima N. Bridging external fixation and supplementary Kirschner-wire fixation versus volar locked plating for unstable fractures of the distal radius: a randomised, prospective trial. J Bone Joint Surg Br. 2008;90(9):1214–21.

Grewal R, MacDermid JC. The risk of adverse outcomes in extra-articular distal radius fractures is increased with malalignment in patients of all ages but mitigated in older patients. J Hand Surg Am. 2007;32(7):962–70.

Handoll HHG, Huntley JS, Madhok R. Different methods of external fixation for treating distal radial fractures in adults. Cochrane Database Syst Rev. 2008;

(1):CD006522. doi: 10.1002/14651858.CD006522.pub2.
Koval KJ, Harrast JJ, Anglen JO, Weinstein JN. Fractures of the distal part of the radius. The evolution of practice over time. Where's the evidence? J Bone Joint Surg Am. 2008;90(9):1855–61.
Mattila VM, Huttunen TT, Sillanpa P, Niemi S, Pihlajama H, Kannus P. Significant change in the surgical treatment of distal radius fractures: a nationwide study between 1998 and 2008 in Finland. J Trauma. 2011;71:939–43.
Rozental TD, Blazar PE, Franko OI, Chacko AT, Earp BE, Day CS. Functional outcomes for unstable distal radial fractures treated with open reduction and internal fixation or closed reduction and percutaneous fixation. A prospective randomized trial. J Bone Joint Surg Am. 2009;91(8):1837–46.
Shyamalan G, Theokli C, Pearse Y, Tennent D. Volar locking plates versus Kirschner wires for distal radial fractures–a cost analysis study. Injury. 2009;40(12):1279–81.
Wei DH, Raizman NM, Bottino CJ, Jobin CM, Strauch RJ, Rosenwasser MP. Unstable distal radius fractures treated with external fixation, a radial column plate, or a volar plate. J Bone Joint Surg Am. 2009;91(7):1568–77.
Wilcke M, Abbaszadegan H, Adolphson PY. Wrist function recovers more rapidly after volar locked plating than after external fixation but the outcomes are similar after 1 year. Acta Orthop. 2011;82(1):76–81.
Wilcke M, Hammarberg H, Adolphson PY. Epidemiology and changed surgical methods for fractures of the distal radius. A registry analysis of 42,583 patients in Stockholm county, Sweden 2004–2010. Acta Orthop. 2013;84:292–6.

21 Combined External Fixation and Internal Fixation

Ola-Lars Hammer

Contents

O.-L. Hammer, MD
Department of Orthopaedic Surgery,
Akershus University Hospital, University of Oslo,
Oslo, Norway
e-mail: olalarsh@broadpark.no

21.1 Summary

Fractures with severe comminution of the joint surface and with little metaphyseal support to the volar rim fragments may benefit from a volar buttress plate in addition to ligamentotaxis served by an external fixator. The most severe, comminuted fractures however should be subject to augmented external fixation. If a CT-scan reveals bone fragments of a size that can be captured by (multidirectional) screws, plate fixation is an alternative. If not, these fragments may be fixated by K-wires through an open approach, or simply left in place. The documentation is poor, but the combination of plate fixation and external fixator can produce a satisfactory outcome in the most comminuted fractures. Given the possible, combined complications of the two methods, it should be an option only when adequate reduction and stability cannot be achieved by one method alone.

External fixation augmented by K-wires provides stability comparable to plate fixation, and reduction of difficult fragments can be achieved through an open approach to the fracture.

21.2 Introduction

Advances in implant technology have left the surgeon with many options when managing fractures of the distal radius. Prior to the introduction of locking plates, external fixation augmented by K-wires was often the method of choice for the most comminuted fractures, as were different

L.M. Hove et al. (eds.), *Distal Radius Fractures*,
DOI 10.1007/978-3-642-54604-4_21,

combinations of volar and dorsal plates. With the introduction of precontoured volar and dorsal locking plates and customized plates, as well specialized volar rim plates, all with locking screw technology, the surgeon has an unprecedented variety of options in the toolbox.

Faced with a high-energy wrist trauma resulting in a comminuted and dislocated fracture, it is tempting to reach into the toolbox and hope that using both external fixation and internal plate fixation will provide you with the best of both worlds, given that complications can be avoided.

21.3 The Theoretical Benefits of a Volar Locking Plate

- In theory a volar locking plate provides a stable, subchondral fixation and a good restoration of articular congruity and extra-articular alignment.
- Earlier return to pre-injury level of function might be possible since the stable construct usually allows earlier postsurgical wrist motion than other methods.
- The construct of the locking plates, which stabilizes the distal screws against lateral movements, provides additional fixation strength in the metaphysis, especially in osteoporotic bone.
- Complications related to dorsal plates, such as extensor tendon ruptures, are to a certain degree avoided (Wright et al 2005).

As volar fixed angle implants gained popularity, authors such as Orbay and Fernandez (2004) reported that this treatment provided a stable internal fixation in osteoporotic bone, with a low complication rate while allowing early mobilization.

Other authors such as Rozental and Blazar (2006) found a substantial complication rate in a series of unstable fractures treated with volar locking plates, although the number of hardware-related complications was lower compared to previous reports on dorsal plating. The most common problems were loss of reduction and tendon irritation.

21.4 Possible Complications with Volar Plate-and-Screw Fixation

- Median nerve neuropathy (with subsequent need for carpal tunnel release)
- Wound infection
- CRPS (complex regional pain syndrome)
- Tendon irritation and rupture
- Intra-articular penetration of screws (Arora et al. 2007)

With proper placement of hardware, the elimination of dorsal tendinopathy (as compared to dorsal plates) may lead to fewer long-term complications. The new volar plates are also said to have a shape and composition more "friendly" to the soft tissue, supposedly reducing the need for removal of hardware.

21.5 The Advantages of External Fixation

- Ease of application.
- Minimal surgical exposure.
- Reduced surgical trauma.
- Low cost of the procedure.
- Augmented by K-wires it is possible to achieve an adequate and stable reduction, also for intra-articular fractures (Margaliot et al 2005).

21.6 The Disadvantages of External Fixation

- Prolonged immobilization
- Indirect reduction of the fracture fragments
- Loss of ligamentotaxis over time (settling of the fracture after hardware removal)

- Radial sensory nerve problems
- Pin-related complications such as infection, loosening of hardware and tenosynovitis

21.7 Discussion

In theory, the combination of external and internal fixation techniques could offer the combined advantages of the two methods, especially when dealing with the most comminuted fractures (McAuliffe 2005).

Cooney and Berger (1993) advocated this combination, in addition to bone grafting, in young adults who had sustained comminuted intra-articular fractures after high-energy accidents. This, however, was prior to the introduction of locking plate technology.

Rogachefsky et al. (2001) treated 17 AO type C3 fractures with a combination of external fixation and non-locking plates: between 30 and 58 % of the patients had a good or excellent result.

With a similar selection of fractures and using an external fixator in combination with volar and dorsal plates, Bass et al. (1995) found good or excellent results in 10 out of 13 fractures.

These studies all deal with the most severe of the distal radius fractures and have a retrospective design, a heterogeneous selection of implants and few patients. They do however demonstrate that satisfactory results can be achieved when dealing with some of the most challenging wrist fractures.

The majority of other studies mentioning the combination of external and internal fixation note this as a last resort, that is to say, as a salvage procedure when adequate stability cannot be achieved by one method alone.

One must also bear in mind that enjoying the benefits from both principles of fixation also introduces the combined spectrum of possible complications, as listed above.

For example, pin tract infection is usually a fairly benign complication when dealing with external fixation alone. The infection is likely to be self-contained without the use of antibiotics and resolves spontaneously after the removal of the pins after six weeks. With the addition of a plate, the road to a complicated, prolonged deep infection is shorter.

21.8 Indications for the Combined Use of External Fixator and Plate Fixation

21.8.1 A Reduction Tool

- For the most comminuted fractures, an external fixator might be useful as a reduction tool while "puzzling" the bone fragments back together through a volar or dorsal approach.

21.8.2 When Stability Cannot Be Achieved by One Method Alone

- With the locking plate technology and the use of multidirectional screws, most fragments are eligible for stable fixation through a plate.
- The eligibility of a plate could to a certain degree be predicted by a preoperative CT-scan.
- In the event that stable fixation cannot be achieved by using internal fixation, the external fixator may be exactly what you need, that is to say, you can draw the additional benefits of ligamentotaxis on those small, hard to reach, fragments.

21.8.3 Subchondral Volar Fragments

Small fragments of the volar rim may be especially difficult to capture with screws, using the plate as a volar buttress in addition to the external fixator is a valid option for the fractures with severe comminution of the metaphysis adjacent to the volar rim and subchondral bone.

With the advent of locking plate technology and the increased use of an open approach to distal radius fractures, it is worthwhile to remember that external fixation augmented by K-wires is still a good, standalone choice for the most comminuted fractures.

The use of open reduction and supplemental K-wire fixation can expand the indications for external fixation.

21.9 Indications for Open Reduction in Combination with External Fixation Augmented by K-Wires

21.9.1 The Most Severely Comminuted Fractures

K-wire fixation not only enhances the reduction of the fracture fragments but also increases the stability of the entire construct (Slutsky 2007). Especially the smaller, intra-articular rim fragments are often available for fixation by K-wires through an open reduction. They are often too small for the screws to gain purchase, and trying to achieve this will often result in more comminution of these fragments. The result is an even more challenging articular puzzle.

Kreder et al. (2005) compared the results of open reduction and internal fixation (ORIF) versus external fixation and pinning in patients with displaced intra-articular fractures. There was no difference in the radiological restoration of anatomical features.

Short et al. (1987) demonstrated that fragment-specific pinning combined with external fixation was able to maintain articular congruity when exposed to a significant load. These test values compared favourably with the stiffness data of five commercially available distal radius plates (Osada et al 2003).

21.9.2 Open Fractures and Fractures with Loss of Soft Tissue

In some cases, the contamination of the open fracture or the loss of soft tissue coverage simply does not permit plate fixation. The external fixator may then be a graceful solution to a difficult problem. The K-wires may be left flush with the cortex, or protruding through the skin if later removal is desirable.

Probably not completely satisfactory in terms of patient-reported pain, ROM and grip strength, this solution may still produce the best basis for a secondary arthrodesis, compared to plate fixation. Peeling away the soft tissue to achieve fixation through a plate might not be the best course of action. The loss of soft tissue connection often makes these fragments more unstable and even more difficult to capture with a screw, as well as making them avascular.

Faced with the flood of novel plate designs, the orthopaedic surgeon should remember that augmented external fixation is a cheap, predictable and well-documented solution to the most comminuted fractures.

References

Arora R, Lutz M, Hennerbichler A, Krappinger D, Espen D, Gabl M. Complications following internal fixation of unstable distal radius fracture with a palmar locking-plate. J Orthop Trauma. 2007;21(5):316–22.

Bass RL, Blair WF, Hubbard PP. Results of combined internal and external fixation for the treatment of severe AO-C3 fractures of the distal radius. J Hand Surg Am. 1995;20(3):373–81.

Cooney WP, Berger RA. Treatment of complex fractures of the distal radius. Combined use of internal and external fixation and arthroscopic reduction. Hand Clin. 1993;9(4):603–12.

Kreder HJ, Hanel DP, Agel J, et al. Indirect reduction and percutaneous fixation versus open reduction and internal fixation for displaced intra-articular fractures of the distal radius: a randomised, controlled trial. J Bone Joint Surg. 2005;87B:829–36.

Margaliot Z, Haase SC, Kotsis SV, Kim HM, Chung KC. A meta-analysis of outcomes of external fixation versus plate osteosynthesis for unstable distal radius fractures. J Hand Surg Am. 2005;30(6):1185–99.

McAuliffe JA. Combined internal and external fixation of distal radius fractures. Hand Clin. 2005;21(3): 395–406.

Osada D, Viegas SF, Shah MA, Morris RP, Patterson RM. Comparison of different distal radius dorsal and volar fracture fixation plates: a biomechanical study. J Hand Surg. 2003;28A:94–104.

Orbay JL, Fernandez DL. Volar fixed-angle plate fixation for unstable distal radius fractures in the elderly patient. J Hand Surg Am. 2004;29(1):96–102.

Rogachefsky RA, Lipson SR, Applegate B, Ouellette EA, Savenor AM, McAuliffe JA. Treatment of severely comminuted intra-articular fractures of the distal end of the radius by open reduction and combined internal and external fixation. J Bone Joint Surg Am. 2001;83-A(4):509–19.

Rozental TD, Blazar PE. Functional outcome and complications after volar plating for dorsally displaced, unstable fractures of the distal radius. J Hand Surg Am. 2006;31(3):359–65.

Short WH, Palmer AK, Werner FW, Murphy DJ. A biomechanical study of distal radial fractures. J Hand Surg. 1987;12A:529–34.

Slutsky DJ. External fixation of distal radius fractures. Hand Surg. 2007;32A:1624–37.

Wright TW, Horodyski M, Smith DW. Functional outcome of unstable distal radius fractures: ORIF with a volar fixed-angle tine plate versus external fixation. J Hand Surg Am. 2005;30(2):289–99.

Open Reduction and Volar Plating: Surgical Guide

22

Per Hølmer

Contents

P. Hølmer, MD
Department of Orthopedic Surgery, Hand Section, Nordsjelland Hospital, Hillerød, Denmark

Department of Hand Surgery, Rigshospitalet, University of Copenhagen, Copenhagen, Denmark
e-mail: per.holmer@regionh.dk

22.1 Summary

Open reduction and volar plating has become a very common procedure in most orthopedic or hand surgery departments despite lack of hard evidence. The indication for the procedure is to restore the distal radius and especially the joint surfaces to a near anatomical status to facilitate a good recovery and function. In this chapter, a basal surgical technique – step by step – for most distal radius fractures is presented. Incision along the flexor carpi radialis tendon, reduction of the fracture with Kapandji technique, fixation of the plate proximally, final modeling of the distal fragment(s) before insertion of the distal locking screws. Complications are mainly related to the hardware, especially to distally placed plates or misplaced screws.

22.2 Introduction

Open reduction and internal fixation (ORIF) with a volar plate has become the most common alternative to conservative treatment of distal radius fractures (Koval et al. 2008).

The treatment is performed in almost all orthopedic or hand surgery clinics with acute patients, despite weak evidence of superior results compared with other treatments (AAOS guideline 2009). In AAOS' clinical practice guidelines, there is no recommendation "for or against any specific operative method for fixation of distal radius fractures" or "for or against

L.M. Hove et al. (eds.), *Distal Radius Fractures*,
DOI 10.1007/978-3-642-54604-4_22, © Springer-Verlag Berlin Heidelberg 2014

operative treatment for patients over age 55 with distal radius fracture" (AAOS guidelines 2009). Similarly conclusions are reported in Cochrane reviews.

- There are few good randomized controlled trails reported in the literature. In one study they looked at patients over the age of 65 years (mean age 76,7 years) treated with closed reduction and plaster against ORIF with volar locking plate. The results showed an initial better wrist function in the operated group. However, after 6 and 12 months, there was no significant difference, even though radiological results were significant better in the operative group (Arora et al. 2011). The argument for ORIF for the elderly population is mainly – but also important – to let them keep their level of activity and independency after the fracture (Jeudy et al. 2012).
- In the younger age group with displaced distal radius fractures, there is more consensus about the indication for ORIF. The decision for surgery should be balanced with the biological age and functional level of the patient. The choice of treatment should be made in a dialogue with the patient.
- Complication rate has been addressed in a few studies. One study found 8 major early complications (in 594 patients) related to locked volar plate fixation (within 1 month postoperatively). These complications were all intra-articular placed screws. There was one late complication, a flexor tendon rupture (in 321 patients available for late follow-up) – but additional 13 patients had tendon irritation (Song et al. 2011). These complications should be avoided with correct screw and plate position, which emphasizes the importance of meticulous surgery (and education of younger surgeons).

  Infections are rare.
- Recent meta-analysis of randomized controlled trials states that ORIF gives a better functional outcome and faster recovery than external fixation (EF) the first year; later there is no difference. The anatomical result is better in the ORIF group. The infection rate is higher in the EF group (Wang et al. 2013; Xie et al. 2013; Esposito et al. 2013).

There is a large amount of different plates, but the biomechanical principle is the same, a strong volar plate with locking screws often with polyaxial locking. This concept provides angular stability just below the joint surface with exact screw positioning.

The surgical technique is generally identical, with minor variations reflecting traditions and different surgical kits. In the following illustrations, you will find the technique the author finds useful for the majority of distal radius fractures. Example of postoperative plan in Table 22.1.

Table 22.1 Postoperative treatment

0–2 weeks	*Cast below elbow, finger-exercise/ edema-prophylaxis*
2 weeks	*Bandage and sutures are removed* *If X-ray control is satisfactory, unloaded wrist exercises are started*
5 weeks	*Start unrestricted exercises, no splint, X-ray on indication*

22.3 Surgical Technique

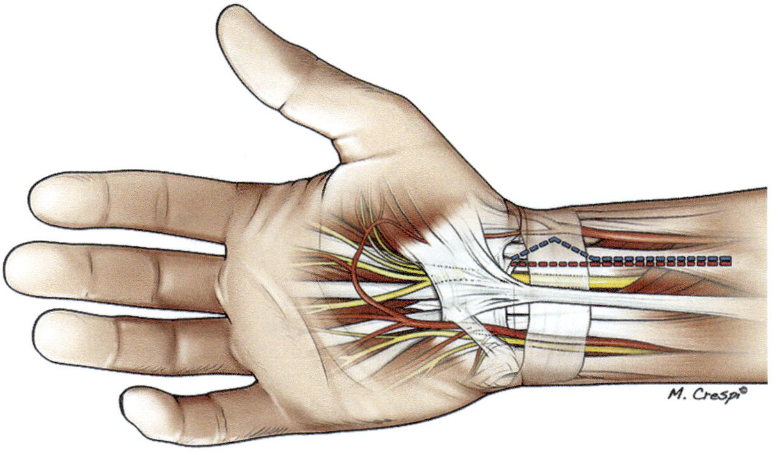

Fig. 22.1 Incision along the FCR tendon, straight or angulated down to the wrist crease; the FCR tendon is pulled ulnarly, protecting the median nerve and its palmar branch; the radial artery is identified and protected and then the fascia incised. The carpal tunnel is not released routinely; if needed, it should be done through a separate incision, preventing injury of the palmar cutaneous branch of the median nerve

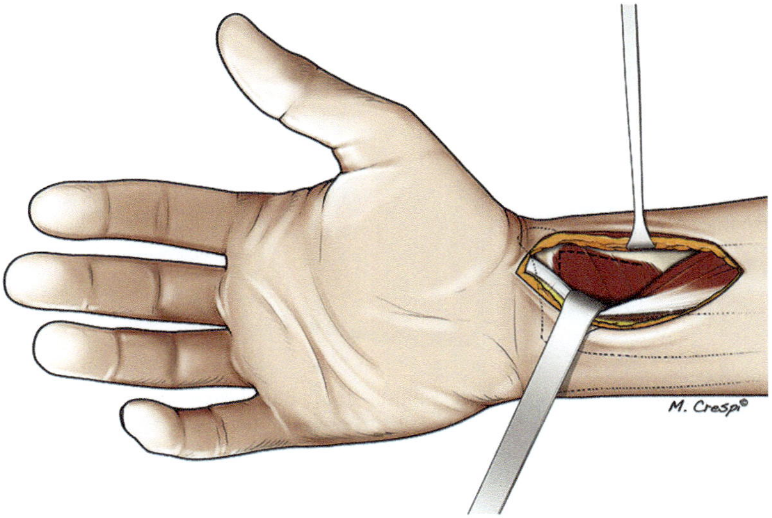

Fig. 22.2 The flexor tendons are retracted ulnarly and the musculus pronator quadratus is exposed; the pronator is released distally at its tendinous portion at "the watershed-line" and radially leaving a small cuff for suturing. The fracture is exposed and is reduced provisionally with traction and manipulation. If needed, the musculus brachioradialis tendon is released from the distal radius, facilitating the reduction

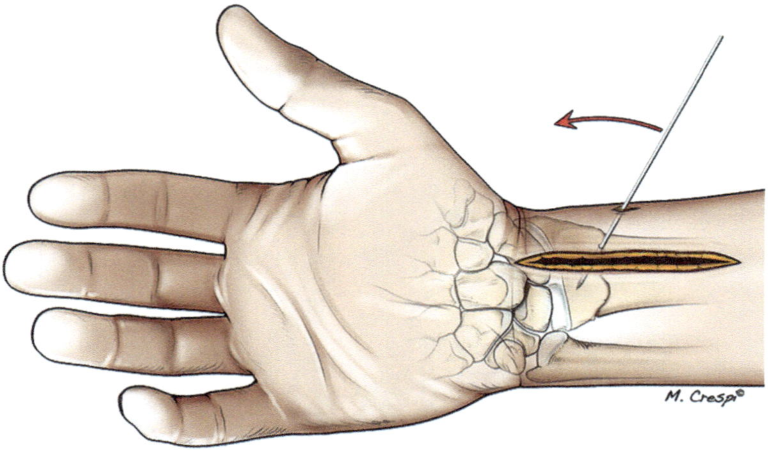

Fig. 22.3 Reduction with 1,6, or 2.0 mm K-wire (Kapandji technique). The first pin is inserted radially into the fracture line, through a small incision (just distal to the fracture line) protecting branches of the radial nerve. The K-wire is advanced in the direction of the distal ulnar corner of the radius, before the tip engages the cortical bone; the shaft of the pin is tipped distally, pressing especially the radial part of the distal fragment back into place. The pin is then advanced until it catches the cortical bone in the proximal part of the radius, stabilizing the fracture. A second pin is inserted into the fracture line dorsally through a small incision just proximal to the Lister's tubercle, advanced distally and tipped so the dorsal angulation is corrected, then the pin is advanced proximally until it engages the cortical bone

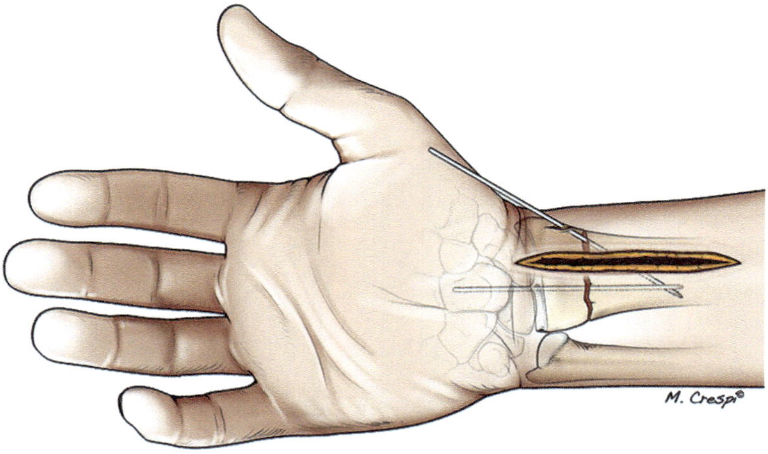

Fig. 22.4 Kapandji pins in place. Occasionally a third pin is needed for reduction of the ulnar corner of the radius. The pin is inserted into the fracture line between 4. and 5. compartments in the direction of the volar edge of the radius; the pin is tipped so the dorsal angulation of the ulnar part is corrected and then the pin is advanced proximally until it stabilizes. Often a near anatomical reduction with normal length can be achieved

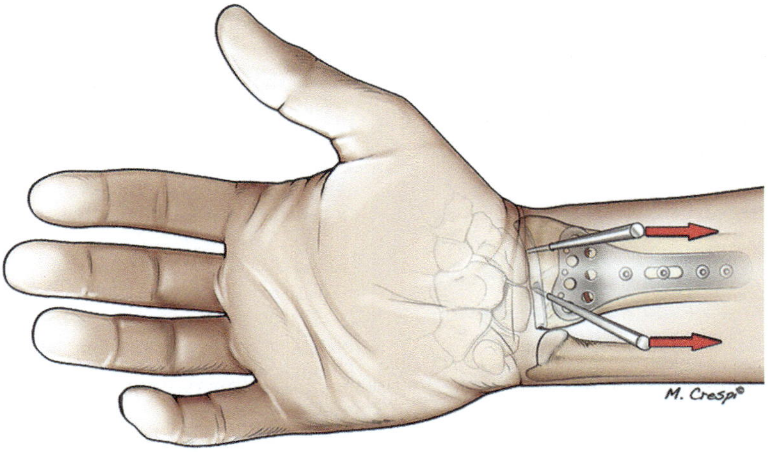

Fig. 22.5 The plate is pushed down to the "watershed-line" and positioned so it supports the ulnar corner of the radius and then aligned over the shaft of the radius. First a cortical screw is placed in the oval hole and a final positioning of the plate is performed under X-ray, and the screw is tightened. If the reduction of the radius is satisfying, the proximal screws are inserted. Optional: In comminuted fractures reduction of residual dorsal angulation can be corrected with two 1.6-mm K-wires inserted into the distal fragment from the volar side just distal to the plate parallel to the joint and then tipping the shaft of the pins proximally forcing the distal fragment distally reducing the dorsal tilt of the joint surface. Holding this reduction, the distal screws can be inserted

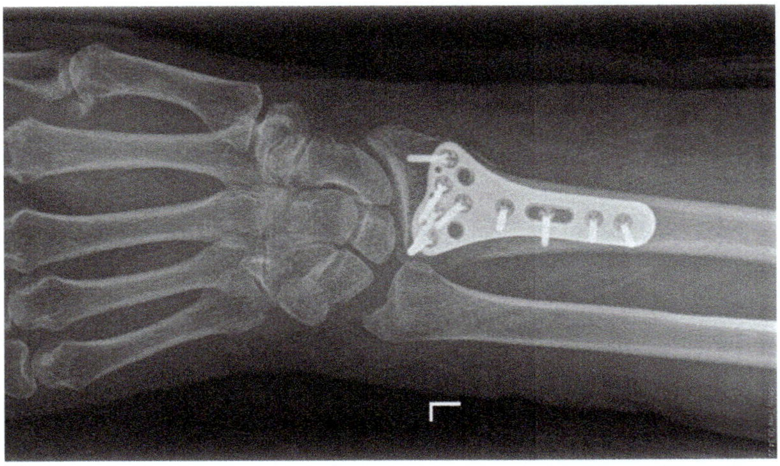

Fig. 22.6 Normally the screw securing the ulnar corner is placed first, and then the rest of the screws in the distal row are placed in the subchondral bone under X-ray evaluation. It is imporftant to insert the drill guide fully in the plate to obtain the correct angulation of the screw for optimal locking in the plate. Do not penetrate the joint surface and go into but not through the dorsal cortex with the screws

Additional Tips

Alternatively an ulnar approach can be used, especially for severe ulnate depression/comminuted fracture or in need for more extensive release of the median nerve.

When dealing with comminuted fractures, a vertical fingertrap traction is beneficial for reduction and maintaining reduction during fixation.

Occasionally, if there are problems with reducing intra-articular fractures especially if they have started to heal, the shaft of the radius can be released and pronated out of the way for exact reduction of the distal fragment and the joint surface (Orbay and Fernandez 2002).

Reinsertion of the musculus pronator quadratus can be difficult; it is helpful to flex the elbow and pronate the forearm.

A different approach to the ORIF is fixation of the plate distally first and using the plate for the reduction, forcing its proximal part down to the shaft of the radius.

References

AAOS. The treatment of distal radius fractures. Guideline and evidence report. 5 Dec 2009.

Arora R, et al. A prospective randomized trial comparing nonoperativ treatment with volar locking plate fization for displaced and unstable distal radial fractures in patients sixty-five years of age and older. J Bone Joint Surg Am. 2011;93:2146–53.

Esposito J, et al. External fixation versus open reduction with plate fixation for distal radius fractures: a meta-analysis of randomized controlled trials. Injury. 2013;44:409–16.

Jeudy J, et al. Treatment of complex fractures of the distal radius: a prospective randomised comparison of external fixation versus locking volar plating. Injury. 2012;43:174–9.

Jupiter J, et al. Operative management of distal radius fractures with 2,4 millimeter locking plates: a multicenter prospective case series. J Bone Joint Surg Am. 2010;92 Suppl 1:96–106.

Koval KJ, et al. Fractures of the distal part of radius. The evolution of practice over time. Where's the evidence? J Bone Joint Surg Am. 2008;90:1855–61.

Orbay JL, Fernandez DL. Volar fixation for dorsally displaced fractures of the distal radius: a preliminary report. J Hand Surg Am. 2002;27A:205–15.

Song M, et al. Fracture of the distal radius: risk factors for complications after locked volar plate fixation. J Hand Surg Am. 2011;36A:3–9.

Wang J, et al. Open reduction and internal fixation versus external fixation for unstable distal radius fractures: a meta-analysis. Orthop Traumatol Surg Res. 2013;99:321–31.

Xie X, et al. Comparison of internal and external fixation of distal radius fractures. A meta-analysis of randomized controlled trials. Acta Orthop Scand. 2013;84:286–91.

When Fixed-Angle Volar Plates Are Not Enough: Alternative Fixation Methods in Problem Fractures

23

Magnus Tägil and Antonio Abramo

Contents

M. Tägil, MD, PhD (✉)
Department of Hand Surgery, Lund's University Hospital, Lund, Sweden

Department of Orthopedics, Skane University Hospital/Lund, Lund, Sweden
e-mail: magnus.tagil@med.lu.se

A. Abramo, MD, PhD
Department of Hand Surgery, Lund University, Skane University Hospital, Malmö, Sweden
e-mail: tony.abramo@med.lu.se

23.1 Summary

The fixed-angle volar plates have revolutionized the treatment of the distal radial fractures (DRF) in the last decade. In particular, the devices have made it possible for the general orthopaedic surgeon to surgically fix almost all fractures, and even the severe DRF is not only for the specialized hand surgeon or high-volume centres. The approach, the technique and the implants have made the operations in many ways simple. However, not all fractures are the same, and there are fractures in which we need alternative treatment and devices. Today, the difficult part of treating DRFs is to recognize the fractures that do need special considerations, to know one's personal ability to master the different techniques and to know the pros and cons of the salvage procedures.

23.2 Plates

With the introduction of implants designed specifically for the distal radius, the open technique has become increasingly popular. Although the newer implants are superior in achieving stability the older concepts are still in use.

- Standard AO-plates and screws can be used with acceptable results in most fractures (Keating et al. 1994). However, to get a good stability compensating for the absent locking capabilities of the screws, usually two or more columns (see below) of the radial cortex have

L.M. Hove et al. (eds.), *Distal Radius Fractures*,
DOI 10.1007/978-3-642-54604-4_23,

to be fixated to achieve the good results. For Smith-Barton fractures, the old volar plates functioned sufficiently as buttress plates supporting the volarly dislocated fragment. With a comminuted fracture and intra-articular extension also in the AP plane, the locking screws definitely have their advantage.

- The pi plate, another older concept, was named after its shape similar to the Greek symbol π and designed to fit on the dorsal side of the radial metaphysis. Good results have been reported but interference with the extensor tendons and high complication rates have been noted (Krukhaug and Hove 2004) and the plate is hardly in use anymore. A change in the design of the dorsal plate has been deemed necessary, and new dorsal plates are being designed and tried in some centres.
- The dorsal nail plate (DNP) is a relatively new implant implanted through a less invasive technique, with a minimum of soft tissue exposure. The plate is inserted through a 3–4-cm long incision on the dorsal side of the wrist and introduced into the medullary canal. It is fixed with screws on the proximal (nail) side of the fracture and threaded or polished locked multidirectional pegs on the distal (plate) side of the fracture. It has been suggested as a good alternative to regular plate fixation when less invasive surgery is desired. Small clinical patient series have been published showing good clinical results on par with the volar plate in a randomized series (Chappuis et al. 2011).

23.2.1 The Three-Column Concept

- The three-column concept was introduced (Rikli et al. 2003) as a helpful biomechanical model for understanding the pathomechanics of wrist fractures. It addresses the individual parts of the fractured wrist separately, "the columns," forming the foundation for the articular surface. The concept is relevant in particular in intra-articular fractures, since these are complex and the treatment sometimes has to be individualized.

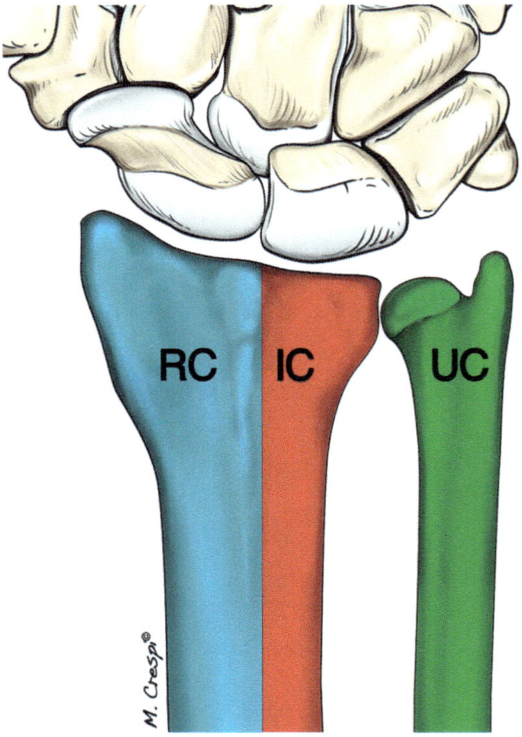

Fig. 23.1 The three-column concept is a helpful biomechanical model for understanding the pathomechanics of wrist fractures. The radial column (*RC*) includes the radial styloid and scaphoid fossa, the intermediate column (*IC*) consists of the lunate fossa and sigmoid notch (distal radioulnar joint, DRUJ), and the ulnar column (*UC*) comprises the distal ulna (DRUJ) with the triangular fibrocartilaginous complex (TFCC)

- Familiarity to the three-column concept helps in visualizing the dislocating forces and patterns and definitely helps in the preoperative appreciation of the fracture and choice of necessary interventions.
- According to the concept, the distal radius and distal ulna form a three-column biomechanical construction (Fig. 23.1):
  - The ulnar column is the distal ulna, the triangular fibrocartilage and the distal radioulnar joint.
  - The intermediate column is the medial part of the distal radius, with the lunate fossa and the sigmoid notch.
  - The radial column is the lateral radius with the scaphoid fossa and the styloid process.
- Analysing a fracture with the three-column concept in mind, stabilization after reduction

requires buttressing of the intermediate column as well as the radial column, and in case of a fractured distal ulna, the ulnar column in some cases needs to be stabilized as well.

- Further, intra-articular fragments once elevated and secured surgically often but not always need to have a bone graft supporting the joint. With the wire form technique, providing a support immediately beneath the subchondral bone, and with the wire form secured by a screw further proximally where the bone quality is better, the graft can be avoided. A step-off in the radiocarpal joint >2 mm will lead to osteoarthritis of the joint in time (Kopylov et al. 1993), which could be painful and lead to compromised function. A step-off in the distal radioulnar joint also will lead to osteoarthritis.
- A step-off of the cortex proximal to the DRUJ does not lead to osteoarthritis but is indicative of a malposition of the radius in the frontal plane. The proximal shaft is always found approaching the ulna with a decreased distance between the two bones. If left unnoticed, a painful and limited rotation of the forearm might be the end result, due to the loss of the curvature of the radius allowing for the full rotation around the ulnar head.
- The ulna is considered to be a separate column, and the ulnar head forms the foundation of the DRUJ upon which the radius bone and the attached hand rotate. The treatment of the distal radius fractures should provide meticulous reconstruction of the DRUJ surface, with stable internal fixation and preferably early functional post-operative treatment. There is a controversy whether a traumatic tear of the TFCC should be repaired or not or if it is enough to restore the anatomy and the articular congruity.

23.3 The Plates Based on the Three-Column Concept

- There are at present two types of plates addressing the surgical solutions from a three-column perspective: the LCP system from Synthes building on the Rikli and Regazzoni ideas and the Fragment-Specific System by Medoff.
  - The Synthes system uses fixed-angle screws and plates with options to secure the position of the separate radial and ulnar columns individually from the radial side as well as ulnar/volar and ulnar/dorsal side. A specific plate is used to handle very distal volar rim fractures.
  - The Fragment-Specific System by Medoff is also based on the three-column concept but also addresses the radial, intermediate and ulnar columns separately, as well as single osteochondral fracture fragments both dorsally and at the volar rim, by a combination of plates, pins and screws. The system is primarily based on pinning of the fracture. Since additional stability is needed to prevent the pins from bending or the fragments from sliding on the pins, a stabilizing plate is added proximally to secure the pins. In addition, wire forms to support the subchondral bone, or small fragments can be used also with a screw fixation proximally. The system is low profile and offers good stability (Konrath and Bahler 2002).
- The fracture by both systems is approached through a radial incision through the first extensor compartment for placement of the pins and fixation with a radial pin plate and secondly through a second incision through the fourth compartment for fixation with wire forms, buttress pins and ulnar pin plate.
- Also a volar approach and a dorsal approach can be performed to secure the fracture with buttress pins. The surgical approach is determined by the type of fracture and the type of fixation needed to address the fragments.

23.4 Volar Locking Plates with Variable Screw Angles

- The newest concept, the volar locking plates with angle stable screws or pegs are becoming widely used as it offers stability and a safe approach to the fracture. The fracture is approached from the volar side using the Henry approach just radially to the flexor carpi radials, ulnarly to the radial artery. This offers an easy access to the volar part of the radius.

  - The volar locking plate has, in biomechanical testing, been shown to be sufficiently stable for fixation of the dorsally comminuted fracture and offer equivalent stability when compared to the fragment-specific fixation (Taylor et al. 2006).
  - The best stability is provided by a combination of a volar locking plate with the Fragment-Specific System (Grindel et al. 2007). Good clinical results have been reported in a few case series. Complications such as tendon ruptures have been reported (Arora 2007). No randomized study has been published yet comparing this concept to conventional DRF fixation in a clinical setting.

23.5 Fractures That Need Special Attention

- When selecting the optimal plate for the special fracture, a biomechanical approach has to be considered at preoperative planning; one has to imagine what the redislocating forces to be neutralized are and customize the choice accordingly.
- The Ulnarization of the Radius Shaft
  - A very common dislocation is the ulnarization of the proximal radius fragment – the shaft – caused by the pulling force of the pronator quadratus. A step-off can be seen (Fig. 23.2a) on the ulnar border of the radius sometimes appearing within the distal radius ulna joint or more common proximal to the joint. Often a rotation of the distal fragment relative to the shaft is also present. Impossible to manipulate using closed reduction, the malposition can be difficult to correct even by open reduction, and in particular, the position once achieved might be difficult to retain by the regular volar plate.
  - A reposition manoeuvre can be attempted and the radius and ulna shaft are spread apart manually using a hook (Fig. 23.2b). Often the dorsal compression and the rotation of the distal fragment are reduced at the same time. The reduced position can be maintained by a temporary pin from the radial styloid directed proximally and ulnarly, and the regular volar fixed-angle plate can be used. The radial approach is superior when an anatomic alignment of the shaft relative to the distal fragment is not possible by the volar approach. Using the Fragment-Specific System, the temporary pin is threaded onto the radial pin plate and the radioulnar malposition corrected as the proximal radial screws of the plate are tightened.
- The Intra-articular Fracture
  - In an intra-articular fracture with an ulnarized proximal radius shaft, the radial pin plate or the radial plate is preferentially supplemented with a fixation device for the lunate fossa fragment.
  - A major advantage with one plate for the radial column and one for the intermediate column is the option to reposition and secure the fragments independently of each other. Even with the radial pin plate fixed to the bone, the lunate fossa fragment can be reduced, and both a rotatory and a die-punch impaction of the fragment can be reduced and secured by a volar buttress pin or an ulnar column plate.
  - Especially in a three-fragment fracture with the ulnar lunate fragment divided in two or more pieces, the position is not possible to maintain from the volar approach, but a separate dorsal approach is needed and a dorsal ulnar pin plate or a dorsal plate is used for dorsal support to stabilize the construct (see figures of authors' preferred method).
- The Watershed Line Fracture
  - In distal volar lip fractures, the regular volar plate is unable to fix the fragment with the distal screws being too proximal not reaching the distal fragment (Fig. 23.3). With a fracture distal to the watershed line, the joint capsule insertion has been disrupted, and the fracture remains unstable and susceptible to secondary dislocation even after volar plate fixation. Alternative solutions must be applied to be able to address and support the distal fragment to avoid a subluxation of the joint.
  - A volar buttress pin can be inserted very distal, juxta-articularily, through the fragment,

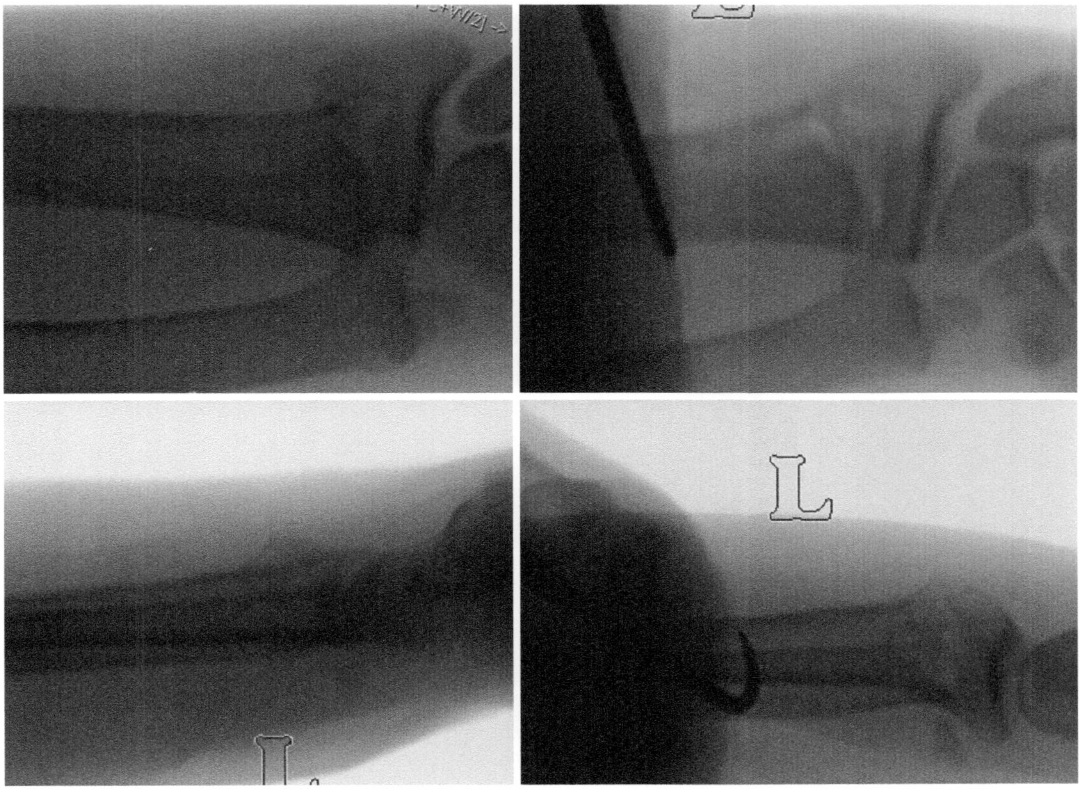

Fig. 23.2 (**a**) The ulnarized radius shaft and B/ the reposition manoeuvre. By the force of the pronator quadratus, the proximal shaft of the radius is converging to the ulna, and in consequence the distal fragment is rotated and angulated dorsally. (**b**) By using a "single-ended hook," the radial shaft and the ulna are separated by force, and often all three malposition components are reduced

and if applied correctly the pin supports the subchondral bone (see figures of authors' preferred method). Alternatively, a plate with adjustable angles of the distal screws can be used allowing for a more distal position of the plate. With this method also comminuted distal fractures can be securely fixated during the healing period.

- The Chauffeur's Fracture Combined with a Dorsal Distal Fragment or Articular Marginal Shearing Fractures
  - The regular two-fragment chauffeur's fracture is benign and can be treated with the regular volar plate or a simple compression screw. However, when combined with a comminuted dorsal fragment, the injury should be regarded as severely unstable (Fig. 23.4).
  - This fracture is often the result of a high-energy injury and is part of a shearing marginal fracture. Intraoperatively it may be difficult to reduce the joint line for congruity, and a combination of a radial pin plate, a volar buttress pin and a dorsal pin plate should preferentially be used. Only exact reposition should be aimed for.
- The Dorsal Ulnar Fragment
  - In some intra-articular fractures, compression forces from the lunate causes the dorsal rim of the radius, consisting of the dorsal part of the lunate fossa, to dislocate dorsally (Fig. 23.5).
  - The fragment is small and often difficult to secure with the standard volar locking plate. Sometimes, the fragment can be reached from the volar side, but the screw length might be difficult to control, on one hand long enough to engage the fragment but at the same time not too long endangering the dorsal tendons. Therefore, a dorsal

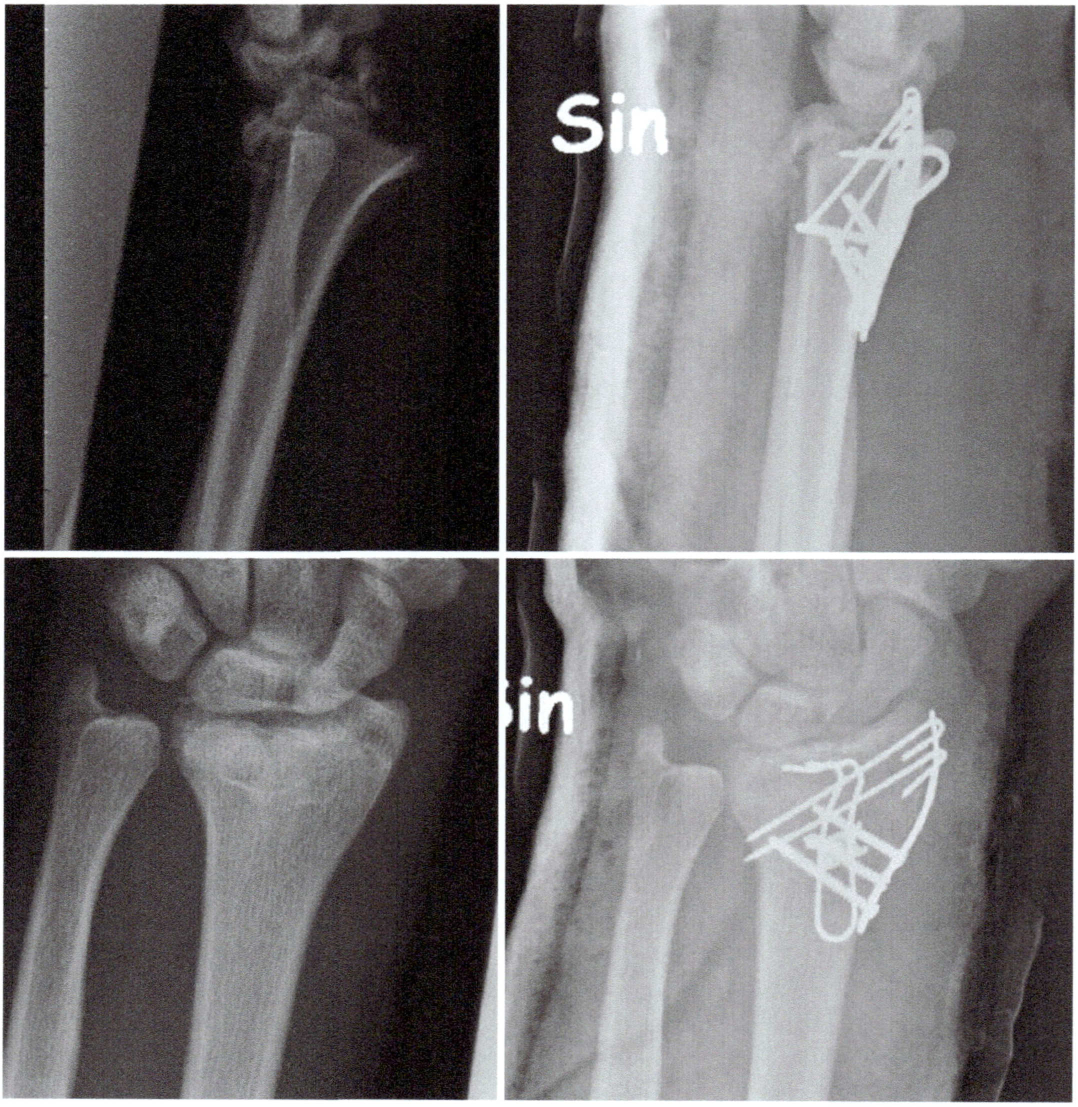

Fig. 23.3 The avulsed volar lip fracture. The volar capsule is avulsed from the volar insertion. The fragment is out of reach for a volar plate and the volar buttress pin is preferred

approach is the preferred method to secure reposition and fixation using a small dorsal plate or an ulnar pin plate.

23.6 Salvage Procedures

23.6.1 When Bony Support is Missing for Screw Fixation

- Still, in the practice of the specialized distal radius fracture surgeon, there will be fractures that are so comminuted that there actually are no possibilities to secure a plate to a comminuted or severely osteoporotic bone. These cases are unusual but alternatives must be mastered intraoperatively when the attempted fixation method fails.
  - *The external fixator* was previously the golden standard to which any new treatment was compared. In comparison, open reduction has been shown to be superior to external fixation regarding both subjective and radiographic results and range of motion (Abramo et al. 2009; Wilcke et al. 2011). However, there are still indications

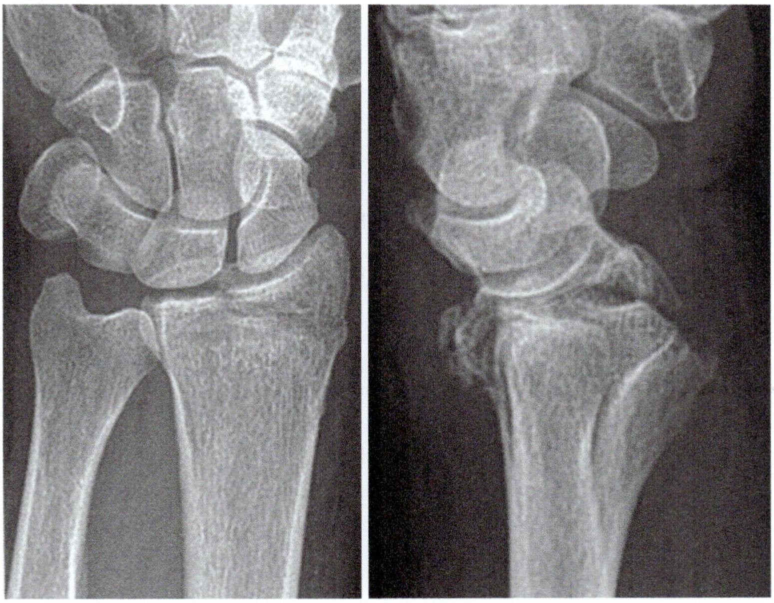

Fig. 23.4 The chauffeur's fracture. The chauffeur's fracture can be the effect of a pure shearing force or a part of a more complex high-energy fracture extending up into the carpal bones. The first is easily managed by a volar plate, whereas the second sometimes is difficult to reduce and fix

for an external fixation (see Chap. 17) in severe comminuted fractures and maybe especially in the very old patient with a bone quality that cannot hold the fixation of the screws.

– *The bridging plate* can be used as an "internal" external fixator. A dorsal 3.5-mm AO/ASIF plate is applied by open surgery extra-articularly from the radius to the third metacarpal under traction. The comminuted segment is bypassed and the articular surface can be anatomically reduced and secured with Kirschner wires or screws. The plate is removed after fracture consolidation and wrist motion initiated. Good/acceptable results have been reported but should only be used as the last resort due to the extreme joint fixation time (Ginn et al. 2006).

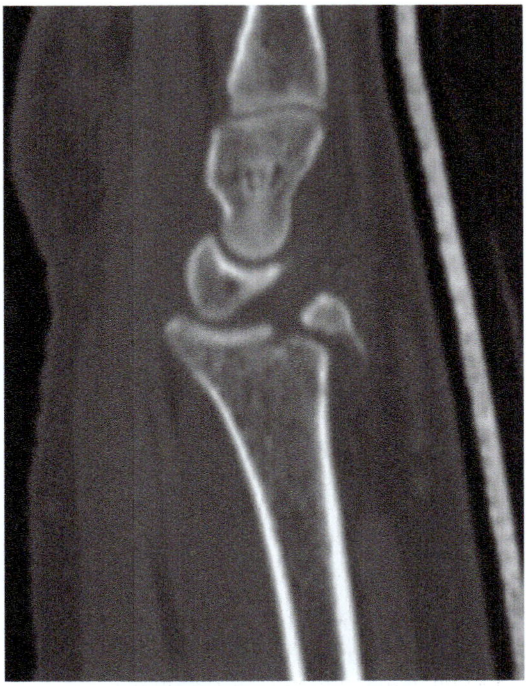

Fig. 23.5 The dorsal ulnar fragment

23.7 Surgical Technique: The Authors' Preferred Method

- Based on the analysis of the fracture and fragments in need of fixation, the approach can and should differ from time to time. We use three standard approaches in the majority of the fracture types above, when the standard fixed-angle volar plate might not be the optimal choice (Fig. 23.6).
- The Radial/Radiovolar Approach
  - A 6–7-cm long incision is made over the first extensor compartment. (Fig. 23.6c, d) Care is taken, not to injure the branches of the radial nerve.
  - After reposition a pin is inserted at the small flat area on the tip of the radial styloid,

dorsal to the first compartment, in a proximal and ulnar direction (Fig. 23.6e–l).
  - The first compartment is opened and the brachioradialis tendon detached to give place for the radial pin plate. The radial pin plate is threaded over the pin (Fig. 23.6m), gently positioned underneath the tendons and secured to the radial shaft proximally with a 2.3-mm screw (Fig. 23.6n, o).
  - The radioulnar malposition as seen in the AP view, mentioned in 1/ above, is often corrected as the screws securing the plate are tightened, thereby repositioning the radial styloid fragment on to the shaft.
  - For the first screw, we use a short screw to make it easier to secure the plate position and thereafter bicortical screws.
  - A second pin is inserted and 2–3 additional screws are inserted and tightened with bicortical fixation. The two pins are retracted, bent and then pushed back into the pinholes in the plate securing the pins (Fig. 23.6s–u).
- The Volar Approach
  - A separate volar incision using a standard FCR approach is preferred, identical to the volar locking plate technique (Fig. 23.6c–f). The volar cortex can be reached by the radial approach, but the FCR approach enables access to the whole volar part of the distal radius especially the lunate facet.
  - For large fragments proximal to the watershed line variable, angle locking plates can be used, but for extreme distal fragments, the volar buttress pin is the fixation device of choice.
  - Two pins are introduced 1 cm apart into the distal fragment immediately proximal to the subchondral bone, guiding for the legs of the volar buttress pin. From the tip of the teardrop of the radial border, the pins should be introduced at an angle of approximately 70° (Fig. 23.6g, h).
  - The volar buttress pin legs are cut, one being longer than the other to ease insertion and not to extend beyond the dorsal cortex. The pins are removed one at a time and replaced by the buttress pin legs introduced under the subchondral bone to support the joint line (Fig. 23.6i, j).
  - The volar buttress pin is finally secured into the radial shaft by 1–2 screws and the washer holding the two legs in compression.
- The Dorsal Approach
  - A straight skin incision and a retinacular incision between the fourth and the third extensor compartment are made. The tendons are retracted and the retinaculum is sharply lifted of the Lister tubercle providing an excellent approach to the major parts of the dorsal radius (Fig. 23.6d, p, q).
  - With this approach it is possible to address the dorsal ulnar fragment of the lunate fossa as well as a dorsally comminuted fracture.
  - For the dorsal ulnar fragment, an ulnar pin plate is preferred with the pins from the distal ulnar corner of the radius reaching the volar intact cortex. The pin plate can be contoured to better fit on the ulnar border of the radius (Fig. 23.6r–t).
  - For a complex, dorsally comminuted fracture, there may be a need to additionally fix the dorsal fragments as well as the intermediate fragments, in between the DRUJ facet fragments and the radial styloid.
  - A dorsal buttress pin positioned underneath the subchondral bone lifts the joint surface and re-establishes a congruent joint line.
  - Two pins 1 cm apart are inserted from the dorsal side subchondrally.
  - The pins are replaced with the legs on the buttress pin, which is inserted fully.
  - The proximal part of the buttress pin is then pushed onto the radial shaft, and this manoeuvre can be used to further lift the joint line in place.
  - The buttress pin is finally secured with one to two screws and a washer.

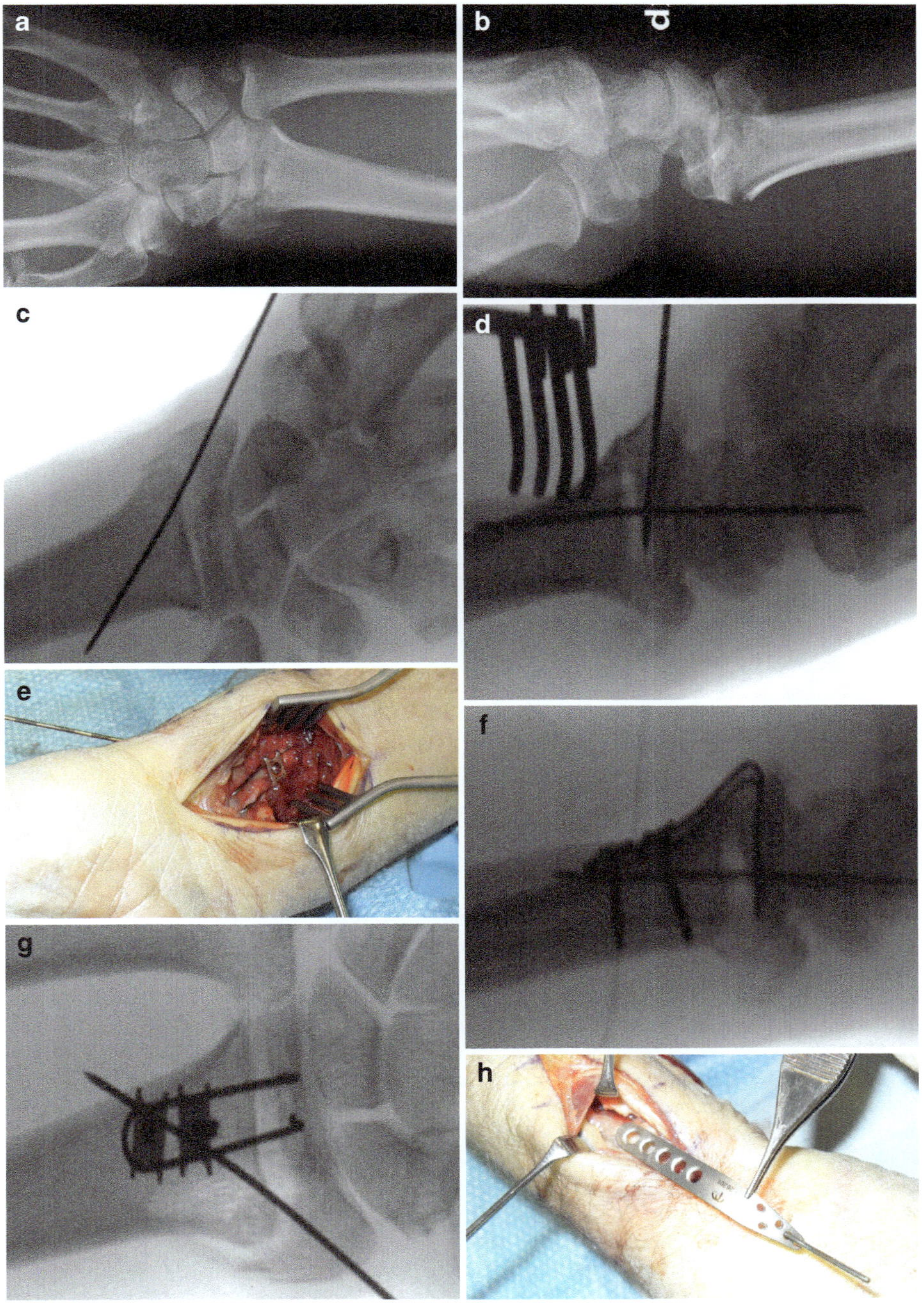

Fig. 23.6 The authors' preferred method. (**a**, **b**) A comminuted fracture showing a distal fracture of the lunate fossa close to the watershed line and a comminuted styloid fragment. (**c**) The fracture is reduced and one or two pins are used for provisional fixation. (**f**); (**d**) With a provisional pin in the styloid, a standard volar FCR approach is established. The distal volar lip fragment is pinned from the tear drop in a dorsal, slightly proximal direction immediately underneath the subchondral bone. A second pin is inserted and exchanged for the final volar buttress pin. (**h**); (**e**, **f**, **g**): The volar buttress pin is secured by screws and washers proximally. (**l**); (**h**, **i**) The radial side is opened and a pin is driven in an ulnar and proximal direction with the insertion point dorsal of the first compartment. The radial pin plate is threaded onto the radial pin and secured with screws. The radial pin plate is secured with screws proximally. (**j**) The dorsal side is opened, the retinaculum divided and the space between the 3rd and 4th compartment developed. A pin is inserted in a volar and proximal direction and an ulnar pin plate threaded onto the pin and secured with screws proximally. (**k**, **l**) The final result with proximal screws inserted into good bone proximally and with the pins and wire form compressing the fracture from three sides against the ulna establishing an adequate stability

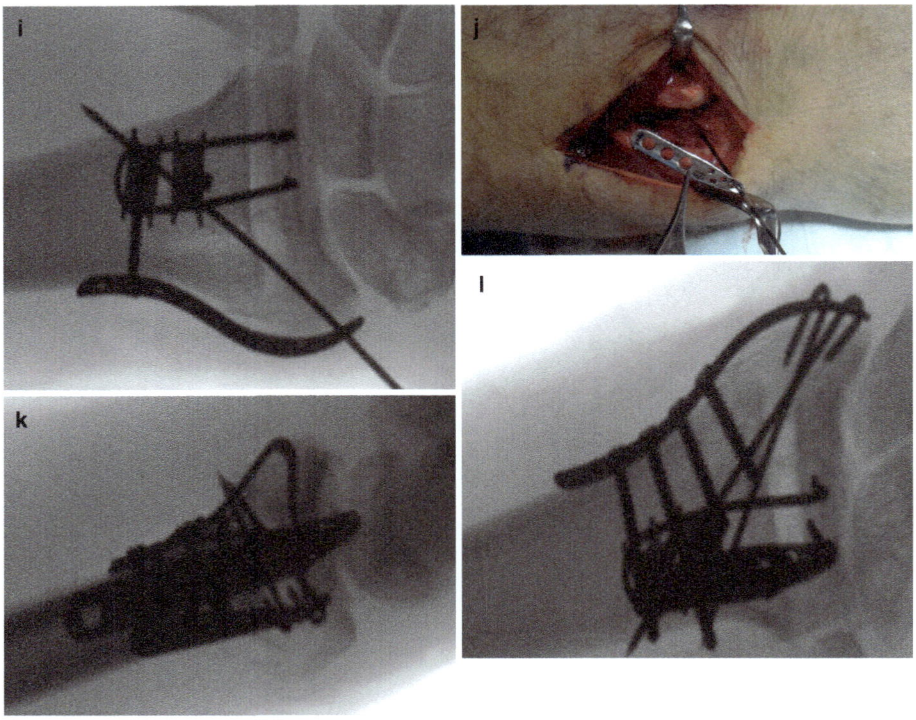

Fig. 23.6 (continued)

References

Abramo A, Kopylov P, Geijer M, Tagil M. Open reduction and internal fixation compared to closed reduction and external fixation in distal radial fractures: a randomized study of 50 patients. Acta Orthop. 2009;80(4):478–85.

Arora R, Lutz M, Hennerbichler A, Krappinger D, Espen D, Gabl M. Complications following internal fixation of unstable distal radius fracture with a palmar locking-plate. J Orthop Trauma. 2007;21(5):316–22.

Chappuis J, Boute P, Putz P. Dorsally displaced extra-articular distal radius fractures fixation: dorsal IM nailing versus volar plating. A randomized controlled trial. Orthop Traumatol Surg Res. 2011;97(5):471–8.

Ginn TA, Ruch DS, Yang CC, Hanel DP. Use of a distraction plate for distal radial fractures with metaphyseal and diaphyseal comminution. Surgical technique. J Bone Joint Surg Am. 2006;88 Suppl 1:29–36.

Grindel SI, Wang M, Gerlach M, McGrady LM, Brown S. Biomechanical comparison of fixed-angle volar plate versus fixed-angle volar plate plus fragment-specific fixation in a cadaveric distal radius fracture model. J Hand Surg Am. 2007;32(2):194–9.

Keating JF, Court-Brown CM, McQueen MM. Internal fixation of volar-displaced distal radial fractures. J Bone Joint Surg Br. 1994;76(3):401–5.

Konrath GA, Bahler S. Open reduction and internal fixation of unstable distal radius fractures: results using the trimed fixation system. J Orthop Trauma. 2002; 16(8):578–85.

Kopylov P, Johnell O, Redlund-Johnell I, Bengner U. Fractures of the distal end of the radius in young adults: a 30-year follow-up. J Hand Surg Br. 1993; 18(1):45–9.

Krukhaug Y, Hove LM. Experience with the AO Pi-plate for displaced intra-articular fractures of the distal radius. Scand J Plast Reconstr Surg Hand Surg. 2004;38(5):293–6.

Rikli DA, Regazzoni P, Babst R. Dorsal double plating for fractures of the distal radius–a biomechanical concept and clinical experience. Zentralbl Chir. 2003; 128(12):1003–7.

Taylor KF, Parks BG, Segalman KA. Biomechanical stability of a fixed-angle volar plate versus fragment-specific fixation system: cyclic testing in a c2-type distal radius cadaver fracture model. J Hand Surg Am. 2006;31(3):373–81.

Wilcke MK, Abbaszadegan H, Adolphson PY. Wrist function recovers more rapidly after volar locked plating than after external fixation but the outcomes are similar after 1 year. Acta Orthop. 2011;82(1): 76–81.

Die-Punch Fractures: Open and Arthroscopy-Assisted Fixation

24

Jarkko Vasenius

Contents

J. Vasenius, MD
Hand Surgery and Therapy, Omasairaala Hospital, Helsinki, Finland
e-mail: jarkko.vasenius@kolumbus.fi

24.1 Summary

Intra-articular compression fractures through the lunate facet of the distal radius are often caused by high-energy trauma. They can cause severe comminution of the joint surface and concomitant ligamentous injuries in extrinsic and intrinsic radiocarpal ligaments as well as distal radioulnar joint. Restoration of the articular surfaces is the most critical factor in achieving good results. In addition to regular radiographs, computed tomograms or cone-beam computed tomogram with or without arthrography is valuable in preoperative planning. Perioperatively the most reliable method in visualization of intra-articular fragments and ligaments is arthroscopy or arthrotomy together with image intensifier irrespective of fixation method used. Concomitant ligamentous injuries are repaired simultaneously with fracture fixation. Substantial experience in other arthroscopic procedures in the wrist is a prerequisite for the arthroscopy-assisted technique.

24.2 Introduction

Intra-articular fractures of distal radius with medial articular (lunate facet, intermediate column) impression were named die-punch fracture first by Scheck in 1962. Today only an impression fracture of dorso-ulnar corner is considered a die-punch fracture (Fig. 24.1). However, lunate facet can be shattered in many other ways, in several

L.M. Hove et al. (eds.), *Distal Radius Fractures*,
DOI 10.1007/978-3-642-54604-4_24, © Springer-Verlag Berlin Heidelberg 2014

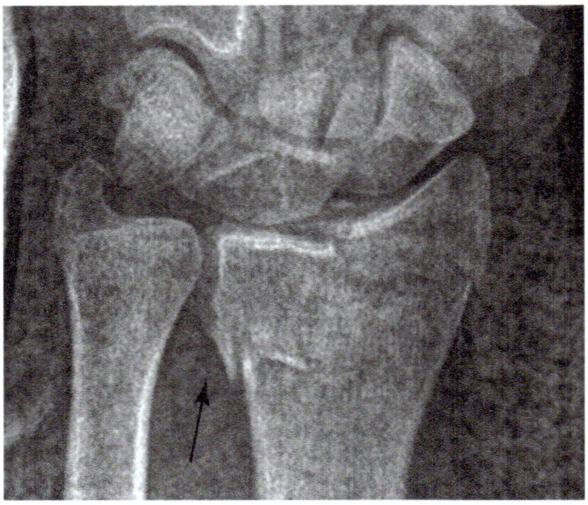

Fig. 24.1 A typical die-punch fragment shown by an *arrow* after insufficient closed reduction and immobilization with dorsal plaster cast

pieces, and in several directions. They are usually caused by a high-energy impact of the carpal bones against the distal joint surface of distal radius causing comminution of radiocarpal and sometimes also radioulnar joints. These fractures are very unstable and concomitant ligamentous injuries such as partial or complete tears of scapholunate ligament or TFCC occur in 30–54 % of intra-articular fractures of distal end of radius (Geissler et al. 1996; Lindau et al. 1997). Patients are often young adults. If residual incongruity is present after fracture consolidation, the occurrence of osteoarthritis is 76–91 % 7 years after injury (Catalano et al. 1997; Knirk and Jupiter 1986). Restoration of articular surface is the most critical factor in achieving good results.

24.3 Pre- and Perioperative Examinations

- Clinical examination of the wrist cannot be done properly in fresh fractures.
- Reliable evaluation of radiocarpal and distal radioulnar joint congruency is not always possible with radiographs or image intensifier.
- Therefore preoperative computed tomograms or cone-beam computed tomogram with or without arthrography is valuable in preoperative planning (Koskinen et al. 2013) (Fig. 24.2).
- Perioperative arthroscopic or open visualization of intra-articular fragments is the most reliable method for good reduction and diagnostics of ligamentous injuries.

24.4 Traditional Open Surgical Techniques

- Kirschner wires + cancellous bone graft + external fixator
- Dorsal fragment-specific plate
  - Before introduction of angular stable volar plates, the reduction and stabilization of intermediate column fractures were usually performed through dorsal open approach with K-wires and cancellous bone graft, which is still a valid method. However, bone grafting causes some donor site morbidity. If the radial column is also fractured, an external fixator is often applied to prevent reimpression of fragments (Fig. 24.3a). In very comminuted intra-articular fractures, an additional volar buttress plate can be applied to support small fragments.
  - By using angular stable plates, a solid die-punch fracture can be stabilized through open dorsal approach with a fragment-specific plate (Fig. 24.3b, c). Reduction of the fracture and repair of possible intercarpal ligament injuries can be done through dorsal arthrotomy, but one should be careful not to cut radiotriquetral ligament. Tethering of this ligament may cause ulnar translocation of the carpal bones. A narrow volar rim fragment that contains insertion of radiolunar ligaments may cause volar dislocation of proximal row. Fixation of this fragment can be very tricky and redislocations occur frequently. Fragment-specific plates with holes for ligament sutures can be utilized for this fracture type (Fig. 24.4).

24.5 Arthroscopy-Assisted Surgical Technique

- Dorso-ulnar fragment fixation with
  - K-wire
  - Dorsal fragment-specific plate or screw

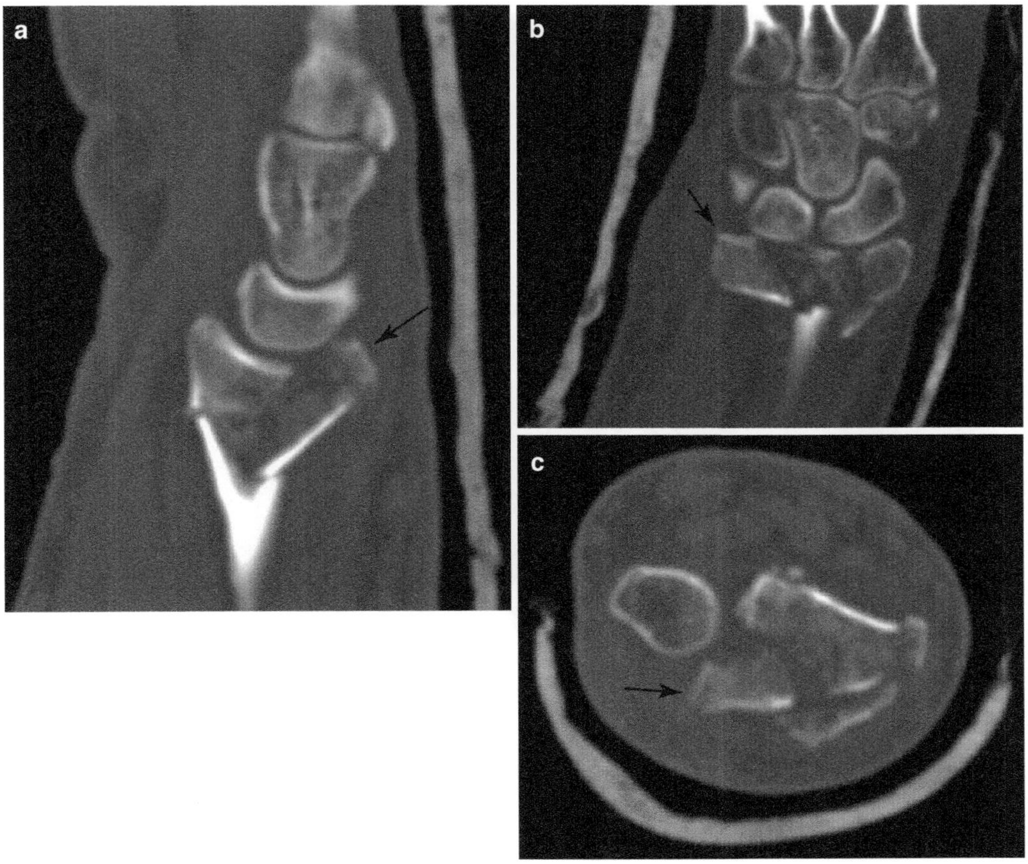

Fig. 24.2 (**a–c**) Preoperative computed tomography gives valuable information of intra-articular fragments for preoperative planning. Dorso-ulnar corner fragment is marked with an *arrow*

- Volar rim fragment fixation with
  - Volar fragment-specific plate or screw
  - Arthroscopic suture technique
- Substantial experience in other arthroscopic procedures in the wrist is a prerequisite for this method. Arthroscopy-assisted technique includes application of volar angular stable plate that is fixed with proximal screws only before introducing the arthroscope.
- A temporary fixation of distal fragments with K-wires inserted through specific plate holes can be done before arthroscopy (Fig. 24.5).
- Then two radiocarpal portals, ¾ and 6R, are established and dry arthroscopy method is used (del Pinal et al. 2007). Under arthroscopic control articular impressions and ligamentous injuries are evaluated. If the primary reduction is insufficient, the K-wires are backed out and impressed fragments are then elevated with an elevator or probe and fixed again with K-wires. During this procedure arthroscope is in the 6R portal, while the probe or elevator are used in the ¾ portal. The reduction is also checked with fluoroscope before precise insertion of distal locking screws.
- A separate narrow dorso-ulnar fragment containing parts of articular facets of distal radioulnar and radiocarpal joints as well as insertion of dorsal radioulnar ligaments of the TFCC may not be sufficiently fixed with distal screws inserted through the volar plate. If it is left insufficiently reduced and fixed, instability of DRUJ occurs.
- Dorso-ulnar corner fragment can be fixed either with percutaneous K-wire inserted by using Kapandji technique (Fig. 24.6), with a dorsal screw or with a fragment-specific dorsal plate (Fig. 24.3).
- An arthroscopic technique to reattach an avulsed volar rim was presented by Del Pinal (2010) (Fig. 24.7).

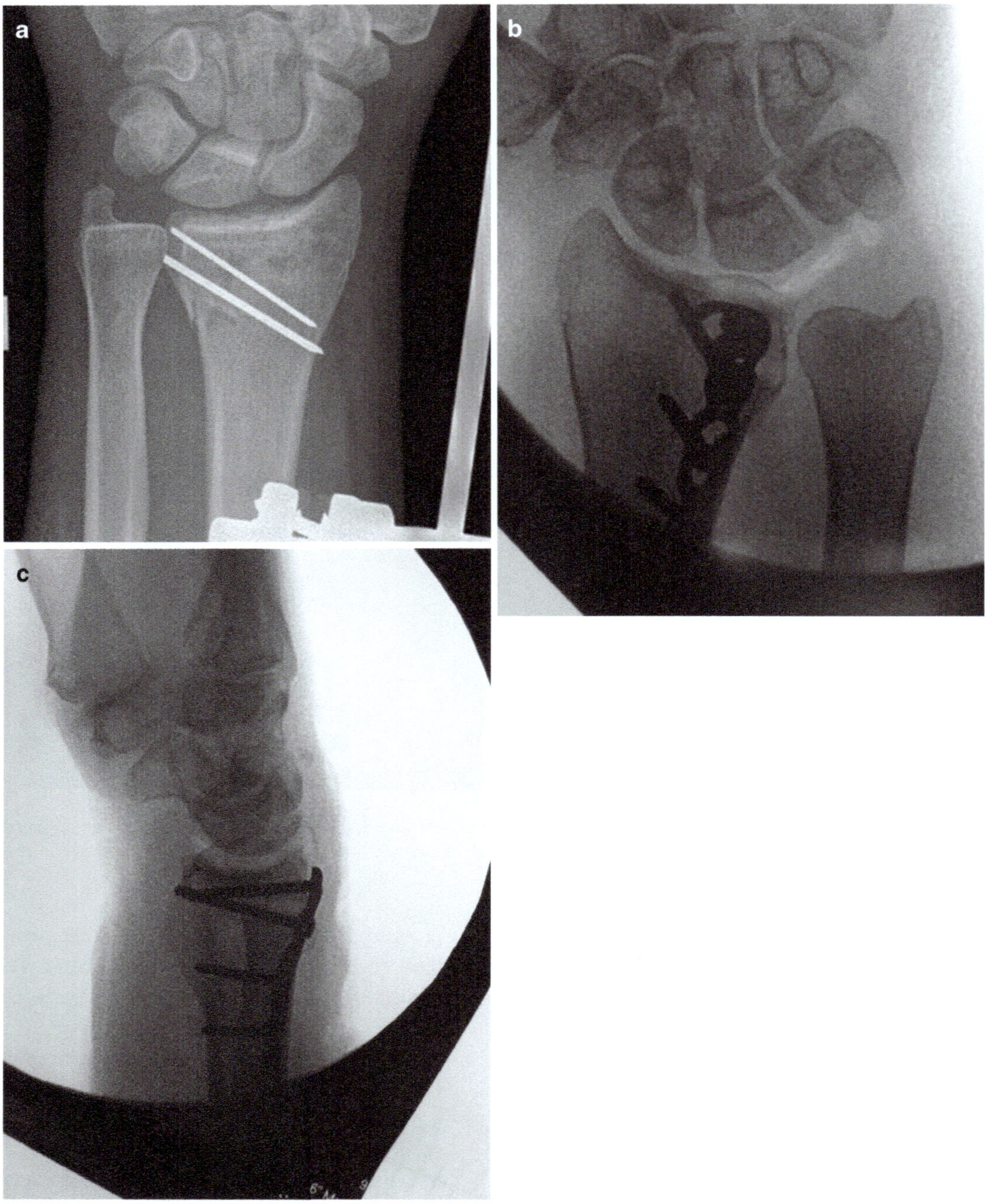

Fig. 24.3 (**a**–**c**) A die-punch fracture fixed with K-wires and external fixator (**a**) or with fragment-specific dorsal angular stable screw plate (**b**, **c**)

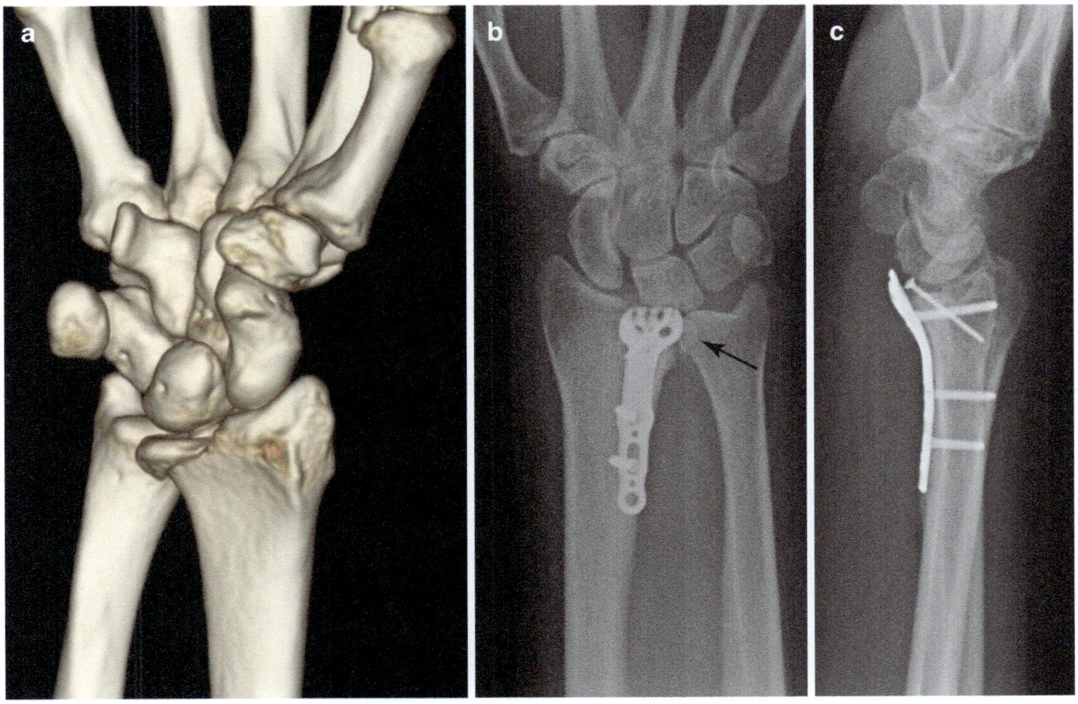

Fig. 24.4 (**a**–**c**) A 3D computed tomography image of a volar rim avulsion fracture (**a**). Redislocation of a volar fragment (*arrow*) after insufficient fixation with a fragment-specific plate and a screw (**b**, **c**)

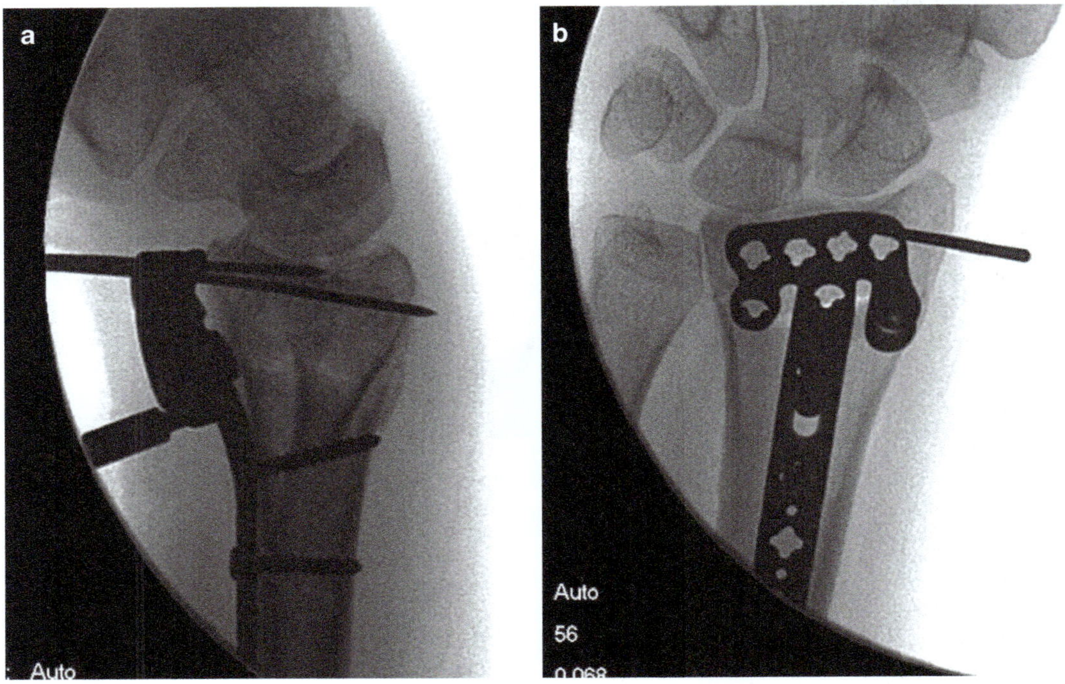

Fig. 24.5 (**a**, **b**) After careful positioning of the plate and insertion of two proximal screws, temporary fixation of distal fragment is done with K-wires inserted through the specific holes in the plate before beginning of the arthroscopy

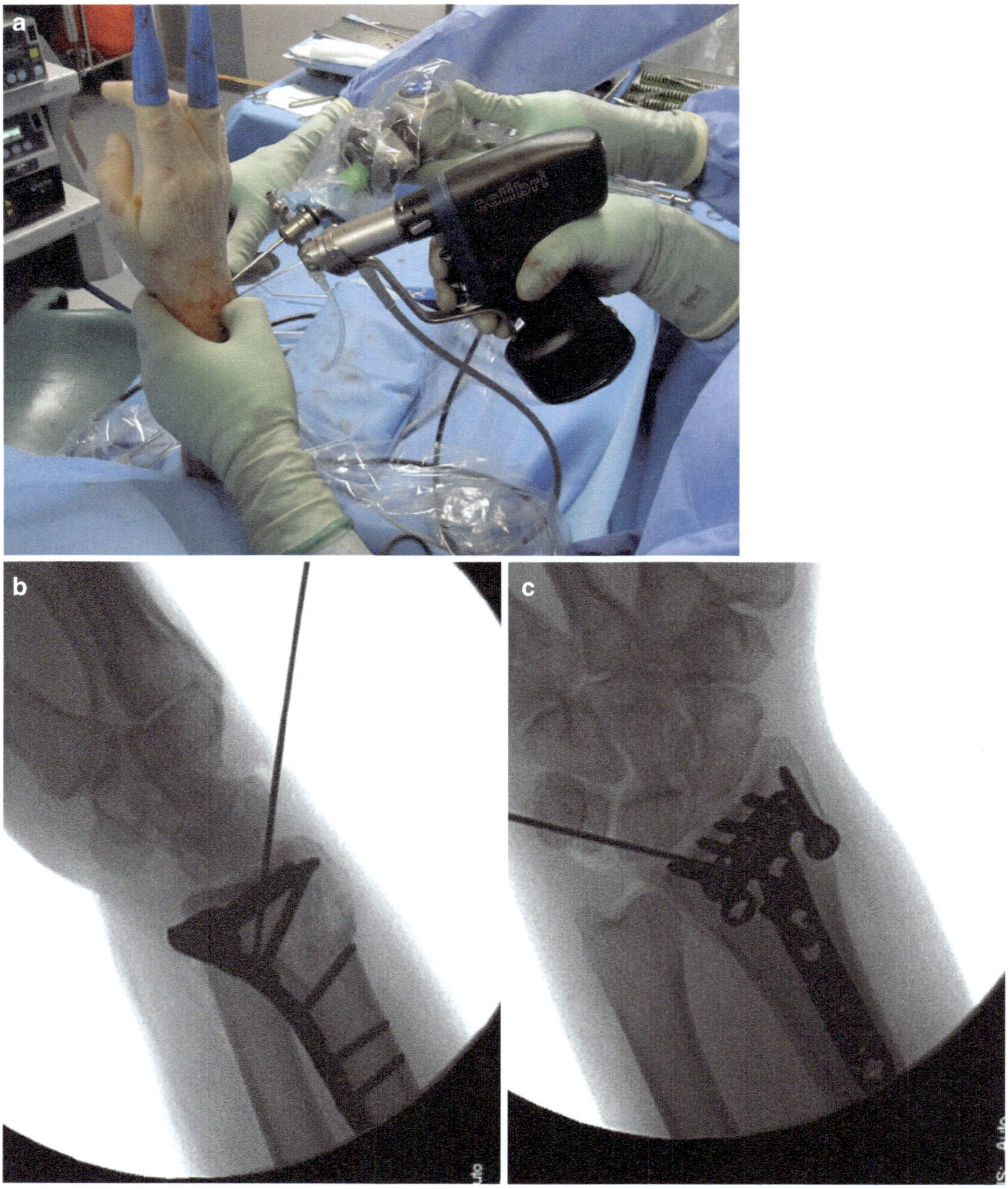

Fig. 24.6 (**a**–**c**) After fixation of other fragments with volar locking screw plate, the dorso-ulnar corner fragment is fixed with an additional K-wire inserted by using Kapandji method and arthroscopy and fluoroscopy control. During reduction the arthroscope is in the 6R portal

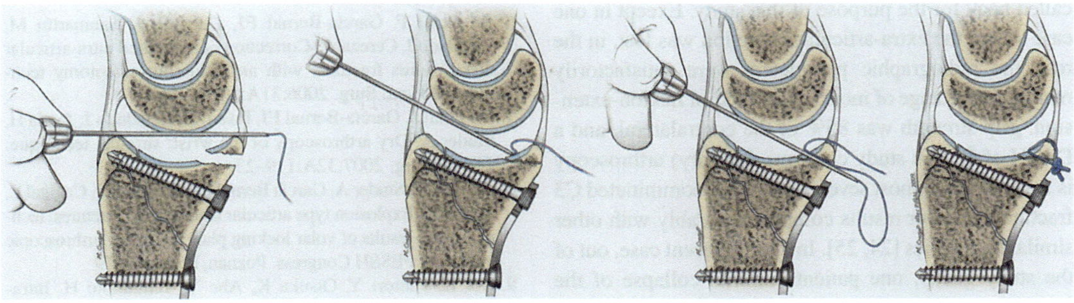

Fig. 24.7 Arthroscopically assisted fixation technique of volar osteochondral avulsion fragment utilizing an epidural-type Touhy or Rodiera's needle (Courtesy of Dr. del Pinal)

24.6 Postoperative Treatment

- A dorsal synthetic short arm cast is worn for 2 weeks if the fixation of all fragments is stable.
- A non-weight-bearing mobilization is begun thereafter and a removable commercial splint is worn between exercises and hand washings for 3 more weeks.
- If there is doubt about the stability of the fixation, short arm cast is worn for 5 weeks, and the mobilization is begun thereafter with guidance of a hand physiotherapist.

References

Catalano 3rd LW, Cole RJ, Gelberman RH, Evanoff BA, Gilula LA, Borrelli J. Displaced intra-articular fractures of the distal aspect of the radius: long-term results in young adults after open reduction and internal fixation. J Bone Joint Surg Am. 1997;79-A: 1290–302.

del Pinal F, Garcia-Bernal FJ, Pisani D, Regalado J, Ayala H, Studer A. Dry arthroscopy of the wrist: surgical technique. J Hand Surg. 2007;32-A:119–23.

del Pinal F. Treatment of explosion-type distal radius fractures. In: del Pinal F, Mathoulin C, Luchetti R, editors. Arthroscopic management of distal radius fractures. Berlin/Heidelberg: Springer; 2010. p. 41–65.

Geissler WB, Freeland AE, Savoie FH, et al. Intracarpal soft tissue lesions associated with an intra-articular fracture of the distal end of the radius. J Bone Joint Surg Am. 1996;78-A:357–65.

Knirk JL, Jupiter JB. Intra-articular fractures of the distal end of the radius in young adults. J Bone Joint Surg Am. 1986;68-A:647–59.

Koskinen SK, Haapamäki VV, Salo J, Lindfors NC, Kortesniemi M, Seppälä L, Mattila KT. CT arthrography of the wrist using novel, mobile, dedicated extremity cone-beam CT (CBCT). Skeletal Radiol. 2013;42(5):649–57.

Lindau T, Arner M, Hagberg L. Intraarticular lesions in distal fractures of the radius in young adults. A descriptive arthroscopic study in 50 patients. J Hand Surg Br. 1997;22(5):638–43.

Scheck M. Long-term follow-up of treatment of comminuted fractures of the distal end radius by transfixation with Kirschner wires and cast. J Bone Joint Surg. 1962;44-A:337–51.

25 Arthroscopy in Distal Radius Fractures

Lars Adolfsson, Peter Jørgsholm, and Francisco del Piñal

Contents

L. Adolfsson, MD, PhD (✉)
Department of Orthopaedics, Linköping University Hospital, University of Linköping, Linköping, Sweden
e-mail: lars.adolfsson@lio.se

P. Jørgsholm, MD
The Hand Unit, Mølholm Private Hospital, Vejle, Denmark

F. del Piñal, MD, Dr Med
Instituto de Cirugia Plastica y de la Mano, Santander, Spain

Unit of Hand-Wrist and Plastic Surgery, Hospital Mutua Montañes, Paseo de Pereda 20-1, E-39004, Santander, Spain

25.1 Summary

The vast majority of fractures of the distal radius can reliably be treated with conventional methods, but for certain intra-articular fractures, especially those with depressed and impacted central fragments, arthroscopy-assisted reduction may significantly reduce the surgical trauma. The arthroscopic examination also allows improved diagnosis and the possibility of treatment of associated soft tissue injuries which may potentially prevent late development of instability problems and osteoarthrosis. The presented results are unanimously good and no adverse effects have been reported. The method is however technically demanding and sometimes time consuming.

25.2 Introduction

- The majority of distal radial fractures are typically dorsally displaced and extra-articular, usually as a result of a low-energy trauma. In most instances, this type of fracture can be adequately diagnosed by conventional radiography, and treatment is usually uncomplicated with the aim to maintain length and anatomical angulation of the radial bone in order to preserve a stable foundation for the hand and a stable, mobile and pain-free distal radio-ulnar joint.
- In intra-articular fractures a further aim is to restore congruent joint surfaces of the distal radial articulations with the carpus and ulnar head. A residual displacement of the joint

L.M. Hove et al. (eds.), *Distal Radius Fractures*,
DOI 10.1007/978-3-642-54604-4_25, © Springer-Verlag Berlin Heidelberg 2014

surfaces will increase the risk of pain and dysfunction and cause osteoarthritis in the long run.

- In the acute phase, intra-articular displacement is sometimes difficult to appreciate on two-dimensional plain radiography, and CT scan is recommended to facilitate institution of an appropriate treatment. This is particularly important in young individuals where high-energy trauma often is involved (Lindau et al. 1999).
- The use of arthroscopy as a tool to assist in reduction of intra-articular distal radius fractures has been advocated in several reports, all in agreement that an improved reduction can be achieved (Adolfsson and Jørgsholm 1998; Doi et al. 1999; Chen et al. 2002; del Piñal et al. 2007). Although it may appear evident that an improved reduction with minimal surgical trauma would be beneficial for the patient, this has however not been clearly demonstrated, and to date only a few studies with controlled design have been published (Doi et al. 1999; Ruch et al. 2004; Varitimidis et al. 2008).
- Arthroscopy has also been used to diagnose associated soft tissue lesions that frequently occur in connection with the fracture. In particular, TFCC lesions are common and can be found in the majority of markedly displaced distal radial fractures. Also scapholunate ligament lesions have been reported to be quite frequent (Geissler et al. 1996; Lindau et al. 1997; Adolfsson and Jørgsholm 1998). The indications for treatment of associated soft tissue injuries are yet to be established.

25.3 Indications

- Most displaced, intra-articular fractures engaging the distal radius are potentially amenable for arthroscopy-assisted reduction. Particularly in instances when an alternative open reduction would include a considerable soft tissue dissection, an arthroscopic approach is an attractive alternative.
- Associated carpal injuries including ligament lesions may be diagnosed and treated as well as TFCC injuries that are frequently seen in combination with displaced distal radial fractures. Certain fractures include fragments of the joint surface that are impacted and not reducible by external manipulation. Typically the lunate facet is engaged with a depressed so-called die-punch fragment or separation of a dorsal and volar fragment carrying the insertions of the radio-ulnar ligaments.
- Displaced fractures of the radial styloid process (Chauffeur's fracture) have also been recommended for arthroscopic reduction and percutaneous fixation, which completely obviates the need of open surgery (del Piñal et al. 2007). Special attention is needed when an intra-articular radial styloid fracture or die-punch fracture of the lunate fossa is found to have major initial displacement (>2 mm) (Fig. 25.1). In these cases an S-L ligament injury must be suspected and ruled out, preferably by an arthroscopy.
- In our experience, young, non-osteopenic patients, injured in a high-energy trauma, are most often considered for an arthroscopy-assisted procedure. Only rarely elderly patients sustain fractures that are difficult to reduce by conventional techniques, but if difficulties are encountered, good results have been reported by using arthroscopic technique also in elderly (Hattori et al. 2007).
- The technique of arthroscopy-assisted reduction is relatively demanding particularly in complex fractures, and it is usually recommended that a novice with the method starts by treating less comminute fractures such as simple articular fractures, according to the AO classification (B1.1, B1.3, B2.1 and B3.1)

25.4 Set-Up

- Standard techniques and set-up for arthroscopy are applied using a traction device and continuous irrigation as necessary. Longitudinal traction is mandatory and should preferably be vertical (Fig. 25.2). A technique using horizontal traction has also been described, but this precludes the use of volar portals, which occasionally are needed, and also any type of volar implant for fracture fixation.

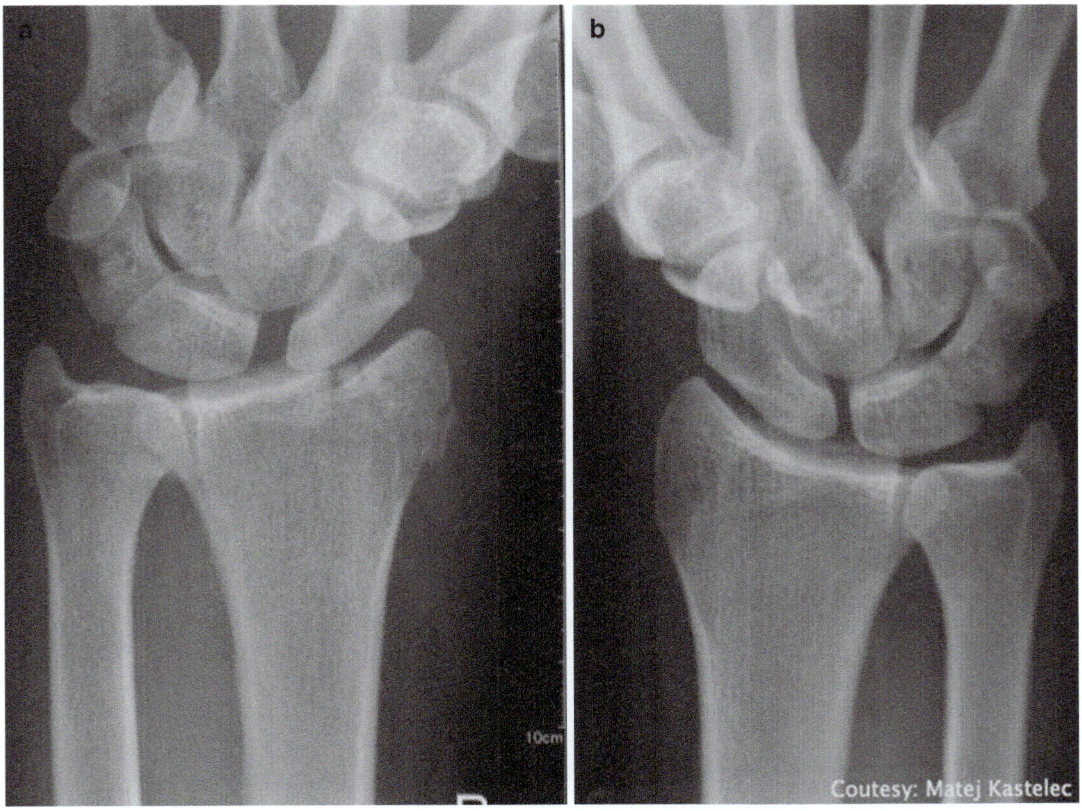

Fig. 25.1 (**a**) Comminuted radial styloid fracture (B1.2) with >2-mm displacement and scapholunar distance. (**b**) Normal contralateral side (Copyright © 2013 by Dr. Kastelec)

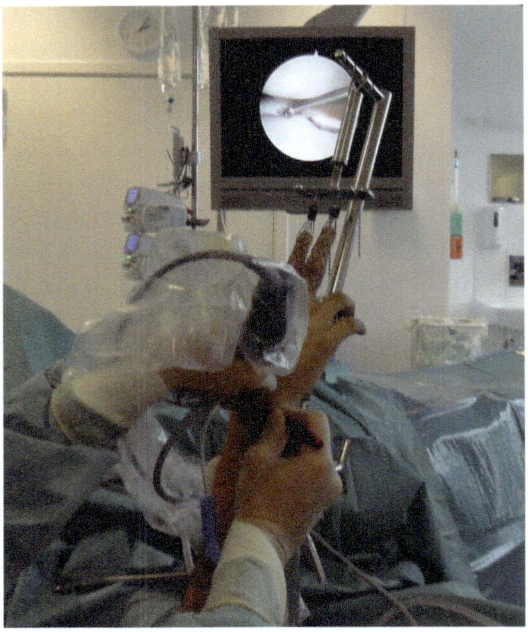

Fig. 25.2 Vertical traction tower

- Shaver equipment is recommended to aid in the removal of debris and blood from the joint.
- Fluoroscopic examination is frequently needed and a device that allows horizontal placement of the c-arm (Fig. 25.3) is helpful when the hand is suspended in vertical traction.
- Arthroscopic probe, small sharp and blunt elevators and K-wires are the most frequently used tools to aid in reduction. Correct wire placement may often be surprisingly difficult but can be facilitated with the use of a drill guide and an oscillating drill (Fig 25.4).

25.5 Techniques

- The first portals to be established are usually the 3–4 and 6R. The 6R is often preferred over the 4–5 portal because of a better view over the entire radial joint surface and also the

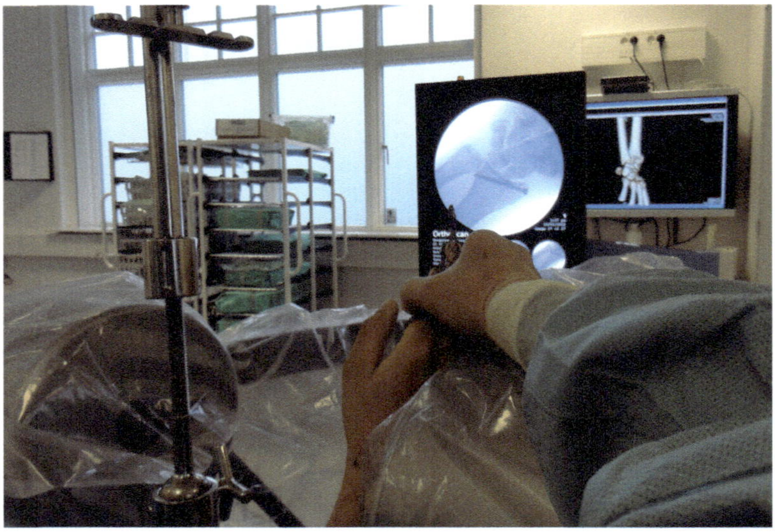

Fig. 25.3 Horizontal fluoroscope

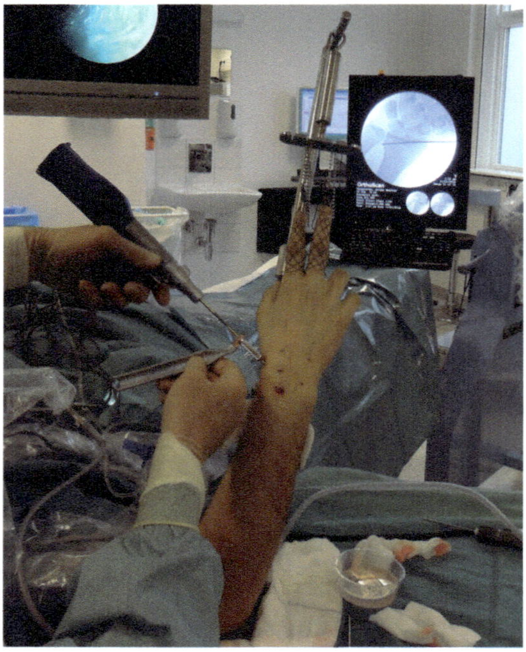

Fig. 25.4 Drill guide to control K-wire insertion

risk that the arthroscope will depress any fracture fragment affecting the lunate fossa or the dorsal rim (Fig 25.5).

- The arthroscope and shaver are alternated between the portals to get a good overview of the fracture extension and to remove blood cloths and debris. A shaver is usually the most efficient tool to clear the joint. Once the view is clear allowing examination of all parts of the joint and all fracture fragments are identified, the irrigation may be stopped and all fluid evacuated from the joint.
- A dry arthroscopy without irrigation is usually feasible and can often be recommended (del Piñal et al. 2007). This reduces the risk of soft tissue swelling around the joint, which at times may make the surgery more difficult and may potentially cause post-operative problems and discomfort. Occasionally, however, the synovium or capsule may obscure the view, making fluid distension of the joint necessary.
- The arthroscopic examination then continues in the mid-carpal space to assess any associated lesions of joint surfaces or ligaments.
- When the fracture and all soft tissues have been assessed, the mode of fixation has to be decided. The 6R portal allows the best overview of the radial joint surface and is then the recommended position for the arthroscope. The 1–2, 3–4 and occasionally 4–5 portals are primarily used as working portals since introduction of the arthroscope in any of these may cause depression of fracture fragments and the short working distance makes reduction difficult to assess.
- Simple intra-articular fractures (type B according to AO classification) with no extra-articular component like the chauffeur's (Fig. 25.6) and the die-punch fracture are

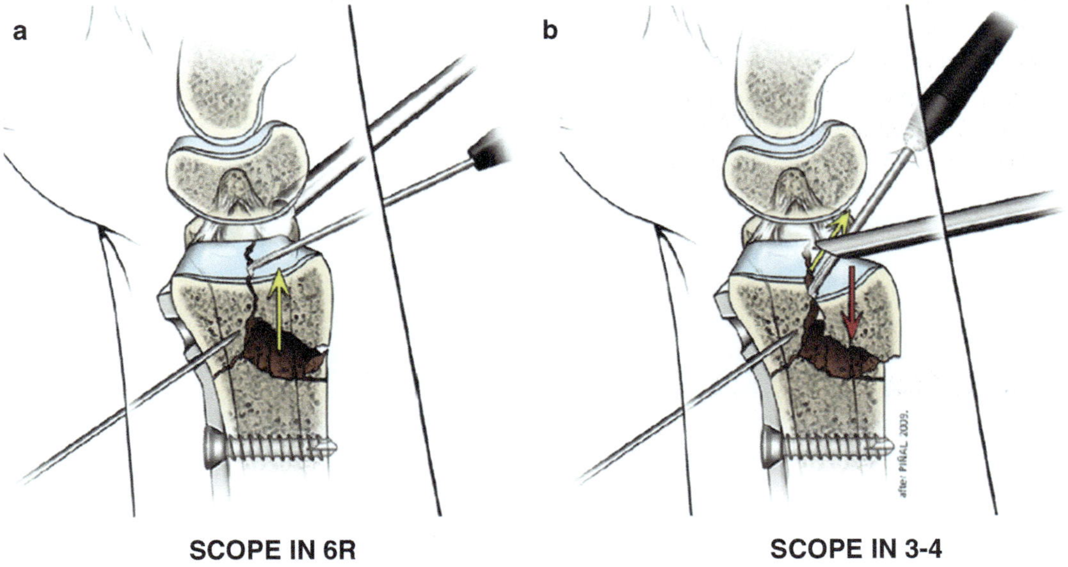

Fig. 25.5 (**a**) Arthroscope in 6R portal facilitates the reduction of dorsal fragments with probes from 3 to 4 portal. (**b**) The scope in portal 3–4 obstacles the reduction of the dorsal fragment (Copyright © 2011 by Dr. del Piñal)

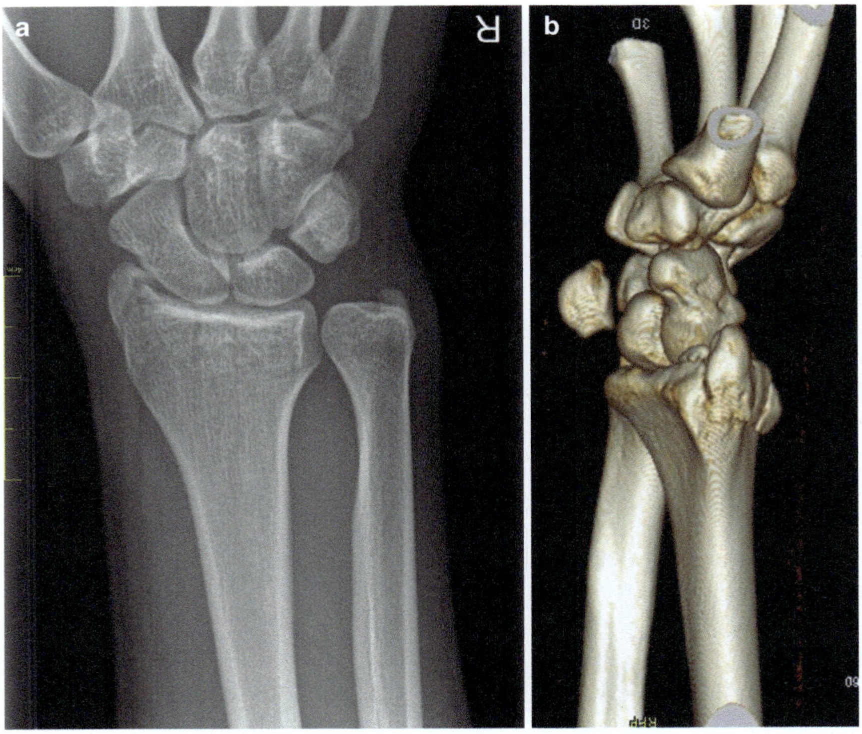

Fig. 25.6 Chauffeur's fracture. Simple intra-articular DRF with multifragmented depressed radial styloid (B1.2). (**a**) x-ray showing a styloid fracture. (**b**) CT scan revealing moderate displacement and comminution of the styloid fracture

stabilised with K-wires or cannulated screws, the latter allowing for immediate mobilisation.

- Radial styloid fractures type B1.1 can easily be reduced by external manipulation, while inspection is carried out from the 6R portal. After appropriate reduction by a thumb or by "fragment joysticking", K-wire fixation from the styloid tip can be performed. Final stabilisation can be achieved with either 1.25 mm K-wires, cannulated screw (Fig. 25.7) or a mini-plate (Fig. 25.8). Depressed and impacted fragments can be disimpacted and reduced with the use of a small osteotome or elevator in the fracture line. In these cases an additional small skin incision may be necessary.
- When an extra-articular component is part of the fracture (type C according to AO classification), a stable internal fixation should be attempted, preferably using screws and plates whenever possible.
- If a plate fixation is to be used from the volar aspect, a conventional open volar approach is performed, and a plate is placed and secured with a proximal shaft screw. The fracture is then provisionally reduced against the plate under fluoroscopic control followed by arthroscopic

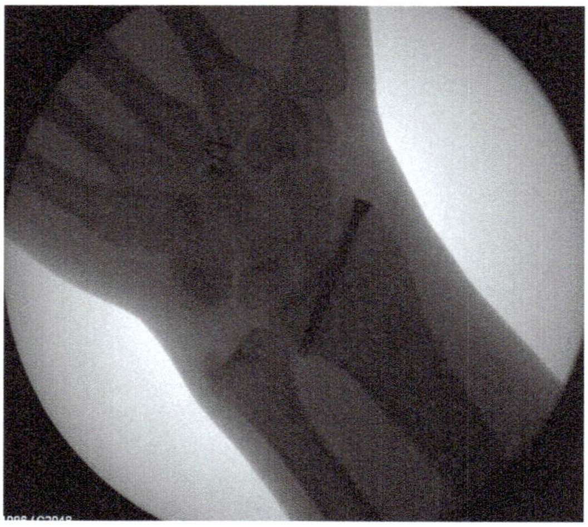

Fig. 25.7 Cannulated screw inserted percutaneously in the patient from Fig. 25.6

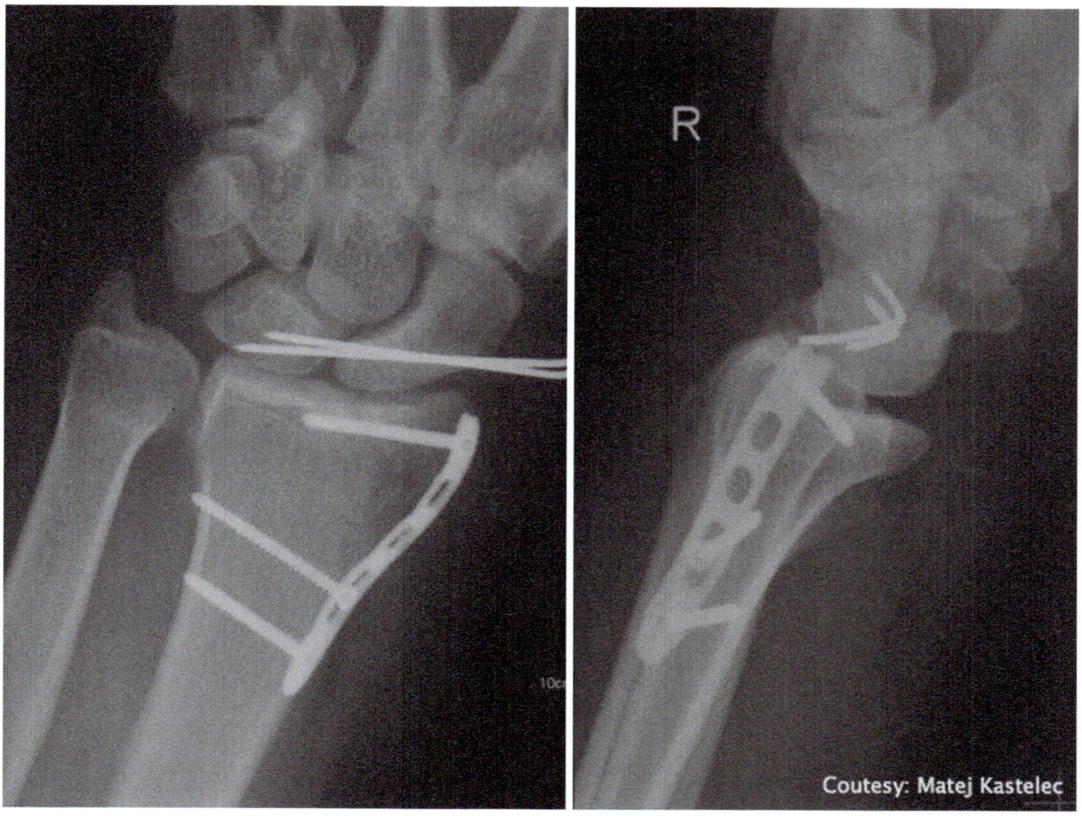

Fig. 25.8 Open reduction and plate fixation and scapholunar K-wire fixation of the patient from Fig. 25.1 (Copyright © 2013 by Dr. Kastelec)

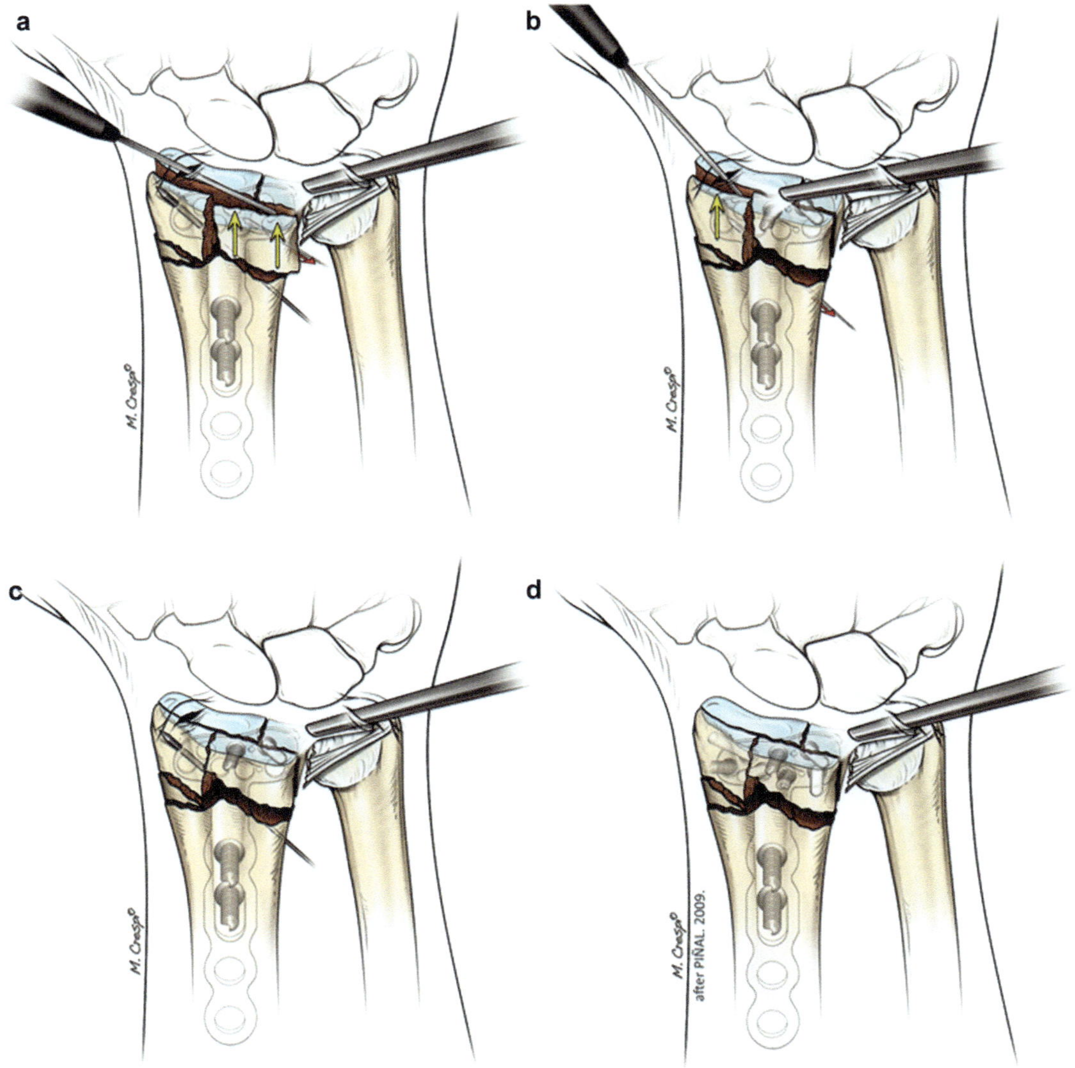

Fig. 25.9 Open volar plating followed by arthroscopic reduction of articular fragments and fixation by locked volar screws. (**a**) following insertion of a volar plate the volar fragments are reduced against the plate and the ulnar fragments are reduced to restore congruence of the DRUJ. (**b**) the dorso-radial fragment is reduced. (**c**) fragments are temporarily fixed with K-wires. (**d**) remaining angle-stable distal screws are inserted via the plate and wires removed (From del Piñal (2010). Copyright © 2009, with permission of Springer Science Business Media)

examination to control and fine-tune the reduction, using K-wires for temporary fixation. After reduction of the joint surface has been assured, the distal fragments are subsequently kept reduced against the distal part of the volar plate and secured with screws after which the wires may be removed (Fig 25.10).

- Depending on the fracture extension, a slightly different order of reduction may be indicated and the fragment-specific techniques as recommended by del Pinal (2010) have often proved helpful (Figs. 25.9, 25.10, 25.11, and 25.12).
- Dorsal plating may occasionally be considered for very distal fractures, and if reduction is to

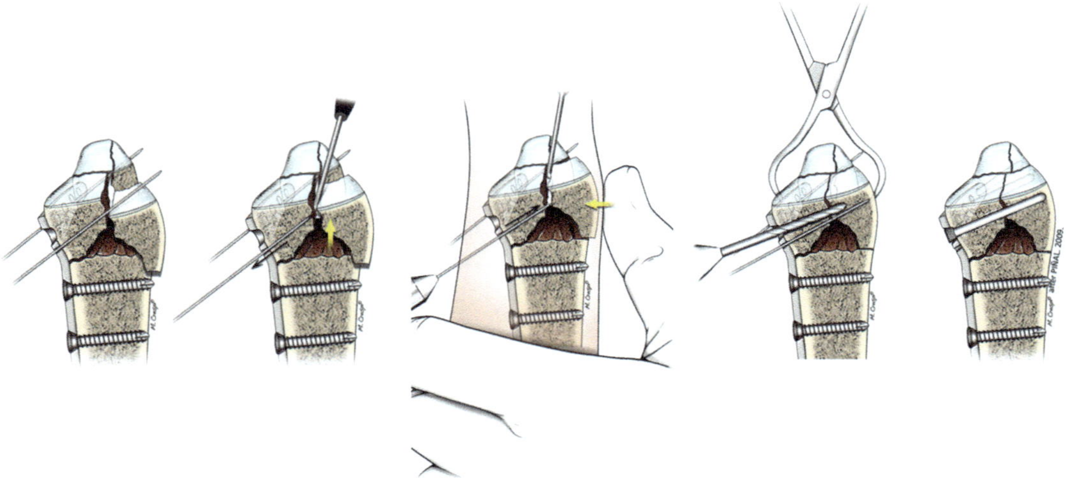

Fig. 25.10 Technique to reduce a dorsal depressed fragment (Copyright © 2011 by Dr. Piñal)

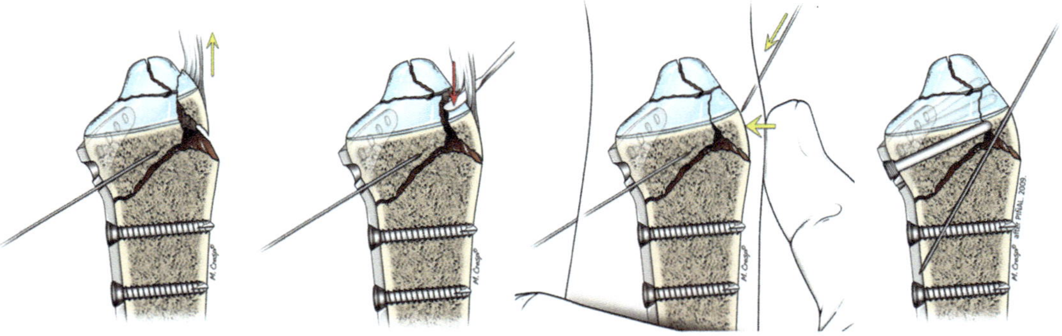

Fig. 25.11 Technique to reduce an elevated dorsal fragment (Copyright © 2011 by Dr. Piñal)

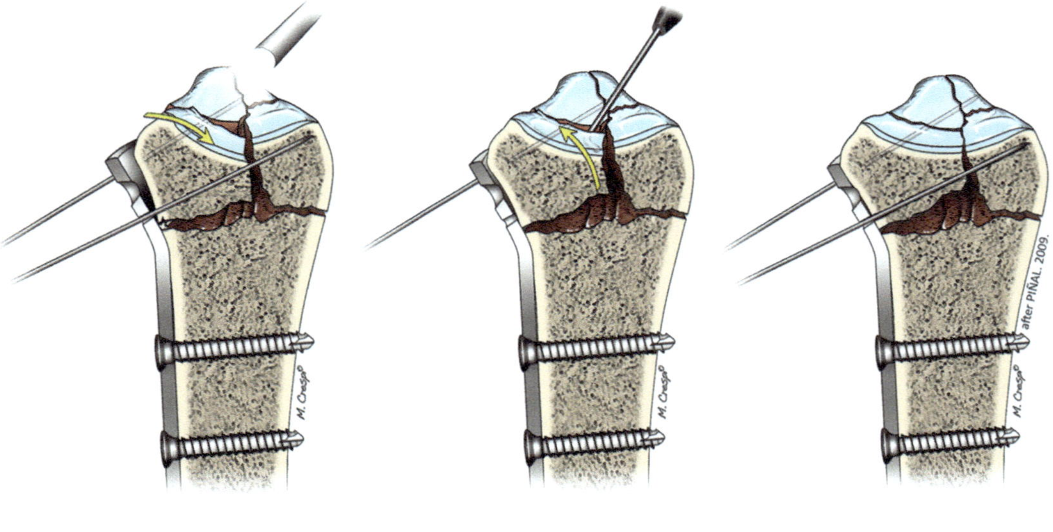

Fig. 25.12 Technique to reduce a volar malrotated fragment (Copyright © 2011 by Dr. Piñal)

be simultaneously controlled, a dorso-ulnar portal or a volar ulnar portal may be utilised.

- A complex fracture pattern often includes fragments of the ulnar part carrying the radio-ulnar ligaments and may also cause incongruence of the DRU joint. Reduction and control of these parts often requires a volar ulnar portal for reduction and fixation, which can be established through a short incision between the ulnar nerve and the finger flexor tendons. If a volar plate is to be used for fracture fixation, the standard incision for the plate is usually sufficient to address any volar fragments.
- In fractures involving the volar lip of the lunate facet, the volar fragment should often be reduced and stabilised first and can then be used as a template for reduction of the rest of the fracture (Figs. 25.13, 25.14 and 25.15).

25.6 Associate Injuries

- Lesions of ligaments and cartilage not visible neither on standard radiographs nor CT scan can be expected. As mentioned above all studies on arthroscopy of patients with acute distal radius fractures demonstrate that soft tissue injuries are found in the majority of cases. For many of the reported lesions, the healing potential and clinical significance remain unclear.
- It however appears reasonable that an observed ligamentous injury that cause displacement or increased laxity between carpal bones, DRUJ and radiocarpal joints should be stabilised and, whenever possible, repaired.

25.7 Post-operative Management

- The post-operative protocol follows conventional principles for distal radius fractures.
- Plaster cast immobilisation is generally recommended for 2 weeks when a stable internal fixation can be achieved. Depending on the mode and reliability of the fixation and the condition of the ligaments and other soft tissues, the period of immobilisation may occasionally be extended up to 6 weeks.

25.8 Results

The current literature suggests that the results are reliably good (Adolfsson and Jørgsholm 1998; Doi et al. 1999; Chen et al. 2002; del Pinal 2010). The few studies comparing conventional techniques with arthroscopy-assisted reduction have reported results favouring the latter. Scientific concerns including selection bias, patient-related factors and varying assessment systems however preclude definitive comparison with conventional techniques.

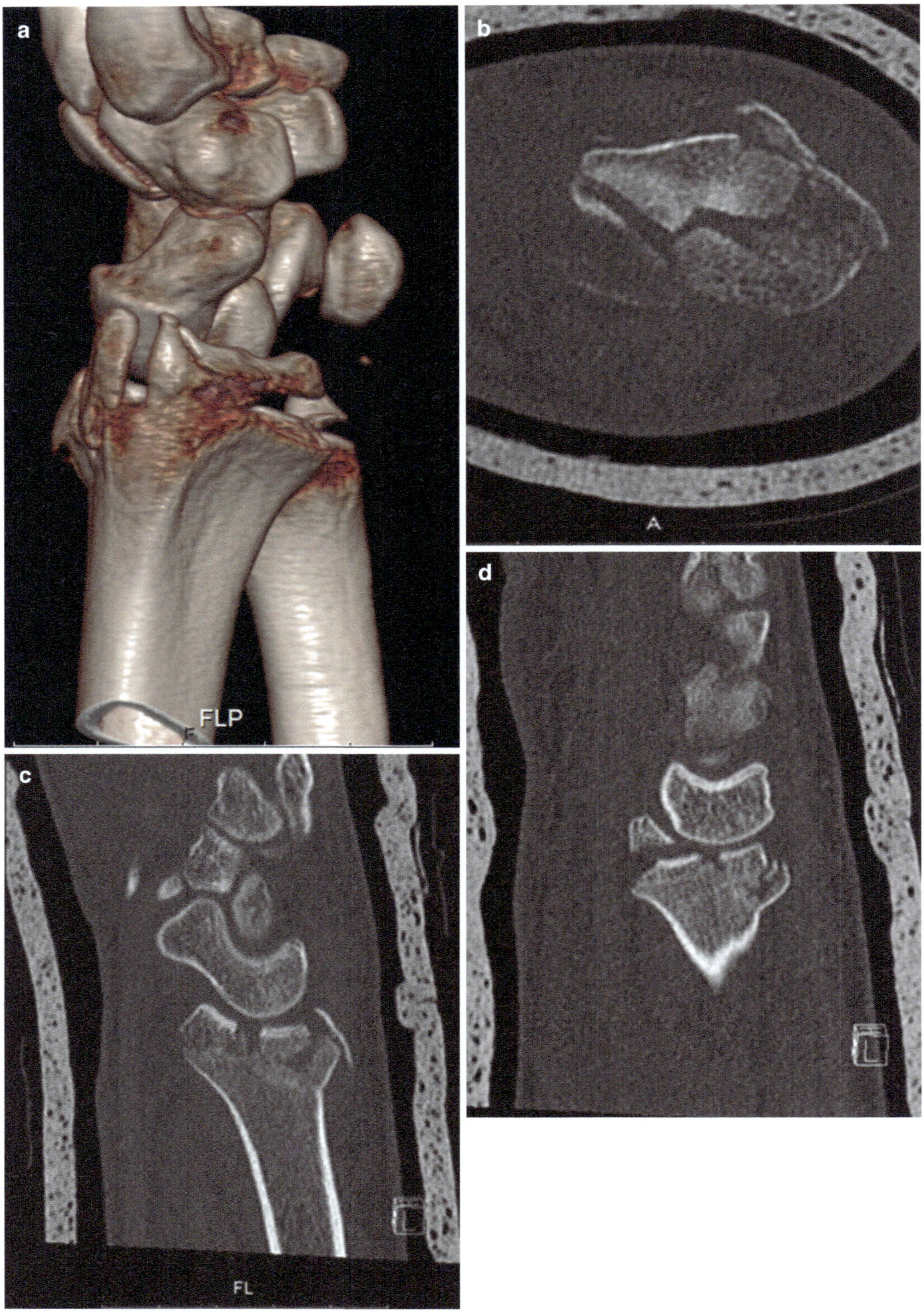

Figs 25.13 (**a**) Fracture of the distal radius and ulna in a 21-year-old male injured in a two-metre fall. (**b**) Horizontal view of radial joint surface. (**c**) Transverse view of scaphoid facet. (**d**) Transverse view of lunate facet

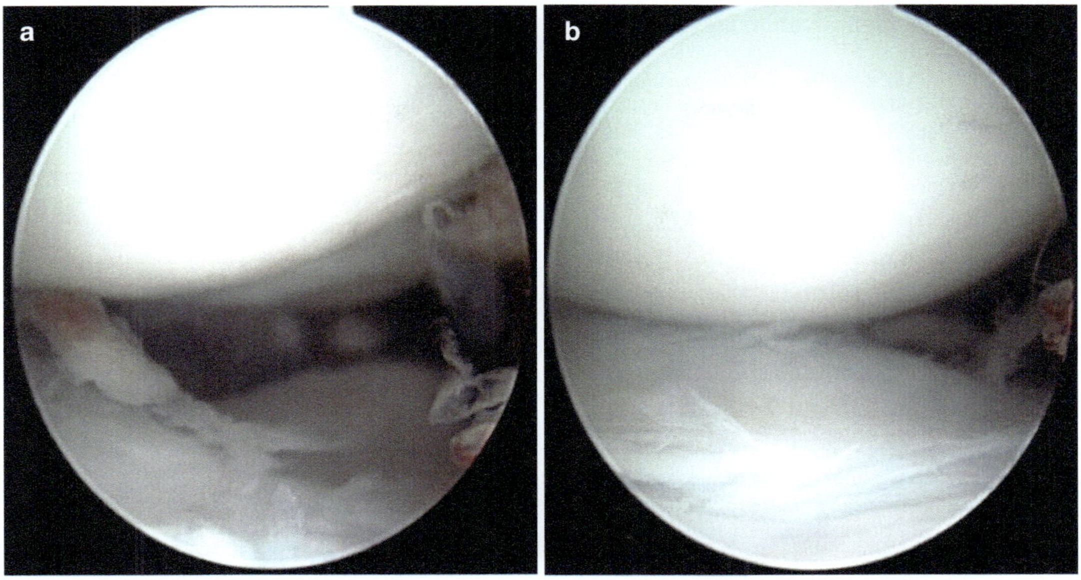

Fig 25.14 Arthroscopic view and reduction of patient in Fig. 25.13. (**a**) Arthroscopic view from the 6R portal. Lunate, S-L joint and scaphoid above. Volar lip fragment partially covered by blood, central fragment depressed. (**b**) The central fragment is reduced in relation to the volar and ulnar fragments, creating a congruent joint surface. The fragment was temporarily stabilised by a K-wire and then definitively using a dorsal plate

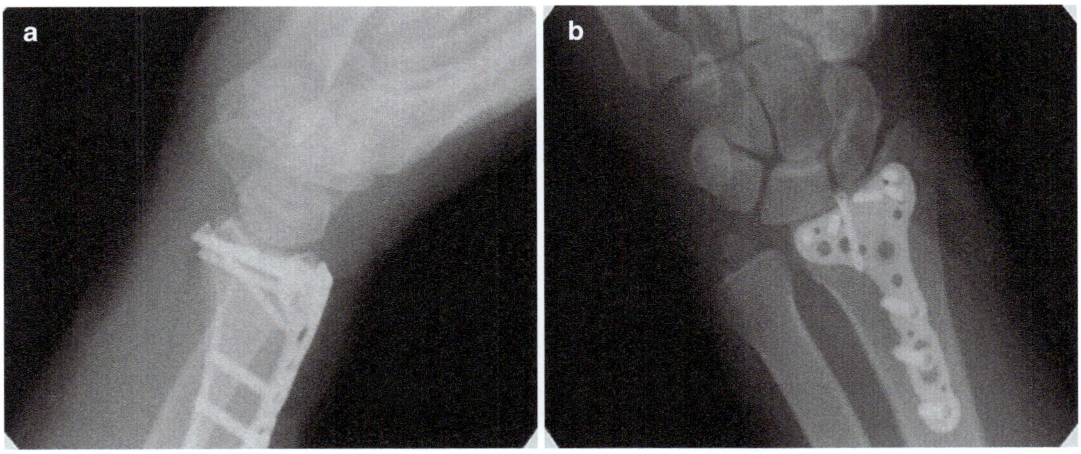

Fig 25.15 Final reduction and fixation of patient in Figs 25.13 and 25.14, using a dorsal plate and a solitary volar screw. (**a**) Perioperative lateral view, the volar lip fragment reduced and stabilised first using a solitary screw, followed by dorsal plate. (**b**) Frontal view. Despite displacement of the ulnar styloid process, there was no markedly increased laxity of the DRUJ and the styloid was left without fixation

References

Adolfsson L, Jørgsholm P. Arthroscopically-assisted reduction of intra-articular fractures of the distal radius. J Hand Surg Br. 1998;23(3):391–5.

Chen AC, Chan YS, Yuan LJ, Ye WL, Lee MS, Chao EK. Arthroscopically assisted osteosynthesis of complex intra-articular fractures of the distal radius. J Trauma. 2002;53(2):354–9.

del Piñal F, García-Bernal FJ, Pisani D, Regalado J, Ayala H, Studer A. Dry arthroscopy of the wrist: surgical technique. J Hand Surg Am. 2007;32(1):119–23.

del Pinal F. Treatment of explosion-type distal radius fractures. In: del Piñal F, Mathoulin C, Luchetti C, editors. Arthroscopic management of distal radius fractures. Berlin: Springer; 2010. p. 41–65.

Doi K, Hattori Y, Otsuka K, Abe Y, Yamamoto H. Intraarticular fractures of the distal aspect of the radius: arthroscopically assisted reduction compared with open reduction and internal fixation. J Bone Joint Surg. 1999;81A:1093–110.

Geissler WB, Freeland AE, Savoie FH, McIntyre LW, Whipple TL. Intracarpal soft-tissue lesions associated with an intra-articular fracture of the distal end of the radius. J Bone Joint Surg Am. 1996;78(3):357–65.

Hattori Y, Doi K, Estrella EP, Chen G. Arthroscopically assisted reduction with volar plating or external fixation for displaced intra-articular fractures of the distal radius in the elderly patients. Hand Surg. 2007;12(1):1–12.

Lindau T, Arner M, Hagberg L. Intraarticular lesions in distal fractures of the radius in young adults. A descriptive arthroscopic study in 50 patients. J Hand Surg Br. 1997;22(5):638–43.

Lindau TR, Aspenberg P, Arner M, Redlundh-Johnell I, Hagberg L. The distal radial fracture in young adults. A population-based epidemiologic description of 341 patients. Acta Orthop Scand. 1999;70:124–8.

Ruch DS, Vallee J, Poehling GG, Smith BP, Kuzma GR. Arthroscopic reduction versus fluoroscopic reduction in the management of intra-articular distal radius fractures. Arthroscopy. 2004;20(3):225–30.

Varitimidis SE, Basdekis GK, Dailiana ZH, Hantes ME, Bargiotas K, Malizos K. Treatment of intra-articular fractures of the distal radius: fluoroscopic or arthroscopic reduction? J Bone Joint Surg Br. 2008;90(6):778–85.

Associated Injuries in Distal Radius Fractures

26

Tommy Lindau and Kerstin Oestreich

Contents

26.1 Introduction

- The outcome of distal radius fracture treatment can still not be fully predicted today. In fact, there is no scientific evidence for anything we do in the management of distal radius fractures (Handoll et al. 2008).
- In addition to the fact that arthroscopic evaluation is superior in assessing the articular step-off as well as the rotation of fractured fragments, it is also possible to recognize chondral and ligament injuries (Geissler et al. 1996; Lindau et al. 1997; Cognet et al. 2008).
- There is a high incidence of soft tissue injuries associated with distal radius fractures, which are frequently missed when the fracture is managed by conventional methods of treatment (Table 26.1) (Geissler et al. 1996; Lindau et al. 1997). These injuries should not be surprising as the radius is involved in the greater arch mechanism described by Mayfield in perilunate dislocations (Mayfield et al. 1980) (Fig. 26.1).
- This is particularly noted in non-osteoporotic patients who more often present with intra-articular fractures caused by a severe, high-energy trauma, whereas in contrast, such

T. Lindau, MD, PhD (✉)
The Pulvertaft Hand Centre, Kings Treatment Centre, Royal Derby Hospital,
Uttoxeter Road, Derby DE22 3NE, UK

University of Derby, Derby, UK
e-mail: tommylindau@hotmail.com

K. Oestreich, MD, MSc
Consultant Paediatric Plastic Surgeon,
Children's Hospital, Steelhouse Lane,
Birmingham B4 6NH, UK

L.M. Hove et al. (eds.), *Distal Radius Fractures*,
DOI 10.1007/978-3-642-54604-4_26, © Springer-Verlag Berlin Heidelberg 2014

Table 26.1 Soft tissue Injuries associated with distal radius fractures

Study (year)	Number and type of injury	TFCC injury (%)	SL injury (%)	LT injury (%)
Fontes (1995)	30, intra- and extra-articular	70	40	17
Geissler et al. (1996)	60, intra-articular	49	32	15
Lindau et al. (1997)	50, intra- and extra-articular	78	54	16
Richards (1997)	118, intra- and extra-articular	35 (intra) 53 (extra)	21 (intra) 7 (extra)	7 (intra) 13 (extra)
Mehta (2000)	3, intra-articular	58	85	61
Hanker (2001)	173, intra-articular	61	8	12

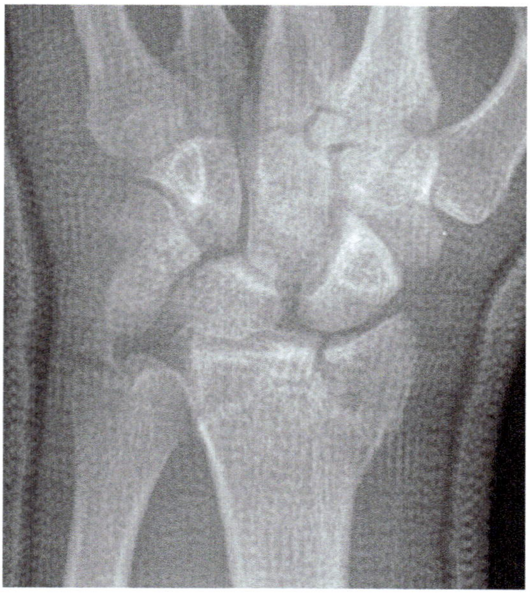

Fig 26.1 Radius fracture with associated scapholunate (*SL*) ligament injury diagnosed with the "ring sign" of the scaphoid

associated injuries are uncommon in osteoporotic patients where most fractures are extra-articular due to low-energy trauma.

- Therefore arthroscopy should be considered in younger patients with a more high-energy trauma, in particular radial styloid fractures in order to detect these injuries in addition to improving intra-articular congruency.

26.2 Indications for Arthroscopy

- The main indication for arthroscopy in the management of distal radius fractures is an intra-articular step-off more than 1 mm after an attempted closed reduction.
- Secondly, fractures with associated scaphoid fractures and/or obvious ligament injuries will benefit from arthroscopic management. Radiological signs may suggest associated soft tissue injuries, such as widening of intercarpal joint spaces and/or radiographic disruption of the carpal arches of the so-called Gilula lines, i.e., the 3 arches that can be drawn along the proximal and distal carpal rows.
- Thirdly, a radiological widening of the distal radioulnar (DRU) joint may be another sign of a ligament injury to the triangular fibrocartilage complex (TFCC) that may need arthroscopic assessment.
- Simple radial styloid fractures are most often 2-part fractures and may be part of an incomplete greater arch injury according to the Mayfield mechanism, but without a dislocation of the lunate (Mayfield et al. 1980) (see Chap. 27).
- Complex, impacted fractures such as the "die-punch" fractures warrant arthroscopic assessment, reduction, and fixation (see Chap. 27) (Fig. 26.1).
- Three- or four-part fractures or even more complex injuries with high-grade intra-articular comminution ("explosion fractures") are challenging but will benefit from arthroscopic management in expert hands (see Chaps. 24, 25, and 39).

26.3 The Arthroscopic Procedure: "Dry" or Wet?

- The "dry" arthroscopic technique will minimize the risk of further soft tissue swelling and consecutive secondary compartment syndrome, compared to the wet technique with continuous saline irrigation, but it may make the procedure slightly more cumbersome (del Piñal 2011).
- "Dry" should not be taken literally, as there might be intra-articular debris and hemarthrosis, which will have to be cleared by irrigating the joint, before continuing with a "dry" arthroscopy technique (del Piñal 2011).
- If a "dry" arthroscopy technique is preferred, the air valve should be kept open to permit free circulation of air through the joint, and the suction should be turned off unless needed.

26.4 The Arthroscopic Procedure: Arthroscopic Assessment

- Safe portals have to be established, occasionally with fluoroscopic assistance.
- The examination starts by assessing the radiocarpal joint surface regarding intra-articular congruency and possible need for optimizing the provisional reduction.
- In this respect, a 2-mm probe is helpful, inserted through the 4–5 or the 6-R portal, to accurately evaluate the gap, separation, and step-off of fragments.
- Once articular congruity is achieved, associated ligament or cartilage injuries are assessed: integrity of the scapholunate (SL) ligament, the luno-triquetral (LT) ligament, and the TFCC or any other intra-articular pathology is visualized and the sequence of surgery can be planned.
- TFCC injuries appear to be the most common associated ligament injury. They are found in around ¾ of the fractures (Table 26.1) (Geissler et al. 1996; Lindau et al. 1997).
- SL ligament injuries are the second most frequent injuries. They are found in between 1/3 and ½ of cases (Table 26.1) (Geissler et al. 1996; Lindau et al. 1997).
- LT ligament tears (Table 26.1) are less common and are seen in about 1/6 of the fractures (Geissler et al. 1996; Lindau et al. 1997).
- Chondral lesions have been found (Lindau et al. 1997) with a possible long-term development of secondary osteoarthritis (Lindau et al. 2003).

26.5 Triangular Fibrocartilage Complex (TFCC) Injuries

- TFCC injuries are the most common associated intra-articular injuries in distal radius fractures in non-osteoporotic patients (Table 26.2) (Geissler et al. 1996; Lindau et al. 1997). Cadaveric studies suggest that a displacement of the distal radius has to be more than 4 mm of radial shortening, down to 0° of radial inclination and a dorsal tilt of minimum 10° in order for an ulnar attachment of TFCC to be compromised.
- One-year outcome study found that peripheral tears to the TFCC will cause instability and subsequent worse outcome (Fig. 26.2) (Lindau 2005). However, in a recent 15-year prospective longitudinal outcome study of untreated TFCC tears, this seems to be less of a problem than anticipated, as only one patient needed a stabilizing procedure due to painful instability (Mrkonjic et al. 2012).
- In the absence of scientific evidence, clinical experience supports the following advice regarding TFCC treatment in association with distal radius fractures (Table 26.2 and Fig. 26.3).

26.6 InterCarpal Ligament Injuries

- Intercarpal ligament injuries to the SL and the LT ligament associated with distal radius fractures can be looked upon as incomplete greater

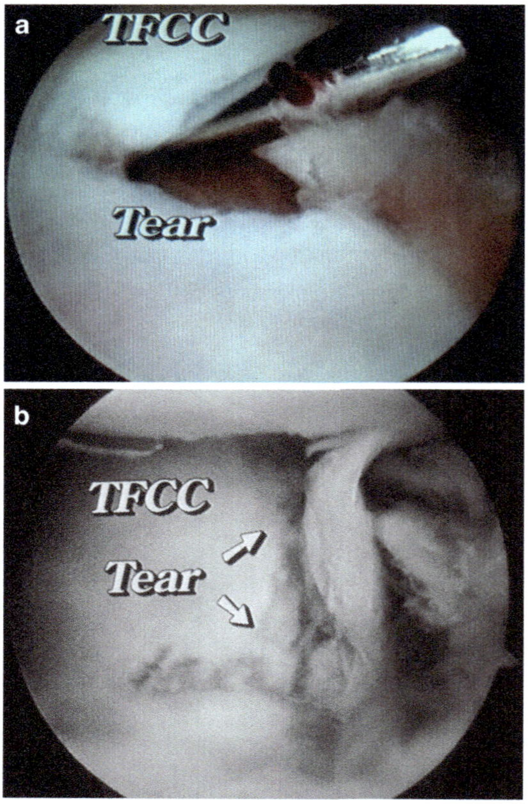

Fig 26.2 (**a**) Central perforation tear of the triangular fibrocartilage (*TFCC*) ligament. This may be painful and debridement should be consistent, but it never leads to instability of the DRU joint (Need permission from Springer Geissler 2008 and 2014) (**b**) Peripheral TFCC tear that 1 year from injury showed increased instability and a worse outcome. 15 years after these injuries, only one patient needed secondary reattachment suggesting that it may not always need repair (Reprinted with permission from Springer)

arch injuries described by Mayfield (Mayfield et al. 1980).

- It is important to assess and diagnose these ligament injuries. In the absence of arthroscopy, fluoroscopic assessment in ulnar and radial deviation will diagnose severe intercarpal ligament injuries. Arthroscopic assessment will not only diagnose them, but also allow grading based on a combined radiocarpal and midcarpal assessment (Geissler et al. 1996; Lindau et al. 1997) (Tables 26.3 and 26.4). Depending on this grading, severity is controlled and further management is decided.
- The ligament injuries are visualized at radiocarpal arthroscopy and are classified as partial or complete (Tables 26.3 and 26.4). The ligaments are examined along their different portions: dorsal, membranous, and palmar portions.
- From the midcarpal joint, the joint space, not the ligament, is assessed for widening and step-off. A probe with known size (e.g., 1 mm thickness and 2 mm tip length) is useful as a template for measurement (Tables 26.3 and 26.4).
- The widening and the step-off reflect the degree of the mobility of the affected intercarpal joint, as a consequence of the ligament injury. This mobility is not necessarily a pathological laxity.
- Once the traction is released, the assessed joint can be tested, by checking signs of pathological excessive mobility with the arthroscope in the midcarpal joint. Thus, the intercarpal ligament injury can be fully classified and graded (Tables 26.3 and 26.4).

26.7 Scapholunate (SL) Ligament Injuries

- SL ligament injuries occur in half of displaced distal radius fractures, at least in the non-osteoporotic population (Lindau et al. 1997). If left untreated, high-grade SL tears are likely to progress first to SL dissociation and symptomatic wrist instability (Forward et al. 2007). This will in the long term further lead to posttraumatic scapholunate advanced collapse (SLAC) osteoarthritis.
- Being aware of the long-term consequences of untreated SL tears, it is important to detect SL tears early and to consider treatment.
- If found and treated early, arthroscopic reduction and percutaneous pinning are the simplest option and has a good outcome in 85 % of the patients.
- It is noteworthy that there is no strong evidence (level 1 or 2) for management of these injuries and recommendations published are mainly experience-based (Chennagiri and Lindau 2013).

Table 26.2 Classification of TFCC tears (15) with explanation on biomechanical problems with the tear and suggested treatment

Type of tear	Understanding the tear	Treatment
Central perforation tears (Palmer 1A)	Stable	Debridement (suction punch, shaver, radiofrequency probe)
	Treatment does not change overall rehabilitation plan	Avoid jeopardizing the stability provided by the important palmar and dorsal radioulnar ligaments
Peripheral tears (Palmer 1B)	May cause DRU joint instability	Distal tears: debride, possibly re-suture to the capsule and ECU subsheath
	Distal tears are avulsed from the capsule and subsheath to ECU	Proximal tears: reattachment to the fovea of the ulna
	Proximal tears are avulsed from the fovea of the ulnar head	Combined tears: reattach
	Proximal tears cannot be seen at radiocarpal arthroscopy	Reattachment with arthroscopy assistance or open technique with similar good outcome
	Combined distal and proximal tears cause instability of the DRU joint	Arthroscopically assisted reattachment:
		2–3 2/0 absorbable (PDS) sutures are passed through the periphery of the TFCC and fixed to the distal ulna, either through drill holes or with any available suture anchor
		Protect repair from supination and pronation for 4 weeks, followed by 2–4 weeks in a short arm cast
Ulnocarpal ligament tears (Palmar 1C)	Very rare	Reinsertion technique:
		Simplest option: directly through the palmar approach in line with the exposure of the critical corner in the intermediate column
		Protect repair for 4 weeks in relation to the rehabilitation for the fracture
Radial avulsion tears (palmar 1D)	Uncommon	Reattachment technique:
	Often associated with a dorso	A dorsal fracture should be fixed
	May cause instability of the DRU ulnar fracture fragment	Due to the distal radius fracture, the technique based on drill holes through the radius is not suitable
		A mini-open dorso-radial approach is done and ligament is reattached, with suture anchors

26.7.1 Grade I–II SL Injuries

- Low-grade injuries are best managed with immobilization, as most patients are asymptomatic at 1 year (Forward et al. 2007). Therefore the protocol for mobilization of the distal radius fracture after volar locking plate fixation may have to be adjusted (Fig. 26.4) (Chennagiri and Lindau 2013).

26.7.2 Grade III-IV SL Injuries

- Radiographic SL dissociation and long-term SLAC wrist are more likely with these injuries, if untreated and consequently early treatment is important (Forward et al. 2007).
- Grade III can be treated with arthroscopic reduction and K-wire pinning (Fig. 26.5). While protecting the sensory branches of the radial nerve, a skin incision is made slightly palmar to the

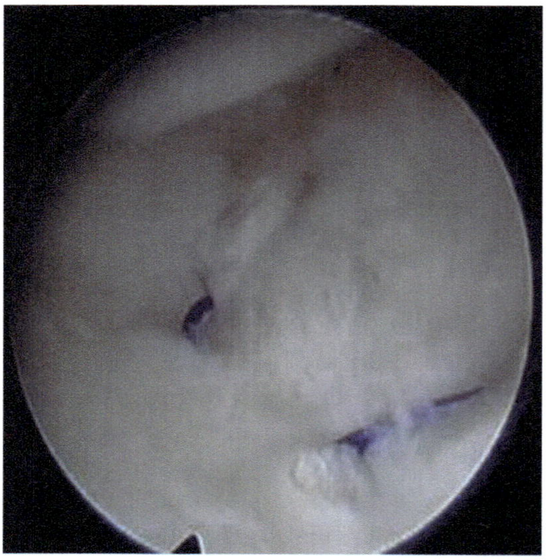

Fig 26.3 Repair of the peripheral tear has to be through the fovea of the ulnar head to regain stability. Suture anchors, drill holes, and other techniques are available

Table 26.3 Arthroscopic classification of scapholunate ligament tears according to Geissler

Grade	Radiocarpal joint	Midcarpal instability	Step-off
1	Hemorrhage of IOL, no attenuation	None	None
2	Incomplete partial or full substance tear, no attenuation	Slight gap (<3 mm)	Midcarpal only
3	Ligament attenuation incomplete partial or small full substance tear	Probe can be passed between carpal bones	Midcarpal and radiocarpal
4	Complete tear	Gross instability 2.7 mm scope can be passed thru (drive-thru sign)	Midcarpal and radiocarpal

Table 26.4 The Lindau classification system for intercarpal SL and LT ligament injuries and mobility of the joints (Lindau et al. 1997)

	Radiocarpal arthroscopy	Midcarpal arthroscopy	
Grade	Ligament appearance	Appearance	
		Diastasis (mm)	Step-off (mm)
1	Hematoma or distension	0	0
2	As above and/or partial tear	0–1	<2
3	Partial or total tear	1–2	<2
4	Total tear	>2	>2

Source: reprinted from Lindau, Arner, and Hagberg [2]

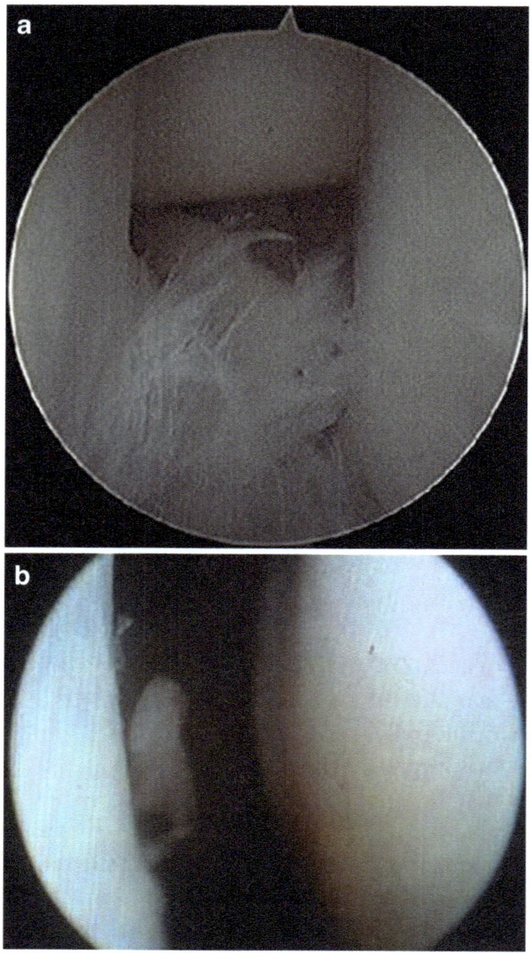

Fig 26.4 (**a**) Arthroscopic view from the radiocarpal portal with a so-called drive through sign; i.e., the scope can be passed through the SL ligament that is completely torn, a Grade IV SL tear (Geissler et al. 1996). (**b**) Midcarpal arthroscopy shows a step and a gap that can be measured for grading, in this case a Grade 3 (Lindau 1997) (Reprinted with permission from Springer)

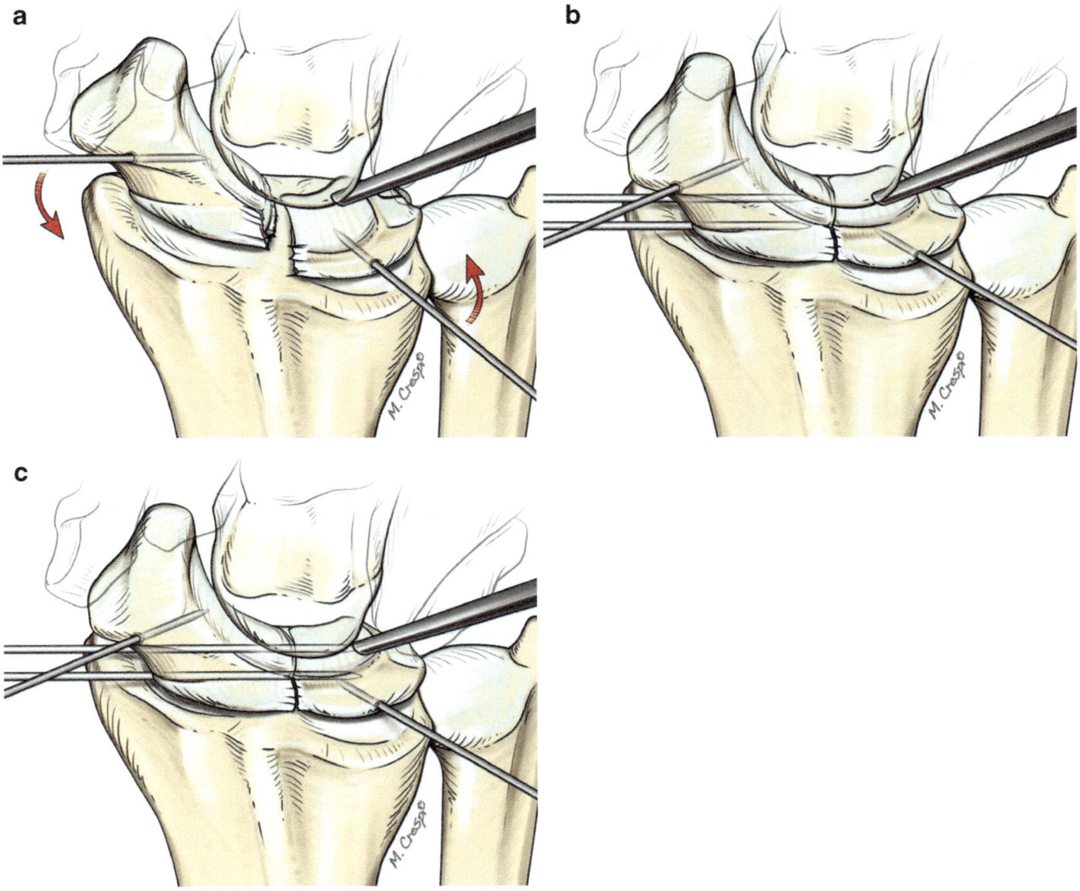

Fig 26.5 Repair of a Grade III–IV SL tears can be done with an arthroscopy-assisted technique. Pinal Arthroscopic management of distal radius fractures 2010. (**a**) One K-wire in the scaphoid and lunate, respectively, is used and a joystick maneuver used with the scope in the midcarpal joint to secure adequate reduction of the joint (**b**). (**b**, **c**). K-wires are inserted into the scaphoid and once reduction has been achieved, the wires are advanced over the SL joint and a final one into the capitate to protect the torn ligament and allow healing. (Reprinted with permission from Springer)

anatomical snuffbox. K-wires into the scaphoid are used as a joystick to achieve arthroscopic reduction, which can be assessed from the midcarpal joint. Once reduction is achieved, the K-wire is advanced into the lunate. An additional K-wire should be inserted into the scapho-capitate (SC) joint. Pins can be removed at 6 weeks (Chennagiri and Lindau 2013).

- Grade IV injuries, especially if found with radiologically visible dissociation already on the trauma films, can be difficult to reduce arthroscopically and should most likely be treated with an open repair (Chennagiri and Lindau 2013). Open direct repair is followed by protective K-wires as described above. During closure, dorsal capsulodesis can be added to augment the repair, which might lead to long-term reduced palmar flexion.

26.8 Luno-Triquetral (LT) Ligament Injuries

- The incidence of LT ligament injuries is about 1/6 (Table 26.1). So far, there is no evidence that LT tears lead to long-term problems when associated with distal radius fractures (Forward et al. 2007).

- Stable LT injuries (Grade I–III) may benefit from immobilization, where again the fracture mobilization protocol needs to be reconsidered.
- Grade IV injuries may need arthroscopic debridement of the tear and pinning of the joint. K-wires are introduced from a dorso-ulnar approach. The LT dissociation is reduced with a joystick maneuver, and two to three wires are advanced across the joint. Wires are kept for 6 weeks.

26.9 Chondral Lesions

- Acute chondral lesions can be seen as:
  - Subchondral hematomas (with or without cartilage cracks)
  - Avulsed cartilage flakes
  - Complete avulsions of the cartilage (Lindau et al. 1997)
- There is some evidence that subchondral hematoma can lead to the development of early-onset of mild, radiographic OA (Lindau et al. 2003).
- There is currently no other treatment option than debridement for these injuries. A tempting, but unproven, option is the micro-fracture treatment as familiar from the knee joint.
- Chondral lesions may lead to treatment changes, as a comminuted intra-articular fracture might be treated with a primary partial wrist fusion instead of a lengthy attempt of reducing a multi-fragmentary joint surface with loss of cartilage, as there is increased awareness of an expected bad outcome with these associated lesions.
- Together with the associated ligament injuries, chondral lesions reflect the complexity of distal radial fractures, especially in the non-osteoporotic population (del Piñal 2011).

26.10 Outcomes

- Currently there is no scientific evidence that arthroscopy is necessary in the management of distal radius fractures. However, there seems to be increasing support regarding the benefit of arthroscopy in the management of distal radius fractures (Mrkonjic et al. 2012; Ono et al. 2012; Scheer and Adolfsson 2012).
- Further, there is limited experience in arthroscopically assisted treatment of associated injuries. However, TFCC repairs in conjunction with distal radius fixation resulted in a high degree of patient satisfaction and good to excellent clinical outcomes (Ruch et al. 2003).

26.11 Summary

- There is an increasing awareness in the complexity of distal radius fracture as it should not only be seen as a bony injury, but rather as a bony consequence of the energy passing the wrist while breaking the radius (Table 26.5).
- The main advantage of arthroscopically assisted management of distal radius fractures is to improve intra-articular accuracy to less than 1 mm of incongruency.
- The second advantage is to combine this with complete assessment, management and treatment of TFCC, intercarpal ligament, and cartilage injuries.
- The third advantage is that the surgeon has complete control of all fracture and treatment-related factors in distal radius fractures by arthroscopic assistance.
- It is our hope that this concept will continue to evolve in future for the benefit of our patients.

Table 26.5 Five top tips in understanding the usefulness of wrist arthroscopy as an adjuvant investigation in the treatment of distal radius fractures

1	There is a wide spectrum of injury pattern after a fall onto the outstretched hand such as: Sprain Radial styloid fracture in isolation Radial styloid fracture as part of the greater arch injury, thereby as part of a complete or incomplete perilunate dislocation mechanism (Mayfield et al. 1980)
2	Displaced fractures in the non-osteoporotic patient have a high incidence of associated soft tissue injuries. Associated injuries will affect the long-term outcome, where arthroscopy plays its role to establish the correct diagnosis and facilitate early treatment
3	Undetected associated injuries may explain the absence of improved outcome after ORIF and early mobilization compared to external fixation. Possibly, further improved outcome may follow if arthroscopy is used in conjunction with volar locking plate fixation
4	Arthroscopy will in falling frequency diagnose: TFCC injuries Intracarpal SL and LT ligament tears Chondral lesions Once diagnosed and graded, the appropriate surgical treatment of these lesions can be added to the fracture fixation
5	Arthroscopy as an adjunct in the management of distal radius fractures has been available for over 20 years, yet still requires experience and management in expert centers

References

Chennagiri RJR, Lindau T. Assessment of scapholunate instability and review of evidence for management in the absence of arthritis. J Hand Surg Eur. 2013;38(7): 727–38.

Cognet JM, Martinache X, Mathoulin C. Arthroscopic management of intra-articular fractures of the distal radius. Chir Main. 2008;27(4):171–9.

Forward D, Lindau T, Melsom D. Intercarpal ligament injuries associated with fractures of the distal radius. Arthroscopic assessment and 12 month follow-up. J Bone Joint Surg Am. 2007;89(11):2334–40.

Geissler WB, Freeland AE, Savoie FH, et al. Intracarpal soft-tissue lesions associated with an intra-articular fracture of the distal end of the radius. J Bone Joint Surg Am. 1996;78:357–65.

Handoll HHG, Madhok R. Conservative interventions for treating distal radial fractures in adults. Cochrane Database Syst Rev. 2003;(2):CD000314. doi: 10.1002/14651858.CD000314.

Lindau T, Arner M, Hagberg L. Intraarticular lesions in distal fractures of the radius in young adults. A descriptive arthroscopic study in 50 patients. J Hand Surg Br. 1997;22:638–43.

Lindau T, Adlercreutz C, Aspenberg P. Cartilage injuries in distal radial fractures. Acta Orthop Scand. 2003;74(3):327–31.

Lindau T. Treatment of injuries to the ulnar side of the wrist occurring with distal radius fractures. Hand Clin. 2005;21:417–25.

Mayfield JK, Johnson RP, Kilcoyne RK. Carpal dislocations: pathomechanics and progressive perilunar instability. J Hand Surg Am. 1980;5:226–41.

Mrkonjic A, Geijer M, Lindau T, Tägil M. The natural course of traumatic triangular fibrocartilage complex tears in distal radial fractures: a 13–15 year follow-up of arthroscopically diagnosed but untreated injuries. J Hand Surg Am. 2012;37(8):1555–60.

Ono H, Katayama T, Furuta K, Suzuki D, Fujitani R, Akahane M. Distal radial fracture arthroscopic intraarticular gap and step-off measurement after open reduction and internal fixation with a volar locked plate. J Orthop Sci. 2012;17(4):443–9.

del Piñal F. Technical tips for (dry) arthroscopic reduction and internal fixation of distal radius fractures. J Hand Surg Am. 2011;36(10):1694–705.

Ruch DS, Yang CC, Smith BP. Results of acute arthroscopically repaired triangular fibrocartilage complex injuries associated with intra-articular distal radius fractures. Arthroscopy. 2003;19(5):511–6.

Scheer JH, Adolfsson LE. Patterns of triangular fibrocartilage complex (TFCC) injury associated with severely dorsally displaced extra-articular distal radius fractures. Injury. 2012;43(6):926–32.

27 Radial Styloid Fractures and Associated Carpal Injuries

Niels Thomsen

Contents

N. Thomsen, MD, PhD
Department of Hand Surgery, Skåne University Hospital, Lund University, Malmø, Sweden
e-mail: niels.thomsen@med.lu.se

27.1 Summary

Fractures of the radial styloid should always be suspected to be part of a progressive perilunate fracture-dislocation injury. Knowledge of the pathomechanism is therefore important in order to detect possible concomitant carpal injuries. A scapholunate ligament disruption and/or a scaphoid fracture are the most commonly associated injuries to the radial styloid fracture. However, correct diagnosis and choice of treatment remain a challenge as various combinations of intrinsic or radiocarpal ligament injuries are known to occur which may lead to late carpal instability. Knowledge of the anatomy and injury patterns is essential to avoid complications and provide optimal treatment. This chapter discusses surgical treatment of radial styloid fractures, concomitant scapholunate ligament tears, and screw fixation of concomitant scaphoid fractures.

27.2 Introduction

Radial styloid fractures have through the last century been synonymous to the term "chauffeur's fracture" (Stephens 1923). The fracture was initially described to occur due to backfire of the automobile crank, hence another synonym to radial styloid fractures, i.e., "backfire fracture." Although this particular trauma mechanism barely is important today, recognition and treatment of the fracture as well as its potentially associated carpal injuries are highly relevant.

L.M. Hove et al. (eds.), *Distal Radius Fractures*,
DOI 10.1007/978-3-642-54604-4_27,

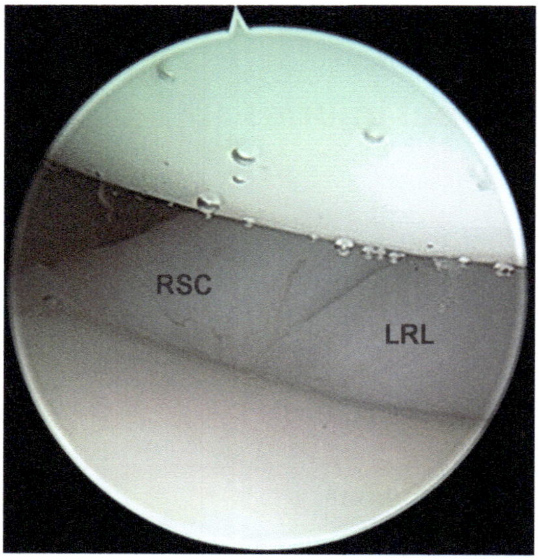

Fig. 27.1 Arthroscopic view of the radial styloid process with the radio-scapho-capitate (*RSC*) and the long radio-lunate (*LRL*) ligament

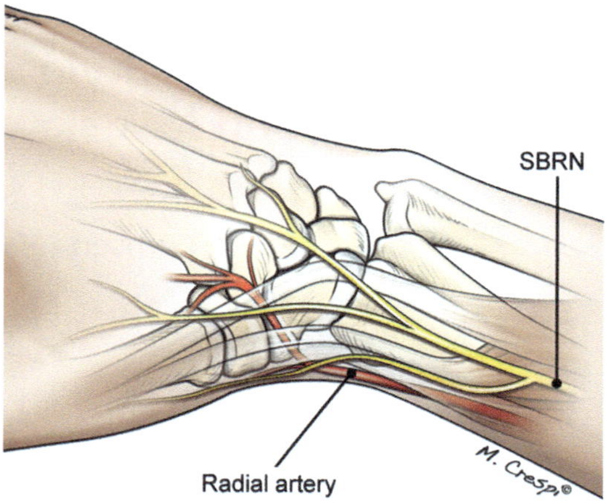

Fig. 27.2 Radial aspect of the wrist demonstrating the course of the superficial branch of the radial nerve (*SBRN*) and the radial artery

27.3 Relevant Anatomy

- The radial styloid mainly serve as a bony buttress for the carpus and provides attachment for two important palmar extrinsic carpal ligaments (Rikli et al. 2007).
- The radio-scapho-capitate (RSC) ligament originates from the radial styloid and the radial most 5–6 mm of the palmar rim of the radius (Fig. 27.1). It constrains against ulnar translocation of the carpus and stabilizes the distal pole of the scaphoid (Berger 1997).
- The long radio-lunate (LRL) ligament originates just ulnar to the RSC from the palmar rim of the scaphoid facet of the distal radius (Fig. 27.1). It further constrains against ulnar translocation of the carpus as well as palmar translocation of the carpus relative to the radius (Berger 1997).
- The brachioradialis tendon inserts at the base of radial styloid about 17 mm from the tip and continues 15 mm further proximally (Koh et al. 2006).
- Several subcutaneous structures are at risk when performing surgery in the radial styloid area (Chia et al. 2009).
- Abductor pollicis longus (APL) and extensor pollicis brevis (EPB) in the 1st extensor compartment run past the volar lateral aspect of the radial styloid process.
- The superficial branch of the radial nerve (SBRN) courses toward the thumb and first dorsal webspace. At the level of the extensor retinaculum, it further branches to innervate the dorsal and dorsoradial aspect of the index and middle finger, respectively (Fig. 27.2) (Steinberg et al. 1995).
- The dorsal branch of the radial artery passes deep to the APL and EPB tendons when it crosses dorsally in the anatomic snuffbox close to the scapho-trapezial-trapezoidal (STT) joint (Fig. 27.2).
- Due to the proximity of these anatomic structures, percutaneous pinning of radial styloid fractures carries a risk for iatrogenic injury. No reliable safe zone exists. It is therefore strongly advocated to make a small incision and do a blunt dissection down to the bone. K-wires should always be inserted using an oscillating drill and through a protective drill sleeve.

27.4 Pathomechanism

- The majority of radial-sided wrist injuries occur from a fall onto an outstretched hand.

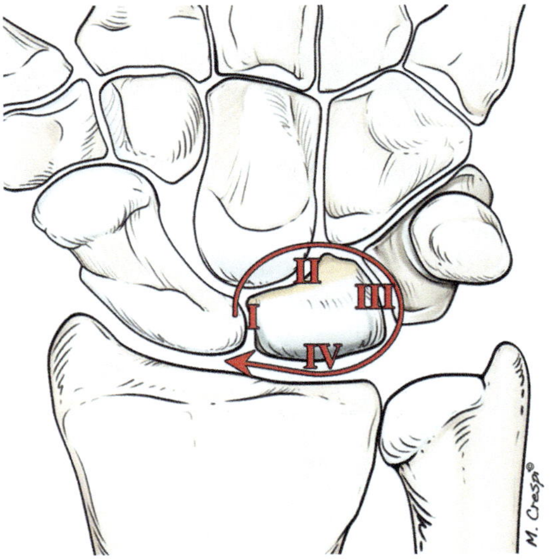

Fig 27.3 Stages of progressive perilunate instability according to Mayfield. Stage *I*: palmar radiocarpal and scapholunate ligaments tear. Stage *II*: lunocapitate tear. Stage *III*: lunotriquetral tear. Stage *IV*: complete palmar lunate dislocation

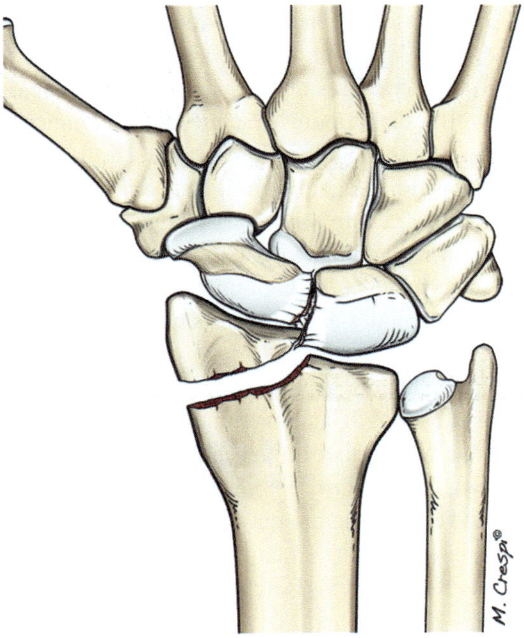

Fig 27.4 SL ligament rupture should always be considered in patients with a radial styloid fracture

- The subsequent axial load and hyperextension force may result in a distal radius fracture or a carpal fracture such as that of the scaphoid.
- If the injury mechanism combines hyperextension with ulnar deviation and intercarpal supination, a progressive perilunate fracture-dislocation injury pattern has been demonstrated to occur (Mayfield et al. 1980).
- The "lesser arc injuries" represent perilunate dislocations with a ligament-only injury. The sequential ligament disruption results in palmar radiocarpal and scapholunate (SL) ligaments tears (stage I), lunocapitate tear (stage II), and lunotriquetral (LT) tear (stage III), and finally a complete palmar lunate dislocation may occur (stage IV) (Fig. 27.3).
- When perilunate carpal bone fractures occur, instead of ligament tears, it is called a "greater arc injury." It may in its complete form incorporate a transradial styloid, trans-scaphoid, trans-capitate, trans-hamate, and trans-triquetrum fracture-dislocation (Johnson 1980).
- If the force extends through the tip of the radial styloid, it may involve an avulsion or disruption of the RSC ligament. Total RSC ligament avulsions should be suspected if the radial styloid fragment involves more than 6–8 mm of the volar joint surface. The load may then continue according to "the greater arc mechanism" or alternatively continue ulnarly in the radiocarpal joint across the extrinsic radiocarpal ligaments and the long and short radio-lunate ligament, with a risk of ulnar carpal translation and dorsal radiocarpal subluxation. This later form is called "radiocarpal fracture-dislocation."
- If, however, the load extends through the base of the radial styloid and continues onto the ridge between the scaphoid and the lunate fossa, there is a high risk of SL ligament tears and a more serious, complete or incomplete, perilunate injury should always be suspected (Fig. 27.4). Such an injury could include lunocapitate and LT ligament tears (Mayfield, stage III).
- A radial styloid fracture followed by a trans-capitate fracture is the most common other fracture found in relation to a scaphoid fracture (Jorgsholm et al. 2013).
- Scaphoid fractures are supposed to be found in isolation, but they are surprisingly often

found in combination with a SL ligament injury (Jorgsholm et al. 2010).
- Carpal fractures are found in 7 % of patients with a distal radius fracture, most commonly being a scaphoid fracture (Komura et al. 2012).
- Suspicion of a more complex, combined distal radius fracture with carpal bony or ligament injuries should always be considered in young male patients, in high-energy trauma, and in partial intra-articular fractures (AO/ASIF type B).
- Other factors such as age, bone quality, ligament strength, and magnitude and direction of load will further influence the injury pattern.
- NB, almost any combination of ligament tear and carpal fracture may occur from a progressive perilunate fracture-dislocation mechanism (Fig. 27.5) (Reichel et al. 2012).

27.5 Radiographic Imaging

- PA X-ray of the wrist makes it possible to evaluate radioulnar length, radial inclination, and articular congruity. Check for disruption of the carpal lines of Gilula, which outlines the proximal and distal articular surfaces of the proximal row as well as the proximal line of the capitate and hamate in the distal row. Ulnar translation of the carpus should be suspected if the lunate is >40 % uncovered by the radius with the wrist in neutral position (Fig. 27.6) (Gilula and Weeks 1978).
- True lateral, as opposed to a standard wrist lateral, is also named "articular views" due to the forearm being tilted about 20° to neutralize the radial angulation of the distal radius. This allows visualization of the lunate facet of the articular surface of the radius and can reveal loss of colinearity between the radius, lunate, and capitate. The center of the capitate's proximal pole should line up with a line parallel to the volar surface of the radius shaft.
- Oblique radiograph of the wrist in 45° of pronation and supination will provide additional information on fracture rotation/displacement of the radial styloid and sigmoid notch, which is not always recognizable on a PA view.
- CT investigation is helpful if a "greater arc" perilunate fracture-dislocation is suspected and will aid the surgeon for preoperative planning due to excellent visualization of the fracture fragments.
- MRI may demonstrate bone bruise, undisplaced carpal fractures, and ligament tears not shown on CT. However, MRI is not recommended as a routine imaging modality in these injuries.
- It is important to diagnose intrinsic carpal ligament injuries, which do not always show at the initial radiographic imaging. Traction fluoroscopy under anesthesia can be helpful to determine carpal instability.
- Arthroscopy is the considered "the gold standard" for diagnosing associated ligament injuries.

27.6 Classification

- The AO/ASIF classification system divides distal radius fractures into extra-articular (type A), partial intra-articular (type B), and complete intra-articular (type C) fractures (Müller et al. 1987) (Chap. 10).
- B 1.1 subclassification refers to a simple radial styloid fracture.
- B 1.2 is a multi-fragmentary styloid fracture.
- B 2.2 represents a more complex radiocarpal fracture subluxation that includes a radial styloid fragment.
- B 2.3 refers to a high-energy radiocarpal dorsal fracture-dislocation with a radial styloid fracture, comminuted dorsal rim, and disruption of the distal radioulnar (DRU) joint.
- Perilunate dislocations and fracture-dislocations have been further classified (Herzberg et al. 1993), where fractures of the tip of the radial styloid are referred to as associated chip fractures and fractures through the base of the radial styloid represents a subgroup of "the greater arc" perilunate fracture-dislocation (Herzberg et al. 1993).

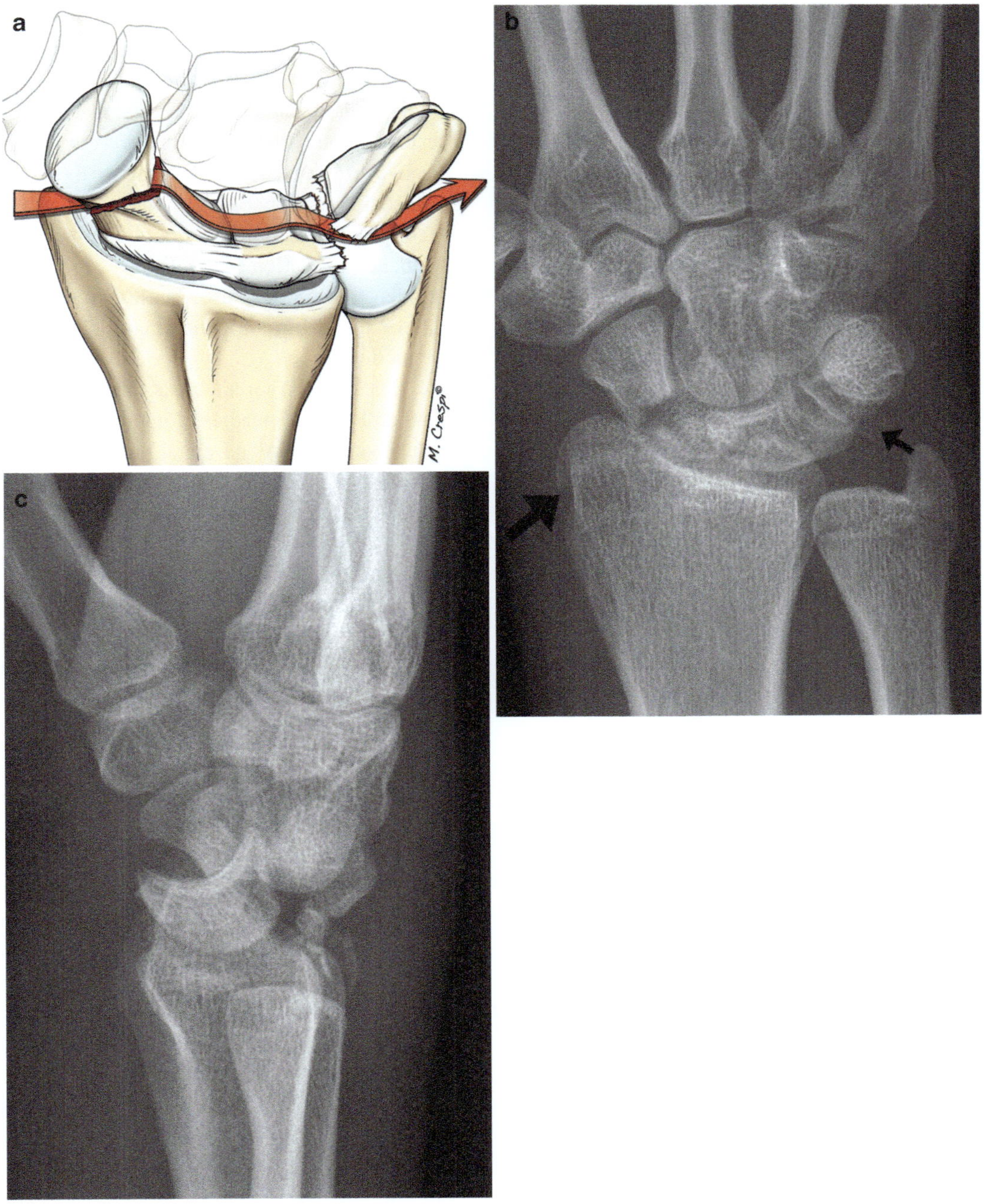

Fig 27.5 (**a**) A radial styloid tip fracture that continues through the waist of the scaphoid and further ulnarly with tearing of the LT ligament. (**b**) AP radiograph which demonstrates a radial styloid (*large arrow*) and scaphoid waist fracture. Small bone fragments are noted at the LT joint (*small arrow*). (**c**) Lateral radiograph reveals it to be part of a dorsal perilunate fracture-dislocation

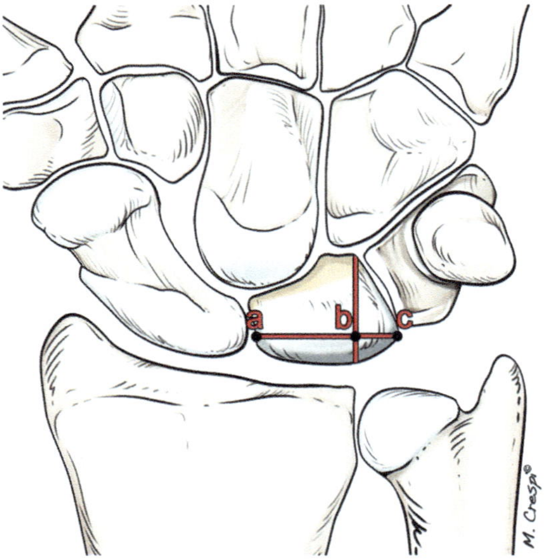

Fig 27.6 Ulnocarpal translation is estimated by calculating the lunate uncovering (distance *b to c*, divided by the distance of *a to c*)

27.7 Surgical Treatment

27.7.1 Radial Styloid Tip Fracture/Fragment

- Radial styloid tip fractures should always be evaluated for radiocarpal instability.
- If the fracture involves more than 6–8 mm of the styloid tip, the RSC ligament is avulsed and may potentially cause ulnar translocation of the carpus.
- Anatomic reduction and osteosynthesis of the fracture fragment will establish the necessary radiocarpal stability.
- K-wire pinning followed by cannulated screw fixation is recommended.
- Principles of surgical treatment are the same as for styloid base fractures (below).

27.7.2 Simple Radial Styloid Fracture at the Base

Open Procedure

- Make a longitudinal incision along the palmar part of the radial styloid.
- Use blunt dissection with attention to the SBRN and relevant anatomy as previously described.
- Use an oscillating drill to insert a K-wire into the radial styloid fragment on each side of the first extensor compartment. Alternatively, use a protective drill sleeve to avoid damage to the SBRN.
- Closed reduction of the fracture is usually achieved by longitudinal traction, ulnar deviation, and pronation of the hand.
- Under fluoroscopy, use the K-wires as joysticks to perform fracture manipulation and reduction.
- Advance the K-wires across the fracture site and replace with headless compression screws.
- Make sure there is no metal prominence over the cortical bone. This will reduce the risk of tendon attrition or nerve irritation.

Arthroscopically Assisted Treatment

- A radial styloid base fracture always carries a high risk for associated intrinsic ligament tears as part of a progressive perilunate "greater arc" pattern.
- Arthroscopy is highly recommended as it provides direct fracture visualization, ensures more accurate fracture reduction, and allows detection of associated intrinsic and extrinsic ligament injuries.
- Arthroscopy is technically demanding and requires surgical experience. However, its use in two- or three-part distal radius fractures is ideal.
- After placement of the K-wires into the radial styloid fragment, as described above, suspend the arm in a traction tower.
- Establish the 3–4 portal for instrumentation and the 6R portal for visualization of the fracture site.
- Irrigation of the joint is necessary to wash out fracture blood clots and improve visualization. Use a needle in the 6U portal for outflow.
- If dry arthroscopy is performed, use the shaver to aspirate fluid through the joint from a syringe connected to the valve of the sheath of the arthroscope.
- Compared to reduction based on fluoroscopy only, arthroscopy will often demonstrate rotation of the fracture fragment.

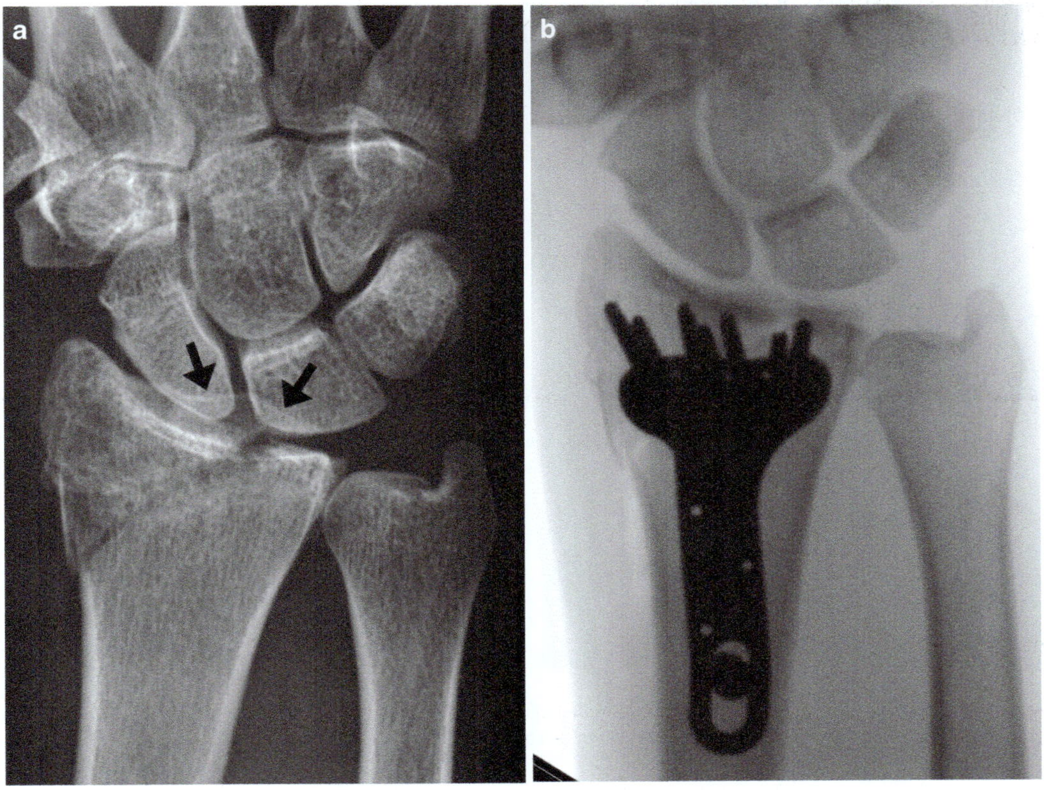

Fig. 27.7 (**a**) A three-part radial styloid fracture with a dislocated dorsal fragment (*arrows*). (**b**) Volar plating was performed in order to stabilize the dorsal fragment

- Under direct arthroscopic vision, combine fracture manipulation using the K-wires with a trochar, probe, or small periosteal elevator introduced through the 3–4 portal.
- After anatomic reduction, advance the K-wires over the fracture site.
- Finally, insert cannulated screws over the guide wires.

27.7.3 Comminuted Radial Styloid Fracture

- Surgical approach depends on fracture geometry and whether additional volar or dorsal fixation is required.
- If additional volar plating is planned, use the distal Henry approach between the radial artery and flexor carpi radialis (FCR) tendon (Fig. 27.7).
- If additional dorsal plating is planned, make the incision over Lister's tubercle.
- Otherwise, make the incision palmar radial between the radial artery and the first extensor compartment. NB! SBRN – blunt dissection!
- Slightly pronate the forearm.
- Make a sharp dissection of the interval between the first and second extensor compartment.
- Open the first extensor tendon compartment, but leave the distal one cm intact to prevent palmar tendon subluxation. Retract the tendons volarly or dorsally as preferred.
- Release of the distal insertion of the brachioradialis tendon often facilitates reduction of the styloid fragment.
- Initial fracture reduction is done by longitudinal traction, ulnar deviation, and pronation of the hand.
- Use a small periosteal elevator to reduce impacted fragments and align the articular surface. This procedure is best done under arthroscopic assistance, but alternatively a dorsal arthrotomy can be used.

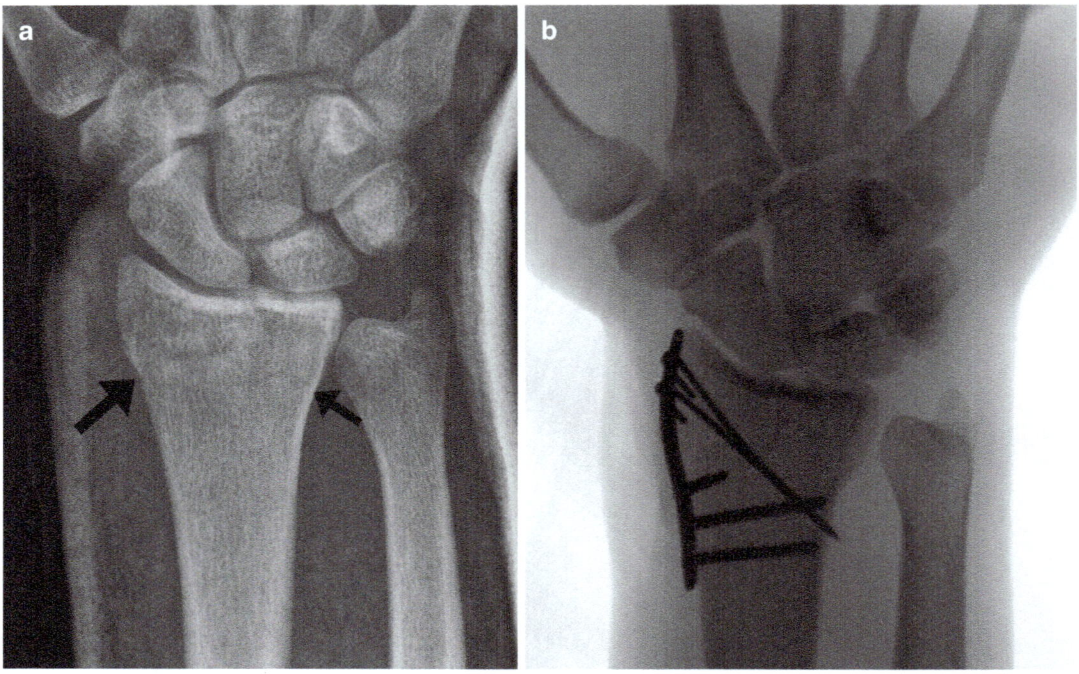

Fig. 27.8 (**a**) A radial styloid (*large arrow*) and lunate fossa (*small arrow*) fracture (Courtesy of Antonio Abramo). (**b**) Radial plating osteosynthesis (Courtesy of Antonio Abramo)

- Secure the fracture temporarily with one or two K-wires depending on fracture pattern. One K-wire inserted through the distal tip of the styloid will hold the length of the radial fragment. Another K-wire parallel to the joint surface can support reduced articular fragments.
- Apply a pre-contoured radial column plate and make sure it is correctly placed on the lateral, and not on the dorsal side of the radial column (Fig. 27.8).
- Prominent parts of the plate or screw heads will cause tendon attrition. Consider covering part of the plate with a slip of the retinaculum.

27.7.4 Concomitant SL Ligament Tears

- SL ligament tears are the most common intrinsic carpal ligament injury found in combination with a radial styloid fracture (Fig 27.9).
- SL ligament repair can be done open, as described here, or with arthroscopic assistance (Chap. 26). In these cases the fixation of the radial styloid fracture is done from dorsal, within the same approach.

Open SL Ligament Repair

- Make an incision centered over Lister's tubercle.
- Open the third extensor retinaculum and retract the EPL tendon radially.
- Subperiosteally, elevate the 4th extensor compartment onto the level of the 5th compartment.
- Elevate the 2nd extensor compartment and retract the ERCL/B together with the EPL in radial direction.
- Open the joint with a ligament-sparing capsulotomy. i.e., with an incision along the dorsal radiocarpal ligament (midpoint between Lister's tubercle and the sigmoid notch toward the dorsum of triquetrum) and dorsal intercarpal ligament (triquetrum to STT joint)

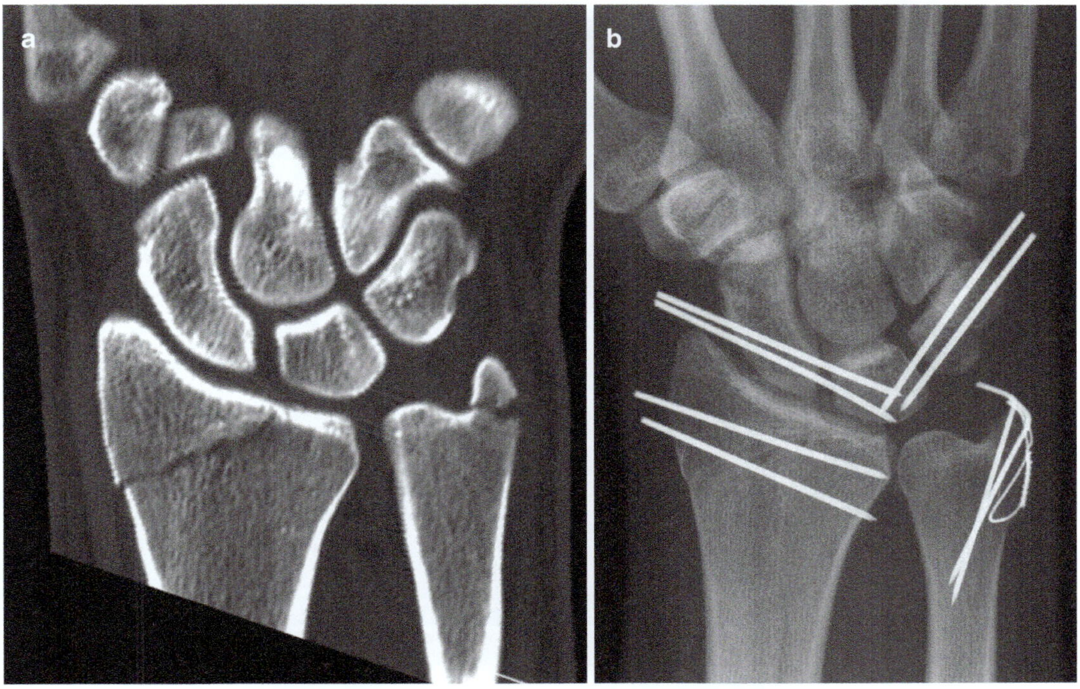

Fig. 27.9 (**a**) The radial styloid fracture line ends at the ridge between the scaphoid and the lunate fossae. Furthermore, an ulnar styloid base fracture is noted. (**b**) Arthroscopy revealed a Mayfield type III perilunate injury with disruption of the SL and LT ligaments. Reduction and pinning were done. Cannulated screw fixation of the radial styloid fragment was not performed, as mobilization of the wrist still had to await removal of the K-wires supporting the SL and LT joints

(Fig 27.10a). Complete the capsulotomy by dividing the radiocarpal capsule radially toward the tip of the styloid process.

- Carefully elevate the radially based capsular flap in order not to damage cartilage or intrinsic ligaments (Fig. 27.10b).
- If supported reduction of the SL joint is required, K-wires can be used as joysticks. Insert one K-wire into the scaphoid in proximal direction and another into the lunate in distal direction. Keep 5 mm distance from the SL articular surface.
- Hold the reduction with a Kocher clamp on the joystick K-wires.
- Under fluoroscopic control, insert two, 1.2- or 1.4-mm K-wires across the SL joint.
- Add another K-wire across the scapho-capitate joint to secure rotational stability of the scaphoid.
- Cut the K-wires subcutaneously, and beware that the cut ends do not impinge on the radial styloid process or important soft tissues structures.
- The SL ligament is often avulsed from the scaphoid but may be avulsed from the lunate (Fig. 27.10c). Ligament reattachment is done with the use of mini suture anchors after the insertion site has been prepared with a small curette.
- If the ligament is avulsed with a bone fragment, then either fix the fragment with a small screw or alternatively remove the fragment and reattach the ligament with a small bone anchor.
- A dorsal intercarpal capsulodesis is often done to augment the SL ligament repair.
- Detach the dorsal intercarpal ligament from the elevated capsular flap while maintaining its distal insertion to the STT joint.
- Fix the dorsal intercarpal ligament strip to the dorsum of the lunate either by using the inserted mini suture anchor (Fig. 27.10d) or by suturing it to the SL ligament.
- Make sure that passive extension of the wrist is possible.
- Close the dorsal capsule and suture the extensor retinaculum with absorbable sutures.

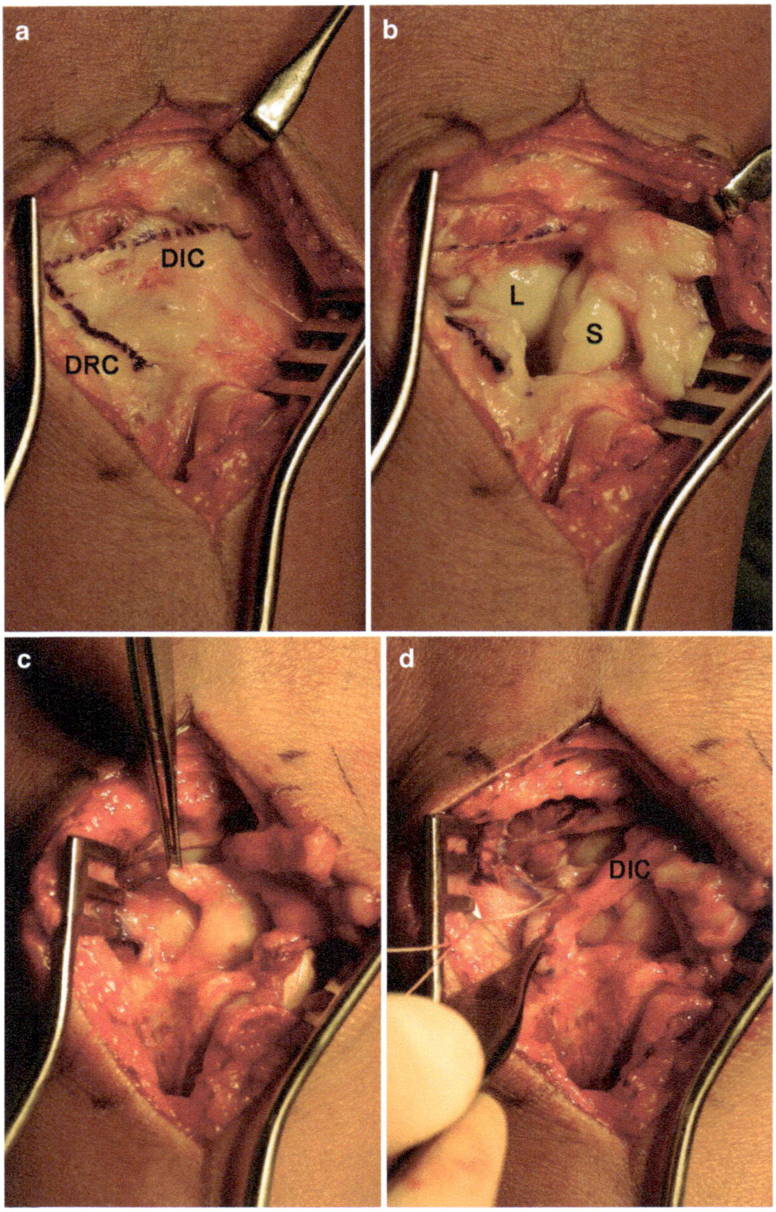

Fig. 27.10 (**a**) Intraoperative photo demonstrating the ligament-sparing capsulotomy. Incision is planned along the dorsal radiocarpal ligament (*DRC*) and the dorsal intercarpal ligament (*DIC*). (**b**). Complete scapholunate ligament rupture is demonstrated after elevation of the capsular flap. Scaphoid (*S*), lunate (*L*). (**c**) After reduction of the scapholunate joint, the avulsed scapholunate ligament, held by the forceps, is ready to be inserted onto the lunate using a mini suture anchor. (**d**) The dorsal intercarpal ligament (*DIC*) is included into the repair as a capsulodesis

27.7.5 Concomitant Scaphoid Fractures

The most common carpal fracture found in combination with a radial styloid fracture or perilunate fracture-dislocation is that of the scaphoid (Fig. 27.5b, c). Volar percutaneous fixation is recommended for minimally displaced scaphoid waist fractures. Dorsal approach to the scaphoid is suitable, for percutaneous fixation of scaphoid proximal pole fractures, although rare in perilunate injuries, or when additional intrinsic ligament repair is required.

Volar Retrograde Percutaneous Screw Fixation

- Access to the distal pole of the scaphoid is achieved with the wrist in extended position with some ulnar deviation.

- Use fluoroscopy to identify correct guidewire entrance point at the scaphoid tubercle, which should be central or slightly radial.
- Make a small 5–8-mm longitudinal incision and perform blunt dissection down to the STT joint.
- If required, a small periosteal elevator could help mobilize the scaphoid volarly, in order to allow the guidewire entrance point somewhat deeper in the joint than otherwise possible.
- Aim and insert the guidewire in approximately 45° dorsal and 30–45° ulnar direction toward the proximal pole of the scaphoid.
- Use fluoroscopy to secure guidewire placement along the central axis of the scaphoid.
- Minor fracture displacement can often be corrected by longitudinal traction and ulnar deviation of the carpus. Alternatively, use a small periosteal elevator to manipulate the distal fragment. Otherwise, use K-wires as joysticks to assist manipulation and reduction of the proximal and distal fragments.
- After reduction of the fracture, advance the guidewire to the subchondral bone of the proximal pole. Use fluoroscopy at multiple angles to confirm that the guidewire does not penetrate into the radiocarpal joint. It can be tricky due to the conic shape of the proximal pole.
- Measurement of the screw length is done either by the fixation system or by holding a guidewire parallel to the guidewire used for fixation, and then calculate the length of the guidewire within the scaphoid. Correct screw length is 4–5 mm shorter than measured to avoid protrusion of the screw.
- Additional K-wire stabilization is only needed for unstable fractures.
- Ream using a drill and not by hand, as torque, is less.
- A headless compression screw is passed over the guidewire and inserted until it cross the fracture line.
- Withdraw the guidewire to the fracture line before final tightening of the screw. A bent wire will block compression.
- Finally, confirm alignment and screw position by fluoroscopy (Fig. 27.11) and check that passive motion of the wrist can be done without hindrance.

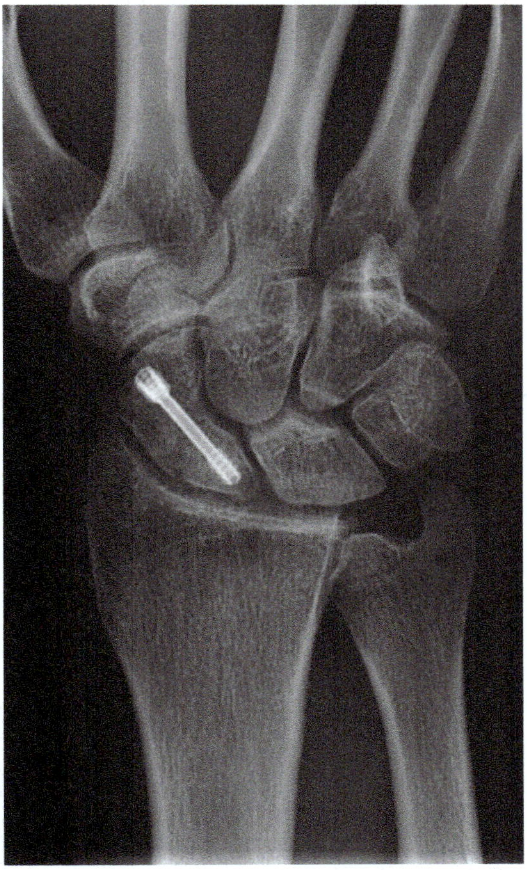

Fig. 27.11 Scaphoid screw fixation from distal to proximal

Dorsal Antegrade Percutaneous Screw Fixation

- Make a small skin incision over the radiocarpal joint 5–10 mm distal to Lister's tubercle.
- Flex the wrist and identify the central axis of the scaphoid by directing the guidewire toward the base of the thumb, parallel to the EPL tendon. Alternatively, pronate and flex the wrist until the "ring sign," which indicates the central axis of the scaphoid appears during fluoroscopy.
- Correct guidewire entrance point is usually 2 mm radially to the SL ligament insertion. Identify and confirm with fluoroscopy.
- The procedure follows the stepwise advice regarding reaming for volar percutaneous screw fixation.

Open Reduction and Internal Fixation: Dorsal Approach

- Make a slightly curved incision from the proximal aspect of Lister's tubercle and toward the STT joint.
- Incise the distal part of the 3rd compartment of the extensor retinaculum.
- Retract the EPL and the extensor carpi radialis brevis (ECRB) and longus (ECRL) tendons radially while retracting the extensor digitorum communis (EDC) tendons ulnarly.
- Make an incision at the edge of the SL articulation for your capsulotomy and extend along the axis of the scaphoid. For wider exposure divide the radiocarpal capsule radially toward the tip of the styloid process as necessary.
- If intrinsic ligament repair is considered, then the ligament-sparing capsulotomy, is recommended.
- Elevate the capsular flap but avoid compromising the blood supply that enters at the dorsal ridge of the scaphoid.
- Longitudinal traction will in many cases improve the reduction of the fracture. If necessary, use K-wires as joysticks in the proximal and distal scaphoid fragments.
- Inspect the radio-scaphoid and scapho-capitate articulation to assess and confirm reduction of the fracture.
- Insert a temporary fixation 1.2-mm K-wire within the dorsal aspect of the scaphoid.
- Flex the wrist and, from a starting point 1–2 mm radially to the SL ligament insertion on the scaphoid, use fluoroscopic guidance to insert a guidewire in the central axis of the scaphoid, similar to the percutaneous technique. Advance the guidewire to the subchondral bone of the distal fragment.
- Use fluoroscopy from multiple angles to verify correct guidewire placement. Screw length is determined by subtracting 4–5 mm from the length of the guidewire within the scaphoid.
- Advance the guidewire over the STT joint to achieve further stability.
- Use the drill when reaming down to the subchondral bone of the distal scaphoid.
- A headless compression screw is passed over the guidewire and inserted until it cross the fracture line.
- Retrieve the guidewire and the provisional K-wire fixation toward the fracture line as they otherwise could prevent compression or even cause distraction of the fragments.
- Advance and tighten the compression screw. Make sure that it sufficiently crosses the fracture line and does not protrude the articular surface of the proximal pole or penetrate into the STT joint.
- Check that passive motion of the wrist is unrestricted.
- Close the dorsal capsule and suture the extensor retinaculum with absorbable sutures.

27.8 Postoperative Care

This is most often high-energy trauma with a lot of swelling due to both the injury and also the surgical procedure. Therapy therefore becomes a very important part of early postoperative care. Active finger range of motion is initiated from the first postoperative day. Hand therapist support may be indicated if the fingers are swollen or if range of motion is restricted.

27.8.1 Radial Styloid Fracture

- For patients with a fracture that has been rigidly fixed with cannulated screws or a dedicated radial column plate mobilization of the wrist can begin 1–2 weeks after surgery.
- If pinning has been performed, the wrist should be immobilized in a cast for 4–6 weeks until removal of K-wires.

27.8.2 Scapholunate Ligament Injury

- K-wires will loosen or break if range of motion exercises are initiated before their removal. Therefore, the wrist should be immobilized in a cast for 8 weeks until removal of K-wires.

27.8.3 Scaphoid Fracture

- For patients with a minimally displaced fracture that has been rigidly fixed, mobilization can begin 2 weeks after surgery. A removable splint is used between exercises.
- If the fracture was severely displaced or unstable, then immobilization should be continued for 4–6 weeks after surgery.
- Follow the patient until fracture healing has been verified. Standard X-rays are not always reliable; hence, CT should be considered.

27.9 Complications

- Missed diagnosis of concomitant ligament injuries!
- Pin tract infection
- Injury to the superficial radial nerve branch
- Painful neuroma
- Protrusion of hardware
- Extensor tenosynovitis due to attrition
- Late presentation of carpal instability
- Nonunion

References

Berger RA. The ligaments of the wrist. A current overview of anatomy with considerations of their potential functions. Hand Clin. 1997;13:63–82.

Chia B, Catalano 3rd LW, Glickel SZ, Barron OA, Meier K. Percutaneous pinning of distal radius fractures: an anatomic study demonstrating the proximity of K-wires to structures at risk. J Hand Surg Am. 2009;34:1014–20.

Gilula LA, Weeks PM. Post-traumatic ligamentous instabilities of the wrist. Radiology. 1978;129:641–51.

Herzberg G, Comtet JJ, Linscheid RL, Amadio PC, Cooney WP, Stalder J. Perilunate dislocations and fracture-dislocations: a multicenter study. J Hand Surg Am. 1993;18:768–79.

Johnson RP. The acutely injured wrist and its residuals. Clin Orthop Relat Res. 1980;(149):33–44.

Jorgsholm P, Thomsen NO, Bjorkman A, Besjakov J, Abrahamsson SO. The incidence of intrinsic and extrinsic ligament injuries in scaphoid waist fractures. J Hand Surg Am. 2010;35:368–74.

Jorgsholm P, Thomsen NO, Besjakov J, Abrahamsson SO, Bjorkman A. The benefit of magnetic resonance imaging for patients with posttraumatic radial wrist tenderness. J Hand Surg Am. 2013;38:29–33.

Koh S, Andersen CR, Buford Jr WL, Patterson RM, Viegas SF. Anatomy of the distal brachioradialis and its potential relationship to distal radius fracture. J Hand Surg Am. 2006;31:2–8.

Komura S, Yokoi T, Nonomura H, Tanahashi H, Satake T, Watanabe N. Incidence and characteristics of carpal fractures occurring concurrently with distal radius fractures. J Hand Surg Am. 2012;37:469–76.

Mayfield JK, Johnson RP, Kilcoyne RK. Carpal dislocations: pathomechanics and progressive perilunar instability. J Hand Surg Am. 1980;5:226–41.

Müller ME, Nazarian S, Koch P, Schatzker J. AO classification of fractures. Berlin: Springer; 1987. p. 106–15.

Reichel LM, Bell BR, Michnick SM, Reitman CA. Radial styloid fractures. J Hand Surg Am. 2012;37:1726–41.

Rikli DA, Honigmann P, Babst R, Cristalli A, Morlock MM, Mittlmeier T. Intra-articular pressure measurement in the radioulnocarpal joint using a novel sensor: in vitro and in vivo results. J Hand Surg Am. 2007;32:67–75.

Steinberg BD, Plancher KD, Idler RS. Percutaneous Kirschner wire fixation through the snuff box: an anatomic study. J Hand Surg Am. 1995;20:57–62.

Stephens P. So-called chauffeur's fracture. Cal State J Med. 1923;21:115–7.

Acute Injuries Around the Distal Ulna

28

Lars Adolfsson and Johan Scheer

Contents

L. Adolfsson, MD, PhD (✉)
Department of Orthopaedics, Linköping University Hospital, University of Linköping, Linköping, Sweden
e-mail: lars.adolfsson@lio.se

J. Scheer, MD, PhD
Department of Orthopaedics, Linköping University Hospital, Linköping, Sweden

28.1 Summary

Soft tissue lesions around the distal ulna as well as fractures of the styloid process are common in association with dorsally displaced distal radius fractures. A majority of the ligamentous injuries appear to affect the triangular fibrocartilage complex (TFCC) in varying degrees. Dorsal fracture displacement more than 34° from anatomic position has been found impossible with intact TFCC attachment. The injury may cause ulno-carpal or distal radio-ulnar joint (DRUJ) instability. In low-demand patients, this however appears well tolerated. Early repair in the acute stage is recommended with severe instability, particularly in high-demand patients. Concomitant fractures of the ulnar styloid process have not, in adults, been found to affect outcome, and early repair is not recommended if sufficient wrist stability can be achieved by treatment of the radius fracture.

28.2 Introduction

Displaced fractures of the distal radius are frequently associated with fractures of the ulnar styloid process or soft tissue lesions around the distal ulna (Geissler et al. 1996; Lindau et al. 1997; Adolfsson and Jörgsholm 1998). The soft tissue component may engage the triangular fibrocartilage complex (TFCC) as well as the volar and dorsal capsule and extrinsic capsular ligaments of the ulno-carpal joint, the distal radio-ulnar joint (DRUJ) and the deep layers of

L.M. Hove et al. (eds.), *Distal Radius Fractures*,
DOI 10.1007/978-3-642-54604-4_28, © Springer-Verlag Berlin Heidelberg 2014

the extensor carpi ulnaris tendon sheath (Scheer and Adolfsson 2011). Frequencies between approximately 45 and 75 % of TFCC lesions have been reported and found associated with both intra- and extra-articular fractures (Geissler et al. 1996; Lindau et al. 1997; Richards et al. 1997; Adolfsson and Jörgsholm 1998).

28.3 Pathomechanisms

The vast majority of distal radius fractures are likely to be caused by a fall on an outstretched hand. Previous reports on epidemiology have demonstrated that postmenopausal women are mostly affected and the majority of fractures are low-energy injuries causing a fracture of the dorsal bending type (O'Neill et al. 2001). With this type of fracture, experimental work has demonstrated that a dorsal displacement of more than 34° from the anatomic position cannot occur with intact ulnar soft tissues (Scheer and Adolfsson 2011).

- The first associated lesion observed to occur due to a dorsal bending force was a separation of the ECU subsheath from the dorso-ulnar part of the TFCC. Sasao et al. (2003) described a ligament running deep to the ECU subsheath which in this scenario obviously also is separated from the TFCC (Figs. 28.1 and 28.2).
- With progressive dorsal angulation, the volar structures, ulno-capitate ligament, volar DRU joint capsule and the volar attachment of the TFCC on the base of the styloid process become gradually loaded and may eventually fail (Fig. 28.3).
- The injury then appears to progress from volar to dorsal affecting the deep TFCC insertion into the pre-styloid fovea and styloid base (Fig. 28.3).
- Probably depending on the force transmission and the resistance of the TFCC insertion, the ulnar styloid process may be affected, resulting in a fracture at varying locations. Four separate patterns of lesions of the soft tissues around the styloid were observed in a cadaver study (Fig. 28.3) (Scheer and Adolfsson 2011). A fracture through the base of the styloid process produced a different lesion in which the volar capsule and the deep foveal insertion of the TFCC were affected but the soft tissues inserting on the styloid process left intact (Fig. 28.4).
- A fracture through the base was not found to be associated with an ECU subsheath avulsion but rather displaced dorsally with the entire soft tissue envelope.

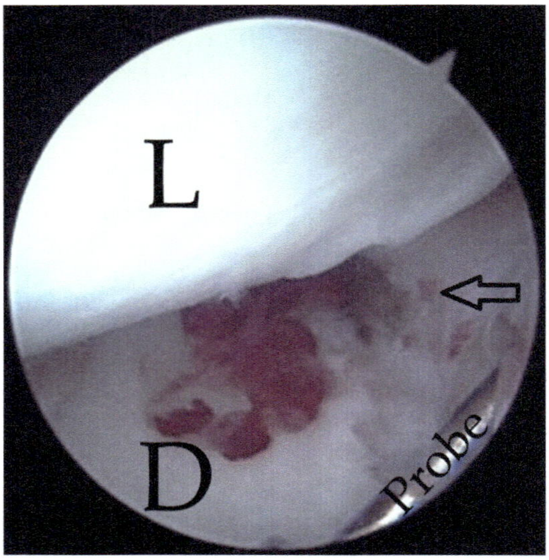

Fig. 28.1 This arthroscopic photo shows a right wrist with dorso-ulnar peripheral acute separation between the TFCC and ECU subsheath (*arrow*) associated with a dorsally displaced distal radius fracture (Reprinted from Scheer and Adolfsson (2012))

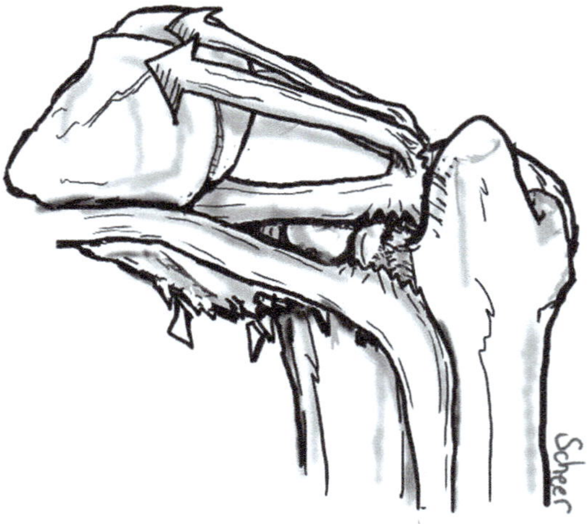

Fig. 28.2 Schematic drawing of the pathomechanism of an ECU subsheath tear (Reprinted from Scheer and Adolfsson (2012))

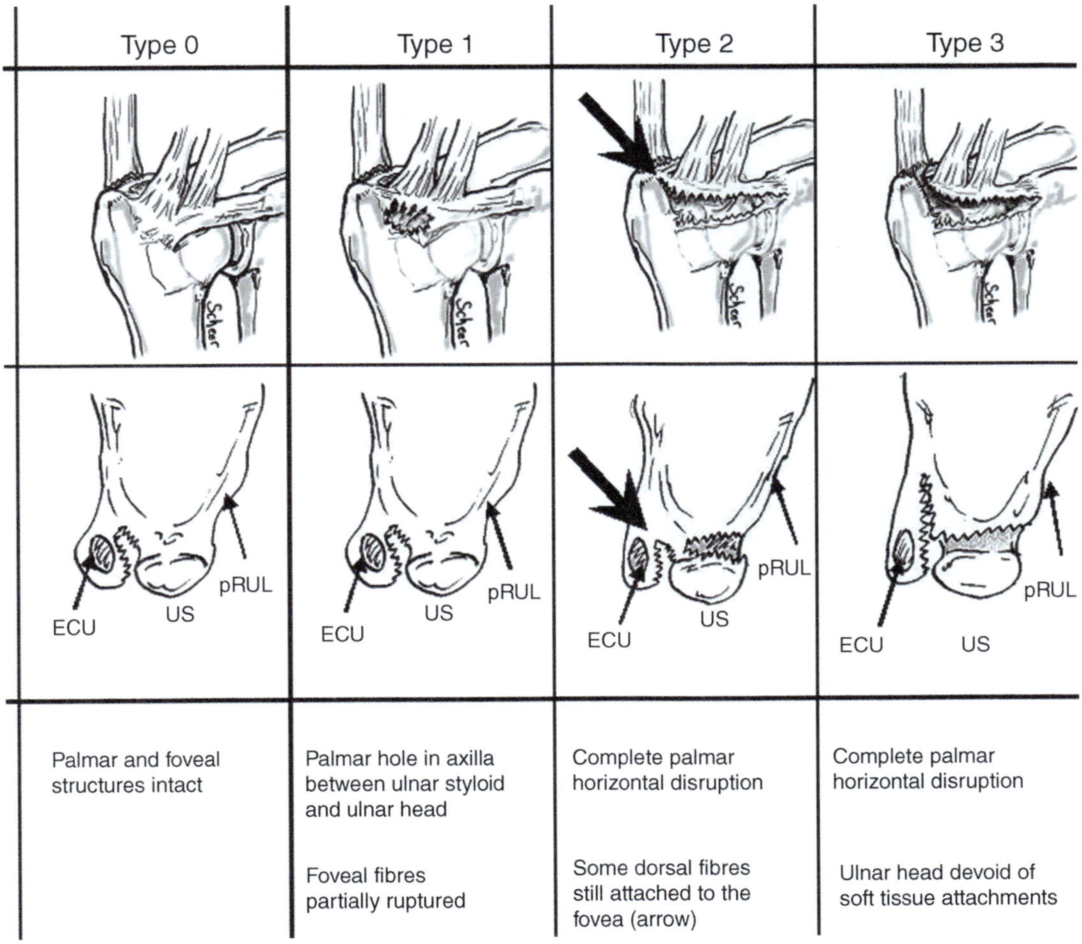

Fig. 28.3 Four stages of ulnar soft tissue affection with increasing dorsal angulation of the distal radius (Reprinted from Scheer and Adolfsson (2012))

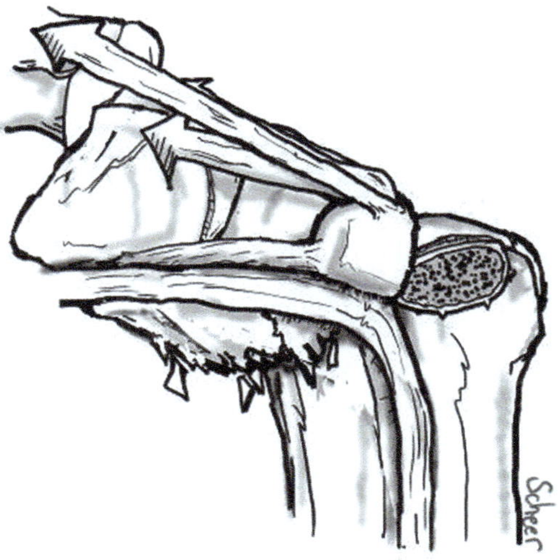

Fig. 28.4 Drawing of the findings associated with a ulnar styloid base fracture

- The first sequence of the peri-ulnar injury only affected the ECU subsheath and some of the volar soft tissue attachments on the styloid process. In a manual laxity test, this produced increased laxity of the ulno-carpal joint but no DRU instability. When the deep fibres of the TFCC are concomitantly avulsed, an increased laxity of the DRU was observed. This complete displacement of the entire soft tissue envelope allowed the ulnar head to protrude through the volar capsule to be subcutaneous during displacement of the fracture. This finding was later confirmed clinically and referred to as a "bald ulnar head" (Fig. 28.5) (Scheer and Adolfsson 2012).

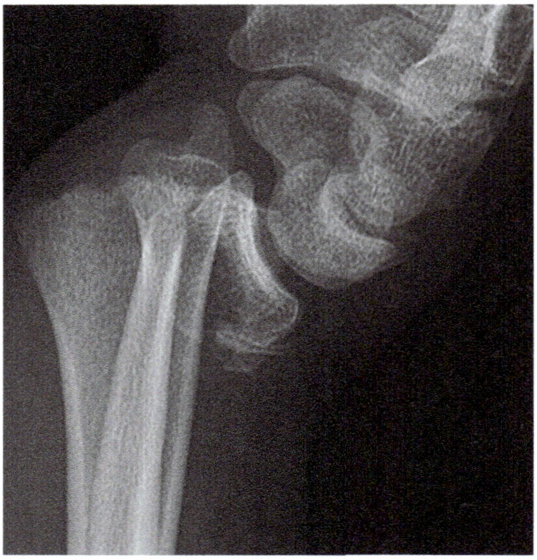

Fig. 28.5 The "bald ulnar head". With severe dorsal displacement of the distal radius, all soft tissues are dorsally displaced with the distal radius fragment leaving the ulnar head subcutaneously (Reprinted from Scheer and Adolfsson (2012))

28.4 Diagnosis

- The displacement observed at the initial x-rays at presentation has probably been more pronounced at the time of impact. Some degree of spontaneous reduction is likely to occur with extra-articular fractures. In intra-articular fractures and fractures following a high-energy trauma, the degree of initial displacement may be more difficult to assess, but high suspicion of associated lesions is warranted.
- If initial x-rays demonstrate a marked displacement between the fractured fragment of the distal radius and the ulnar head, this is indicative of a pronounced soft tissue affection. Since lateral views are often taken with the aim to have the styloid processes of the radius and ulna aligned, a displacement may easily be overlooked. If instead the shafts of the bones are parallel and aligned, the displacement is often evident.
- At clinical examination, swelling and tenderness around the distal ulna obviously indicate an associated injury. Palpation of the area may reveal fractures of the ulna and assessment of ECU stability in its groove. Clinical laxity testing may be indicated in this situation and can be performed if the fractured fragment of the distal radius is manually stabilised after anaesthesia. In the instance that the distal radius fracture is to be treated by internal fixation, the laxity test is performed after the distal radius has been stabilised. With conservative treatment, laxity testing can be performed after infiltration with local anaesthesia in the fracture haematoma followed by reduction as necessary. After closed reduction, the fracture can be stabilised manually, and using the other hand, the examiner may assess ulno-carpal and DRU laxity. The uninjured wrist is always used for comparison.

28.5 Indications for Treatment

- A pronounced, untreated ulno-carpal or DRU laxity may cause ulnar-sided wrist pain as demonstrated by several reports on late repair (Haugstvedt and Husby 1999).
- In a recent long-term follow-up of TFCC lesions diagnosed in the acute stage, a correlation was found between laxity and inferior grip strength. In the majority of cases, most lesions were however well tolerated, and in this study late surgery was only rarely needed (Mrkonjic et al. 2012).
- A pseudarthrosis of the ulnar styloid process may also be symptomatic. Frykman in his classic study found inferior outcome in patients with associated ulnar styloid fractures (Frykman 1967). The impact of ulnar styloid fractures has since then been frequently investigated, and apart from a recent report on children (Zoetch et al. 2013), none of the relatively large studies published in recent years could demonstrate that acute repair of ulnar styloid fractures would be beneficial (Krämer et al. 2013; Zenke et al. 2012; Reichl et al. 2011; Souer et al. 2009; Sammer et al. 2009).
- It is apparent that residual symptoms are unacceptable to some patients, but presently there are no guidelines to which lesions and patients that would benefit from acute repair. The published results of late repair have been encouraging

which makes late reconstruction in patients with intolerable symptoms a reasonable alternative. It however appears likely that in the rare instance of an acute, complete dislocation of the DRU joint, stabilisation and repair should be performed. Most series of late repairs include relatively young patients in whom increased laxity around the ulnar head appears less well accepted. It may therefore be possible that acute repair could be considered in young, high-demand individuals with pronounced laxity. In severely comminuted fractures of the distal radius following a high-energy trauma or concomitant carpal injuries, a stabilisation of a displaced ulnar styloid fracture may be indicated to enhance stability of the wrist.

28.6 Methods of Treatment

- Fractures of the ulnar styloid are often classified according to the location. There are no reports on fixation of tip fractures which are mainly considered as avulsion injuries with a good prognosis.
- Displaced fractures in the proximal third or at the base are believed to be more often associated with instability problems, and fixation may occasionally be indicated as discussed above. Large fragments may be reduced and fixed with screw, but fracture of the styloid during screw insertion is always a concern. Most reports on fixation have been using a modified tension band technique with two K-wires on either side of the styloid tip and a cerclage wire or large-diameter suture around the wires, underneath the ECU tendon sheath in an 8-configuration (Fig. 28.6).
- The repair of TFCC lesions is dependent on the extent of the injury. In the majority of cases, the dorsal displacement of the radius fracture inflicts a peripheral tear causing ulnocarpal laxity. The defect between the dorsal radio-ulnar ligament and the ECU subsheath can be sutured back to the capsule. Arthroscopy-assisted repair is most frequently adopted, and several reports with varying methods have been described.

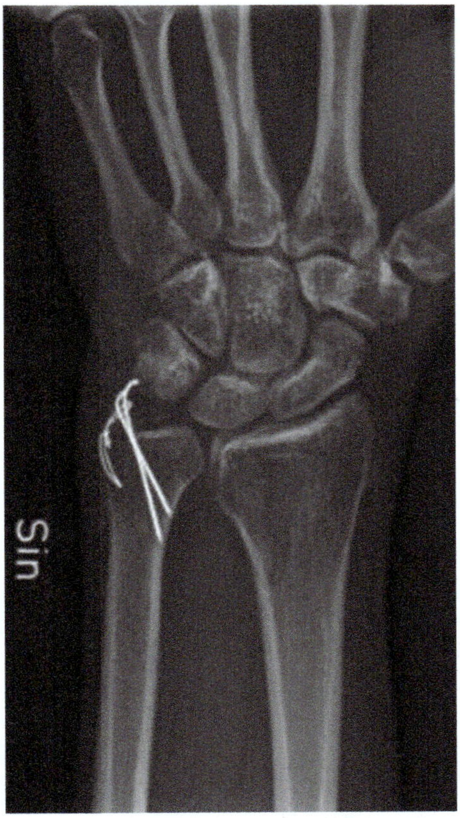

Fig. 28.6 An ulnar styloid fracture repaired with tension band technique

- More pronounced injuries, affecting the deep fibres of the TFCC causing increased DRU laxity, require bony reattachment of the TFCC to the ulna (Fig. 28.5).
- This may also be accomplished using arthroscopic assistance, but since the lesion often involves the volar capsule and ligaments that are usually not visible from inside the joint, open repair from a volar approach has been advocated (Moritomo 2009; Scheer and Adolfsson 2012) (Fig. 28.7).
- In cases where internal fixation or suture is found indicated, the repair is protected in a below-elbow plaster splint for 5 weeks. After removal of the plaster, active exercises are allowed, but an orthotic brace is used between exercises during 3 weeks. Eight weeks after the operation, normal activities of daily living are allowed without brace. Heavy load is avoided until 12 weeks postoperatively.

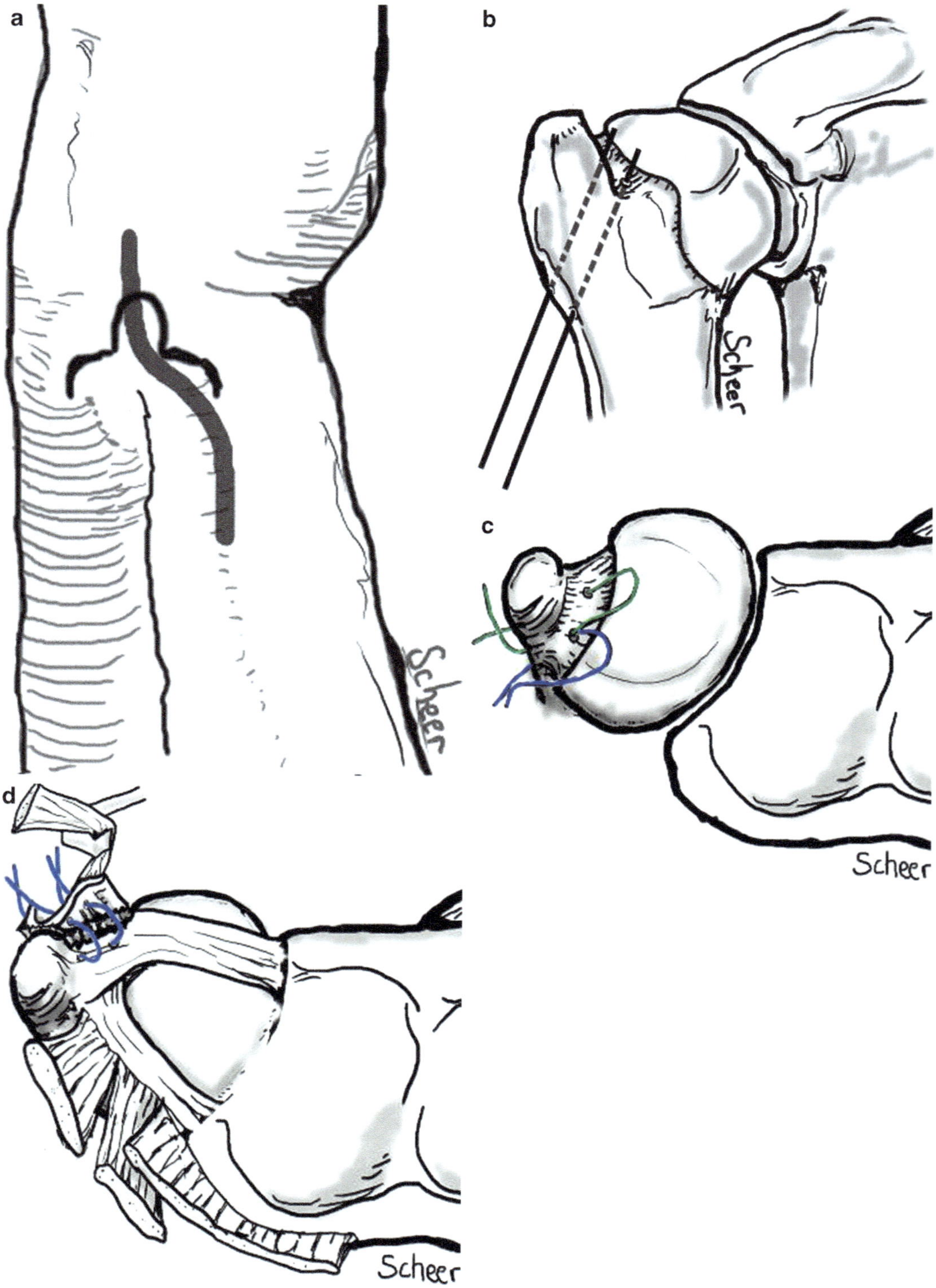

Fig. 28.7 Drawing of methods for TFCC repair including trans-osseous sutures and repair of a dorsal separation. (**a**) Skin incision. (**b**) Drill holes aiming at the pre-styloid fovea. (**c**) Two sutures placed where one is allowed to engage the volar capsule. (**d**) Final sutures of the dorsal peripheral sub-sheath separation (Reprinted from Scheer and Adolfsson (2012))

28.7 Results

- Presently, on a group level, there is no evidence to suggest that primary fixation of an ulna styloid fracture is beneficial. The available data however suggest that if such a treatment, for reasons discussed above, is instituted, the results are usually good.
- Sutures of TFCC lesions resulting in moderate ulno-carpal or DRU instability have uniformly been reported to produce acceptable results, in both the acute and late stages. In the more unusual instance of a severe DRU instability, a direct suture in the late stage may however not be sufficient, and ligament reconstructions may be required. In acute lesions with severe instability or complete dislocation of the DRU joint, a primary stabilisation and repair are most likely warranted.

References

Adolfsson L, Jörgsholm P. Arthroscopically-assisted reduction of intra-articular fractures of the distal radius. J Hand Surg Br. 1998;23:391–5.

Frykman G. Fracture of the distal radius including sequelae-shoulder hand finger syndrome, disturbance in the distal radio-ulnar joint and impairment of nerve function. A clinical and experimental study. Acta Orthop Scand. 1967;Suppl 108:3.

Geissler WB, Freeland AE, Savoie FH, et al. Intra-articular soft-tissue lesions associated with an intra-articular fracture of the distal end of the radius. J Bone Joint Surg Am. 1996;78:357–65.

Haugstvedt JR, Husby T. Results of repair of peripheral tears in the triangular fibrocartilage complex using an arthroscopic suture technique. Scand J Plast Reconstr Surg Hand Surg. 1999;33:439–47.

Krämer S, Meyer H, O'Laughlin PF, Vaske B, Krettek C, Gaulke R. The incidence of ulnocarpal complaints after a distal radial fracture in relation to the fracture of the ulnar styloid. J Hand Surg Eur Vol. 2013;38:710–7.

Lindau T, Arner M, Hagberg L. Intraarticular lesions in distal fractures of the radius in young adults. A descriptive arthroscopic study in 50 patients. J Hand Surg Br. 1997;22:638–43.

Moritomo H. Advantages of open repair of foveal tear of the triangular fibrocartilage complex via a palmar surgical approach. Tech Hand Up Extrem Surg. 2009;13:176–81.

Mrkonjic A, Geijer M, Lindau T, Tägil M. The natural course of traumatic triangular fibrocartilage complex tears in distal radial fractures: a 13–15 year follow-up of arthroscopically diagnosed but untreated injuries. J Hand Surg Am. 2012;37:1555–60.

O'Neill TW, Cooper C, Finn JD, Lunt M, Purdie D, Reid DM, Rowe R, Woolf AD, Wallace WA. UK Colles' Fracture Study Group. Incidence of distal forearm fracture in British men and women. Osteoporos Int. 2001;12:555–8.

Reichl M, Piatek S, Adolf D, Winckler S, Westphal T. Unrepaired fracture of the styloid process of the ulna: not a bad treatment result at distal radius fracture. Unfallchirurg. 2011;114:1099–104.

Richards RS, Bennett JD, Roth JH, Milne Jr K. Arthroscopic diagnosis of intra-articular soft tissue injuries associated with distal radial fractures. J Hand Surg Am. 1997;22:772–6.

Sammer DM, Shah HM, Shauver MJ, Chung KC. The effect of ulnar styloid fractures on patient-rated outcomes after volar locking plating of distal radius fractures. J Hand Surg Am. 2009;34:1595–602.

Sasao S, Beppu M, Kihara H, Hirata K, Takagi M. An anatomical study of the ligaments of the ulnar compartment of the wrist. Hand Surg. 2003;8:219–26.

Scheer JH, Adolfsson LE. Pathomechanisms of ulnar ligament lesions of the wrist in a cadaveric distal radius fracture model. Acta Orthop. 2011;82:360–4.

Scheer JH, Adolfsson LE. Patterns of triangular fibrocartilage complex (TFCC) injury associated with severely dorsally displaced extra-articular distal radius fractures. Injury. 2012;43:926–32.

Souer JS, Ring D, Matschke S, Audige L, Marent-Huber M, Jupiter JB. AOCID Prospective ORIF Distal radius Study Group. Effect of an unrepaired fracture of the ulnar styloid base on outcome after plate-and-screw fixation of a distal radial fracture. J Bone Joint Surg Am. 2009;91:830–8.

Zenke Y, Sakai A, Oshige T, Moritani S, Nakamura T. Treatment with or without internal fixation for ulnar styloid base fractures accompanied by distal radius fracture fixed with volar locking plate. Hand Surg. 2012;17:181–90.

Zoetch S, Kraus T, Weinberg AM, Heidari N, Lindtner RA, Singer G. Fracture of the ulnar styloid process negatively influences the outcome of paediatric fractures of the distal radius. Acta Orthop Belg. 2013;79:48–53.

Bone Substitutes, Grafts and Cement

29

Magnus Tagil

Contents

M. Tagil, MD
Department of Hand Surgery,
Lund's University Hospital, Lund, Sweden

Department of Orthopedic Surgery,
University of Lund, Lund, Sweden
e-mail: magnus.tagil@med.lu.se

29.1 Summary

Bone is a unique tissue for all members of "the vertebrate family" and necessary for us to be able to walk upright. Bone is the only tissue capable to fully regenerate. Injured bone is able to heal and form bone again with the full function of the original tissue. All other tissues will undergo some degree of scar or fibrous tissue formation with an impaired function compared to the original tissue. However, there are times when this regenerative process fails or when we rapidly need to form large quantities of bone.

29.2 Introduction

29.2.1 When Do We Need to Replace Bone?

Bone is a paradox material. Dead bone is practically as strong as living bone, but fatigue fractures would rapidly occur without an elegant maintenance and repair system.

Bone is a living material in a living organism but consists mainly of dead inorganic mineral arranged in hydroxyapatite crystals. About 2/3 of the weight consists of minerals and 1/3 of organic material, mainly collagen, but also other important proteins involved in the regulation of bone repair and formation.

- The bone cells produce osteoid, which is basically a collagen mass. The osteoid subsequently becomes mineralised, and the bone-

L.M. Hove et al. (eds.), *Distal Radius Fractures*,
DOI 10.1007/978-3-642-54604-4_29, © Springer-Verlag Berlin Heidelberg 2014

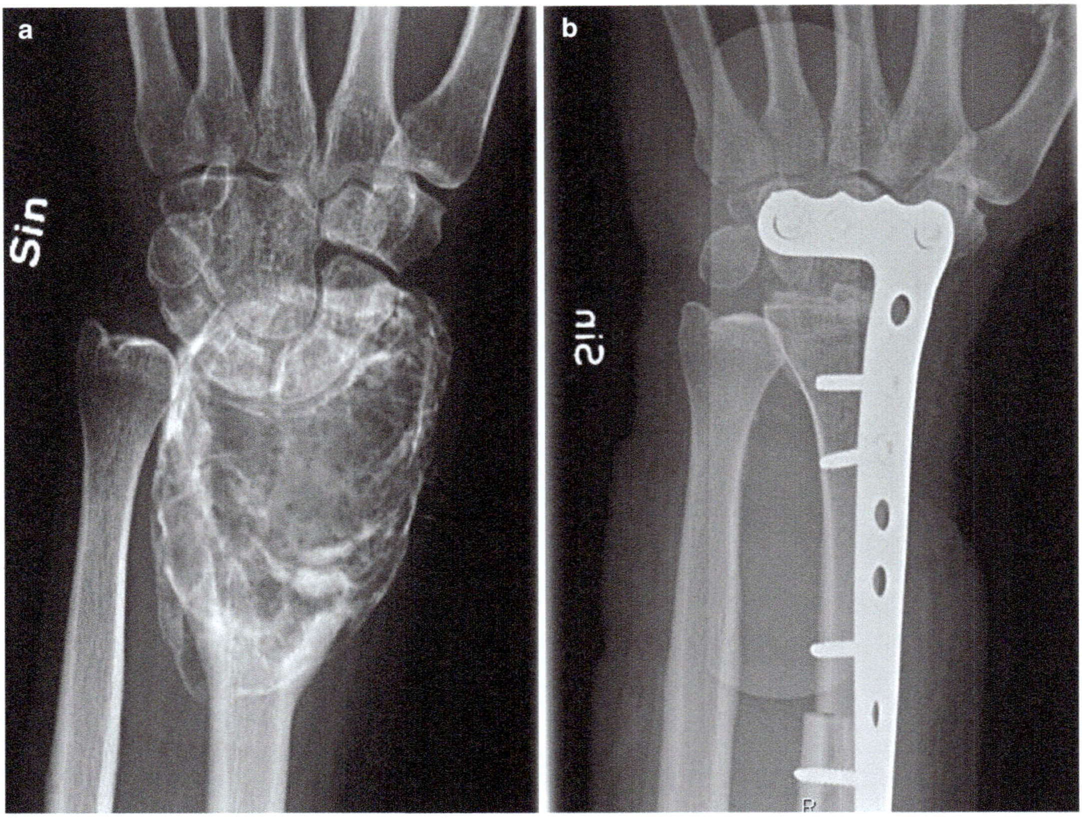

Fig. 29.1 (**a**, **b**) A bone allograft is used in a large defect after an osteolytic giant cell tumour

forming cell eventually becomes buried in its own osteoid.

- Most of the bone-forming cells undergo apoptosis, programmed cell death, after being active, but some survive as osteocytes with an important function of sensing deformation.
- The bone-resorbing cells, the osteoclasts, work tightly with the bone-forming cells to keep the bone mass and structure optimised in function regarding strength vs. weight (Dimitriou et al. 2011).

There are two main reasons to interfere with nature in order to make bone: firstly to restore the *mechanical support* or secondly to *initiate bone healing*:

Mechanical Support

- In the first case, bone is to a larger or lesser extent missing, and the distance between the living bone ends is too long for the patient's own bone-forming capacity to fill the void. This may be the case in a segmental bone defect after a tumour resection or a reconstructive osteotomy with a "bone loss" that would not fill spontaneously by normal callus (Figs. 29.1 and 29.2).
- The need is obvious from a mechanical point of view, and we have to replace the missing bone as otherwise the extremity would be too short after fixation in the tumour case, or we would have a metal fatigue fracture of the plate fixing the osteotomy.
- For immediate fixation, we can use a bone graft to fill the defect or a bone substitute or even polymethylmethacrylate (PMMA or "bone cement"). For the immediate fixation properties, the choice of material is not essential, but during the healing and remodelling period, all those materials will behave differently and affect the end result (Fig. 29.2).

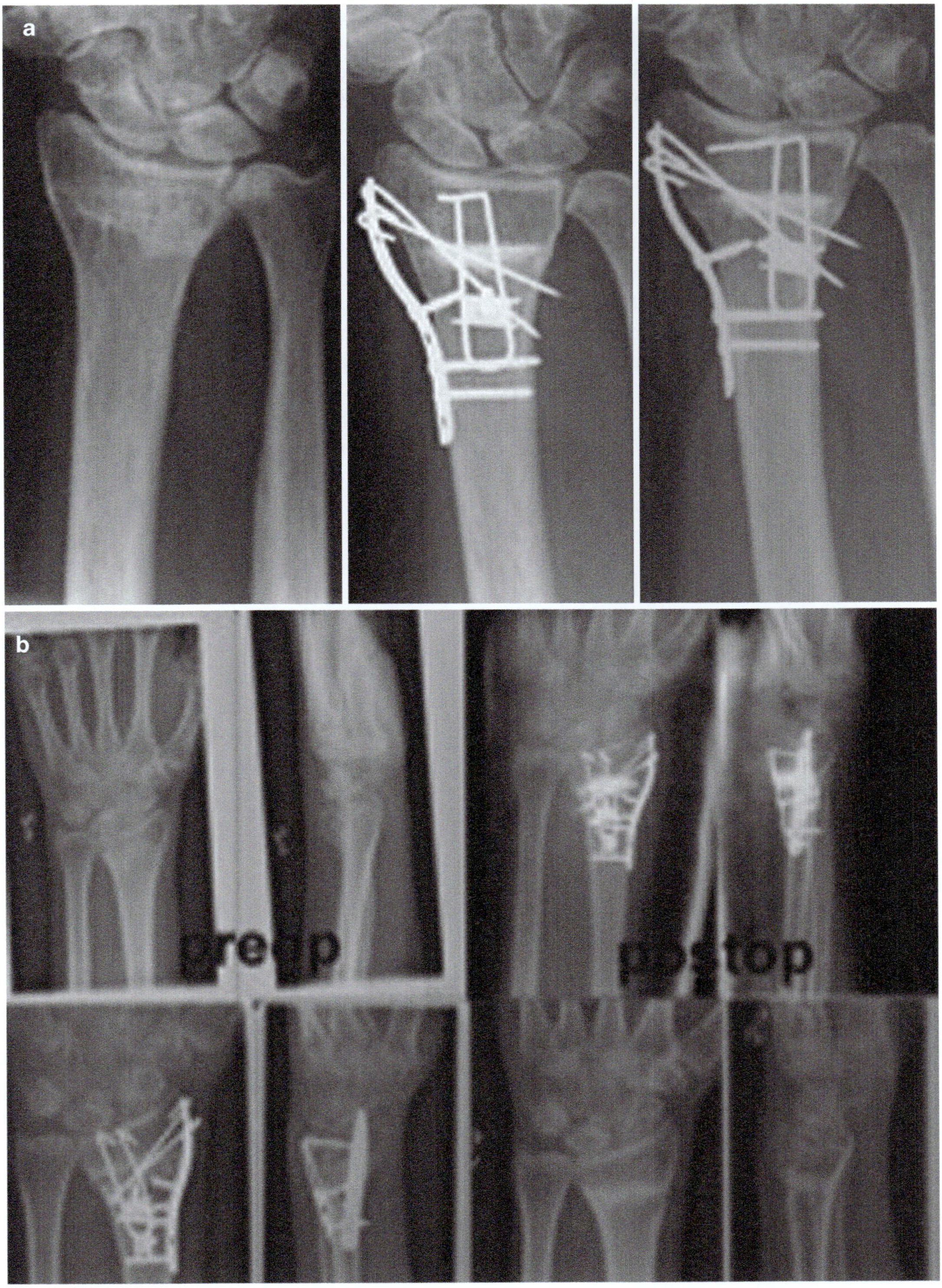

Fig. 29.2 (**a**, **b**) A radius corrective osteotomy is done due to malunion after fracture. In the left panel, an unresorbable apatite (Norian) was used, and the bone substitute is practically unremodelled but well integrated after 2 years. In the right panel, a composite containing both a fast-resorbing calcium sulphate and a slower-resorbing calcium phosphate (Cerament) was used which was remodelled into bone already after 1 year

Biological Support: Healing Stimulation

- Another important reason for using bone graft is to induce bone formation. Some fractures are known to have a high rate of non-union, like open tibial fractures where the primary cell source, the periosteum, is absent due to devascularisation. To prevent non-union, a bone graft can be applied to the fracture gap already at the time of primary fixation to increase the biological response, regarding both chemical signals like the bone morphogenetic protein (BMP) and to some extent living progenitor cells capable of proliferation and differentiation into bone-forming cells (Bauer and Muschler 2000).
- In an established non-union, we need some biological aid to initiate the healing cascade, and at present, preferably autograft should be used for biological support, i.e. to induce bone healing.
- Bone substitutes do not initiate bone healing and do not at present replace autograft but, on the contrary, act as a hinder for living bone to form.

29.3 Building Materials to Replace Lost Bone

29.3.1 Autograft

Autograft bone is harvested from the patient and contains some living cells at least initially. Autograft bone is the "gold standard" to which all methods are compared. Autograft bone is superior to allograft to induce healing and is used in fractures that are difficult to heal, as well as in delayed healing or established non-unions. Autograft by definition is non-immunogenic. It should be handled with care and not be allowed to dry.

- Autograft bone is by far most used as a particulate but can be structural and thereby also contribute to the mechanical support, for example, as a tricortical iliac crest graft to protect and support an opening wedge radial osteotomy, to maintain the reduction in a severely compressed distal radial fracture or to be impacted in the void to stabilise a die punch fragment.
- The importance of the mechanical support provided by bone graft in radial fractures has become less important as the implants, such as the volar plates, have improved mechanically, allowing the implant to support the subchondral bone with screws.
- However, the benefits of an autograft, i.e. the absence of an immune reaction and a rapid revascularisation of the graft, also mean a rapid remodelling, which might not be entirely beneficial. With the osteoclasts preceding the osteoblasts in bone graft healing, there will be a temporary decrease of the mechanical integrity of the graft and a risk of loss of reduction if the implant is not rigid enough during healing.
- Cortical allograft revascularises and remodels more slowly, which then on the other hand might be an advantage in some situations. The major drawback with autograft is the shortage of bone and the morbidity at the donor site.
- Vascularised autograft is the most physiological and immediate way of treating large bone defects but is rarely used in the radius except in some tumour cases and long-standing, particularly infected, non-unions.

29.3.2 Allograft

Allogenic bone from other individuals has the main benefit of avoiding pain at the donor site. In addition, the amount of bone is basically unlimited.

The use of allograft has been popular, but allograft is still second to autograft to replace bone. Almost exclusively, frozen allograft is used and taken from diseased donors as strut graft with inherent mechanical support or as morsellised bone graft from living donors undergoing a primary hip arthroplasty.

- Compared to other transplanted organs or tissues, the immune reaction is less pronounced in bone, making it possible to use allogenic tissue without controlling the immune reaction by drugs.

- The results of using allograft to induce bone formation are inferior compared to autograft, probably due to the relatively small amount of living cells and the immune reaction. To some extent, it is possible to decrease the immune reaction by freezing the tissue before being transplanted. Still, enough foreign protein is present to make it inferior to the patient's own bone.
- The handling procedures using allograft are somewhat time-consuming and include besides freezing also handling permissions from the donors and taking cultures to rule out blood-borne diseases, which all makes allograft less accessible.

29.3.3 Bone Substitute

Due to the problems with auto- and allografts, the need for alternatives has therefore arisen, and various bone substitutes have been developed (Bhatt and Rozental 2012; Kurien et al. 2013). Synthetic bone substitutes can be designed to have comparable mechanical properties as the bone grafts. However, just as the allografts, they lack the osteoinductive properties.

- *Calcium sulphate* (plaster of Paris, PoP) was one of the first bone substitutes and was first used in the late nineteenth century. It has the disadvantage of having poor mechanical resistance and fast resorption rate. It resorbs by dissolution during a period of approximately 4–6 weeks. An advantage of a material resorbing by dissolution is its ability to act as a drug carrier. However, in a clinical setting, a short resorption time could be a drawback when ingrowth of bone and bony union in a fracture or osteotomy might not be completed before the material has lost its strength. Therefore, substitutes with slower resorption and better strength have been developed.
- To mimic bone, various bone substitutes using *calcium phosphate*, the major mineral component of bone, have been developed. It is used as *hydroxyapatite*, which is practically non-resorbable, and as *tricalcium phosphate*, which is relatively soluble, or a combination of both. These substitutes can be obtained in granules or mono-blocks, but to facilitate minimal invasive surgery, injectable substitutes have been developed.
- The injectable calcium phosphates form either apatite or brushite in vivo. The apatite is more osteoconductive and has better mechanical properties but resorbs slowly over years, while brushite normally resorbs over a few months.
- Combinations of calcium sulphate and calcium phosphates also exist to capture the osteoconductivity of the calcium phosphate and the solubility of calcium sulphate.
- All the above-mentioned types of bone substitutes are highly biocompatible but have no osteoinductive properties in contrast to bone graft. This can, however, be dealt with when designing composite grafts and in the future combining bone substitute with either substances increasing ingrowth such as osteogenic proteins (BMP) or bone marrow aspirate or substances reducing resorption such as bisphosphonates (Table 29.1).

29.4 Drugs and Growth Factors

Demineralised bone matrix (DBM) is popular in some countries. It is made from bovine bone and contains proteins from the osteoid, which are released by the demineralising process (Dinopoulos and Giannoudis 2006).

- The graft cannot be used for any mechanical support due to the processing and is meant to be osteoinductive, but due to the remaining trabecular form, it can be considered osteoconductive.

Bone morphogenetic protein (BMP) induces differentiation of osteoprogenitor cells into active secreting osteoblasts. BMP is commercially available as BMP 7 (Osigraft) or BMP 2 (Infuse), roughly similar in clinical efficacy (Calori et al. 2009).

- In clinical randomised studies, BMP has never been proven superior to autograft in non-union healing, presumably due to an induction not only of bone formation but also of bone resorption.
- BMP is rarely used in distal radius fractures, but in one small series of radius osteotomies fixed by pins, the rate of non-unions was surprisingly high (Ekrol et al. 2008) by

Table 29.1 The various types of bone substitutes and a rough estimate of the remodelling time

Type	Application options	Resorption time	Commercial product
Apatite	Blocks/granule	Years/months	Actifuse
			Allogran-N
Apatite	Injectable	Years/months	Norian
			HydroSet
			Calcibon
Brushite	Injectable	Months	ChronOs Inject
Tricalcium phosphate	Blocks/granule	Months	Vitoss
			ChronOs
			Allogran-R
Apatite/tricalcium phosphate	Blocks/granule	Years/months	BoneSave
Calcium sulphate	Blocks/granule	Weeks	Osteoset, Stimulan
Calcium sulphate	Injectable	Weeks	MIIG
Apatite/calcium sulphate	Injectable	Months/weeks	Cerament
Tricalcium phosphate/calcium sulphate	Injectable	Months/weeks	GeneX
			Pro-Dense

speculation due to the combination of the protein and a non-rigid fixation.

Parathyroid hormone PTH and derivates increase both the formation and resorption of forming bone with a net increase of bone. It has been shown to decrease the time to healing moderately (see Chap. 11).

Platelet-derived growth factors (PDGF) and platelet concentrate are general wound healing response inducers and induce chemotaxis, angiogenesis and proliferation of the cells already present (Alsousou et al. 2009). They cannot differentiate osteoprogenitor cells to go into the osteoblastic lineage.

29.5 Bone Graft and Bone Substitutes in the Treatment of Distal Radius Fractures

Non-unions are rare in the treatment of distal radius fractures (Prommersberger and Fernandez 2004). In our prospective register (University of Lund, Sweden) of 4,000 patients, we have not had any non-unions so far.

- The prerequisites for bony healing are optimal in the distal radius if surgery is not performed.
- The fracture occurs in metaphyseal well-vascularised trabecular bone and even in the elderly still with a red marrow and an abundance of progenitor cells.
- In an open fracture with devascularisation of the periosteum, the secondary cell source of progenitor cells, the surrounding muscle satellite cells, is present in the nearby pronator quadratus (PQ).
- Even if torn, as often seen also in low-energy fractures, the chance for the PQ muscle to stay attached and adhere at some point to the fracture gap is still high.
- With the leaking BMP from the fracture ends, the progenitor/satellite cells in the muscle are likely to start to differentiate into the osteoblastic lineage.
- When shifting the surgical approach from the dorsal side to the volar with the introduction of the volar fixed angle plates, the operative technique has changed the secondary local support of progenitor cells.
- Hence, in the standard FCR (flexor carpi radialis) approach technique, the PQ is divided, risking losing the progenitor muscle cells, with a theoretical risk of causing a non-union (Table 29.2).

Table 29.2 Top tips when using bone grafts and substitutes!

All bone grafts and bone substitutes can be used for mechanical support, but only autograft can be used for biological support to induce bone formation
Always consider which of the mechanical or the biological support is most important and make an educated choice of which material to use. Once decided, consider what mechanical environment the graft is inserted into, to make it withstand the forces during the full length of the healing period
Bone substitute has no biological activity! If healing the fracture might be a problem, the material of choice should be autograft
All bone substitutes have sufficient strength immediately after insertion. However, the strength between the various materials differs a few weeks into the healing period. Choose a material that is slower to remodel if a less stable situation is accomplished by the fixation implant. A quick resorption is never desired except if the bone substitute is used as a carrier for antibiotics
The use of bone substitutes in distal radius
Allograft has no place in the treatment of distal radial fractures
The rate of non-union in DRF is extremely low but does exist. Always treat the PQ with care when dividing it as it provides secondary progenitor cells
Do not fill the whole deficit when doing a radial osteotomy, but rather leave space for bone to grow above the substitute to bridge the osteotomised bone ends. Remember that all bone substitutes are rather a barrier to healing and has to be removed by the resorbing cells before healing and substitution of newly formed bone

References

Alsousou J, Thompson M, Hulley P, Noble A, Willett K. The biology of platelet-rich plasma and its application in trauma and orthopaedic surgery: a review of the literature. J Bone Joint Surg Br. 2009;91(8):987–96.

Bauer TW, Muschler GF. Bone graft materials. An overview of the basic science. Clin Orthop Relat Res. 2000;371:10–27.

Bhatt RA, Rozental TD. Bone graft substitutes. Hand Clin. 2012;28(4):457–68.

Calori GM, Donati D, Di Bella C, Tagliabue L. Bone morphogenetic proteins and tissue engineering: future directions. Injury. 2009;40 Suppl 3:67–76.

Dimitriou R, Jones E, McGonagle D, Giannoudis PV. Bone regeneration: current concepts and future directions. BMC Med. 2011;9:66. doi:10.1186/1741-7015-9-66.

Dinopoulos HT, Giannoudis PV. Safety and efficacy of use of demineralised bone matrix in orthopaedic and trauma surgery. Expert Opin Drug Saf. 2006;5(6):847–66.

Ekrol I, Hajducka C, Court-Brown C, McQueen MM. A comparison of RhBMP-7 (OP-1) and autogenous graft for metaphyseal defects after osteotomy of the distal radius. Injury. 2008;39 Suppl 2:73–82.

Kurien T, Pearson RG, Scammell BE. Bone graft substitutes currently available in orthopaedic practice: the evidence for their use. Bone Joint J. 2013;95-B(5):583–97.

Prommersberger KJ, Fernandez DL. Nonunion of distal radius fractures. Clin Orthop Relat Res. 2004;419:51–6.

The Elderly Osteoporotic Patient

30

Rakel Sif Gudmundsdottir

Contents

R.S. Gudmundsdottir, MD
Department of Orthopaedic Surgery,
Haukeland University Hospital, Bergen, Norway
e-mail: rakel.gudmundsdottir@helse-bergen.no

30.1 Summary

Distal radius fractures are one of the most frequent fractures in the elderly. With the growing population of older people, the incidence of distal radius fractures will increase as well. The treatment of those fractures, as well as means to prevent them, has become of great interest. The two most important factors of prevention are prevention of falls and treatment of osteoporosis, as those are the two strongest predictors for sustaining a distal radius fracture in this age group. Osteoporosis does not only increase the risk of a fracture but also places a challenge in the treatment as it contributes to delayed healing, secondary displacement and problems regarding choice of osteofixations. With a growing age, there is a general increase in co-morbidity, and the functional demands tend to be lowered. Nevertheless, increased number of today's elderly is remaining active, and the choice of treatment requires individual evaluation. Even though there is evidence showing correlation between anatomical outcome and functional outcome in younger patients, this does not seem to be the case for the elderly. This is the main reason why the choice of treatment for this age group is so highly controversial. In fact, there seems to be no consensus in the orthopaedic society regarding treatment methods. Large systematic reviews of the literature have failed to reveal strong evidence for or against any known treatment in this age group. Pending good-quality evidence, the treatment will remain controversial and surgeon dependent.

L.M. Hove et al. (eds.), *Distal Radius Fractures*,
DOI 10.1007/978-3-642-54604-4_30, © Springer-Verlag Berlin Heidelberg 2014

30.2 The Elderly Patient

- Distal radius fractures are one of the most frequent fractures in the elderly. With the growing population of older people, the incidence of distal radius fractures will increase as well. In the year 2000, there were estimated to be 574,000 new fractures of the forearm in people over 50 years of age in Europe. The frequency of these fractures raises a significant public health concerns with a substantial economic consequences and a relevant impact on health in general for the elderly population (Kanis et al. 2013).
- When considering the elderly patient, one has to bear in mind that the way the term is defined creates a greatly heterogeneous group of patients. The definition often takes stand in the age of onset of osteoporosis, including patients in their early 1950s and older with a great difference in general health and functional demands of individuals within the group.

30.2.1 Falls and Fall Prevention

- The propensity to falling increases with age. It is greater in elderly women than in elderly men and greater among those living in a long-term institution than those living at home. Studies have shown that as much as 40 % of women over the age of 70 years report history of falling in a course of 1 year, increasing to over 50 % for women older than 80 years. Falls in the elderly result in fracture in 2–6 % of the cases, fractures of the distal radius accounting for about 20 % of all fractures (Geusens et al. 2002; Rubenstein 2006).
- Most falls in the elderly can be associated with identifiable risk factors. These risk factors are either "patient related" or "environmental related", and most often the fall is a combination of risk factors.
- The risk of falling increases linearly with the number of risk factors, from being less than 10 % with none present to almost 80 % with four or more risk factors present.
- Patient-related factors include mobility impairments with unsteady gait, slower reflexes, joint stiffness and reduced strength. Other patient-related factors are medications and drug side effects, cognitive impairment and diseases such as arthritis, disorders of the central nervous system, cardiovascular diseases and visual disorders.
- Environment-related factors include everything in the surroundings that can provoke a fall in an individual with diminished protective responses. Rugs, thresholds and electrical cords are only few of the environmental hazards found in almost every home, whereas icy, wet or uneven terrain is an example of outdoor hazards (Stalenhoef et al. 2002; Rubenstein 2006).
- Preventative intervention is a challenge because of the complex nature of falls and the involvement of multiple risk factors.
- The main aspects of interventions are various exercise programmes, education for the elderly regarding risk factors, home assessments and education pointed at primary physicians and other health-care professionals, to identify the elderly patient of risk of falling and the necessity to intervene.
- Single intervention and programmes for prevention of falls in unselected groups of older people living in the community have not shown to be effective. On the other hand, multifactorial interventions targeting the high-risk patient, assessing the risk factors or the causes of falling and then developing an individual intervention plan have been proven to decrease falls.
- As mobility impairment is one of the most important predisposing factors for falls, most high-risk patients will benefit from intervention to improve balance gait, such as exercise programmes and walking aids. This should be combined with home safety evaluation and modifications to eliminate hazards that can provoke falls in addition to medical assessment and subsequent rationalisation of drugs and optimisation of medical conditions (Feder et al. 2000; Rubenstein 2006).
- Despite well-recognised predictors of falls, fall prevention intervention has not gotten the attention it should in clinical settings. There seems to be a great potential for improvement in most sectors of the health-care system involved in the treatment of the elderly patient at risk of falling.

30.2.2 Osteoporosis and Distal Radius Fractures

- Osteoporosis affects over 200 million people worldwide (Gullberg et al. 1997), and its involvement in low-energy distal radius fractures in elderly patients is well established, osteoporosis being the single most important predictor of future fracture (Geusens et al. 2002; Øyen et al. 2011; Bouxsein 2011).
- Osteoporosis is not merely a contributing factor to the high incidence of fragility fractures of the distal radius but is relevant in number of other aspects regarding those fractures.
- Both biomechanical and clinical studies have revealed correlation between low bone mineral density and increased probability of severe dislocation after low-energy trauma, such as decreased radial length and increased dorsal angulation as well as metaphyseal comminution. The clinical consequences reflect in early instability with secondary displacement, carpal malalignment and malunion (Clayton et al. 2009).
- Furthermore, osteoporosis contributes to delayed fracture union. Although the healing of an osteoporotic fracture processes through a natural course, this process is prolonged in the elderly patient as callus formation is influenced by both less active and decreased number of osteoblasts, their biological activity being negatively influenced by age (Bouxsein 2011).
- Biomechanical studies have demonstrated an increased fixation failure related to surgical treatment of osteoporotic distal radius fractures. Even though there seems to be a general opinion in the orthopaedic society that osteoporosis is related to increased risk of complications, this has not yet been reproduced in clinical studies (Goldhahn 2008).
- Effectiveness of osteoporosis treatment to prevent fragility fractures is widely recognised, as is the fact that previous fracture in the elderly osteoporotic patient is a major risk factor for future fracture. Despite this knowledge, only a minority of elderly people are being screened and treated for osteoporosis following a fragility fracture, in order to reduce the risk of future fracture.
- Reported prevalence of intervention postfracture, with evaluations and treatment of osteoporosis, is as low as 3 % to about 25 %.
- Studies aimed to improve follow-up rate of elderly fracture patients and to improve the quality of osteoporosis care have only partly succeeded when directed solely at primary care physicians, only increasing appropriate intervention rate to close to 40 %.
- Including the orthopaedic surgeon treating the fracture can dramatically improve the osteoporosis evaluation and treatment rate. Simple intervention as ordering the bone mineral density examination in the orthopaedic clinic and forwarding the results to the primary care physician has shown to improve the evaluation rate and the initiation of treatment at least threefold (Rozental et al. 2008).
- Orthopaedic surgeons have a unique opportunity to address this problem as often being the only physicians to see the elderly patient with fragility fracture. This is particularly true for distal radius fractures, as those tend to occur 10–15 years before other fragility fractures and are often the first sign of underlying osteoporosis.
- Thus, all men and women aged 50 years and older with distal radius fracture should be referred to osteoporosis evaluation by their treating orthopaedic surgeon or emergency/fracture clinic physician and, if indicated, then treated (Rozental et al. 2008; Majumdar et al. 2008; Øyen et al. 2011; Bouxsein 2011).

30.3 Treatment of Distal Radius Fractures in the Elderly

- The management of distal radius fractures in the elderly has received substantial attention in the literature. However, the lack of good-quality trials and the heterogeneity of available trials make it difficult to extract practical conclusions and properly assess the outcome of a particular treatment method. Large systematic reviews of the literature have failed to reveal strong evidence for or against any known treatment in this age group, and the management of this common injury remains without consensus in the orthopaedic society.

- The elderly osteoporotic patients differ from younger patients. There is good evidence showing correlation between anatomical outcome and functional outcome in younger patients. This, however, is much more controversial regarding the elderly. Especially in the low-demand elderly patient, poor anatomical outcome does not seem to translate into poor functional or clinical outcome. Nevertheless, an increased number of the elderly of today are remaining healthier, living more active lifestyle, and are more likely to be affected by inadequate anatomical outcome. This is probably the main reason why the choice of treatment for this age group is so highly contentious.
- Hence, pending good-quality evidence, the decision-making will be opinionated and surgeon dependent but should be made with due consideration for the general condition of the patient and medical co-morbidity as well as the patient's preference. The primary treatment goal must be a wrist without pain and with satisfactory functional outcome for each individual patient (Blakeney 2010; Arora et al. 2011).

30.3.1 Closed Reduction and Immobilisation

- Closed reduction and immobilisation in a plaster cast is a convenient, safe and cost-effective treatment for distal radius fractures in the elderly. The patient can be treated ambulatory and rarely requires hospitalisation.
- There are a number of different methods of conservative treatment, none proven better than the other (Handoll and Madhok 2003).
- Commonly used protocol includes reduction of displaced fractures in local anaesthesia and immobilisation in a below-elbow splint. Above-elbow cast does not improve outcome. Radiographic follow-up is recommended weekly for 2–3 weeks, to detect eventual secondary displacement, and at cast removal at 6 weeks. In case of redisplacement, decision must be made whether to convert to surgery or to accept the displacement. Repeated manipulation is of no value, as it will not improve the final anatomical outcome, especially in osteoporotic bone (Hove et al. 1995).
- When anatomical reduction is not the goal of the treatment, cast is applied for pain relief. In these cases, there is no need for radiographic follow-up, and closed reduction should be restricted to severely displaced fractures where there is a risk of nerve entrapment (Makhni et al. 2008; Blakeney 2010; Arora et al. 2011).
- Conservative treatment is widely accepted and regarded adequate treatment method for undisplaced fractures and for displaced fractures after successful reduction efforts, where the likelihood of secondary displacement is considered small.
- However, fracture instability is strongly associated with growing age, dorsal comminution and the severity of initial displacement. As this applies to majority of distal radius fractures in the elderly patient, those are, per definition, instable and tend to lose reduction (Hove et al. 1994).
- Trials on anatomical outcome after conservative fracture management have revealed secondary displacement in 30–90 % of the cases. Both incidence and the severity of redisplacement correlate with increasing age. Even fractures with minimal initial displacement tend to lose reduction in older people, often to a greater displacement than at the time of injury (Fig. 30.1) (Makhni et al. 2008; Blakeney 2010).
- Even though there seems to be some support in the literature indicating discrepancy between anatomical outcome and functional outcome in older people, this is both inconclusive and controversial.
- Conservative management should therefore be reserved for patients with less ambitious functional demand and patients regarded too fragile for surgery or those who deny surgery.
- For the healthy high-demand elderly patient, treatment aimed at anatomical reduction might be more likely to give adequate functional outcome.

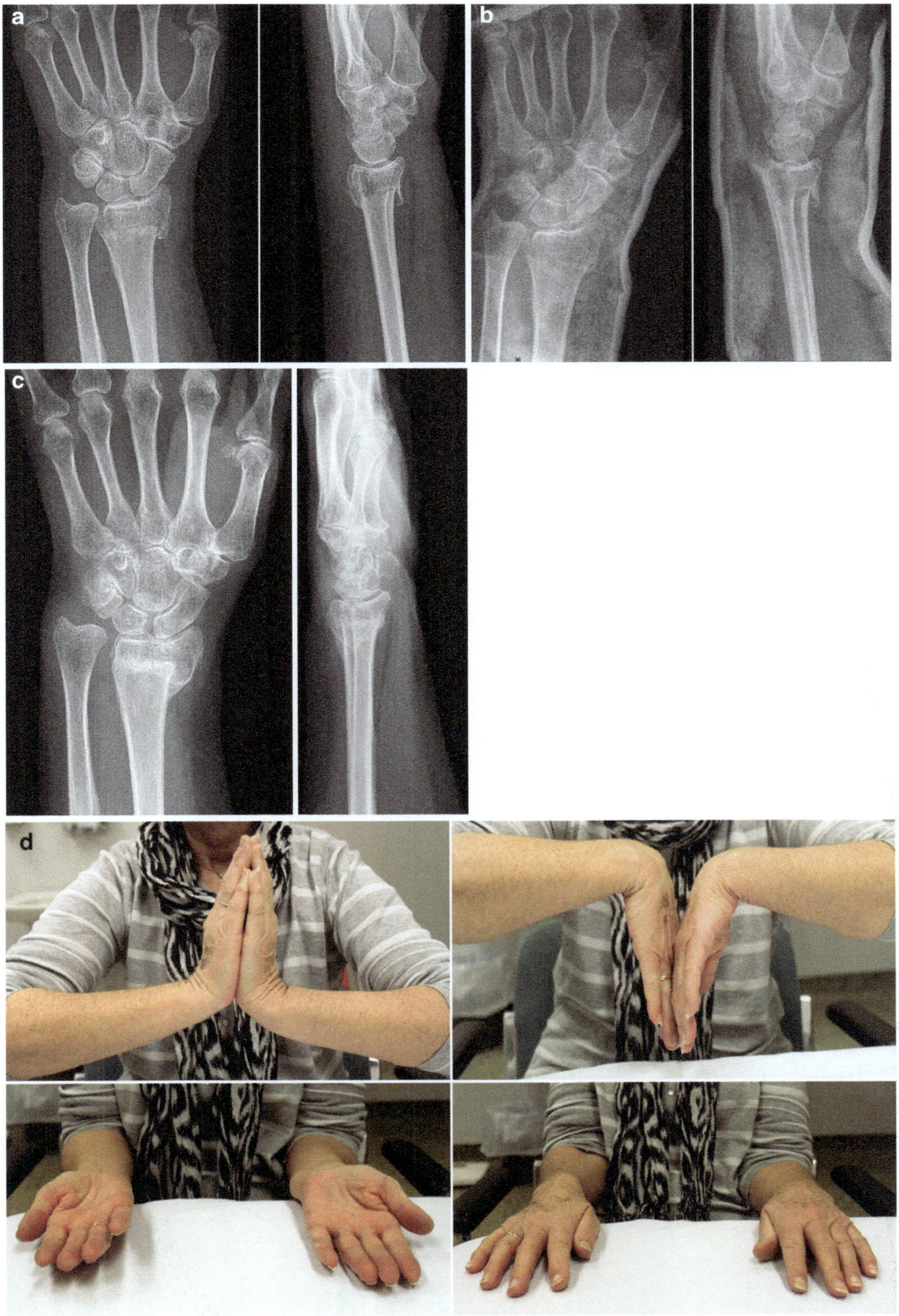

Fig. 30.1 A dorsally angulated extra-articular distal radius fracture in an active 70-year-old woman treated conservatively with a closed reduction and cast immobilisation. Posteroanterior (PA) and lateral views. (**a**) Before reduction, (**b**) after reduction and (**c**) at 3 months. (**d**) Wrist motion attained at 3 months. Note prominent ulna on the left side. Patient reported that she had no pain

30.3.2 External Fixation

- External fixation is a well-established treatment method that has been used since the 1940s.
- A variety of devices have been developed, but all use one of two techniques, either wrist bridging or non-bridging, both intended to hold the position of a closed reduced fracture while it heals.
- Using external fixation in the elderly patient has shown to give better anatomical results, compared to closed reduction and immobilisation. The functional benefits are controversial (Fig. 30.2).
- This surgical method has the advantage above open reduction and internal fixation that it is easy, rapid and less invasive with compatible anatomical and functional outcome.

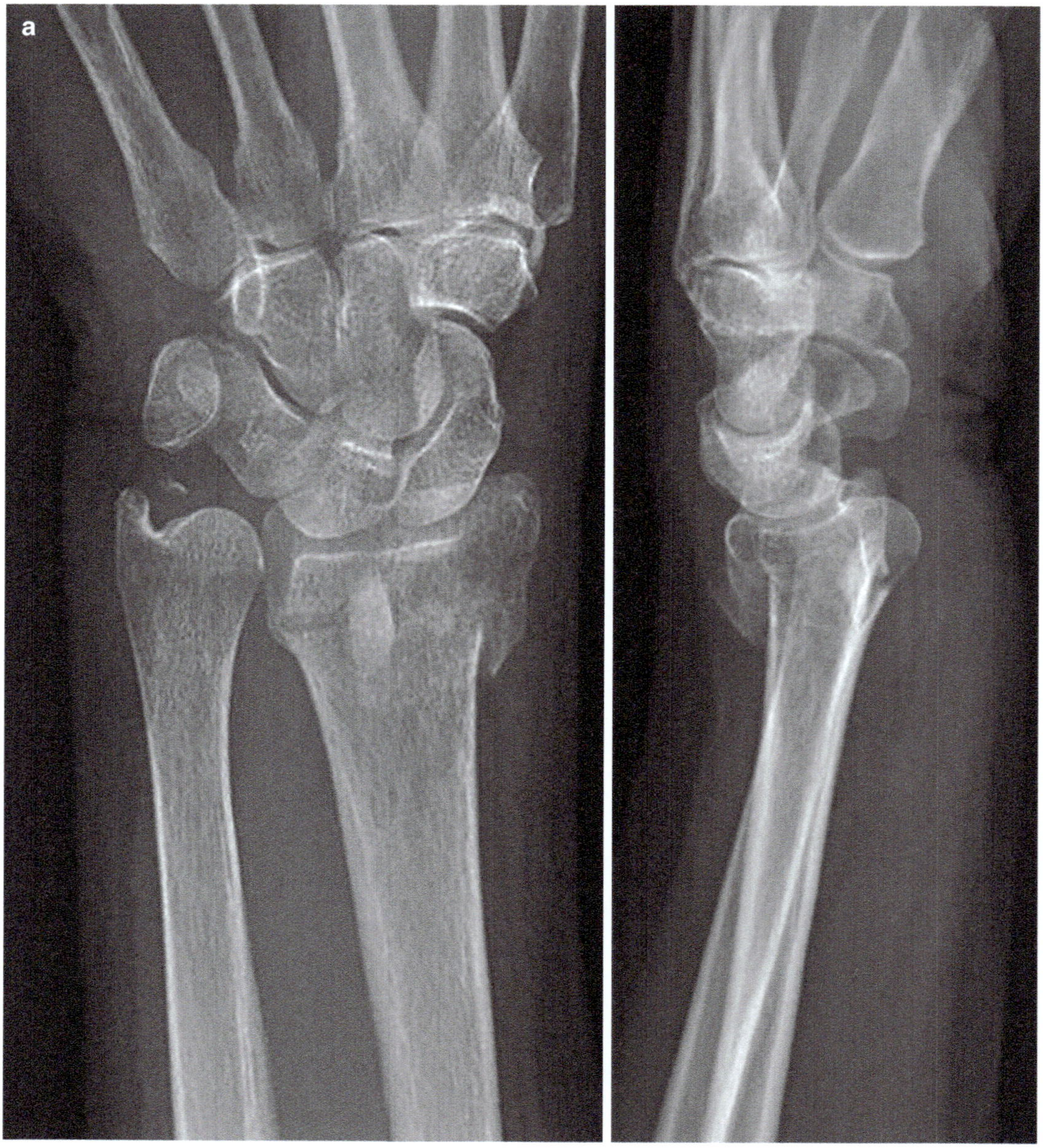

Fig. 30.2 A dorsally angulated extra-articular distal radius fracture in an active 71-year-old woman treated with external fixation. PA and lateral views. (**a**) Before reduction, (**b**) after operation and (**c**) at 3 months. (**d**) Wrist motion attained at 3 months

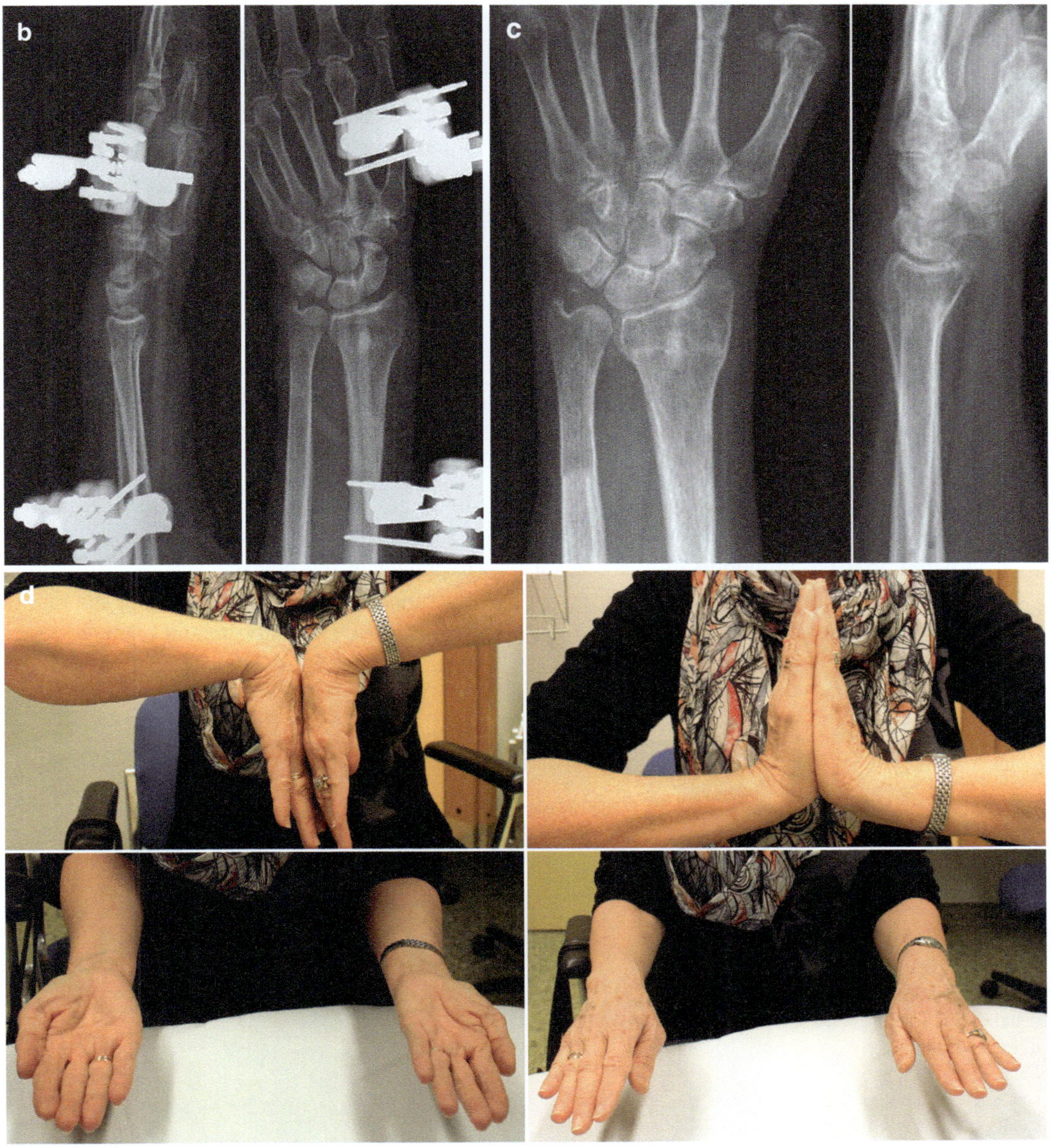

Fig. 30.2 (continued)

- The drawback of this method in the elderly patient is loosening of the pins resulting from inadequate hold in poor-quality osteoporotic bone, leading to removal of the devise before solid sign of bone healing.
  - Other common complications to using external fixation are pin-track infections and damage to the superficial radial nerve and digital nerves. Incidence of complex regional pain syndrome (CRPS) has been reported, possibly due to over-distraction of the wrist joint using bridging technique, as well as joint stiffness resulting from immobilisation. These complications are general and do not only apply to the elderly (Blakeney 2010; Arora et al. 2011; Schneppendahl et al. 2012).

30.3.3 Percutaneous Pinning

- Percutaneous pinning is used to supplement closed reduction and cast immobilisation or external fixation, in order to maintain reduction.
- Percutaneous pinning with cast immobilisation is recommended for fractures without metaphyseal comminution and articular involvement and thus only rarely indicated for distal fractures in the elderly, especially not those with underlying osteoporosis.
- The majority of trials with elderly people reveal high incidence of secondary displacement as poor bone quality makes pins more likely to loosen and less likely to maintain fracture alignment.
- Compared to cast immobilisation alone, it is only marginally superior for anatomical outcome with no correlation to functional outcome.
- Percutaneous pinning is, however, indicated in combination with bridging external fixation in comminuted intra-articular distal radius fractures in the elderly as it helps maintain fracture reduction by providing an inter-fragmentary support.
- Commonly reported complications include pin-track infections and damage to the superficial radial nerve (Blakeney 2010; Arora et al. 2011; Schneppendahl et al. 2012).

30.3.4 Open Reduction and Internal Fixation (ORIF)

- In the last decade, open reduction and internal fixation has become an increasingly popular treatment in the management of distal radius fractures in the elderly, increasing the rate of surgical procedures for fractures that have been managed conservatively in the past (Fig. 30.3).

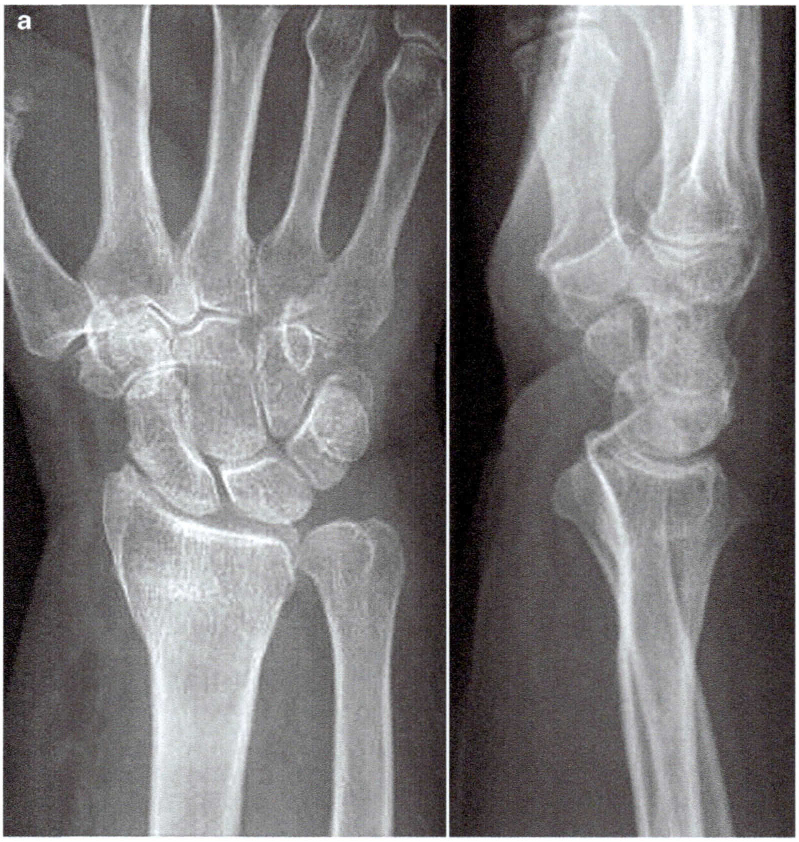

Fig. 30.3 A 77-year-old woman who previously had bilateral extra-articular distal radius fractures treated conservatively. Nine years later, she sustained yet another extra-articular fracture in her right wrist which was treated with open reduction and a volar locking plate. (**a**) Healed fracture in the right wrist, PA and lateral views. (**b**) Healed fracture in the left wrist, PA and lateral views. (**c**) Right wrist after ORIF with a volar locking plate. Reduced to the anatomical position as it was at time of injury without further correction of previous maluninon. (**d**) Wrist motion attained at 6 weeks

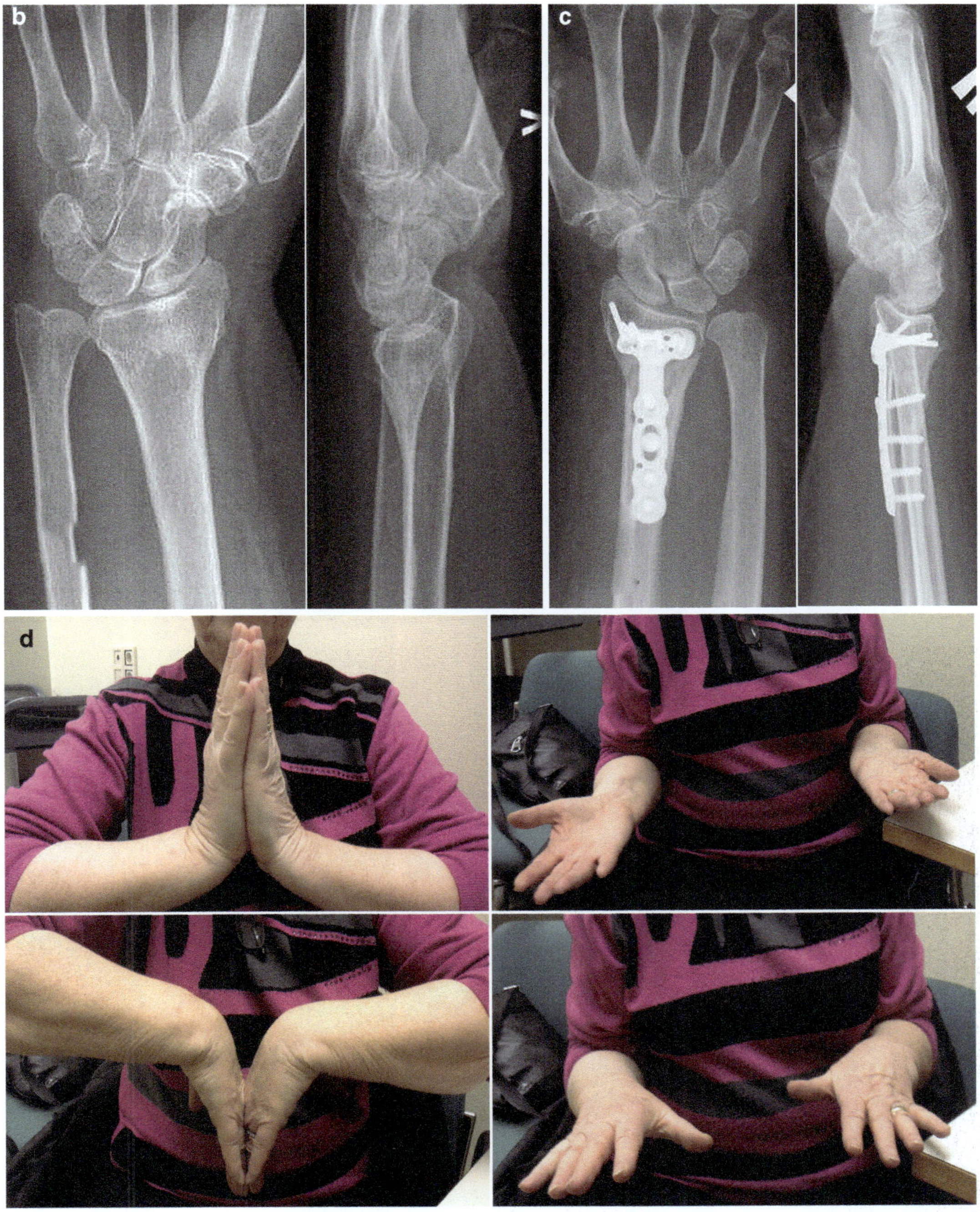

Fig. 30.3 (continued)

- This change in the treatment is due to the introduction of locking plates. Before the locking plate system, internal fixation was considered too unstable and prone to fail when used on osteoporotic bone.
- There are countless variations of plates available based on the locking screw principle, and the volar fixed-angle plate is most widely used. In biomechanical studies, the volar fixed-angle plate has shown excellent stability,

even in osteoporotic bone compared to non-locking osteofixations (Fig. 30.4).

- The fixed-angle screws lock into the plate, and the construction transfers forces from the subchondral bone away from the weaker dorsal metaphysis towards the stronger diaphysis, unloading the fracture.
- In the osteoporotic bone, the placement of the distal locking screws immediately under the subchondral plate is important. A considerable gap between the distal locking screws and the subchondral plate can lead to a collapse of cancellous bone until the distal locking screws reach the supporting subchondral plate, reducing radial length. This phenomenon has been associated with increasingly poor bone quality in the elderly and can be avoided with proper screw positioning (Blakeney 2010; Arora et al. 2011; Schneppendahl et al. 2012; Rhee et al. 2013).
- Open reduction and volar plating are not free from complications. Tendon irritation and ruptures from screw penetration and plate interference are reported and, to a lesser extent, osteosynthesis failure, carpal tunnel syndrome, CRPS and infections, pointing out the drawbacks of internal fixation. Overall complication rate as high as 27 % has been reported (Fig. 30.5) (Arora et al. 2011).

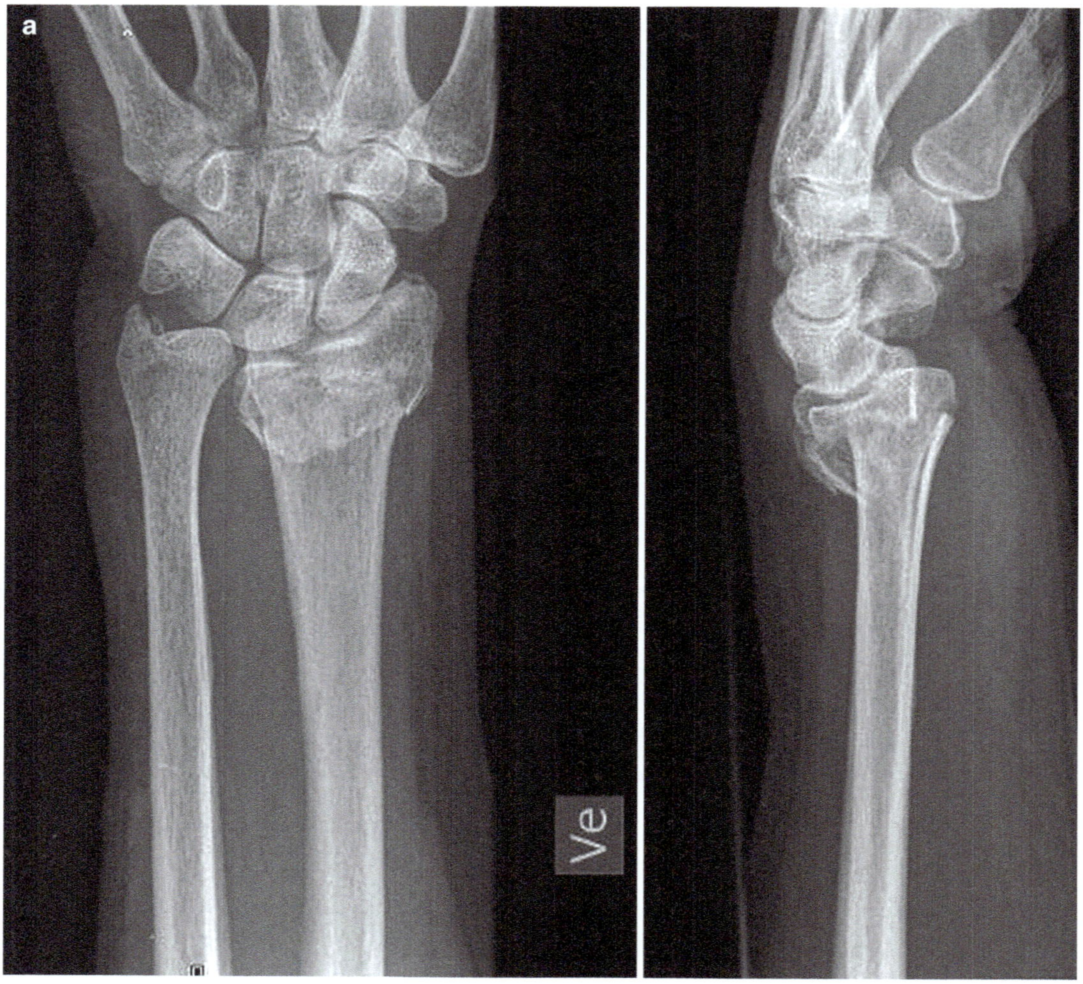

Fig. 30.4 A dorsally angulated intra-articular distal radius fracture with a metaphyseal comminution in a healthy and active 63-year-old woman. PA and lateral views. (**a**) Before reduction, (**b**) at 6 weeks and (**c**) Wrist motion attainded at 3 months

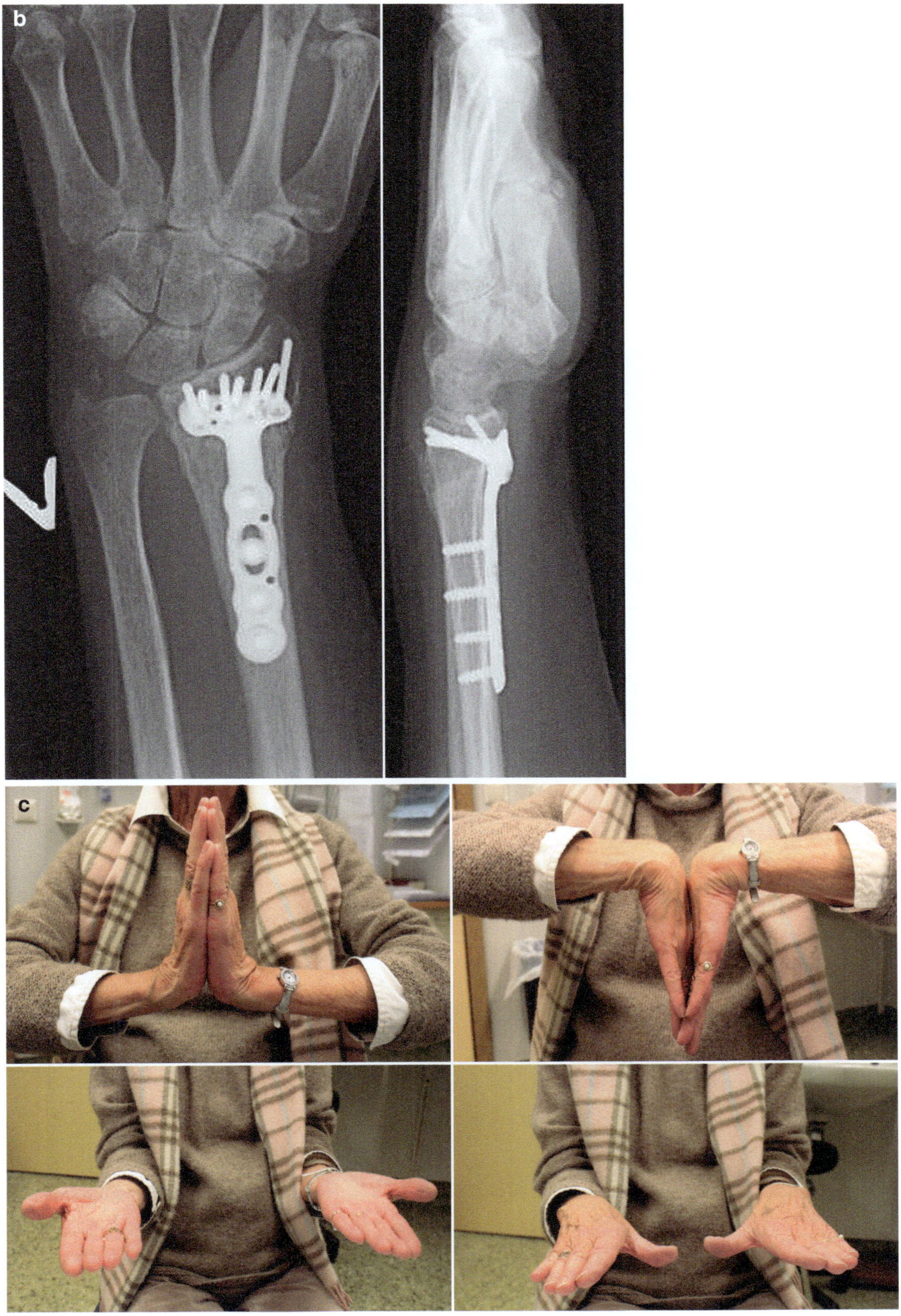

Fig. 30.4 (continued)

- The theoretical advantage of open reduction and internal fixation is the consistently good anatomical outcome as well as stable and reliable fixation that allows for early mobilisation and rehabilitation. In the elderly, these benefits must be weighed against the increased risk of both aesthetical- and surgical-related complications, the cost of surgical invention and hospitalisation as well as the fact that for the elderly patient it remains highly controversial if the biomechanical advantages of internal fixation translate into better functional and clinical outcome (Blakeney 2010; Arora et al. 2011; Schneppendahl et al. 2012).

30.4 Discussion

- Elderly people are the fastest growing group in the world, and the burden of osteoporotic fractures is increasing worldwide. This chap-

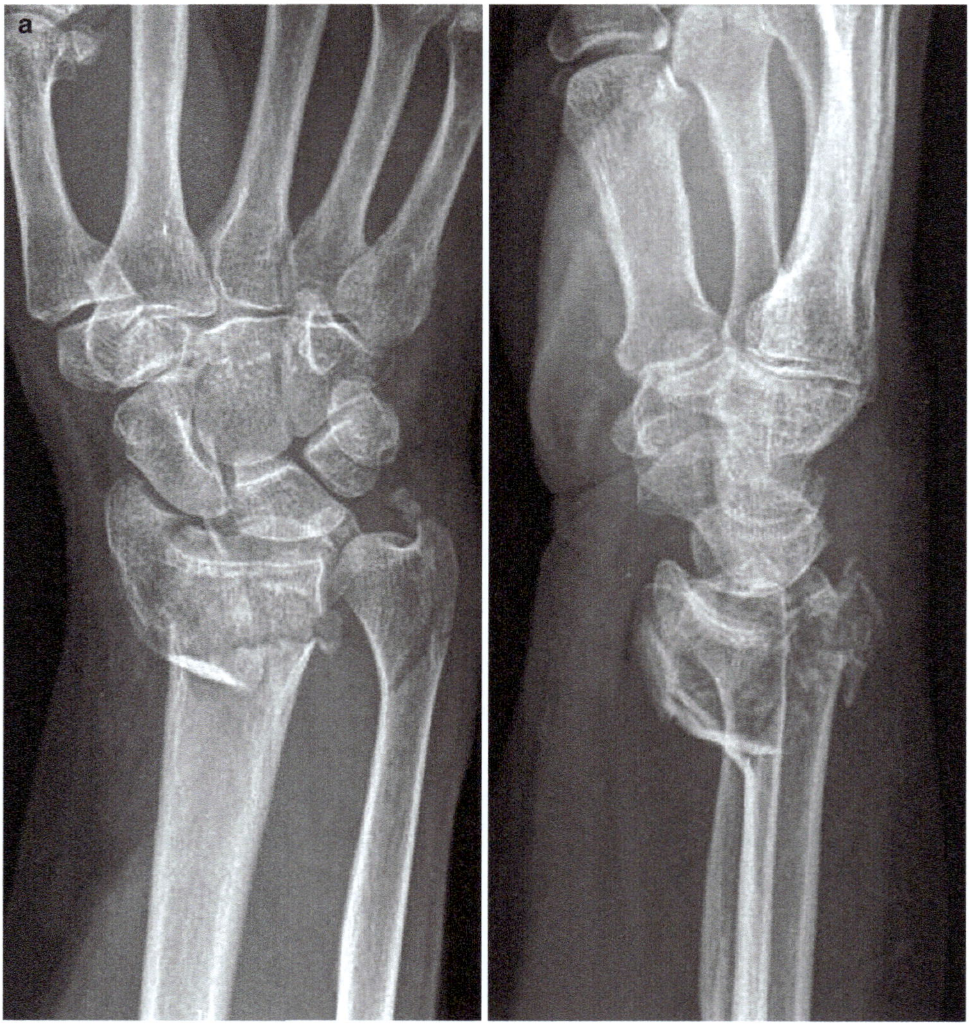

Fig. 30.5 A comminuted intra-articular distal radius fracture in a 68-year-old healthy but inactive woman treated with a volar locking plate. PA and lateral views. (**a**) Before reduction and (**b**) immediately after ORIF with volar locking plate. (**c**) Six weeks after surgery showing dorsal collapse and screw penetration. (**d**) After removing the distal locking screws. The patient had no extension in her wrist and only 30° flexion. She had no pain and was satisfied with the result despite limited range of motion

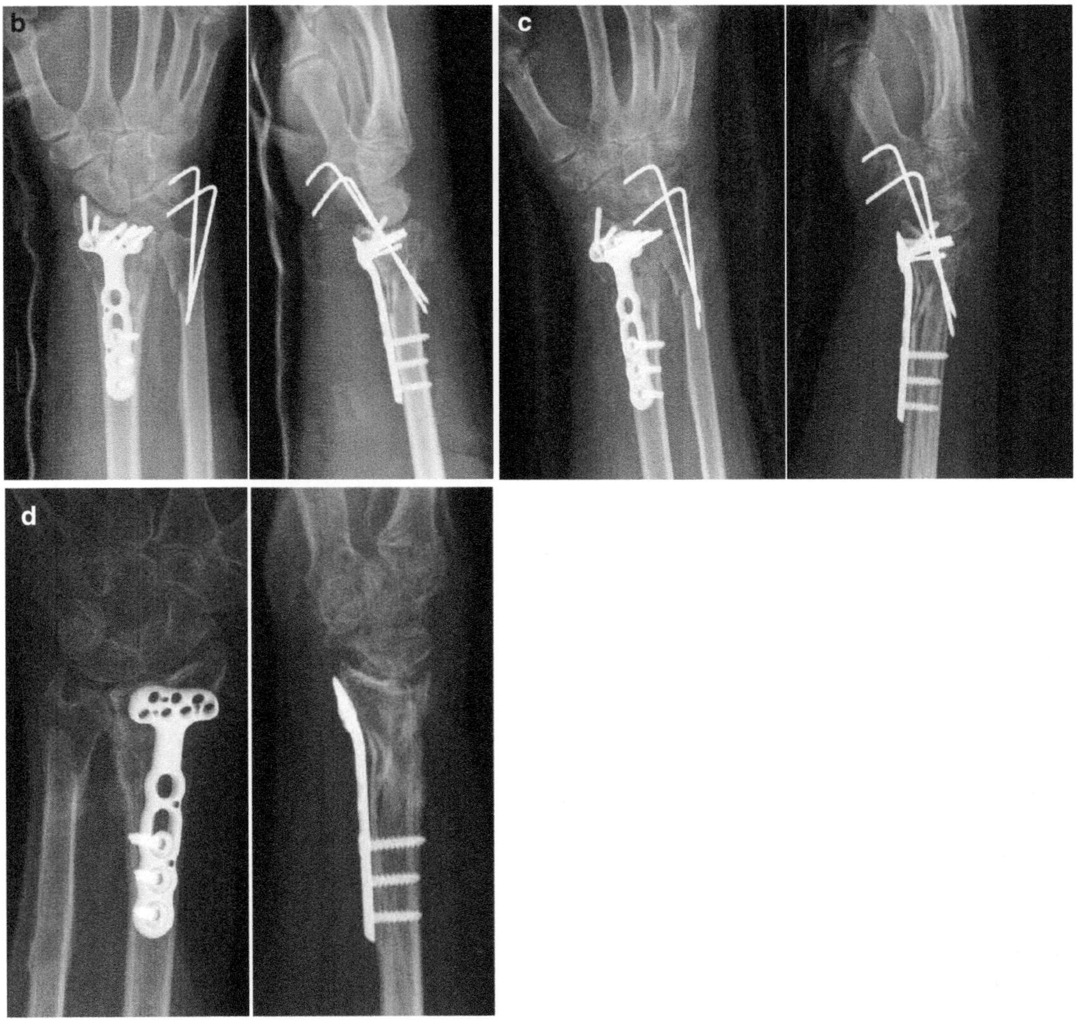

Fig. 30.5 (continued)

ter is meant to emphasise two important issues related to the elderly osteoporotic patient: first, the necessity of fracture prevention and, second, the poverty of clinical evidence regarding the management of distal radius fractures in this patient group.

- The consistent risk factors for distal radius fractures across ethnicity include older age, history of falls, low bone mineral density and previous history of fractures. Systematic attention to early identification of elderly people that would benefit from preventative interventions is essential in the attempt to reduce this significant health hazard.
- The question of economic burden of both osteoporosis and fall-related health problems versus the cost-effectiveness of preventions programmes has been raised and not yet fully answered. However, an interdisciplinary approach to treatment of osteoporosis and prevention of falls and fall-related health challenges such as fractures should be, despite costs, self-evident and prioritised.
- Even though distal radius fractures in the elderly patients are one of the most common injuries treated by orthopaedic, trauma and hand surgeons, the treatment is without consensus. The poor bone quality represents

a problem regarding choice of treatment. Various treatment methods are reported and conducted. Conservative treatment with closed reduction and a plaster cast of an unstable fracture tend to result in malunion. Open/closed reduction and internal/external fixation are widely used to ensure best possible anatomical results. Obtaining a reliable stable fixation in an osteoporotic bone can however be a challenge.

- Giving the lack of evidence supporting any decision-making faced by physicians encountering this patient group, this will be a judgement call that needs to be based on the general condition of the patient as well as the surgeons and the patient's preferences.
- It can be argued that the surgeon should have a lower threshold for surgical intervention in high-demand, healthy and active elderly patients. One important argument is that even though there is a lack of evidence supporting a correlation between anatomical outcome and functional outcome in the elderly, it does not mean that the correlation does not exist; it merely means that there is a lack of evidence.

References

Arora R, et al. Aspects of current management of distal radius fractures in the elderly individuals. Geriatr Orthop Surg Rehabil. 2011;2(5–6):187–94.

Blakeney WG. Stabilization and treatment of Colles' fractures in elderly patients. Clin Interv Aging. 2010;5: 337–44.

Bouxsein ML. Bone structure and fracture risk: do they go arm in arm? J Bone Miner Res. 2011;26(7):1389–91.

Clayton RAE, et al. Association between decreased bone mineral density and severity of distal radial fractures. J Bone Joint Surg Am. 2009;91:613–9.

Feder G, et al. Guidelines for prevention of falls in people over 65. BMJ. 2000;321:1007–11.

Geusens P, et al. The relationship among history of falls, osteoporosis, and fractures in postmenopausal women. Arch Phys Med Rehabil. 2002;83:903–6.

Goldhahn J. Influence of osteoporosis on fracture fixation – a systematic literature review. Osteoporos Int. 2008;19:761–72.

Gullberg B, et al. World-wide projections for hip fracture. Osteoporos Int. 1997;7(5):407–13.

Handoll HHG, Madhok R. Conservative interventions for treating distal radial fractures in adults. Cochrane Database Syst Rev. 2003;2, CD000314.

Hove LM, Solheim E, Skjeie R, Sørensen FK. Prediction of secondary displacement in Colles' fracture. J Hand Surg Br. 1994;19B:731–6.

Hove LM, Fjeldsgaard K, Skjeie R, Solheim E. Anatomical and functional results five years after remanipulated Colles' fractures. Scand J Plast Reconstr Surg Hand Surg. 1995;29:349–55.

Kanis JA, et al. European guidance for the diagnosis and management of osteoporosis in postmenopausal women. Osteoporos Int. 2013;24:23–57.

Majumdar SR, et al. Multifaceted intervention to improve diagnosis and treatment of osteoporosis in patients with recent wrist fracture: a randomized controlled trial. CMAJ. 2008;178(5):569–75.

Makhni EC, et al. Effect of patient age on the radiographic outcome of distal radius fractures. Subject to nonoperative treatment. J Hand Surg. 2008;33A: 1301–8.

Øyen J, Brudvik C, Gjesfal CG, Tell GS, Lie SA, Hove LM. Osteoporosis as a risk factor for distal radial fractures. J Bone Joint Surg Am. 2011;93:348–56.

Rhee SH, et al. Factors affecting late displacement following volar locking plate fixation for distal radial fractures in elderly female patients. J Bone Joint. 2013;95-B:396–400.

Rozental TD, et al. Improving evaluation and treatment for osteoporosis following distal radial fractures. A prospective randomized intervention. J Bone Joint Surg Am. 2008;90(5):953–61.

Rubenstein LZ. Falls in older people: epidemiology, risk factors and strategies for prevention. Age Ageing. 2006;35(S2):ii37–41.

Schneppendahl J, et al. Distal radius fractures: current concepts. J Hand Surg Am. 2012;37A:1718–25.

Stalenhoef PA, et al. A risk model for the prediction of recurrent falls in community-dwelling elderly: a prospective cohort study. J Clin Epidemiol. 2002;55:1088–94.

Rehabilitation

31

Kerstin Runnquist

Contents

K. Runnquist, Msc (Orthopedics)
Department of Orthopedics,
Lunds University Hospital, Lund, Sweden
e-mail: runnquist.kerstin@gmail.com

31.1 Summary

There is insufficient evidence from randomised controlled trials to determine how to manage the rehabilitation of adults with distal radius fractures. General advice and instruction on mobilisation should be given to all patients. A home-exercise programme is adequate rehabilitation for most patients, and the main role for the physiotherapist is to motivate the patient to independent exercise. Additional therapy may be necessary for patients with complications or serious functional impairment. The challenge is to identify these patients in due time. This is easier if there are "departmental protocols for therapy" and established routines. Early control of oedema and pain and early mobilisation and use of the hand are of paramount importance in preventing and eliminating long-term dysfunction and a bad outcome.

31.2 Introduction

> Some knowledge comes from books, more comes from experience; in the case of the hand most comes by touch, by skin-to-skin, eye-to-eye dynamic interaction, whereby a good therapist comes to know just how a patient feels and react. (Hunter et al. 1990)

L.M. Hove et al. (eds.), *Distal Radius Fractures*,
DOI 10.1007/978-3-642-54604-4_31, © Springer-Verlag Berlin Heidelberg 2014

31.2.1 "The Hand Is the Extension of the Brain to the Outer World" (Lundborg 1990)

- The hand is one of the most important motor and sensory organs in the body and combines very fine tactile sense with great mobility, coordination and power.
- This is demonstrated by the homunculus representation in the motor and sensory cortex.
- The hand is important in the individual's gesturing body language and in human contact.
- Its function is dependent on the whole upper extremity, but the wrist and forearm play a key role in normal hand balance regarding both the hand position and its ability to power transmission.

31.2.2 Does Distal Radius Fracture Treatment Include Physiotherapy?

- Colles' fracture is one of the most common fractures and is often minimally displaced, extra-articular and stable.
- Residual deformity is minimal, complications are unusual and full function generally returns.
- It is necessary to have a realistic view on the value of more extensive and time-consuming treatment, as physiotherapeutic resources are not infinite.
  - A meta-analysis of randomised controlled trials done by the Cochrane Institute found no scientific support that physiotherapeutic interventions accelerate the functional recovery or improve the functional outcome (Handoll et al. 2006). The physiotherapeutic interventions investigated were:
  - Passive mobilisation
  - Ice packs
  - Pulsed electromagnetic field
  - Whirlpool immersion
  - Continuous passive motion (CPM)
  - Intermittent pneumatic compression
  - Ultrasound
- In conservatively treated cases, it did not appear to matter whether the doctor or the physiotherapist gave instructions for home exercises or if the physiotherapist gave information combined with several follow-ups. The outcome regarding mobility and grip strength in these cases was the same.
- Prescription of formal occupational therapy did not improve the average motion or disability score compared to patients who received surgeon-directed independent exercises (Souer et al. 2011). In fact, formal occupational therapy was only comparable or slightly inferior to surgeon-directed independent exercises.
- Patients guided by physiotherapists compared to self-training after conservatively treated Colles' fracture were all satisfied with the treatment, but no functional advantages could be discerned (Oskarsson et al. 1997).
- Physiotherapy cannot be expected to counterbalance unsatisfactory primary treatment or complications caused by a difficult fracture, and only patients with severe stiffness and those who for any reason cannot execute their self-training programme should be referred to a physiotherapist (Oskarsson et al. 1997).
- It is not possible to establish what kind of rehabilitation is necessary for an acceptable functional recovery, who should provide this care, when or for how long this care should be provided or indeed in what circumstances it should be provided!
- This evidence-based statement should not be construed as a basis for the non-provision of any rehabilitation intervention. Clearly, general advice and instructions on mobilisation should be given to all patients with radius fractures.
- The physiotherapeutic contribution should normally be minimised and to the greatest part be advisory, aiming at getting the patients' full cooperation in a rehabilitation process that normally should be done by the patients themselves.
- Additional therapy may be necessary and essential for patients with complications or serious functional impairment.
- The aim must be to devote the therapist's time and energy to the patients that really need our help.

31.3 Background Knowledge for Hand Rehabilitation

31.3.1 Wrist Motion

- The wrist joint consists of multiple complex joint systems with equally complex biomechanics to provide a substantial range of motion (ROM).
- ROM in normal extension and flexion is approximately 120° (85–160°).
- ROM in radial and ulnar deviation is approximately 65° (15–25° in radial deviation and 30–45° in ulnar deviation).
- ROM in normal supination and pronation is approximately 150°.
- A functional ROM for most of the daily activities requires:
  - 40° wrist extension and flexion, respectively
  - 50° supination and pronation, respectively
  - 15° radial and ulnar deviation, respectively
- It has been found that a much greater wrist ROM (95 % of the arc of motion) must be recovered for patients to be fully satisfied than what is needed to perform activities of daily life (Chung and Haas 2009).

31.3.2 Wrist Stability

- Wrist stability is of utmost importance in load transmission from the hand to the forearm. It is the compression force in the long finger flexor and extensor contraction that together with the position of the carpal bones and supported by intact ligaments contribute to wrist stability.
- Once the fracture is sufficiently healed in an accurate position, the bony part of the wrist stability is restored, and adequate rehabilitation should not be a problem, unless there are additional, possibly unknown, ligament injuries.

31.3.3 Grip Strength

- Grip strength is primarily dependent on the strength in extrinsic muscles, i.e. the finger flexors, especially the little and ring fingers.
- The strength in thumb adductors and short flexors reinforces the pressure from the fingers supported by well-functioning ligaments to stabilise the grip.
- The interosseus muscles, which flex the MCP joints and rotate the phalanges, further adjust the shape of the hand to the object that is gripped.
- Optimal wrist position for maximum grip strength is 30–40° extension, with neutral rotation (pronation vs supination) and neutral ulnar and radial deviation.
- Grip strength is an important function in daily life activities and is often used as an outcome measure of the functional recovery of patients with distal radius fractures, as it is correlated to functional ability and request of pain relief.
- Recovering 65 % of grip strength has been associated with satisfied patients (Chung and Haas 2009).
- In order to generate a powerful grip, the finger flexor grip has to be counterbalanced by strong wrist extensors (extensor carpi radialis longus ECRL and brevis ECRB) (Fig. 31.1). The finger flexors pass the wrist, and when activated they would also flex the wrist if this was not simultaneously stabilised by the wrist extensors. A volarly flexed wrist combined with maximum finger flexion results in nonoptimal tendon length where finger flexors become too long (active insufficiency) and finger extensors become too short (passive insufficiency). The result is an ineffective grip with low strength (Fig. 31.2).
- It is most important to get a functional and stable wrist position as soon as possible in order to get an effective "oedema pump" and a useful grip.
- A splint can be useful to stabilise the wrist in the early rehab phase.
- Patients often have difficulties in activating the wrist extensors (m extensor carpi) and therefore try to extend the wrist with the help from the finger extensors (EDC). The EDC muscle is inactivated by keeping the wrist extended during simultaneously static or dynamic finger flexion.

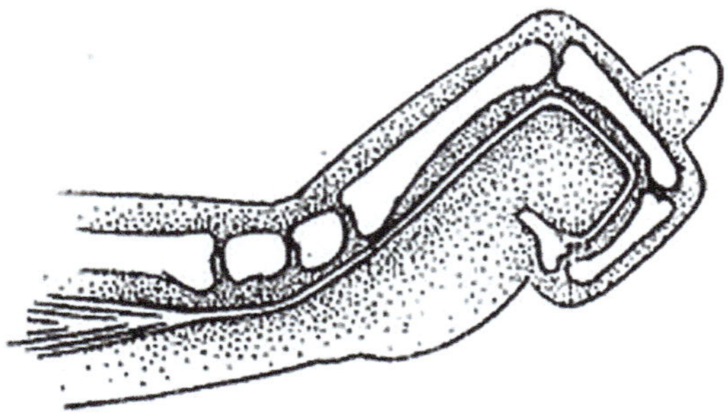

Fig. 31.1 Optimal wrist position for maximum grip strength

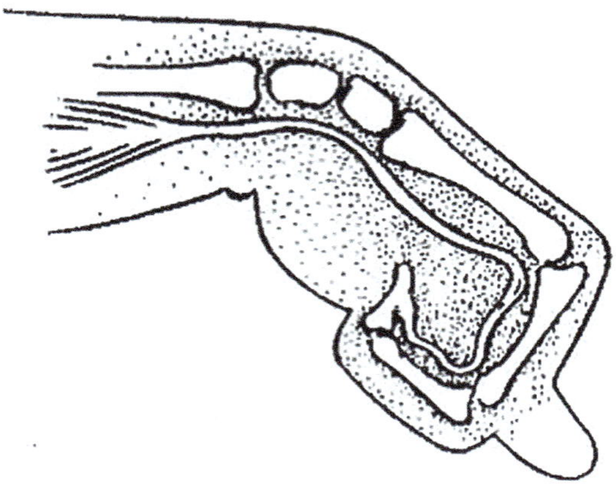

Fig. 31.2 Flexed wrist position results in an ineffective grip

- The prerequisite for good hand function is that the shoulder, elbow and wrist can be placed into positions that optimise the hand function. Physiotherapy intervention thus sometimes requires engagement of the whole upper extremity.

Normal hand function requires (in falling ranking):

- Freedom from pain. Pain is the dominant predictor of upper extremity-specific health status. Sensitivity. Numbness, hyposensitivity, paraesthesia or hypersensitivity makes the hand difficult to use even if motion and strength are normal.
- Stability. Instability is painful and prevents forceful griping.
- Mobility.
- Strength.

31.4 Priorities in Rehabilitation to Restore Good Hand Function

- Freedom from exaggerated pain gives highest priority since pain prevents the hand from being used. Try to evaluate whether pain is related to the restriction in joint movement, is sympathetically mediated or possibly stems from nerve compression problems. Adequate pain relief should be organised.
- Treatment of oedema takes priority before wrist exercises, as residual swelling increases the tension in the tissues and causes ischemic pain. It impairs the circulation and delays the healing process. It increases the friction of the tissues and gradually transforms into a diffuse, nonelastic scar tissue.
- Finger and thumb motion takes priority to wrist exercises, as good wrist function is useless if the fingers and thumb are stiff.
- Rotation gives priority to wrist exercises, as supination is often the most restricted missed mobility around the wrist.

31.5 Effects of Immobilisation

- A short period of immobilisation facilitates wound healing and reduces pain but has negative effects on different structures.
- The tendon's gliding ability and tenacity are reduced after 2 weeks.
- Ligaments lose 40 % of their strength after 6–8 weeks.
- Muscles lose in volume after 1 week. After 6 weeks, their strength has diminished by 40 %.
- Bone mass decreases with 50 % during 12 weeks without loading.

31.6 Effects of Early Mobilisation

- Early mobilisation is the best method to avoid joint contracture, to moisturise articular cartilage and to restore joint proprioception. The restoration of joint mobility is inversely proportional to the length of the immobilisation within the first 6–8 weeks after which the changes may become irreversible. Later mobilisation (over 6 weeks) should start carefully due to the weakness in the various tissues described above. Consequently, recovery may deteriorate if mobilisation is done too aggressively.

- Collagen tissue that is moved or stretched will adapt to the new demands by lengthening and growth. Appropriately timed application of moderate stress can actually enhance tissue strength.
- Immobilisation for 1–2 weeks: during this inflammatory phase, the tissue has approximately 20 % of its normal strength.
- Light stress after 2–6 weeks: during the repair phase, the tissue has approximately 30 % of its normal strength.
- Moderate to normal stress after 6–12 weeks: during the remodelling phase, the tissue has approximately 50 % of its normal strength.
- After 3 months, there are no restrictions.

• In the absence of scientific knowledge, clinical experience suggests that joint tightness is improved by controlled physical stress over significant periods rather than by intensity. In other words, low-load, prolonged stretch/stress is more effective than high-load, brief stretch stress.

31.7 Departmental Protocol for Therapy (Table 31.1)

Table 31.1 Departmental protocol for therapy intervention and time frames for observations by all members of the treatment pathway

Acute care
Plaster immobilization
Only immobilize what is necessary. MCP-joints must be free. Full finger flexion creates tension in the skin on the dorsal part of the hand, which helps to compress the underlying venous and lymphatic system.
Do not press the hand into a bowl-shape. This hinders the intrinsic-muscles important function in minimizing edema.
Do not press the thumb into an adduction-position (NB: Many patients suffer from arthritis in the base of the thumb).
Ensure that the cast is comfortable and well padded over the distal ulna.
Do not immobilize the arm in an arm-sling.
Be generous about changing the plaster when the patient says that the cast does not feel comfortable.
Adequate analgesia should be prescribed.
Written information in lay-mans words about the injury, healing process and its regime is handed out.
Contact telephone number
7–10 days post-injury
Decision about further treatment–conservatively or surgically.
Physiotherapy if the patient presents with high level of pain, edema and/or stiff fingers.
Conservatively treated patients without complications are discharged from the orthopedic unit. Referral to a physiotherapist in primary care 4 weeks post-injury.
Surgically treated patients are referred to a physiotherapist at the orthopedic clinic 2 weeks post-surgery
Removal of the plaster. If surgically treated a nurse removes the sutures.
A *wrist brace* is trialed if surgically treated to be used for 2–3 weeks and only when the patient feels unprotected or as an occasional relieve.
General information about the injury, healing process and regime. Start to use the hand for light daily tasks are a prerequisite for recovery and should be given priority before more specific practice.
Instructions in specific independent home-exercise regarding wrist motion and strengthening.
Follow-up visits when needed.

Summary 1

The therapist's main role is to motivate the patient to exercise independently with advice and instructions on:

- The importance of using the hand in daily activities
- Positive effects of early motion
- The healing-process and the strength in the tissues
- Tissue-load, activities and exercises
- Expected outcome

Summary 2
The clinical difficulty lies in the ability to correctly identify:
- Which patients demand more extensive supervised therapy
- Which degree of exercise intensity is the optimal
- When changes in the hand status require a change in exercise or other actions
- What normal recovery is
- What a good result is

Summary 3
What predicts the final outcome?
- Type of fracture and fracture-position?
- Treatment – surgery/conservative, early/late surgery, surgical technique?
- Immobilization – plaster alignment, period?
- Rehabilitation – early motion, physiotherapeutic capacity?
- Routines – early identification of patients with complications?
- Patient-related factors – motivation, optimism, expectations, compliance?

- The physiotherapist intervention for *non-operated* patients normally consists of 1–2 follow-ups.
- For *operated* patients, 3–4 follow-ups (after 2, 4, 6, 10/12 weeks).
- Patients can normally be discharged when they use the hand spontaneously.

31.8 Complications Requiring More Extensive Rehabilitation

- Complex fracture
- Immobilisation during a long time and/or in a poorly fitted plaster cast.
- Oedema
- High level of pain/inappropriate amount of pain
- Stiffness of fingers and thumb
- Signs of increased sympathetic reactivity
- Signs of nerve involvement
- Reluctance to use the hand due to exaggerated fear of moving the hand and/or pain anxiety
- Ineffective home exercise

31.9 CRPS (Complex Regional Pain Syndrome)

- The most dreaded complication after wrist fracture is residual pain, oedema and finger stiffness, which can lead to a more or less advanced CRPS (complex regional pain syndrome) with devastating functional limitation as a result.
- Warning signs and potential causes of CRPS relate to:
  - Poorly fitted plaster or a tight elastic bandage on top of the plaster
  - Inadequate pain relief
  - Not having received written information
  - Not having been informed about how to prevent complications
  - Not having been referred to a physiotherapist during immobilisation
  - Failure to identify the symptoms and/or to understand the seriousness
- CRPS can be prevented:
  - Immediately involve the physiotherapist when needed.
  - Establish a well-functioning "departmental protocol for therapy" (Table 31.1).
  - Well-educated staff and cooperation between all members of the team.

31.10 Special Problems After Open Reduction and Internal Plate Fixation (ORIF)

- Tethered flexor tendons
- Pins/screws that are too proud and cause attrition wear on either extensor or flexor tendons
- Hypersensitivity of the scar
- Numbness in the area dorsally/radially on the back of the thumb and hand (sensory branch of the radial nerve)
- Carpal tunnel syndrome

31.11 Special Problems After External Fixation (EF)

- Difficulties in regaining a normal hand position due to the immobilisation position.
- Difficulties in reducing swelling due to immobilised wrist position in flexion.
- Difficulties flexing the MCP joint to the index finger due to the distal pins.
- Difficulties moving the thumb in radial deviation and extension due to the distal pins.
- Carpal tunnel syndrome due to wrist immobilisation in a flexed position.
- Adherence around the pins.
- Patients operated with EF usually have more limitations and need more rehabilitation during the first few months.

31.12 Prevention of Falling Is Better than Cure

- Almost all distal forearm fractures are sustained by a fall on an outstretched hand.
- One of the risk factors of falling is impaired balance, which occurs in women after menopause.
- It is proven that exercise to increase muscle strength and balance improves those functions and therefore reduces the risk of falling (Nordell 2003), estimated to a reduction in the frequency of falling with 32 % (Karlsson 2004).
- All members of the health-care team, i.e. doctors, nurses and especially physiotherapists, carry a responsibility in identifying patients with fall-related fractures and low bone mineral density so that preventive measures can be taken.

31.13 Summary

- Treating patients with distal radius fractures and other injuries of the hand is a skill that calls for an understanding of the functional anatomy and the physiological healing processes. That means taking into consideration the different healing phases, the knowledge about the positive effects of early mobilisation and above all the early use of the hand.
- There is no scientific benefit in using different modalities like thermotherapy, ultrasound, short wave, iontophoresis and laser (Handoll et al. 2006).
- Early control of swelling and pain, as well as early active motion, is of paramount importance in eliminating and preventing dysfunction.
- We have to be realistic about our ability to affect the functional outcome and setting reasonable goals, which are different in a simple undisplaced, extra-articular fracture in an osteoporotic patient as opposed to a displaced intra-articular fracture in a young active high-demanding person.
- We should not ask ourselves what we can do to the patient, but what the patient can do for himself or herself to achieve a satisfactory end result. A positive relationship was found between primarily home-exercise adherence and short-term outcomes (Lyngcoln et al. 2005).
- We have to apply a holistic view of the patient and his/her injury, where consideration is taken to each patient's special problems, comorbidities and general condition.
- In the absence of scientific support for therapy, we have to apply a professional skill in increasing motivation and give patients confidence in their own ability to influence their own recovery.

References

Chung KC, Haas A. Relationship between patient satisfaction and objective functional outcome after surgical treatment for distal radius fractures. J Hand Ther. 2009;22:302–8.

Handoll HHG, Madhook R, Howe TE. Rehabilitation for distal radial fractures in adults. Cochrane Database Syst Rev. 2006;3:1–63.

Hunter S, et al. Rehabilitation of the hand: surgery and therapy. Philadelphia: Mosby; 1990.

Karlsson M. Has exercise an antifracture efficacy in women? Scand J Med Sci Sports. 2004;14:2–15.

Lundborg G. The hand – extension of the brain reaching out to the world. Lakartidningen. 1990;87(1–2):42–4.

Lyngcoln A, Taylor N, Baskus K. The relationship between adherence to hand therapy and short-term outcome after distal radius fracture. J Hand Ther. 2005;18(1):2–8.

Nordell E. Falls, fractures and function, – focus on women with a distal forearm fracture. Dissertation Lund University, Sweden; 2003.

Oskarsson GV, Hjall A, Aaser P. Physiotherapy: an over-estimated factor in after-treatment of fractures in the distal radius? Arch Orthop Trauma Surg. 1997;116:373.

Souer JS, Buijze G, Ring D. A prospective randomized controlled trial comparing occupational therapy with independent exercises after volar plate fixation of a fracture of the distal part of the radius. J Bone Joint Surg Am. 2011;93(19):1761–6.

Part IV

Complications and Their Treatment

Complications: An Overview

32

Per-Olof Josefsson, Björn E. Rosengren,
and Magnus K. Karlsson

Contents

P.-O. Josefsson, MD, PhD (✉)
Department of Clinical Sciences,
University of Lund, Lund, Sweden

Department of Orthopedics, Skåne
University Hospital, Malmö, Sweden
e-mail: perolof.josefsson@skane.se

B.E. Rosengren, MD • M.K. Karlsson
Department of Orthopedics and Clinical Sciences,
Skåne University Hospital, Lund University,
Malmö, Sweden
e-mail: magnus.karlsson@med.lu

32.1 Summary

Complications are common with distal radius fractures. The complications can in general be divided into those primarily related to the injury and those related to the choice of treatment. The most common of complications related to the injury are malunions, tendon injuries, neurological disturbances and complex regional pain syndrome (CRPS). Malunions are seen more often after nonsurgical than after surgical treatment. The clinical relevance of the entity is however ambiguous, as there, in spite of concomitant radiological degenerative changes following a malunion, often also is a gradual improvement in clinical symptoms during the subsequent years. The expected spontaneous improvement, the functional demands of the patient and the predicted result of surgery must therefore all be taken into consideration in the decision-making process preceding any surgery of an established malunion.

The most common complications related to surgery are superficial wound infections and superficial radial nerve lesions. These complications are therefore mostly seen after unstable distal radius fractures that are in need of surgery. Unstable and displaced fractures are in most patients treated with reduction of the displacement while the choice of fixation varies. The type of fixation with the lowest complication rate, malunions excluded, seems to be cast immobilisation. The type of fixation with the highest rate of complications, most often superficial infections and superficial radial nerve lesions, seems

L.M. Hove et al. (eds.), *Distal Radius Fractures*,
DOI 10.1007/978-3-642-54604-4_32, © Springer-Verlag Berlin Heidelberg 2014

to be external fixation. The type of fixation with the highest rate of complications that necessitate second surgery seems to be plate fixation.

32.2 Introduction

Fractures of the distal radius are in most cases the result of indirect trauma after a fall on the outstretched hand. However, a fracture at this site may also occur after high-energy trauma and is then often only one among several other injuries.

- Irrespective of the trauma type, a distal radius fracture in adults is often followed by residual clinical symptoms.
- The most common treatment of choice for this type of fracture, both non-displaced and displaced, has since long been nonoperative.
- During the recent decades, there have been several shifts in treatment strategies, in search for better clinical outcome and reduction of rate and severity of complications.
- There is heterogeneity in the use of the term complication after a distal radius fracture.
- Some authors include a malunion; others regard this as an expected result following some fracture types.
- Some refer a long duration of symptoms and unexpected problems as a complication, while others do not.
- Finally, in some reports, the term complication is used when two or more injuries follow the fracture, while others do not define this as a complication. Partly due to this, there is no gold standard of treatment, since it is difficult to compare complication rates of each specific treatment.

32.3 Non-unions and Malunions

Non-union of distal radius fractures is rare independent of fracture type.

Symptomatic malunion probably is the most common complication after a distal radius fracture.

- Malunions can be classified as extra-articular and/or intra-articular. Extra-articular malunions involve distorted angulation and a shortening of the distal radius, whereas intra-articular malunions result in nonanatomical surfaces in the radio-carpal or the radio-ulnar joint.
- Malunions can be seen as nascent malunions, i.e. within weeks from expected healing or as mature malunions after 6 months.
- Malunions are often followed by residual symptoms. The most common complaints are pain, weakness or loss of mobility.
- Most studies indicate a gradual improvement of symptoms by time, and 2–4 years after the fracture, there is usually a significant improvement in the clinical presentation compared to baseline (Brogen et al. 2011). The improvement can often be expected to continue further, even up to 30 years after a fracture, where 2/3 had no discomfort at all compared to the contralateral wrist and the remaining 1/3 reported only minor complaints despite obvious radiological degenerative changes (Kopylov et al. 1993).
- It is difficult to predict the long-term outcome after a malunion.
- In general, a significant deformity is usually associated with lower subjective residual complaints and lower functional loss in older than younger patients.
- The degree of displacement of the malunion can also be important for the outcome. Large observational studies have reported a correlation between the degree of angulation or shortening of the radius following a malunion and the rate of residual symptoms (Lidström 1959; McQueen and Caspers 1988). This may partially be the result of soft tissue damage at the injury with the most displaced fractures, often undiagnosed at the time of the trauma (Lindau et al. 1997; Spence et al. 1998).
- The treatment of choice for a malunion should primarily be chosen depending on the functional loss in relation to functional demands of the specific patient, rather than on the absolute degree of the deformity.
- The success of any surgical intervention of malunions depends on patient age, functional demands and type and extent of deformity.
- The predicted gain in function by surgery must be taken into consideration when deciding treatment.

32.4 Neurological Complications

A severely displaced distal radius fracture is sometimes accompanied by neurological deficits from the nerve branches around the wrist.

- The most common neurological complication involves the median nerve with radiating pain or sensory deficit in the volar aspect of three radial fingers. This can be caused by a temporary injury to the nerve, neurapraxia, resulting either from the initial impact or from compression in the carpal tunnel.
- Relief of symptoms is achieved by reducing the fracture as soon as possible to the best possible, preferably anatomical, position. The reduction is often followed by a marked improvement or complete recovery of the neurological symptoms.
- In those patients with remaining severe symptoms after the reduction, an acute decompression of the carpal tunnel is recommended.
- Neurological symptoms may also develop later in the posttraumatic period, usually due to hematoma, oedema and general swelling.
- Compression neuropathy caused by late swelling can be seen in 5 % of conservatively treated fractures: 4 % affects the median nerve, 1 % the ulnar nerve and 0.5 % the radial cutaneous nerves.
- Most of these late compression neuropathies recovered spontaneously within 3 months leaving only 0.5 % of all conservatively treated patients for surgical nerve decompression (Hove 1995).

32.5 Pain Versus Complex Regional Pain Syndrome (CRPS)

Pain is expected with distal radius fractures, but it should settle after the first week. Prolonged pain should be carefully assessed as it may be a sign of a complication:

- The plaster and dressing may be too tight and may need to be refitted.
- Swelling may have caused a CTS.
- Re-displacement of the fracture should be checked with an updated x-ray.
- Prolonged disproportionate pain may be an early sign of CRPS.
- It is contraindicated to simply prescribe stronger painkillers!

The term complex regional pain syndrome (CRPS) type 1 was launched by the group "International Association for the Study of Pain" in 1994. CRPS was then defined as a syndrome which usually develops after an initial traumatic event, trauma or immobilisation and results in pain and tenderness disproportionate to the degree of the injury not limited to the territory of a single peripheral nerve and additional symptoms of vasomotor instability. No other condition which could account for the degree of pain and dysfunction should be present (Stanton-Hicks et al. 1995).

- In CRPS type 1, no demonstrable nerve lesion should be present in contrast to CRPS type 2 where there is nerve involvement such as a carpal tunnel syndrome.
- CRPS is currently the recommended term, but other descriptions are being used such as finger–hand–shoulder syndrome, causalgia, algodystrophy, reflex sympathetic dystrophy (RSD) and, when associated with radiological changes, Sudeck's atrophy.
- CRPS is maybe the most severe complication to a distal radius fracture as it has a high risk to result in chronic impairment.
- CRPS has in some reports been associated with psychological and social patient factors.
- CRPS is found in both nonsurgically and surgically treated patients, and the incidence after a distal radius fracture has been reported between 1 % (Hove 1995) and 28 % (Birkensatff and Kanis 1994), depending on how CRPS was defined.
- It is essential to have all members of the team involved in the assessment and management of CRPS, i.e. intense physiotherapy of all mobile parts of the extremity including the finger, elbow and shoulder joints, for both prevention and treatment of established symptoms.
- Occupational therapy deals with oedema control, adequate splints, etc.
- Other interventions with preventive effects include appropriate pharmacological pain

control and in CRPS 2 also active treatment of the underlying neurological symptom such as surgery of a carpal tunnel syndrome.
- Treatment is probably more effective if initiated in an early stage of the disease.
- As the aetiology of CRPS has not yet been clearly demonstrated, it is difficult to find a specific therapy, but the condition seems to involve both the autonomic and the central nervous systems. Different drugs that modify these systems have therefore been tested.
- Stellate/lumbar sympathetic blocks, mannitol, gabapentin and physio-/occupational therapy are all interventions that have been shown with some effects (Tran et al. 2010).
- Improvements have also been found in some studies with bisphosphonates, dimethyl sulfoxide, steroids, epidural clonidine, intrathecal baclofen, spinal cord stimulation and mental practice by motor imagery (mirror therapy), but there is currently no consensus on when or how these treatments should be used.
- Other drugs have also been tested, and some recommend calcitonin, vasodilators or sympatholytic and neuro-modulative intravenous regional blockade, but none of these have consistently been shown with significant beneficial effects.

32.6 Tendon Injuries

Another common complication following a distal radius fracture is tendon rupture. Most ruptures are, however, not seen at the fracture event but weeks after the fracture.
- The most common is late rupture of the extensor pollicis longus (EPL) tendon.
- EPL rupture is most often seen after a non- or minimally displaced distal radius fracture, in a range from 0.3 % of all distal radius fractures (Hove 1994) to 5 % (Roth et al. 2012).
- Ruptures of other tendons near the wrist are rare and are usually only found after high-energy trauma with open fractures and additional soft tissue injuries.

32.7 Complications Related to the Method of Treatment

Cast, external fixation and open reduction and internal fixation are methods used to retain the reduction of displaced distal radius fractures.
- The highest treatment-related complication rate (both minor and major complications) that did not require surgery was found in patients treated with bridging external fixation (Table 32.1) (Diaz-Garcia et al. 2011). Sixteen percent of the patients in this group developed a superficial infection, and 6 % developed CRPS (Table 32.1).
- The highest rate of major complications that required further surgery was found in patients treated with volar plating. Six percent of the patients in this group required additional surgery due to tendon rupture/adhesion and 3 % due to hardware problems (Table 32.1).
- The lowest rate of any treatment-related complication was found in patients immobilised in a cast (Table 32.1).

32.8 Tricks and Tips

- Be aware of possible complications and their course.
- Analyse the cause of pain by reassessing all aspects of the fracture, patient and treatment modality! Then treat pain with adequate painkillers!
- Recommend active motions of all mobile parts of the extremity from day one.
- Natural improvement of symptoms after a malunion can be expected to continue several years after the fracture.
- Treatment of malunions should not be based on the degree of displacement alone.
- Treatment of malunions must include evaluation of the functional demands of the patient in relation to risks and expected outcome after surgery.
- Symptoms of CRPS, i.e. disproportionate pain, should immediately involve the entire team with emphasis on improved pain control and intensive physio- and occupational therapy.

Table 32.1 Rate of complications in relation to treatment for unstable distal radius fractures

	Volar plates (*n*=298)	Non-bridging ex-fix (*n*=83)	Bridging ex-fix (*n*=249)	Percut. K-wire fixat (*n*=163)	Cast immobilisation (*n*=239)	*p*-value
Minor complications						
Superficial infection	0 (0 %)	25 (30 %)	39 (16 %)	2 (1 %)	0 (0 %)	
Others	2 (0.5 %)	0 (0 %)	0 (0 %)	9 (6 %)	0 (0 %)	
Total (%)	2 (0.5 %)	25 (30 %)	39 (16 %)	11 (7 %)	0 (0 %)	<0.001
Major complications not requiring surgery						
Nerve lesion	6 (2 %)	1 (1 %)	10 (4 %)	4 (2 %)	4 (2 %)	
CRPS	9 (3 %)	0 (0 %)	16 (6 %)	2 (1 %)	11 (5 %)	
Early hardware removal	0 (0 %)	0 (0 %)	6 (2 %)	3 (2 %)	0 (0 %)	
Others	3 (1 %)	0 (0 %)	2 (1 %)	0 (0 %)	0 (0 %)	
Total (%)	18 (6 %)	1 (1 %)	34 (14 %)	9 (6 %)	15 (7 %)	<0.001
Major complications requiring surgery						
Tendon rupture/adhesion	18 (6 %)	2 (2 %)	0 (0 %)	3 (2 %)	3 (1 %)	
Nerve lesion	2 (0.5 %)	0 (0 %)	2 (1 %)	0 (0 %)	0 (0 %)	
Infection	2 (0.5 %)	0 (0 %)	1 (1 %)	0 (0 %)	0 (0 %)	
Hardware loosening, failure or removal	8 (3 %)	0 (0 %)	0 (0 %)	0 (0 %)	0 (0 %)	
Others	2 (0.5 %)	0 (0 %)	2 (1 %)	0 (0 %)	0 (0 %)	
Total (%)	32(11 %)	2 (2 %)	5 (2 %)	3 (2 %)	3 (1 %)	<0.001

Data are reported as numbers and proportions (%) (Diaz-Garcia et al. 2011)
Group differences were estimated by chi-square test. Significant differences were found when comparing all the treatment groups except the following pairs: (i) Major complications not requiring surgery: percutaneous Kirschner wire fixation versus cast immobilisation; (ii) Major complications requiring surgery: non-bridging external fixation versus percutaneous Kirschner wire fixation; and (iii) Major complications requiring surgery: bridging external fixation versus percutaneous Kirschner wire fixation

References

Birkensatff DR, Kanis JA. Algodystrophy: an under-recognised complication of minor trauma. Br J Rheumatol. 1994;33:240–8.

Brogen E, et al. Fractures of the distal radius in woman aged 50 to 75 years: natural course of patient reported outcome, wrist motion and grip strength between 1 year and 2–4 years after fracture. J Hand Surg Eur Vol. 2011;36(7):568–76.

de Tran OH, et al. Treatment of complex regional pain syndrome, a review of the evidence. Can J Anaesth. 2010;57(2):149–66.

Diaz-Garcia RJ, et al. A systematic review of outcomes and complications of treating unstable distal radius fractures in the elderly. J Hand Surg Am. 2011;36(5):824–35.

Hove LM. Delayed rupture of the thumb extensor tendon. A 5-year study of 18 consecutive cases. Acta Orthop Scand. 1994;65(2):199–203.

Hove LM. Nerve entrapment and reflex sympathetic dystrophy after fractures of the distal radius. Scand J Plast Reconstr Surg Hand Surg. 1995;29(1):53–8.

Kopylov P, et al. Fractures of the distal end of the radius in young adults: a 30-year follow-up. J Hand Surg Br. 1993;18B:45–9.

Lidström A. Fractures of the distal end of the radius. A clinical and statistical study of end results. Acta Orthop Scand. 1959;41 suppl 36:1–118.

Lindau T, Arner M, Hagberg L. Intraarticular lesions in distal radius fractures in young adults. A descriptive arthroscopic study in 50 patients. J Hand Surg Br. 1997;22(5):638–43.

McQueen MM, Caspers J. Colles' fracture; does the anatomical result affect the final function? J Bone Joint Surg Br. 1988;70(4):649–51.

Roth KM, et al. Incidence of extensor pollicis longus tendon rupture after nondisplaced distal radius fractures. J Hand Surg Am. 2012;37(5):942–7.

Spence LD, et al. MRI of fracture s of the distal radius: comparison with conventional radiographs. Skeletal Radiol. 1998;27(5):244–9.

Stanton-Hicks M, et al. Reflex sympathetic dystrophy: changing concepts and taxonomy. Pain. 1995;63:127–33.

Nerve Entrapments and Nerve Injuries in Distal Radius Fractures

33

Adalsteinn Odinsson

Contents

A. Odinsson, MD
Section of Hand Surgery,
Department of Orthopaedic Surgery,
St Olav's University Hospital, Trondheim, Norway
e-mail: adalsteinn.odinsson@stolav.no

33.1 Summary

There are four main nerves in the distal forearm and wrist: *the median nerve*, *the ulnar nerve*, *the superficial radial nerve*, and *the posterior interosseous nerve*. The most commonly affected nerve in distal radius fractures is the median nerve.

The nerves may be damaged at the time of injury or in treatment of the fracture. This emphasizes the importance of a thorough examination and documentation of the neurovascular status prior to any treatment of the fracture and also after the treatment. This includes evaluation of sensibility and motor function. Nerve conduction studies can be of help in diagnosing and evaluating the nerve injury.

In the acute phase, the nerve is affected by either a direct injury or an entrapment. Late nerve dysfunction is most often an entrapment of the nerve.

In patients with a distal radius fracture and acute carpal tunnel syndrome, the fracture must be reduced and stabilized. Then the concomitant nerve compression syndrome will generally improve substantially over 24–48 h. If neurological symptoms increase or show no improvement after 1 or 2 days, carpal tunnel release is recommended with inspection of the nerve. It is important to remember that the compression or injury to the nerve may be in the carpal tunnel or 3 cm proximally, at the fracture site. An extended approach with adequately visualization and decompression at both sites is therefore recommended.

L.M. Hove et al. (eds.), *Distal Radius Fractures*,
DOI 10.1007/978-3-642-54604-4_33, © Springer-Verlag Berlin Heidelberg 2014

33.2 Anatomy

There are four main nerves in the distal arm and wrist: *the median nerve*, *the ulnar nerve*, *the superficial radial nerve*, and *the posterior interosseous nerve* (Figs. 33.1 and 33.2). The most commonly affected in distal radius fractures is the median nerve (Aro et al. 1988). Several authors have reported injury to the ulnar nerve in distal radius fractures, but the nerve is more at risk in distal forearm fractures when both radius and ulna are fractured than in isolated distal radius fracture (Clarke and Spencer 1991; Hove 1995). Although posterior interosseous nerve is at the risk of injury in distal radius fracture, there seems to be very few rapports of this in the literature. The superficial radial nerve is at risk of injury when treating distal radius fracture with K-wires or external fixation (Chen et al. 2010).

33.3 Median Nerve

The median nerve is commonly entrapped or injured in distal radius fractured, causing nerve dysfunction. The reported incidence varies in the literature from 0.07 to 17 % (Hove 1995).

- The most commonly affected nerve in distal radius fracture.
- Contusion, stretching, or compression can cause the dysfunction.
- Thorough clinical examination with documentation of neurological status prior to and after treatment is important.
- Concomitant nerve compression syndrome will generally improve substantially over 24–48 h.

33.3.1 Acute Median Nerve Entrapment or Injury

The nerve is often contused by the trauma, stretched over the dislocated fracture, or entrapped in the fracture. The fracture hematoma or swelling may increase the pressure in the carpal tunnel causing an acute carpal tunnel syndrome (Bienek et al. 2006).

Some authors have described median nerve dysfunction after volar incision and volar plating of this fracture:

- The dysfunction after operation can be caused by direct injury to the nerve or
- By prolonged use of self-retaining wound retractors during the operation (Nourbakhsh and Tan 2010)

Diagnosis

The nerve can be damage at the time of injury or in treatment of the fracture. This emphasizes the importance of a thorough examination and documentation of the neurovascular status prior to any treatment of the fracture and also after the treatment. This includes careful measurements of the two-point discrimination and the thenar motor function. Nerve conduction studies can be of help in diagnosing and evaluating the nerve injury.

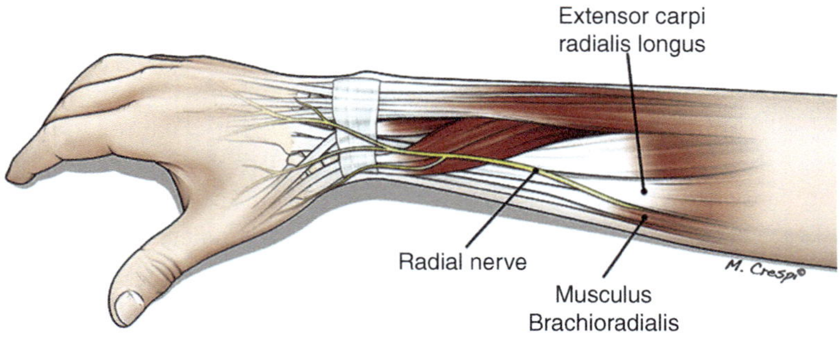

Fig. 33.1 The picture shows the location of the radial superficial nerve in the forearm

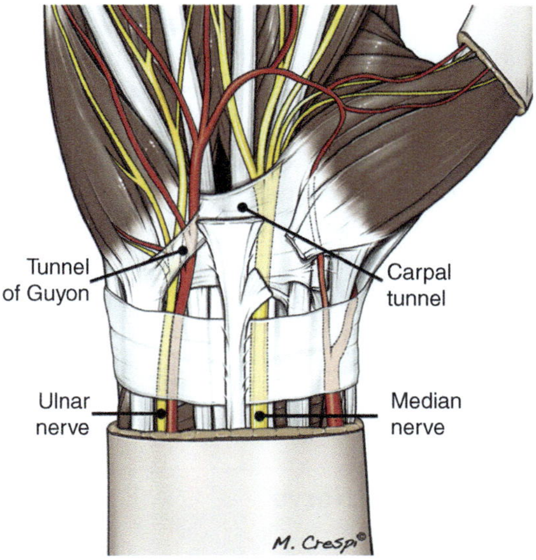

Fig. 33.2 The picture shows the location of the median and ulnar nerves in the distal forearm and wrist

Treatment

Most distal radius fractures are managed conservatively with or without closed reduction and cast treatment.

- The majority of distal radius fractures have no neural complications.
- There is no indication for routine or prophylactic release of the carpal ligament.

The incidence of acute post traumatic carpal tunnel syndrome which requires carpal tunnel release in operatively treated fractures is estimated to 5.5–9 %. This type of Carpal tunnel syndrome is associated with high-energy trauma and multifragmentary or intra-articular fracture types (Bienek et al. 2006).

- After reduction and stabilization of the fracture, the concomitant nerve compression syndrome will improve substantially over 24–48 h.
- If neurological symptoms worsen or show no improvement after this time, an operation is recommended with reduction and stabilization of the fracture and carpal tunnel release with inspection of the nerve.
- It is important to remember that the compression or injury to the nerve can be in the carpal tunnel or 3 cm proximally at the fracture site. An extended approach which adequately visualizes and decompresses both sites is therefore recommended (Campbell 2007).

33.3.2 Late Median Nerve Entrapment

The incidence of late carpal tunnel syndrome, or a more proximal entrapment of the nerve in the distal forearm, occurring several months or years after injury, varies from 0.5 to 22 % in different reports.

- It is considered to be associated with malunion.
- Residual palmar displacement of distal fragment.
- Chronic inflammation and edema of the tenosynovium.
- Prolonged immobilization of the limb with the wrist flexed.
- Encroaching callus (Bienek et al. 2006).

Diagnosis

The diagnosis is made by clinical examination, testing the sensibility in the fingers, Phalen's test, and Tinel's sign. Numbness in the three radial fingers and positive clinical tests confirm the diagnosis. Nerve conduction studies can be of help especially when the clinical examination is unclear and when a thorough documentation is needed.

Treatment

The treatment is carpal tunnel release. Our standard method is open surgery and incision of the transverse carpal ligament. The nerve is visualized and inspected for injury or deformity.

33.3.3 Superficial Radial Nerve Injury

This nerve lies on the posterior and radial aspect of the forearm and wrist. It supplies sensibility to the dorsum of the hand and fingers. Injury to this nerve in distal radius fracture is very rare, occurring in only 1 % of cases and is usually iatrogenic. The nerve can be injured when treating the distal radius fracture either with percutaneous K-wires and external fixation or by a tight cast (Chen et al. 2010).

- Injury to this nerve is usually iatrogenic.
- Causing loss of sensation distally or pain from neuroma.
- The best treatment is to avoid injuring the nerve.
- Loss of sensation and painful neuroma are indications for surgery with exploration of the injured nerve.

Diagnosis

The patient complains of reduced sensibility on the radial and dorsal side of the wrist and hand. This can be verified by clinical examination and two-point discrimination. Later on this nerve injury may cause painful neuroma in the forearm at the site of injury, where only a light touch may give severe and radiating neuropathic pain.

Treatment

The best treatment is *prevention*:

- Make sure that the cast in conservatively treated patients is not too tight and inform the patient to return to the clinic if there is any numbness or excessive pain.
- When external fixation is used, we recommend a proper incision for the proximal pins, and the soft tissue is carefully dissected down to the bone, making sure that the nerve is not injured.
- In cases of K-wire fixation, we may reduce the danger of damaging the superficial branch of the radial nerve by inserting the K-wires in the tip of the radial styloid process or only 1 cm proximally from the tip (Chen et al. 2010).

When a *nerve injury* has occurred, we must evaluate the extent of the injury and the symptoms of the patient.

- If the symptoms are only sensory loss in a small area on the back of the hand, the most likely cause is an injury to a small branch of the nerve. This is best treated conservatively and may reside over time.
- If there is a large area with sensory loss, or the patient complains of pain when touching the injured nerve and often radiating proximally or distally, an operation with exploration of the nerve is warranted.
- On exploring the nerve it may be embedded in a scar tissue, making it necessary for neurolysis and, if possible, nerve relocation out of the scared area.

Painful neuroma is very difficult to treat and vary from conservative treatment with padding the area, physiotherapy with desensitization and functional training, to operations. There are a number of operative techniques described for neuromas so it is clear that none of them is reliable. The most usual operations are removal of the neuroma and if possible reconnection of the damage nerve. If reconnection is not possible, the neuroma is removed and the end is then placed in healthy tissue in an area with minimal exposure for touch and pressure.

33.4 Ulnar Nerve

Ulnar nerve injury subsequent to a fracture of the distal radius is rare compared to a median nerve injury, occurring in about 4 % of distal radius fractures (Aro et al. 1988).

- Check for both median and ulnar nerve injury in high-energy and comminuted distal radius fractures.
- The neurapraxia usually recovers to normal or near normal strength and sensation.
- If there is no sign of clinical improvement after 2–3 months, we recommend nerve conduction study and surgical exploration.
- Operation at the time of injury is only recommended when there is a complete ulnar nerve palsy associated with an open wound or an acute carpal tunnel syndrome.

33.4.1 Acute Ulnar Nerve Injury or Compression

Ulnar nerve injury is associated with younger patients with a high-energy trauma, wide displacement of fracture, comminution, combined distal ulna fracture, and open fracture (Cho et al. 2010). The mechanism of injury can be contusion, traction, or a compression on the ulnar nerve. It is recommended that cases with high-energy trauma and widely displaced or comminuted fractures of the distal radius should be evaluated carefully for ulnar nerve injury as well as for median nerve injuries.

Diagnosis

The patient complains of reduced sensibility on the volar side of fourth and fifth fingers. There is reduced two-point discrimination on clinical examination and the abduction and adduction in all the fingers are weakened.

Treatment

The injury usually causes a neurapraxia which usually recovers to normal or near normal strength and sensation.

- Operation with exploration and release of the nerve at the time of injury is only recommended when there is a complete ulnar nerve palsy associated with an open wound or an acute carpal tunnel syndrome.
- Observation without exploration is recommended otherwise (Soong and Ring 2007).

If there is an ulnar nerve injury in a closed distal radius fracture and there is no sign of clinical improvement after 2–3 months

- We recommend nerve conduction study and surgical exploration with decompression and neurolysis of the nerve.

33.4.2 Late Ulnar Compression Neuropathy in Guyon's Canal

This late compression of the nerve occurring several months or years after injury is considered to be associated with residual hematoma, malalignment of the radius after the fracture, or local soft tissue edema (Bienek et al. 2006).

Diagnosis

The diagnosis is made by clinical examination, testing the sensibility in the fingers with two-point discrimination. Numbness in 4 and 5 fingers, increased two-point discrimination, and reduced abduction and adduction in all of the fingers confirms the diagnosis. Nerve conduction studies can be of help especially when the clinical examination is unclear and when a thorough documentation is needed.

Treatment

The treatment is surgical exploration with decompression and neurolysis of the nerve.

33.5 Posterior Interosseous Nerve Injury

The anatomy of the posterior interosseous nerve (PIN), which lies directly on the periosteum of the distal epiphysis of the radius, may predispose to nerve migration between fragments after a fracture. This is especially likely to be the case in a comminuted fracture of the distal radius, when the fragment lines run in the sagittal plane.

These patients have pain syndrome in the narrow fourth extensor compartment of the forearm, which includes extensor indicis proprius and extensor digitorum communis tendons. Good results can be obtained after neurectomy or neurolysis of the posterior interosseous nerve (Baczkowski et al. 2006).

References

Aro H, Koivunen T, Katevuo K, Nieminen S, Aho AJ. Late compression neuropathies after Colles' fractures. Clin Orthop Relat Res. 1988;(233):217–25.

Baczkowski B, Dzwonkowska J, Lorczynski A, Klimek T. Posterior interosseous nerve neuropathy in distal radius fracture. Ortop Traumatol Rehabil. 2006;8:350–5.

Bienek T, Kusz D, Cielinski L. Peripheral nerve compression neuropathy after fractures of the distal radius. J Hand Surg Br. 2006;31:256–60.

Campbell D. Peripheral nerve compression neuropathy after fractures of the distal radius. J Hand Surg Br. 2007;32:233–4.

Chen Y, Zheng X, Wang J, Zhu Y, Zhan C. Reliable techniques to avoid damaging the superficial radial nerve due to percutaneous Kirschner wire fixation of the distal radius fracture through the radial styloid process. Surg Radiol Anat. 2010;32:711–7.

Cho CH, Kang CH, Jung JH. Ulnar nerve palsy following closed fracture of the distal radius: a report of 2 cases. Clin Orthop Surg. 2010;2:55–8.

Clarke AC, Spencer RF. Ulnar nerve palsy following fractures of the distal radius: clinical and anatomical studies. J Hand Surg Br. 1991;16:438–40.

Hove LM. Nerve entrapment and reflex sympathetic dystrophy after fractures of the distal radius. Scand J Plast Reconstr Surg Hand Surg. 1995;29:53–8.

Nourbakhsh A, Tan V. Median nerve fibrosis at the distal forearm after volar plate fixation of distal radius fracture. J Hand Surg Br. 2010;35:768–9.

Soong M, Ring D. Ulnar nerve palsy associated with fracture of the distal radius. J Orthop Trauma. 2007;21:113–6.

Tendon Complications of Distal Radial Fractures

34

Michael A.C. Craigen and Claire K. Simpson

Contents

M.A.C. Craigen, MD FRCS
(Tr Orth) Dipl Hand Surg (✉) • C.K. Simpson,
MD FRCS (Tr Orth) Dipl Hand Surg
The Birmingham Hand Centre, Birmingham, UK

The most commonly affected tendon is the extensor pollicis longus (EPL). This is more frequent after undisplaced fractures of the distal radius. EPL ruptures may be caused by a double insult of increased pressure within an intact tendon sheath resulting in reduced blood flow to an already poorly vascularised tendon lead to tendon rupture. It typically presents at 2–3 weeks after the fracture.

Extensor tendon entrapment at the fracture site occurs more frequently than flexor tendon entrapment. In volarly displace fractures, a visible gap after closed reduction should alert the surgeon to this possibility.

Tendon complications from dorsal plating, extensor tenosynovitis and tendon ruptures, required plate removal and tendon reconstruction.

Several early reports after volar plating have presented 1/3 of patients with tendon complications, most often ruptured flexor pollicis longus (FPL) tendons, or attrition and fraying of the flexor tendons. Ruptures are not always preceded by symptoms. "Technical issues" with the fixation is most often the cause, as either suboptimal positioning of the volar plate or prominent screw heads.

In a meta-analysis of papers describing complications of distal radius fixation, it was suggested that tendon complications are just as common with volar as with dorsal fixation.

L.M. Hove et al. (eds.), *Distal Radius Fractures*,
DOI 10.1007/978-3-642-54604-4_34, © Springer-Verlag Berlin Heidelberg 2014

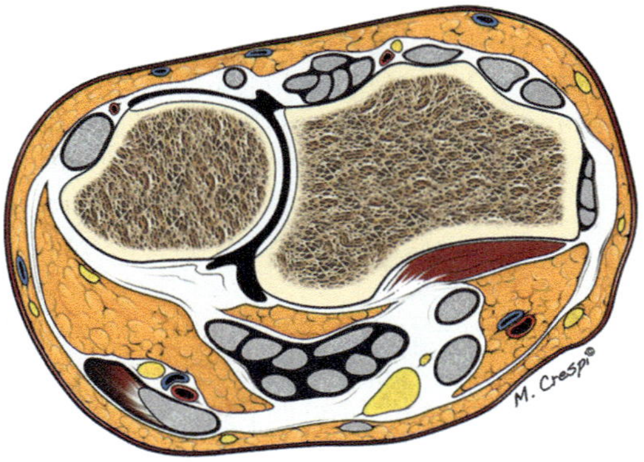

Fig. 34.1 The dorsal tendons are closely applied to the distal radial cortex. Volarly, the pronator quadratus muscle lies adjacent to the bone, with the flexor tendons lying a reasonable distance away. *I–VI*=represent the extensor compartments. *1*=pronator quadratus, *2*=flexor tendon mass

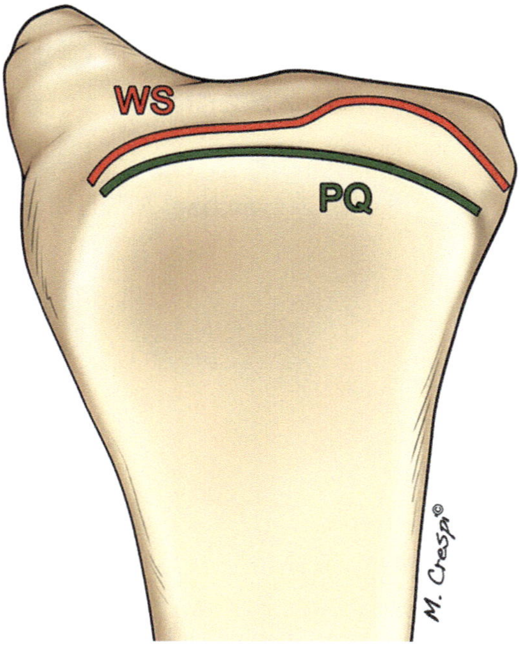

Fig. 34.2 The watershed line (*red*) lies distal to the insertion of pronator quadratus (*green*)

34.1 Introduction

Tendon complications of distal radial fractures have long been recognised, even before the recent marked increase in the use of internal fixation, especially with the vogue for fixed-angle volar implants. This chapter seeks to explore the variety of tendon complications seen with management of distal radial fractures and seeks to offer techniques to reduce the incidence following internal fixation.

34.2 Tendon Anatomy

- When considering internal fixation of distal radius fractures, it is important to appreciate the relationships between the bone contours and the tendon location for both dorsal and volar approaches.
- On the dorsum of the distal radius, the extensor tendons are closely apposed to the bone in separate anatomical compartments (Fig. 34.1). The floor of the compartments is very thin providing little protection from over-long volarly placed screws. The lack of space between the tendons and bones also makes placement of dorsal implants difficult while still protecting the tendons from abrasion on plates and screw heads.
- The pronator quadratus (PQ) muscle covers the volar aspect of the distal radius to near the so-called watershed line (Fig. 34.2). This protects the flexor tendons from over-long dorsal screws. As screw penetration distal to the watershed line usually results in joint penetration, the flexor tendons are usually protected from incorrectly placed dorsal implants. Distal to the watershed line, the flexor tendons come into close contact with the volar rim of the distal radius. Therefore placement of implants volarly distal to this line is likely to irritate or abrade the tendons especially as the distal edge of a distally placed plate projects anteriorly.

34.3 Tendon Complications After Nonoperative Management

- The most commonly affected tendon is the extensor pollicis longus (EPL). This is more frequent after undisplaced fractures of the

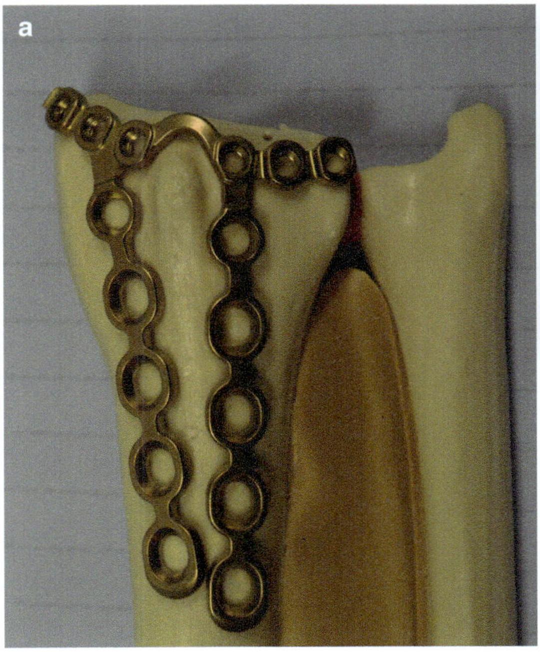

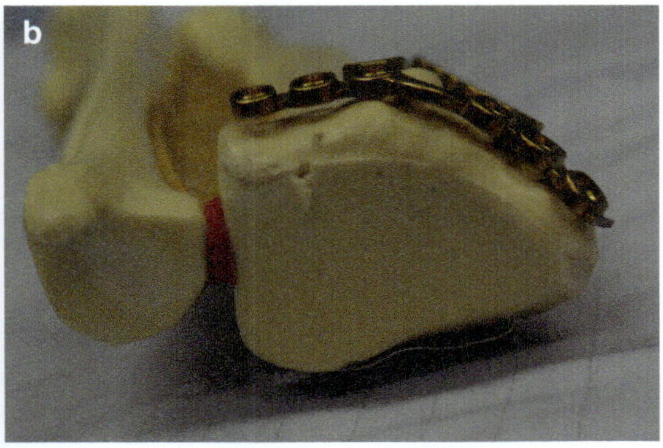

Fig. 34.3 (**a**, **b**) Pi plate has a distal juxta-articular band shaped to accommodate Lister's tubercle and two separate longitudinal proximal limbs. The screws were recessed into the plate and had cruciform heads to reduce the risk of irritation of the extensor tendons. Figures demonstrate positioning of the Pi plate on the distal radius

distal radius. EPL ruptures may be caused by a double insult of increased pressure within an intact tendon sheath resulting in reduced blood flow to an already poorly vascularised tendon lead to tendon rupture (Engkvist and Lundborg 1979). It typically presents at 2–3 weeks after the fracture.

- Extensor tendon entrapment at the fracture site occurs more frequently than flexor tendon entrapment. In volarly displace fractures, a visible gap after closed reduction should alert the surgeon to this possibility. This mainly involves EPL or extensor indicis proprius (EIP) tendons at surgery, with variable involvement of extensor digitorum communis (EDC) and extensor digiti minimi (EDM) (Okazaki et al. 2009). Tendons were then reduced via a dorsal approach and the fractures fixed (Okazaki et al. 2009).
- Flexor tendon entrapment is almost non-existent (Okazaki et al. 2009).

34.4 Tendon Complications After Dorsal Plate Fixation

- The Pi plate (Synthes, PA) was specifically developed to address the problems associated with the management of more complex distal radial fractures (Ring et al. 1997) (Fig. 34.3a, b). Initially produced in titanium, a stainless steel version was also available.
- In their initial series, some developed extensor tendon irritation, requiring removal of the hardware. In order to improve this, a subperiosteal dissection of the fourth compartment, and a suggested retinacular flap to protect the second compartment, was suggested.
- Subsequently there were increasing reports of cases of tendon irritation and even rupture caused by this plate (Chiang et al. 2002).
- Tendon complications, with both the Synthes Pi plate and a dorsal low-profile plate, seen both as extensor tenosynovitis having visible

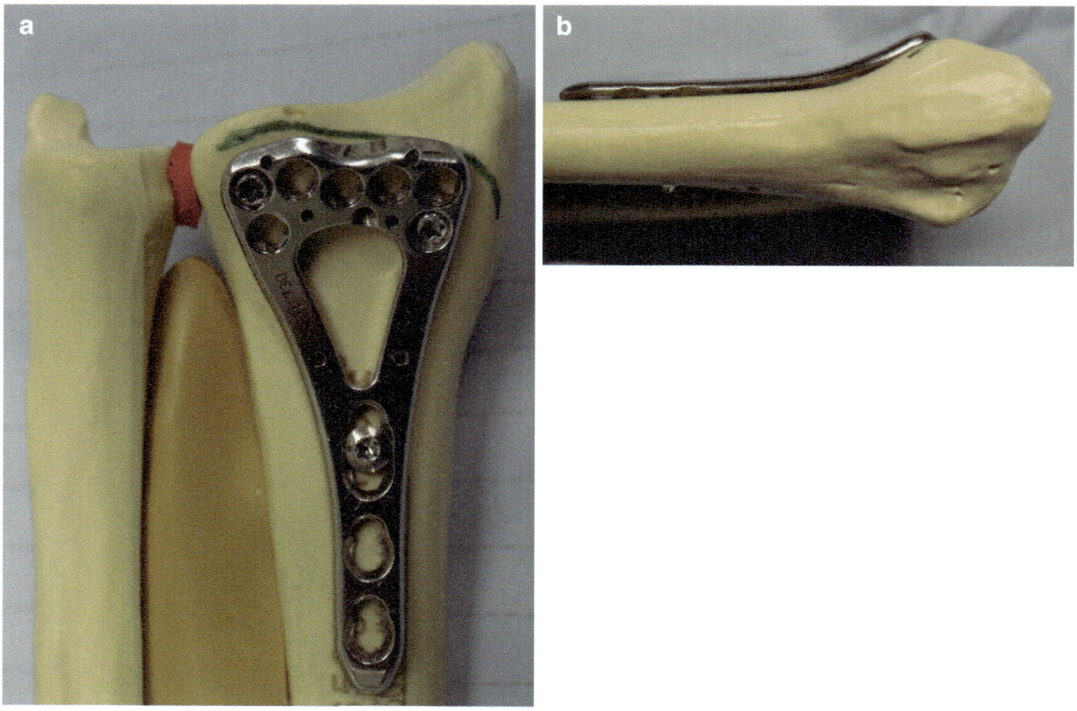

Fig. 34.4 (**a**, **b**) Variable angle LCP two-column volar distal radial plate (DePuy-Synthes). Demonstrates the various design features of the modern volar locking plates (*green line* represents watershed line)

attritional changes of the tendons and tendon ruptures, required plate removal and tendon reconstruction (Rozental et al. 2003).

- In spite of modification of the plate, there was no difference to the tendon complications, and this was an important reason for popularisation of volar-placed fixed-angle plates.

34.5 Paradigm Shift: Volar Plating for Dorsally Displaced Distal Radial Fractures

- Volar plating was popularised following development of the Distal Volar Radius (DVR) plate (DePuy, Warsaw, IN) in an attempt to avoid the high incidence of extensor tendon problems (Orbay et al. 2001).
- The approach released the PQ in an L-shaped fashion from the watershed line of the distal radius, lifting it as a flap to approach the volar fracture site. Reattachment of PQ was advocated to cover the plate to add a layer of protection to the flexor tendons.
- There are recurring themes in the design of the implants; fixed-angle locking screw technology is common to most, anatomic contouring of the plate allows distal placement up to the watershed line, and two rows of screws or pegs allow support of different areas of subchondral bone (Fig. 34.4).

34.6 Tendon Complications After Volar Plate Fixation

- The early use of the DVR plate had no reports of tendon complications (Orbay and Fernandez 2004), but other investigators were already reporting problems with tendons.
- An early report presented 1/3 of patients with tendon complications, most often ruptured flexor pollicis longus (FPL) tendons (Drobetz and Kutscha-Lissberg 2003).

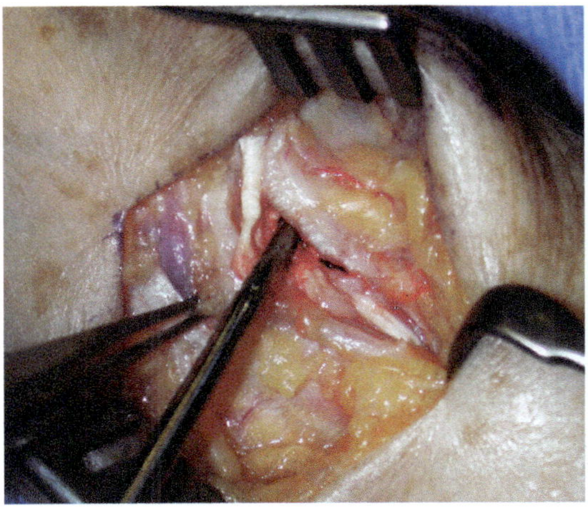

Fig. 34.5 Rupture of EPL tendon after volar fixation of distal radial fracture. An empty screw hole (with scissors in hole) was found at exploration

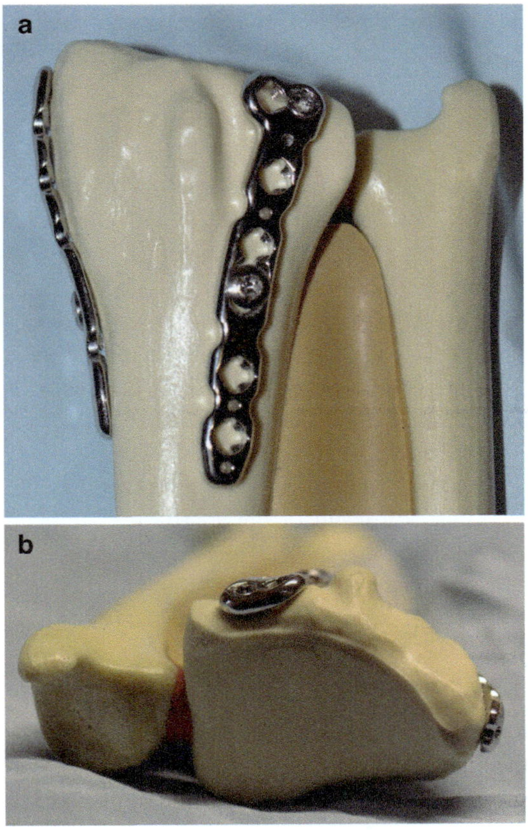

Fig. 34.6 (**a**, **b**) Modern dorsal locking plates. Note the rounded low-profile edges of the plates and anatomic contouring

- There have been further reports of ruptures of flexor tendons since this description (Adham et al. 2009; Casaletto et al. 2009), both with attrition and fraying of the flexor tendons. Ruptures are not always preceded by symptoms.
- "Technical issues" with the fixation is most often the cause (Casaletto et al. 2009), as either suboptimal positioning of the volar plate or prominent screw heads.
- Retention of the angled drill guides after use of the DVR plate can also result in flexor tendon injury.
- Design of the plate and its best fit upon the intact distal radius need to be appreciated by the surgeon as different plate manufacturers aim for different distal positions of the plate (Soong et al. 2011). Flexor tendon ruptures can be avoided by assessing the position of the distal part of the plate in relation to a radiographic "critical line", i.e. the most volar extent of the volar rim, where flexor tendon ruptures occurred in patients whose implants projected volar to the volar rim.
- Further studies imply that the FPL tendon is at risk of attrition rupture secondary to an incorrectly, distally placed volar locking plate (Tanaka et al. 2011).
- Volar plating techniques also cause extensor tendon ruptures, probably iatrogenic in nature given that incidence of extensor tendon rupture in nonoperatively managed fractures is far lower than in series with volar plate fixation (Al-Rashid et al. 2006). In fact, drilling for screw placement may cause direct or indirect tendon ruptures (Fig. 34.5) in addition to the more common cause by prominent over-long screws.
- In a meta-analysis of papers describing complications of distal radius fixation, it was suggested that tendon complications are just as common with volar as with dorsal fixation (Wei et al. 2013).
- Avoiding screw penetration of the dorsal cortex is vital in order to reduce the risk of extensor tendon rupture. However, recognition of perforation of the screw can be difficult, due to the contour of the dorsal distal radius. Overlapping of Lister's tubercle may obscure

a protruding screw on the standard radiographs obtained at the time of surgery, lulling the surgeon into a false sense of security.
- The skyline view technique (Riddick et al. 2012) is a simple new radiographic tangential view of dorsal distal radius, allowing visualisation of the EPL groove in order to avoid complications. When compared to lateral and oblique fluoroscopic views, the skyline technique demonstrated 83 % accuracy for detection of dorsal cortical penetration of the screw. Recognition of protruding screws at the time of fixation allows for timely replacement with more appropriately sized implants.
- Tendon complications from dorsal fixation occur as a result of the approach or implant loosening.
- Complications from volar fixation occur as a result of incorrect hardware placement and failure to be able to visualise prominent screws on the dorsum.

34.7 Assessment of Tendon Complications

- The best form of treatment is prevention using the techniques described earlier.
- If, following fixation, the patient complains of dorsal or volar wrist pain especially when moving the fingers, consider urgent plate removal or exploration. A high index of suspicion should be maintained for patients with pain on the side away from the fixation.
- If the fracture is not united, then CT scanning or ultrasound may give some information as to the fixation prominence or the tendons being irritated.
- If a patient presents with weakness or lack of extension or flexion of the fingers, then rupture is more likely than purely irritation. Urgent exploration may prevent further tendon ruptures that might make reconstruction difficult.
- If tendons have ruptured, then tendon transfer or grafts are usually necessary as the tendon is frequently abraded over a significant length and it is unlikely that primary repair will be possible.

34.8 Extensor Tendon Reconstruction

- EPL is the commonest tendon to be ruptured following operative or nonoperative treatment. Reconstruction using EIP, if intact, is the most effective treatment as it is the most synergistic muscle.
- With multiple ruptures of the EDC tendons, flexor carpi radialis is most synergistic, although will provide mass action. However there may be a problem with length to the most distal tendon ends, and proximal stumps might need to be used as grafts to extend the transfer.
- If EIP is ruptured and one other of the EDC (Extensor digitorum communis) tendons is also ruptured, consider side-to-side anastomosis with the adjacent finger tendon.
- Multiple tendon grafts are rarely used, as multiple grafts will often adhere to each other producing a mass action effect and often more stiffness.
- Rupture of one of the wrist extensors (Extensor carpi radialis brevis ECRB or longus ECRL) may not require treatment especially if the wrist clinically remains balanced. This may be particularly appropriate in the elderly patient.
- If both radial tendons (ECRB or ECRL) are ruptured, an interposition graft using part of the other radial extensor can be utilised. ECRB should probably be reconstructed in preference to ECRL due to its central position.
- Ulnar-sided extensor injuries are extremely rare in association with distal radius fractures as opposed to in rheumatoid arthritis. The same principles apply.

34.9 Flexor Tendon Reconstruction

- The commonest tendon to be affected is FPL. This should be reconstructed using an interposition graft such as palmaris longus (PL) or plantaris. Primary grafting is usually possible as the rupture is outside the fibrous flexor

Table 34.1 Tips and tricks to avoid tendon complications

Dorsal fixation (Fig. 34.6a, b)
Carefully preserve the fourth and second compartments by subperiosteal dissection during the approach
Contouring of the plate to accommodate the desired direction of the screw
Avoid intra-articular placement of screws
Avoid leaving prominent screw heads that are not seated properly into the screw holes
Consider a retinacular flap to reduce contact between the tendons and the plate
Volar fixation
Strive for accurate positioning of the plate in relation to the watershed line
Consider fixing the plate on the distal fragment first to avoid plate lift-off
Extreme care when drilling for screws to avoid penetration and iatrogenic injury to the extensor tendons
Locking screws do not need to perforate the dorsal cortex for fixation; use shorter rather than longer screws
Use smooth pegs to avoid the sharp tip of screws damaging extensor tendons
Obtain skyline view prior to acceptance of completed fixation to ensure no dorsal screw penetration
If possible, reconstruct pronator quadratus over the volar plate
Fixation in general
Use hardware specifically designed for the task
Do not use standard small fragment plates for fixation
Pain or crepitus sited around the metalwork should prompt its removal to avoid potential progression to tendon rupture

sheath. If grafting is not possible, or if the patient refuses, interphalangeal (IP) joint arthrodesis of the thumb can be considered.

- If multiple tendons are ruptured, then flexor digitorum profundus (FDP) is usually affected. This should, in general, be reconstructed using grafts or individual tendons buddied to adjacent intact ones, as the muscle is mass action anyway.
- Other options include distal interphalangeal joint arthrodesis of the affected finger if the flexor digitorum superficialis is intact.
- Rupture of all finger flexors or wrist flexors have not been described.

34.10 Summary

- Internal fixation of dorsally angulated distal radial fractures has become popularised in recent times.
- In order to avoid morbidity to tendons, meticulous surgical techniques should be employed, and follow-up of the patients in the clinic should be rigorous.
- Prodromal symptoms of tendon damage should prompt intervention to avoid the serious complications of tendon rupture, which frequently require tendon reconstruction (Table 34.1).

References

Adham MN, Porembski M, Adham C. Flexor tendon problems after volar plate fixation of distal radial fractures. Hand. 2009;4:406–9.

Al-Rashid M, Theivendran K, Craigen MAC. Delayed ruptures of the extensor tendon secondary to the use of volar locking compression plates for distal radial fractures. J Bone Joint Surg Br. 2006;88(12):1610–2.

Casaletto J, Machin D, Leung R, Brown DJ. Flexor pollicis longus tendon ruptures after palmar plate fixation of fractures of the distal radius. J Hand Surg Eur. 2009;34(4):471–4.

Chiang PP, Roach S, Baratz M. Failure of a retinacular flap to prevent dorsal wrist pain after titanium Pi plate fixation of distal radius fractures. J Hand Surg Am. 2002;27(4):724–8.

Drobetz H, Kutscha-Lissberg E. Osteosynthesis of distal radial fractures with a volar locking screw plate system. Int Orthop. 2003;27:1–6.

Engkvist O, Lundborg G. Rupture of the extensor pollicis longus tendon after fracture of the lower end of the radius – a clinical and microangiographic study. Hand. 1979;11(1):76–86.

Okazaki M, Tazaki K, Nakamura Y, Sato K. Tendon entrapment in distal radius fractures. J Hand Surg. 2009;34E(4):479–82.

Orbay JL, Fernandez DL. Volar fixed-angle plate fixation for unstable distal radius fractures in the elderly patient. J Hand Surg Am. 2004;29:96–102.
Orbay JL, Badia A, Indriago IR, et al. The extended flexor carpi radialis approach: a new perspective for the distal radius fracture. Tech Hand Up Extrem Surg. 2001;5(4):204–11.
Riddick AP, Hickey B, White SP. Accuracy of the skyline view for detecting dorsal cortical penetration during volar distal radius fixation. J Hand Surg Eur. 2012;37(5):407–11.
Ring D, Jupiter JB, Brennwald J, Büchler U, Hastings H. Prospective multicentre trial of a plate for dorsal fixation of distal radial fractures. J Hand Surg Am. 1997;22(5):777–84.
Rozental TD, Beredjiklian PK, Bozentka DJ. Functional outcome and complications following two types of dorsal plating for unstable fractures of the distal part of the radius. J Bone Joint Surg Am. 2003;85(10):1956–60.
Soong M, Earp BE, Bishop G, et al. Volar locking plate implant prominence and flexor tendon rupture. J Bone Joint Surg Am. 2011;93(4):328–35.
Tanaka Y, Aoki M, Izumi T, et al. Effect of distal radius volar plate position in contact pressure between the flexor pollicis longus tendon and the distal plate edge. J Hand Surg Am. 2011;36:1790–7.
Wei J, Tu-Bao Y, Luo W, et al. Complications following dorsal versus volar plate fixation of distal radius fracture: a meta-analysis. J Int Med Res. 2013;41(2):265–75.

Complex Regional Pain Syndrome 35

Niels H. Søe and Lene Buch

Contents

N.H. Søe, MD (✉)
Clinic for Hand Surgery, Gentofte Hospital, University of Copenhagen, Copenhagen, Denmark
e-mail: niels.soee.nielsen@regionh.dk

L. Buch, OT
Clinic for Hand Surgery, Gentofte University Hospital, Copenhagen, Denmark

35.1 Summary

Treatment of complex regional pain syndrome type 1 (CRPS) is still a subject to discussion.

The diagnosis of CRPS is difficult and should only be made when other causes for the symptoms of the patient have been excluded. The diagnosis is only clinical. It is a syndrome that usually develops after an initiating noxious event. The main symptoms are pain out of proportion, oedema, joint stiffness and vasomotor instability. The reported incidences of CRPS after distal radius fracture range widely in sources, everything from less than 2 % to up to 39 %. We have searched the literature (levels 1–3) for guidance to manage the disease and to prevent the occurrence of CRPS after wrist fracture. Vitamin C is recommended together with adequate perioperative analgesia, limitation of operative time and use of tourniquet. Anatomical reduction of the fracture and regional anaesthetic techniques are recommended.

35.2 Background

- After a radius fracture, complex regional pain syndrome (CRPS) may complicate recovery and increase the risk of poor outcome. CRPS has a strong negative impact on health-related quality of life and function (Gradl et al. 2003).
- CRPS is a complicated combination of pain, oedema, movement abnormalities including joint stiffness and vasomotor symptoms, such

L.M. Hove et al. (eds.), *Distal Radius Fractures*,
DOI 10.1007/978-3-642-54604-4_35, © Springer-Verlag Berlin Heidelberg 2014

as discoloration, changes in surface temperature and hair and nail growth in the affected area. Pain is the main problem and is generally out of proportion to the degree of injury.

- The syndrome has been given many names such as reflex sympathetic dystrophy, causalgia, Sudeck's atrophy, algodystrophy and shoulder-hand syndrome as examples.
- CRPS is divided into two different types – type 1 with no identifiable peripheral nerve injury (CRPS) and type 2 with a peripheral nerve injury.
- The exact pathophysiology of CRPS is unknown.
- CRPS is between two to four times more common in women, with a median age of onset between 40 and 53 years. Postmenopausal women appeared to have a higher risk of developing CPRS. The upper extremities are most frequently involved with fractures as the most common causative event. Often cast immobilization appears to be associated with CRPS, with increased pressure and early complaints of tightness as predictive risk factors.
- The exact incidence and prevalence of CRPS after radius fractures are unknown. The reported incidences of CRPS after distal radius fracture range widely in sources, everything from less than 2 % to up to 39 % (Stanton-Hicks et al. 1995; Veldman et al. 1993).
- Theories differ between sources, but compression of the median nerve, injury of median or ulnar nerves, over-distraction, instability of the distal radioulnar joint DRUJ and ulnar fracture may contribute to CPRS after distal radius fractures. Other sources find no evidence that degree of displacement or fracture type appears to make any difference nor do alterations in methods of treatment. New surgical procedures as internal fixation of distal radius fractures may change the risk of CRPS.
- All practitioners and surgeons treating patients with radius fractures should be aware of CRPS as the onset is variable and often delayed.
- To ensure the best possible functionality recovery and pain relief of CRPS, early recognition and management are key factors.

35.3 Classification

- Complex regional pain syndrome (CRPS) is a complicated combination of allodynia, oedema, decreased range of motion, weakness, trophic changes and vasomotor symptoms in an extremity, most often affecting the upper limb.
- The condition frequently appears after minor trauma, such as a distal radius fracture, immobilization, ischemia or nerve compression.
- Coexisting conditions, such as hyperlipidemia, diabetes mellitus, hemiplegia, migraine, osteoporosis and asthma, alcoholism and treatment with ACE inhibitors may increase the risk for CRPS (Goebel 2011).
- There is no evidence of a psychological comorbidity or heredity. The clinical findings are characterized by being disproportionate to the extent of the injury (Fig. 35.1).

35.4 Diagnosis

In 1994, the International Association for the Study of Pain (IASP) made a consensus for the diagnostic criteria of CRPS with the purpose to uniform the criteria and to meet research standards for the syndrome (Harden et al. 2010). The syndrome is now referred to as either type 1 or type 2, respectively. The clinical features of the two types are identical, except that type 2 represents a previous identified peripheral nerve injury and that the pain is usually limited to the distribution of one nerve. The physical appearance may vary from patient to patient, and it may also undergo changes in the same patient over time (Harden et al. 2010).

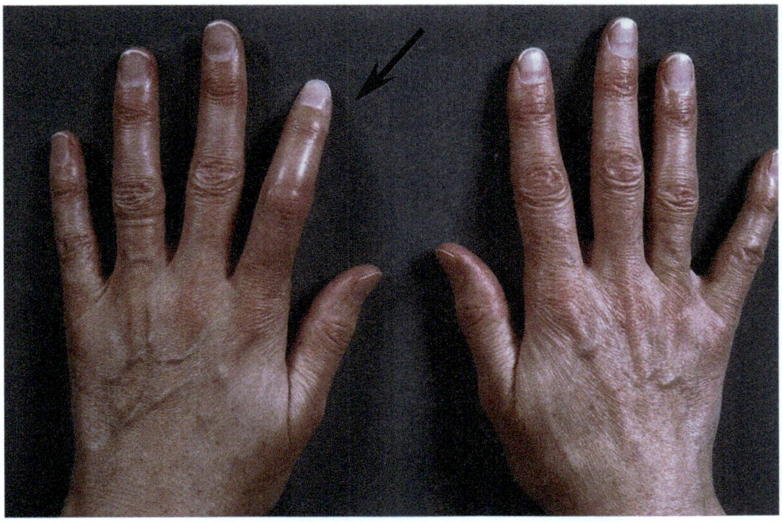

Fig. 35.1 Digital CRPS located to the left index finger

> The diagnosis of CRPS can be made, according to the current Budapest criteria, if the following criteria are fulfilled:
>
> A. Continuing pain, which is disproportionate to any inciting event.
> B. Sensory, vasomotor, oedema or trophic changes, where at least one symptom of these four should be found.
> C. At least one sign at the time of evaluation in two or more of the following categories – sensory, vasomotor, oedema or trophic changes.
> D. There are no other diagnoses that better explain the signs and symptoms.

Because of a low specificity (0.41) of the IASP criteria, the guidelines were further modified in Budapest, in 2003. The Budapest criteria retained the sensitivity of the IASP criteria (0.99) but improved upon the specificity to 0.68. Some research criteria were further modified, resulting in a specificity of 0.79.

Until recently, CRPS progress was considered divided into three stages, each characterized by different symptoms. This division is no longer used as CRPS develops very individually.

The terms warm CRPS and cold CRPS are also being used. Normally, the first symptoms appear within the first month – but sometimes as early as 2 weeks after an injury, with a burning pain, oedema as well as warmth and redness. This is called the warm CRPS. Later may follow joint stiffness and contracture, the cool atrophic limb – called the cold CRPS.

35.5 Epidemiology

Since CRPS is a multifactorial syndrome with many overlying symptoms, there is some uncertainty of the scientific data available.

- The prevalence is estimated to <2–10 %, while the incidence is calculated to 0.8–6.2 per 100,000.
- The female-to-male ratio is 2–4:1, and the upper extremity is most often involved.

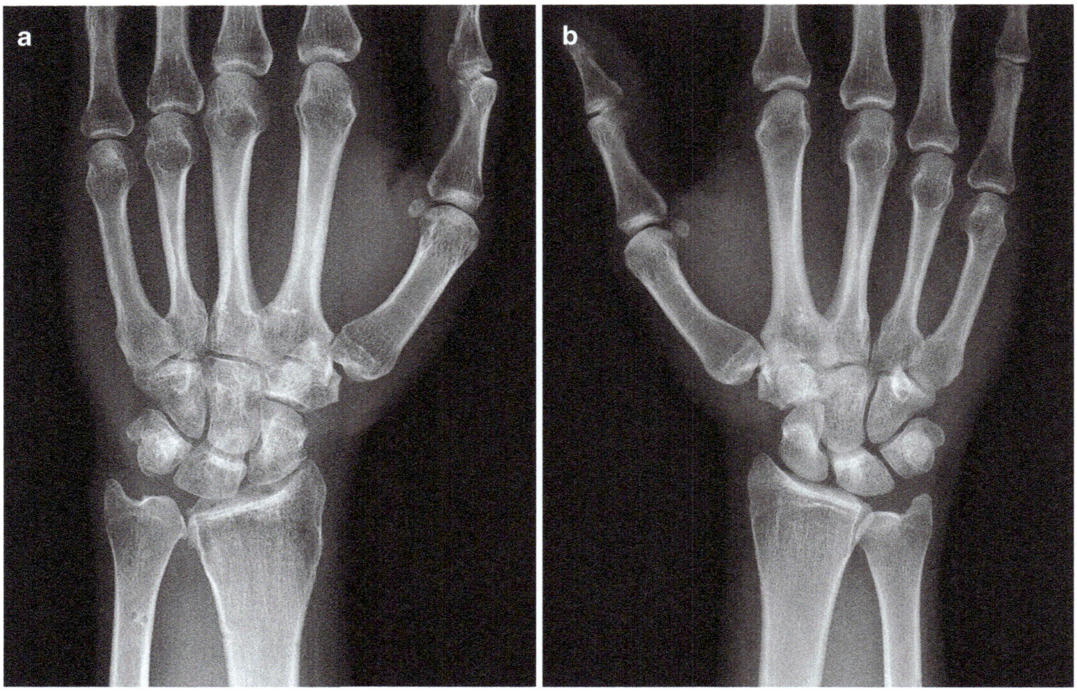

Fig. 35.2 X-ray from a patient with CRPS. (**a**) Halisteresis with decalcification of the wrist. (**b**) The normal wrist of the opposite hand

- Few studies report of the prevalence in children, but the syndrome is believed to be rare in children (De Mos et al. 2007).
- In general, the prognosis seems to be poor, since even 6 years after onset of the syndrome, only 30 % of patients consider themselves completely recovered. Several patients never return to work.
- Treatment is difficult to evaluate since currently a definition of the recovery from CRPS does not exist.

35.6 Diagnostics

It is important to remember that there is no single test, which is validated for the diagnosis of CRPS. There are, however, tools that help practitioners to document their clinical findings of autonomic, sensory and motor function and their dysfunction. Here, we describe various tests that may be useful and their relation to CRPS.

- *Plain radiographs (X-ray)*
  During the first stage of CRPS (0–3 months), the plain radiograph of the extremity usually looks normal, while in later stages (3–12 months) osteopenia appears. According to a German study, specificity is high for plain radiography that facilitates the diagnosis as soon as any changes in the bone develop (De Mos et al. 2007) (Fig. 35.2).
- *Bone scans*
  Bone scanning, used for CRPS, can only detect changes that occur during the first year. The three-phase bone scan, which uses immediate and delayed images to study blood flow, is especially useful to diagnose CRPS, showing increased periarticular uptake around most joint in the hand. Bone density tests have a low specificity and sensitivity for the diagnosis of CRPS (Malis-Gagnon 2005).
- *Magnetic resonance imaging (MRI) and positron emission tomography (PET scans)*

MRI and PET scans that measure the biological activity throughout the body are non-invasive and can be used, but both techniques have a low specificity and a medium sensitivity.

- *Measurement of skin temperature*
  Infrared thermometry/thermography measures differences in skin temperature and blood flow. Any changes are controlled by the sympathetic nervous system. This testing is sensitive to skin temperature changes to one-tenth of one degree centigrade

35.7 Treatment

Several treatments have been described in the literature, but only few methods have been efficient on an evidence-based evaluation. There is a general agreement that multidisciplinary treatment is the most effective way to reduce or, if possible, remove complaints regarding CRPS. Perez et al. have gathered information regarding the treatment in a large review article containing the results of over 150 studies on this topic.

35.8 Occupational Therapy

The treatment of CRPS requires interdisciplinary management. Occupational therapy is essential in treatment of CRPS in patients with radius fractures. Unfortunately, the scientific evidence on the therapy on this area is lacking, and there is no precise recipe for treating CRPS. The occupational therapist must use an in-depth and ongoing knowledge concerning pain, CRPS and rehabilitation of radius fracture to develop an appropriate treatment. The problem-solving should be based on the patient's pain and presenting signs and symptoms. Treatment must be carefully balanced; otherwise, the therapist may cause worsening rather than an improvement of CRPS symptoms. If the treatment is too aggressive, the pain or oedema will increase. Inactivity can further more impact the condition in a negative direction. It is important that the patient becomes an active participant, who is willing and able to participate and take control as well as responsibility in his or her treatment.

The therapy should include education to assist the patient in understanding correlations including what may provoke and relieve pain. It is also important for the patient to understand that moderation is the key, as both too much exercise and too little activity will result in a worsening of the condition. The structure of the patients' daily life and activities of daily living (ADL) may have influence on pains. The patients should know that there may be periods with slow or no progress. The occupational therapist should guide the patient through a programme designed to minimize CRPS symptoms while maximizing functional use of the extremity. In the early stages, the treatment of pain and oedema should be of the top priorities. Also a focus on assisting the patient in increasing his or her ability to perform daily activities should be a high priority. The second priority is to improve the patient's range of motion in the hand and also in the elbow and shoulder if the ranges of motion in these joints are limited. The range of motion exercises should be gentle and must not increase the pain. Treatment on joint stiffness is first approached through an active range of motion programme for the entire upper extremity. Passive range of motion exercises and continuous passive motion on the wrist can be started, when the radius fracture is healed, if the exercises can be done without increasing pain and other CRPS symptoms.

In summary, the occupational therapy should include a thorough assessment of symptoms, the active and passive range of motion, movement disorders, pain patterns during activities and general CRPS impact on daily routines and activities. This assessment should be the base for the occupational therapy intervention, which may include education, oedema control, pain management including desensitization, mirror visual feedback, exercises with active range of motion, activities of daily living (ADL), exercises with gentle passive range of motion and continuous passive motion and splinting.

- *Oedema-control*
  Treatment of oedema includes elevation, compression, massage and active exercise.
- *Mirror visual feedback/Mirror therapy*
  By mirror therapy, a mirror is placed with the mirrored side towards the healthy hand, while the afflicted hand is hiding behind the mirror. The patient is not allowed to see the afflicted hand, but most keep attention to the mirror image of the healthy hand while exercising the healthy hand. This can provide pain relief, as the brain is tricked into believing that the afflicted hand is moved freely and without pain.
- *Desensitization*
  Desensitization is a process of adjusting the hand to an increasing level of stimulation. It can be accomplished by stimulating the affected area with texture of different roughness. From soft, begin rubbing the affected area with softer tissue, like silk, and then increase the roughness of the material – from silk, to cotton, to towel. Another option is to immerse the hand in a material like sand, rice, etc. Massage may also be a part of the desensitization programme. Desensitization is targeted to normalize sensation through stimulus to the affected area for shorter periods of time frequently throughout the day. It is the intention to affect the brain with sensory input and then to acclimate it to the sensation, with a gradually decreased response to the pain to those particular stimuli.

Early recognition is essential to relieving most CRPS symptoms. An occupational therapist rehabilitates many patients with radius fracture, and the occupational therapist has the opportunity to recognize the symptomatology early. Early treatment of these symptoms increases the chance of resolving them and preventing a downward spiral (Veizi et al. 2012; Harden and Swan 2006; Hove 1995; Field 2013).

35.9 Regionally Applied Drugs

- *Spinal cord stimulation (SCS) and percutaneous sympathetic block (PSB)*
  Spinal cord stimulation (SCS) consists of implantation of stimulating electrodes in the epidural space; an electrical pulse generator, which is implanted in the lower abdominal area or in the gluteal region; conducting wires connecting the electrodes to the generator; and a generator remote control. This can result in a significant decrease in pain and increase in quality of life, but no improvement in function of the affected limb is observed (Perez et al. 2010).
- *Intravenous sympathetic block*
  Ketanserine, administered intravenously in doses of 10–20 mg, has a slight effect on the reduction of pain among patients with type 1 CRPS. However, treatment with guanethidine or lidocaine has no pain-reducing effect in patients with type 1 CRPS (Perez et al. 2010).
- *Percutaneous sympathetic block (PSB)*
  Treatment with percutaneous sympathetic block (PSB) has no effect on patients with type 1 CRPS. One study, with a total of 1,144 patients included, showed a temporary effect in pain reduction in less than a third of the patients, and the results were considered to be caused by a placebo effect (Perez et al. 2010).

35.10 Systemically Administrated Drugs

- *Vitamin C*
  Prophylactic treatment with vitamin C may reduce the development of type 1 CRPS in patients with a distal radius fracture (Perez et al. 2010).
- *Corticosteroids*
  Several trials have shown a beneficial effect by using corticosteroids in the treatment of type 1 CRPS, but the evidence level is considered to be low. A Danish study, including 23 patients, demonstrated a pronounced effect in

pain reduction (Field 2013). However, dosage and duration of the treatment with the drug are still uncertain (Hove 1995; Harden and Swan 2006; Perez et al. 2010).

- *N-acetylcysteine*
  Treatment with *N*-acetylcysteine is effective in oral doses of 600 mg three times a day for 2 months.
- *Bisphosphonates*
  Treatment with bisphosphonates does have a beneficial effect on signs of inflammation, such as tenderness, swelling and increased temperature of the affected limb in patients with CRPS 1. The optimal dosage, the frequency and the duration of treatment are yet to be explored. It is recommended to administer 40 mg orally per day (Perez et al. 2010).
- *Paracetamol, NSAIDs and opioids*
  Treatment with paracetamol and NSAIDs has a pain-relieving effect and should be used as a supplement to other treatments (Hove 1995).
- *Others*
  Calcium channel blockers, oral muscle relaxants (OMR) and anticonvulsants have insufficient evidence of use in patients with CRPS. Treatment with calcium channel blockers may have some effect on type 1 CRPS in the acute phase, but the specific effect is not described or defined (Perez et al. 2010).
  Gabapentin has only a limited effect on other symptoms, such as allodynia and hyperaesthesia (Perez et al. 2010). Carbamazepine, pregabalin and phenytoin have not been proven to reduce symptoms of CRPS.
  Intraoperative IVRA with clonidine on patients with a history of CRPS can significantly reduce the recurrence rate (Reuben et al. 2004).

References

De Mos M, de Bruijn AG, Huygen FJ, Dieleman JP, Stricker BH, Sturkenboom MC. The incidence of complex regional pain syndrome: a population-based study. Pain. 2007;129(1–2):12–20.

Field J. Complex Regional Pain Syndrome: a review. J Hand Surg Eur. 2013;38(4):330–4.

Goebel A. Complex regional pain syndrome in adults. Rheumatology. 2011;50(10):1739–50.

Gradl G, Steinborn M, Wizgall I, Mittlmeier T, Schurmann M. Acute CRPS I (morbus sudeck) following distal radial fractures–methods for early diagnosis. Zentralbl Chir. 2003;128(12):1020–6.

Harden RN, Swan M. King Amie, Costa B, Barthel J. Treatment of Complex Regional Pain Syndrome, Functional Restoration. Clin J Pain. 2006;22(5):420–4.

Harden RN, Bruehl S, Perez RS, Birklein F, Marinus J, Maihofner C, et al. Validation of proposed diagnostic criteria (the "Budapest Criteria") for Complex Regional Pain Syndrome. Pain. 2010;150(2):268–74.

Hove LM. Nerve entrapment and reflex sympathetic dystrophy after treatment of distal radius fracture. Scand J Plast Reconstr Surg Hand Surg. 1995;29:53–8.

Malis-Gagnon A. How are bone scans used in the diagnosis and treatment of CRPS? Reflex Sympathetic Dystrophy Assoc. 2005;18(2):11.

Perez RS, Zollinger PE, Dijkstra PU, Thomassen-Hilgersom IL, Zuurmond WW, Rosenbrand KCJ, Geertzen JH. Evidence based guidelines for complex regional pain syndrome type 1. BMC Neurol. 2010;10:20.

Reuben SS, Rosenthal EA, Steinberg RB, Faruqi S, Kilaru PA. Surgery on the affected upper extremity. Patients with a history of complex regional pain syndrome: the use of intravenous regional anesthesia with clonidine. J Clin Anesth. 2004;16:517–22.

Stanton-Hicks M, Janig W, Hassenbusch S, Haddox JD, Boas R, Wilson P. Reflex sympathetic dystrophy: changing concepts and taxonomy. Pain. 1995;63:127–33.

Veizi E, Chelimsky TC, Janata JW. Chronic Regional Pain Syndrome: What Specialized Rehabilitation Service Do Patients Require? Curr Pain Headache Rep. 2012;16:139–46.

Veldman PHJM, Reynan HM, Arntz IE, Goris RJA. Signs and symptoms of reflex sympathetic dystrophy. Prospective study of 829 patients. Lancet. 1993; 342:1012–6.

Compartment Syndrome of the Forearm

36

Leiv M. Hove and Christina Brudvik

Contents

L.M. Hove, MD, PhD (✉)
Department of Orthopaedic Surgery,
Haukeland University Hospital,
N-5021 Bergen, Norway

Department of Surgical Sciences,
University of Bergen, Bergen, Norway
e-mail: leiv.hove@k1.uib.no

C. Brudvik, MD, PhD
Department of Surgical Sciences, University of Bergen,
Bergen, Norway

Accident and Emergency Department,
Bergen, Norway

36.1 Summary

Compartment syndrome is a group of symptoms associated with elevated interstitial tissue pressure within a limited space of fascial compartments. The forearm is divided into two main compartments, the dorsal and the volar compartments. Further, the dorsal compartment can be subdivided into the extensor compartment and the mobile wad compartment, and the volar compartment into the superficial and the deep components. Unlike the fascial compartments of the leg, the forearm compartments are interconnected. These interconnections are of importance in that a release of the volar compartment alone may sufficiently decompress the dorsal compartment.

Fortunately, compartment syndrome is a rare complication after distal radius fractures and occurs in less than 1 % of the cases. The diagnosis of compartment syndrome is primarily a clinical one, based on symptoms of muscle and nerve ischemia. Persistent, increasing pain, usually out of proportion to that expected from the injury, is the most important finding. A tense, swollen and tender compartment is present. The most typical sign is increasing pain with passive stretch of the muscles within the compartment: Thus move the patients wrist and fingers!

Sensory disturbances in the nerve distribution are intermediate findings. Motor paralysis and pulselessness are late findings. The diagnosis may be verified by intra-compartmental pressure measurements. If this pressure is

L.M. Hove et al. (eds.), *Distal Radius Fractures*,
DOI 10.1007/978-3-642-54604-4_36, © Springer-Verlag Berlin Heidelberg 2014

above 30–45 mmHg and concomitant clinical findings are present, fasciotomy should be performed. Start the incision distally like in an ordinary carpal tunnel decompression procedure. Release the skin, volar fascia and transverse carpal ligament. Continue the incision proximally and over the most prominent forearm muscles, forming a lazy-S, up to the antecubital fossa.

36.2 Definition

Compartment syndrome is a group of clinical signs and symptoms associated with elevated interstitial tissue pressure within a rigid, limited space of fascial compartments (Matsen 1975; Naido and Heppenstall 1994; Botte 1998).

36.3 Anatomy

The forearm is divided into two main fascial compartments:

- The *dorsal compartment*, which is subdivided into the extensor compartment (extensor muscles) and the "mobile wad of three" (the brachioradialis, extensor carpi radialis longus and extensor carpi radialis brevis).
- The *volar compartment*, which is subdivided into the superficial components (the flexor carpi ulnaris, palmaris longus, pronator teres and flexor carpi radialis) and the deep components (the flexor digitorum superficialis and profundus, and the flexor pollicis longus) (Fig. 36.1).
- The forearm compartments are interconnected, unlike the fascial compartments of the leg. These interconnections are of importance in that a release of the volar compartment alone may sufficiently decompress the dorsal compartment (Gelberman et al. 1981).

36.4 Aetiology

Acute compartment syndrome in the forearm is usually secondary to high-energy trauma.

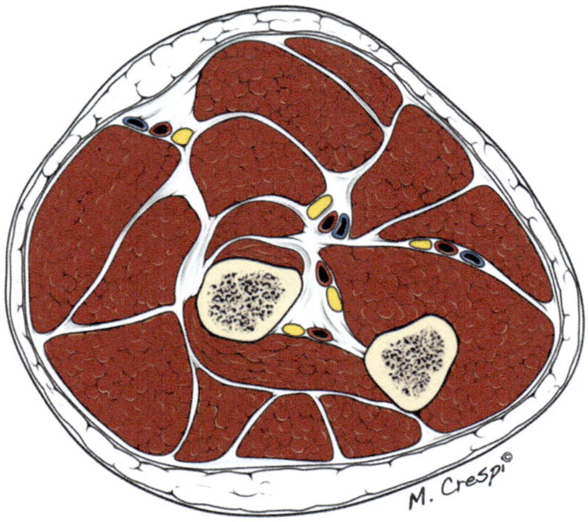

Fig. 36.1 Cross section of the forearm showing the different muscles

- Forearm fractures located in the proximal one third of the forearm is a high-risk group (Broström et al. 1990; Gulgonen and Ozer 2011; Styf 2003).
- Compartment syndrome is a rare complication (<1 %) after distal radius fractures.
- Patients younger than 50 years with comminute and displaced fractures of the distal radius may be at risk (Stockley et al. 1988; Soong et al. 2011).

In an eight-year series of 164 patients with acute compartment syndrome (McQueen et al. 2000), 29 patients (18 %) had concomitant fractures of the distal radius or the forearm. In a personal four-year series, nine of 17 patients with compartment syndrome of the forearm had fractures of the forearm or distal radius (Hove et al. 2004).

36.5 Pathogenesis

Increased pressure within a compartment decreases the blood supply to the soft tissues, resulting in tissue hypoxia and damage. The blood flow is determined by several factors, including arterial pressure, venous pressure, resistance within the vessel and local tissue pressure. Increased capillary permeability results from muscle ischaemia and leads to intramuscular oedema which again leads to increased tissue pressure and decreases blood flow and oxygen transport, causing even more tissue damage. This vicious cycle escalate the development of the compartment syndrome.

- Conditions that decrease compartment volume, i.e. tight casts or dressings, application of traction and increased external pressure on forearm from prolonged weight, are associated with compartment syndrome.
- Conditions that increase compartment contents, i.e. bleeding from arterial or venous injury, anticoagulation or trauma, oedema, injection of infusions and infections, are risk factors for the development of compartment syndrome.

36.6 Natural History

Functional changes from hypoxic cell damage occur in muscles after 2–4 h of total ischemia. Hypoxia to nerves causes hypoesthesia within 30 min of ischemia. However, irreversible nerve damage may not occur until 12 h or more of total ischaemia (Szabo and Gelberman 1984; Jones et al. 2011).

36.7 Diagnosis

The diagnosis of compartment syndrome is primarily a clinical one, based on symptoms of muscle and nerve ischemia. The classic signs are pain, pallor, paralysis and pulselessness, although all of these are not always present.

- Disproportionate pain relative to the physical findings is the most important sign.
- A tense, swollen and tender compartment is present.
- Pain with passive stretch of the muscles within the compartment: *Move the patient's wrist and fingers*!!
- Sensory disturbances in the nerve distribution are intermediate findings. This can be accompanied by motor weakness.
- Motor paralysis is a later finding.
- Pallor and pulselessness are late findings.

Intra-compartmental pressure measurements in the forearm are measured in the volar muscle wad and in the dorsal compartment.

There is no absolute level of compartment pressure that warrants fasciotomy. However, if the pressure is above 30–45 mmHg (or above the diastolic pressure minus 30 mmHg) and concomitant clinical findings are present, a fasciotomy should be performed.

Anyway, the clinical examination is the cornerstone to the diagnosis. If a compartment pressure measurement is not available, an immediate fasciotomy should still be performed based on the signs of disproportionate pain, a tense compartment and pain with passive stretching of wrist and fingers.

36.8 Fasciotomy of the Forearm

Several different *volar* incisions have been recommended. A practical technique is to make a single, curvilinear incision from the carpal tunnel to the antecubital fossa (Friedrich and Shin 2007; Styf 2003).

- Start the incision distally as in an ordinary carpal tunnel decompression. Release the skin, volar fascia and transverse carpal ligament. Continue the incision proximally and over the most prominent forearm muscles, forming a lazy-S (Fig. 36.2).
- Release the fascia covering the superficial and deep compartment as well as the mobile wad compartment, through this incision.
- In the forearm, a release of the volar compartment and the mobile wad compartment may decrease the pressure in the dorsal (extensor) compartment (Fig. 36.3).
- After the volar fasciotomy, the pressure in the dorsal compartment is remeasured if it was elevated initially. If the pressure remains elevated or the compartment remains tight, a dorsal fasciotomy is performed. A dorsal fasciotomy almost always lowers the pressure to normal in the mobile wad compartment (Gelberman et al. 1981).
- Make a longitudinal *dorsal* incision, starting just ulnar to Lister's tubercle, and extend it proximally toward the lateral epicondyle. Release the fascia over the extensor compartment. A straight linear scar on the dorsum of the forearm will not cause a contracture

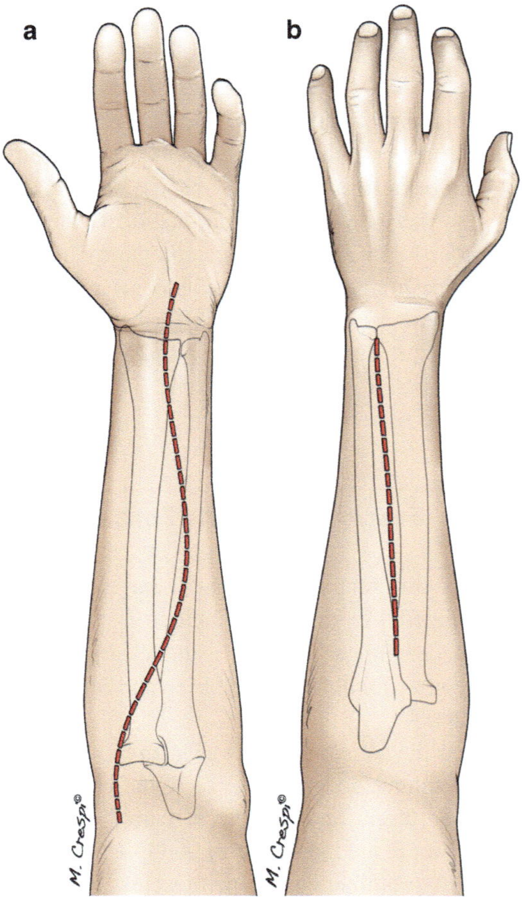

Fig. 36.2 (a) Volar incision for decompression of the volar compartment. (b) Dorsal incision for decompression of the dorsal compartment

problem and is preferred because fewer veins will be damaged than with a curving incision.
- The skin edges may be gradually approximated with the vessel loop-stapling technique.

36.9 Postoperative Care

The first postoperative day, an inspection, looking for devitalized tissue, is performed.
- Gradually, the approximation of the skin edges (but not the fascia!!) may start.
- The vessel loop-stapling technique is used in this delayed primary closure of the entire incision.
- If significant soft tissue has been lost with exposed tendons, nerves or bone, flap coverage is planned.
- Split-skin grafting is performed to cover possible remaining defects.
- The extremity is elevated, and active range of motion of the hand, wrist and elbow should be initiated as soon as possible.

36.10 Outcome

In general, patients with prompt diagnosis and treatment have favourable outcomes.

Patients with severe initial injuries, delayed treatment or extensive tissue necrosis have a more uncertain prognosis for functional recovery.

In our personal series, the time from initial symptoms of compartment syndrome to fasciotomy varied from 3 to 24 h. The postoperative DASH scores varied from 1 to 31 and correlated with the time delay before treatment.

36.11 Complications

Volkmann's ischemic contracture is the results of untreated acute compartment syndrome.

Necrosis and fibrosis of the muscle occur, with a resultant claw hand deformity.

36.12 Pearls and Pitfalls

Early symptoms:
- Disproportionate pain relative to the physical findings
- A tense, swollen and tender compartment
- Pain with passive stretching of the muscles within the compartment: Move the patient's wrist and fingers!

Intermediate symptoms:
- Sensory disturbances in the nerve distribution area
- This can be accompanied by motor weakness.

Later findings:
- Motor paralysis

Late findings:
- Pallor and pulselessness

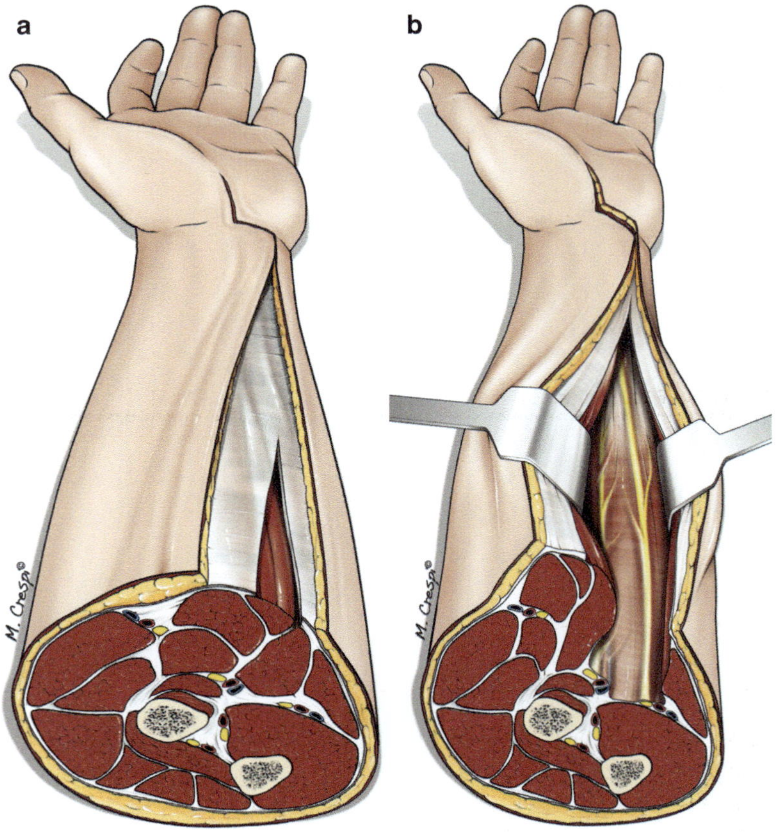

Fig. 36.3 (**a**) Opening of the volar fascia. (**b**) Decompression of the volar compartment, the superficial and deep portion and the mobile wad through the same incision

References

Botte MJ. Compartment syndrome and Volkmann's ischemic contracture. Hand Clin. 1998;14:331–510.

Broström LA, Stark A, Svartengren G. Acute compartment syndrome in forearm fractures. Acta Orthop Scand. 1990;61:50.

Friedrich JB, Shin AY. Management of forearm compartment syndrome. Hand Clin. 2007;23:245–64.

Gelberman RH, Garfin SR, Hergerroeder PT, et al. Compartment syndromes of the forearm: diagnosis and treatment. Clin Orthop. 1981;161:252–61.

Gulgonen A, Ozer K. Compartment syndrome. In: Wolfe H, Pederson K, editors. Green's operative hand surgery. Philadelphia: Elsevier Churchill Livingstone; 2011. p. 1929–48.

Hove LM, Krukhaug Y, Schrama J. Compartment syndrome of the forearm. Proceedings of the Norwegian Hand Society 2004; 225.

Jones MD, Santamarina R, Warhold LG. Surgical decompression of the forearm, hand, and digits for compartment syndrome. In: Wiesel SW et al., editors. Operative techniques in orthopaedic surgery. Philadelphia: Lippincott Williams Wilkins; 2011. p. 2875–81.

Matsen FA. Compartment syndrome: a unified concept. Clin Orthop. 1975;68:1103–8.

McQueen MM, Gaston P, Court-Brown CM. Acute compartment syndrome: who is at risk? J Bone Joint Surg. 2000;82B:200–3.

Naidu SH, Heppenstall RB. Compartment syndrome of the forearm and hand. Hand Clin. 1994;10:13–27.

Soong M, var Leerdam R, Guitton TG, et al. Fracture of the distal radius: risk factors for complications after locked volar plate fixation. J Hand Surg. 2011;36A: 3–9.

Stockley I, Harvey IA, Getty CJ. Acute volar compartment syndrome of the forearm secondary to the fractures of the distal radius. Injury. 1988;19:101.

Styf J. Kompartment syndrom. Lund: Studentlitteratur; 2003. p. 1–187.

Szabo RM, Gelberman RH. Peripheral nerve compression – etiology, critical pressure threshold and clinical assessment. Orthopedics. 1984;7:1461.

37 Extra-articular Malunion of the Radius; Osteotomy of the Radius

Leiv M. Hove

Contents

L.M. Hove, MD, PhD
Department of Orthopaedic Surgery, Haukeland University Hospital, Bergen N-5021, Norway

Department of Surgical Sciences, University of Bergen, Bergen, Norway
e-mail: leiv.hove@k1.uib.no

37.1 Summary

The most common radial deformity includes loss of palmar tilt, loss of inclination, loss of radial length, and a supination deformity of the distal fragment relative to the proximal diaphysis. In addition, the distal fragment may be displaced in a radial or ulnar translation and in a dorsal or palmar shift.

Operative treatment is appropriate when the radiographic deformity correlates with a specific and anatomically correctable problem and if the deformity is associated with a substantial risk of dysfunction.

The indication for operative correction is based on the combined appreciation of functional wrist impairment, the severity of pain, the grip strength, the degree of cosmetic deformity, and the radiographic findings.

The planning of angular, rotational, and length corrections are based on preoperative radiographs of both wrists.

Because radial shortening is a constant component of the deformity in both dorsal and volar malunion, an opening wedge osteotomy is recommended. This osteotomy should be transverse in the frontal plane and oblique (i.e. parallel to the joint surface) in the sagittal plane.

In nascent malunion the intention is to "take down" the maturing callus and the "osteotomy" is performed at the site of the original fracture. After removing the callus, the fracture site is exposed, and the "osteotomy" may be performed with the knife or a small chisel into the fracture line.

L.M. Hove et al. (eds.), *Distal Radius Fractures*,
DOI 10.1007/978-3-642-54604-4_37, © Springer-Verlag Berlin Heidelberg 2014

37.2 Introduction

Impaired function and pain after extra-articular malunion of distal radius fractures may be caused by derangements of the radiocarpal, ulnocarpal, and radioulnar joints.

- Mal-alignment does not always result in dysfunction. In particular, the vast majority of older and physically low-demanding patients may function well with a wrist deformity.
- In younger and active patients, especially in those who engage in heavy manual work or who require a normal range of motion of the wrist, the deformity may become symptomatic shortly after healing of the fracture (Fernandez 1993; Ekenstam et al. 1985; Amadio and Botte 1987; Posner and Ambrose 1991).

37.3 Definition

In this setting, malunion of the radius is defined as mal-alignment associated with dysfunction (Ring et al. 2011).

37.4 Anatomical Variables

The normal anatomical variables of the distal radius have been described in Chap. 9.

- A mal-united extra-articular fracture is most often a complex deformity in more than one plane.
- Radiographic comparison with the uninjured wrist is useful and serves as a template for operative correction.
- The most common radial deformity includes loss of palmar tilt, loss of inclination, loss of length, and a supination deformity of the distal fragment (Fig. 37.1a, b).
- In addition, the distal fragment may be displaced in a radial or ulnar translation or in a dorsal or palmar shift (Fernandez et al. 2002).

37.5 Preoperative Evaluation

In a large number of clinical studies, it has been observed that in young and active patients, there is a correlation between the quality of the anatomic result and the overall wrist function (Aro and Koivunen 1991; McQueen and Caspers 1988; Flinkkila et al. 2000).

Restoration of the anatomical variables may improve the biomechanics of the wrist, resulting in improved grip strength, improved movements of the wrist and forearm, and reduced pain (Fernandez 1982, 1993; Krukhaug and Hove 2007)

- The indication for operative treatment is based on the combined appreciation of the loss of

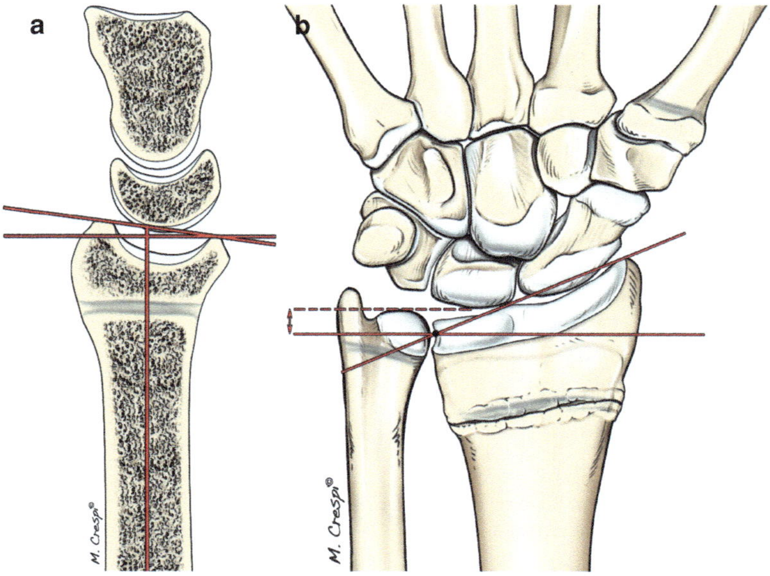

Fig. 37.1 (**a**) How to measure the palmar tilt. (**b**) How to measure the radial inclination and ulnar variance

wrist function, the severity of pain, the grip strength, the degree of cosmetic deformity, and the radiographic findings.

- Operative treatment is appropriate when a radiographic deformity correlates with a specific anatomically correctable problem, and the deformity is associated with a substantial risk of dysfunction.
- From a radiographic point of view, there are no fixed parameters to determine the surgical indication for correction.
- The functional problems are more important and include painful or limited movement of the wrist and limited rotation of the forearm.
- Lack of motion should be clearly due to mal-alignment and not due to pain, capsular contracture, or instability of the distal radioulnar joint (DRUJ).
- Loss of grip strength may be an additional indication for osteotomy. Grip strength can be an indicator of wrist dysfunction, but loss of strength is largely determined by pain.
- Pain should be very discrete and specific, such as the discomfort associated with a substantial ulnocarpal impingement. Diffuse or disproportionate pain should not be treated with osteotomy (Ring et al. 2011).
- Any signs and symptoms of complex regional pain syndrome is a relative contraindication for corrective osteotomy.

37.6 Preoperative Planning

The goals of radial osteotomy are to restore function and improve the appearance of the wrist by correcting the deformity at the level of the old fracture site.

The osteotomy should accomplish the reorientation of the joint surface to guarantee normal load distribution, reestablish the mechanical balance of the midcarpal joint, and restore the anatomic relationship of the distal radioulnar joint (DRUJ) (Fernandez 1993; Fernandez et al. 2002).

The operative approach may be either dorsal or volar or combined, depending on the deformity and the chosen surgical technique (Shea et al. 1997).

- The osteotomy permits radial lengthening of as much as 10–15 mm and corrects the radial tilt in the sagittal plane, the inclination in the frontal plane, and the rotational deformity in the horizontal plane.
- The planning of angular, rotational, and length corrections should be based on preoperative radiographs of both wrists.

37.7 Timing

Early reconstruction is recommended in patients with radiographic characteristics that are predictive of persistent functional limitations (Jupiter and Ring 1996).

- In cases with substantial mal-alignment, such as cases with both extra-articular and intra-articular malunion, it may be indicated to do an early operative intervention.
- Anatomic corrections should be done through an immaturely healed fracture site in order to limit the soft-tissue contracture and the radio-ulnar joint dysfunction.
- Corrective osteotomy of such "nascent malunion" (usually within 2–4 months post injury) facilitates both radial realignment and realignment of the distal radioulnar joint (DRUJ).
- The duration of disability and time out of work are considerably decreased in these cases.

37.8 Technique for "Nascent" Malunion

A volar approach may be useful in extra-articular fractures that have healed with shortening and angular deformity of the distal fragment.

- The intention is to "take down" the maturing callus and perform the "osteotomy" at the site of the original fracture.
- After removing the callus, the fracture site is exposed. Often, the "osteotomy" may be performed with the knife or a small chisel directly into the fracture line.
- If the ulnar variance can be restored with angular realignment alone, the volar cortex can be cracked and hinged open in an attempt to maintain some stability of the osteotomy.

- The removed callus should combined with cancellous bone be placed in the defect caused by the realignment of the distal fragment.
- The previous technique with the use of a corticocancellous bone graft (a "pre-shaped" bone block with three cortices) as an extra stabilizer is not necessary when using distal radius locking plates (plates with fixed angle screws or blades).

In case of dorsal mal-angulation of the distal fragment, a volarly placed distal radius locking plate may be fixed at the distal fragment prior to the osteotomy. The proximal part of the plate will then have a position of 20–50° off the shaft of the radius. After the osteotomy, the plate may be used as a "joystick" to reduce the distal fragment and finally be fixed to the radius shaft.

Even if the fracture is solidly healed, an attempt should be made to identify the prior fracture site. However, if impossible, choose a site that creates a distal fragment that is large enough to facilitate manipulation and internal fixation, but stay distal enough to take advantage of the healing capacity of metaphyseal bone.

37.9 Technique for "Mature" Extra-articular Malunion

The osteotomy should reorient the distal articular surface to improve normal load distribution, reestablish the kinematics of the midcarpal joint, and restore the anatomic relations of the distal radioulnar joint (DRUJ).

- Because radial shortening is a constant component of the deformity in both dorsal and volar malunion, an opening wedge osteotomy is recommended that is transverse in the frontal plane and oblique (i.e. parallel to the joint surface) in the sagittal plane.
- Nowadays, we often use a volar approach.
- Release of the radial and dorsal soft tissues facilitates realignment in the dorsally angulated malunions.
- If needed, the brachioradial tendon may be released from the distal radius, facilitating the reduction.
- In most cases, the volarly angulated malunions do not need extensive soft-tissue release.
- The distal radius volar locking plate can facilitate realignment by pushing the distal fragment into position as the proximal screws are tightened (Fig. 37.2a).
- Once the radius is realigned, a cancellous bone graft is inserted though the excellent radial access available (Fig. 37.2b, c).
- In volarly displaced fractures (Smith's type), a K-wire into the distal fragment may be used like a "joystick" til reduce the mal-angulation (Fig. 37.3a–c).

37.10 Outcome

In most published series, the majority of patients had improved their range of motion, grip strength, cosmetic score, and subjective assessment of function after anatomic correction. However, the objective function of the wrist is not fully restored in all patients (Pommersbergen et al. 2002; Krukhaug and Hove 2007).

37.11 Pearls and Pitfalls

- A mal-united extra-articular fracture is most often a complex deformity in more than one plane.
- The goals of radial osteotomy are to restore function and improve the appearance of the wrist by correcting the deformity at the level of the old fracture site.
- A detailed plan based on radiographic findings should be made preoperatively.
- Early reconstruction is recommended in patients with radiographic characteristics that are predictive of persistent functional limitations….
- In "nascent malunion" the intention is to "take down" the maturing callus with a knife or a little chisel and perform the "osteotomy" at the site of the original fracture.
- Radial shortening is a constant component of the deformity in both the mature dorsal and volar malunion. Thus, an opening wedge osteotomy is recommended that is transverse in the frontal plane and oblique (i.e. parallel to the joint surface) in the sagittal plane.
- Cancellous bone graft and removed callus can be filled in the defect from the osteotomy.

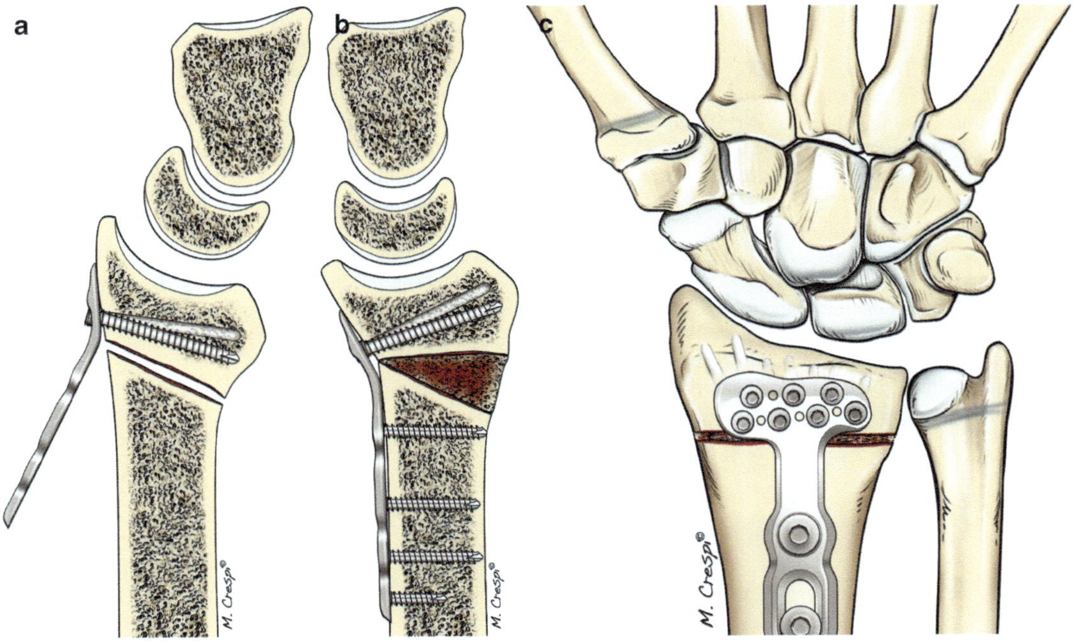

Fig. 37.2 (**a**) The distal volar locking plate can facilitate the realignment of the distal fragment by pushing the proximal part of the plate into position. (**b**) Once the radius is realigned, cancellous bone graft is inserted through the radial access. (**c**) Volar view with the plate in position

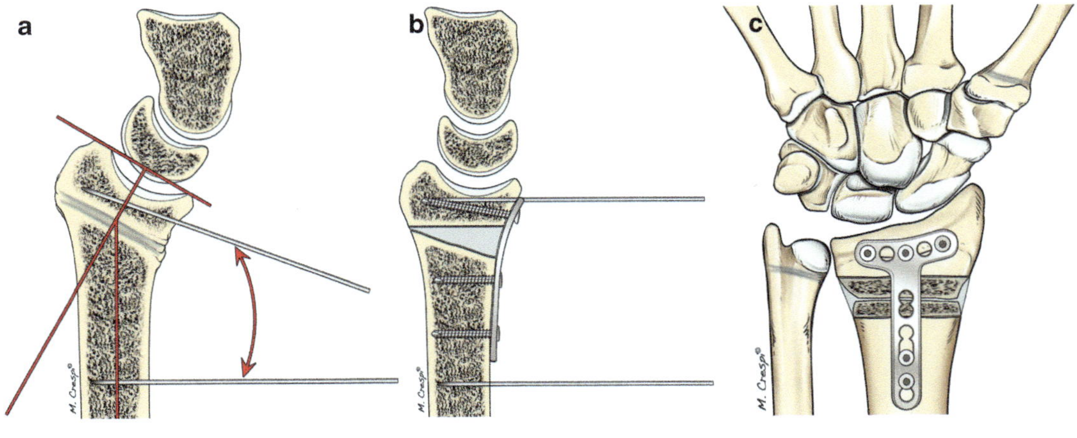

Fig. 37.3 (**a**) In cases with volar mal-angulation, a K-wire can be used as a joystick in the distal fragment. (**b**, **c**) The volar locking plate is fixed before the osteotomy-gap is filled with cancellous bone

References

Amadio PC, Botte MJ. Treatment of malunion of the distal radius. Hand Clin. 1987;3:541–61.

Aro HT, Koivunen T. Minor axial shortening of the radius affects outcome of Colles' fracture treatment. J Hand Surg. 1991;16A:392–8.

Ekenstam F, Hagert CG, Engkvist O, Tornvall AH, Wilbrand H. Corrective osteotomy of malunited fractures of the distal end of the radius. Scand J Plast Reconstr Surg. 1985;19:175–87.

Fernandez DL. Correction of post-traumatic wrist deformity in adults by osteotomy, bone-grafting, and internal fixation. J Bone Joint Surg. 1982;64A:1164–78.

Fernandez DL. Reconstructive procedures for malunion and traumatic arthritis. Orthop Clin North Am. 1993;24:341–63.

Fernandez DL, Jupiter JJ, Nagy L. Malunion of the distal end of the radius. In: Fernandez DL, Jupiter JB, editors. Fractures of the distal radius. A practical approach to management. New York: Springer; 2002. p. 289–344.

Flinkkila T, Raatikainen T, Kaarela O, Hamalainen M. Corrective osteotomy for malunion of the distal radius. Arch Orthop Trauma Surg. 2000;120:23–6.

Jupiter JB, Ring D. A comparison of early and late reconstruction of malunited fractures of the distal end of the radius. J Bone Joint Surg. 1996;78A:739–48.

Krukhaug Y, Hove LM. Corrective osteotomy for malunited extra-articular fractures of the distal radius: a follow-up study of 33 patients. Scand J Plast Reconstr Surg Hand Surg. 2007;41:303–9.

McQueen M, Caspers J. Colles fracture: does the anatomical result affect the final function? J Bone Joint Surg. 1988;70B:649–51.

Posner MA, Ambrose L. Malunited Colles' fractures: correction with a biplanar closing wedge osteotomy. J Hand Surg. 1991;16A:1017–26.

Prommersberger KJ, Van Schoonhoven J, Lanz UB. Outcome after corrective osteotomy for malunited fractures of the distal end of the radius. J Hand Surg. 2002;27B:55–60.

Ring D, Fernandez DL, Jupiter JB. Corrective osteotomy for distal radius malunion. In: Wiesel SW et al., editors. Operative techniques in orthopaedic surgery. Philadelphia: Lippincott Williams Wilkins; 2011. p. 2234–43.

Shea K, Fernandez DL, Jupiter JB, Martin Jr C. Corrective osteotomy for malunited, volarly displaced fractures of the distal end of the radius. J Bone Joint Surg. 1997;79A:1816–26.

Ulnar Shortening Osteotomy After Distal Radius Fracture

38

Peter Jørgsholm

Contents

38.1 Summary

Ulnar positive variance is common after malunited distal radius fracture. This can lead to an excessive load bearing across the ulnar side of the wrist resulting in an impaction of the ulnar head on the carpus primarily the lunate and has been termed ulnocarpal impaction syndrome. This condition can ultimately give raise to localized osteoarthritis between the ulnar head and the lunate and cause chronic ulnar-sided wrist pain. It is one of the most common complains after distal radius fracture.

In patients presenting with only minor angular deformity or solely axial shortening of the radius, ulnar shortening is the preferred treatment. The results are good after the introduction of rigid fixation and precise oblique or step-cut osteotomies and non-union rates has almost been eliminated. The procedure is simpler than radius osteotomy, which often needs bone grafting, and postoperative immobilization.

Smoking and NSAID increase the risk of non-union. Early DRUJ osteoarthritis is not a contra-indication to ulnar shortening.

The goals of the shortening procedure are to relieve pain and prevent arthritis by reestablishing a neutral or slightly negative ulnar variance.

P. Jørgsholm, MD
Hand Unit, Mølholm Private Hospital,
Vejle, Denmark
e-mail: jorgsholm@mac.com

L.M. Hove et al. (eds.), *Distal Radius Fractures*,
DOI 10.1007/978-3-642-54604-4_38, © Springer-Verlag Berlin Heidelberg 2014

38.2 Introduction

Pain-free forearm rotation is vital for normal function of the hand. Loaded forearm rotation is often impaired when DRUJ has been involved in a distal radius fracture.

- For almost a century the Darrach (1992) procedure or excision of the ulnar head has been recommended for problems in the distal radioulnar joint (DRUJ) or for ulnocarpal impaction after fractures of the distal radius. Generally pain reduction and improved range of movement (ROM) can be expected in elderly low demanding individuals, but radioulnar impingement and instability are common (Field et al. 1993). Particularly in the young or physically demanding patient, correction of the malunited distal radius has been advocated to restore length as well as angular deformity (Hove and Molster 1994).
- Ulnar positive variance is common after distal radius fracture. Ulnar positive variance exists when the distal ulnar articular surface is being more distal than the ulnar articular surface of the distal radius (Fig. 38.1). This can lead to an overload between the ulnar head and the carpus often the lunate and has been termed ulnocarpal abutment or ulnocarpal impaction syndrome (Chun and Palmer 1993). This will in long term give raise to chondromalacia of the ulnar part of the lunate and ulnar head, degenerative tear of the triangular fibrocartilage complex, and ultimately localized osteoarthritis first in the lunate and later even in the ulnar head.
- The symptoms of ulnocarpal impaction are ulnar-sided wrist pain, ulnar swelling and decreased ROM and grip force.
- Diagnosis can be confirmed by radiography, bone scan, MRI, SPECT/CT scan and ultimatively arthroscopy (Uschiyama 1991; Imaeda et al. 1996; Krüger et al. 2011; Tatebe et al. 2005).
- Ulnar shortening is a well-accepted treatment in patients with symptomatic idiopathic ulnar positive variance but less so in patients with a shortened malunited distal radius although described as early as 1941 by Milch.
- The reported relatively high rates of nonunion in ulna osteotomies (Köppel et al. 1997) have been reduced to acceptable levels, particularly after the introduction of rigid fixation and step-cut or oblique osteotomy the latter performed with one of the commercially available sawing jigs.
- In patients presenting with solely axial shortening of the radius or only minor angular deformity, results are good after ulnar shortening (Petersen et al. 2005). The procedure is also thought to stabilize the DRUJ by tightening the ulnocarpal ligaments, which deals with many of the biomechanical problems after distal radius fractures.
- The goals of the shortening procedure are to relieve pain, improve ROM and grip strength and prevent arthritis by reestablishing a neutral or slightly negative ulnar variance.

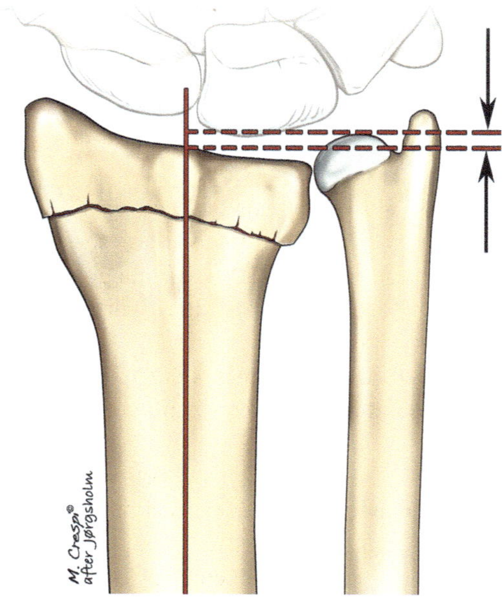

Fig. 38.1 Ulnar positive variance after distal radius fracture

Pain-free forearm rotation is vital for normal function of the hand.

Loaded forearm rotation is often impaired when DRUJ has been involved after distal radius fracture.

Ulnar positive variance is common after distal radius fracture (Fig. 38.2).

Ulnar positive variance can lead to an overload between the ulnar head and the carpus often the lunate and has been termed ulnocarpal impaction syndrome.

Ulnocarpal impaction will in long term give raise to chondromalacia of the ulnar part of the lunate and ulnar head, degenerative tear of the triangular fibrocartilage complex, and ultimately localized osteoarthritis first in the lunate and later even in the ulnar head.

In patients presenting with ulnar-sided wrist pain and solely axial shortening of the radius or only minor angular deformity, results are good after ulnar shortening.

Diagnosis can be confirmed by radiography, bone scan, MRI and ultimately by arthroscopy.

Non-unions are rare after the introduction of rigid fixation and step-cut or oblique osteotomy the latter performed with a sawing jig.

The goals of ulnar shortening procedure are to relieve pain, improve ROM and grip strength and prevent arthritis.

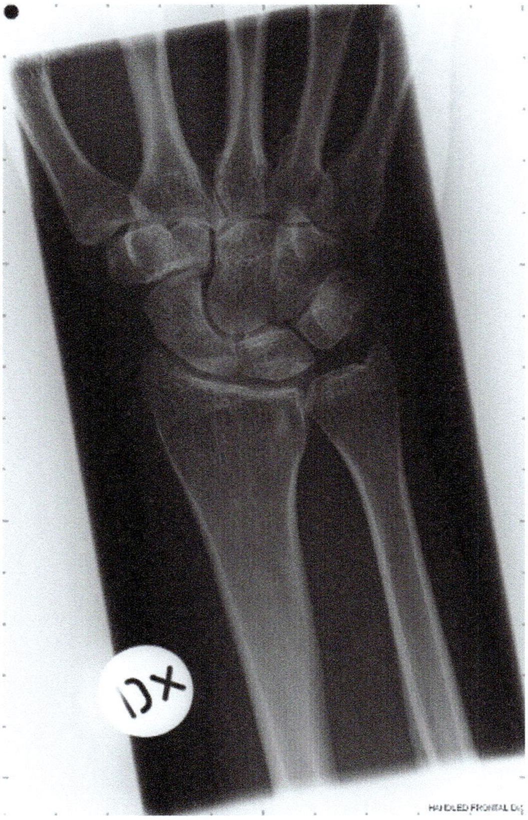

Fig. 38.2 Ulnar positive variance after distal radius fracture

38.3 Biomechanics

- 2-mm shortening of the radius will double the force through ulna from 20 to 40 % (Fig. 38.3).
- Ulnocarpal impaction will in long term give raise to chondromalacia of the ulnar part of the lunate and ulnar head and degenerative tear of the triangular fibrocartilage complex and ultimately localized osteoarthritis first in the lunate and later even in the ulnar head (Uschiyama 1991).
- Late manifestation will include lunotriquetral ligament tear and possible proximal hamate osteoarthritis.
- If the dorsal tilt of the manumitted distal radius is >15°, incongruity of the DRUJ is a concern.
- The inclination of the sigmoid notch (Fig. 38.4) (Tolat et al. 1992) may have effect on the development of osteoarthritis in the DRUJ after ulnar shortening but not the clinical outcome (Baek et al. 2011).
- Instability of the DRUJ can affect the symptoms of impaction.

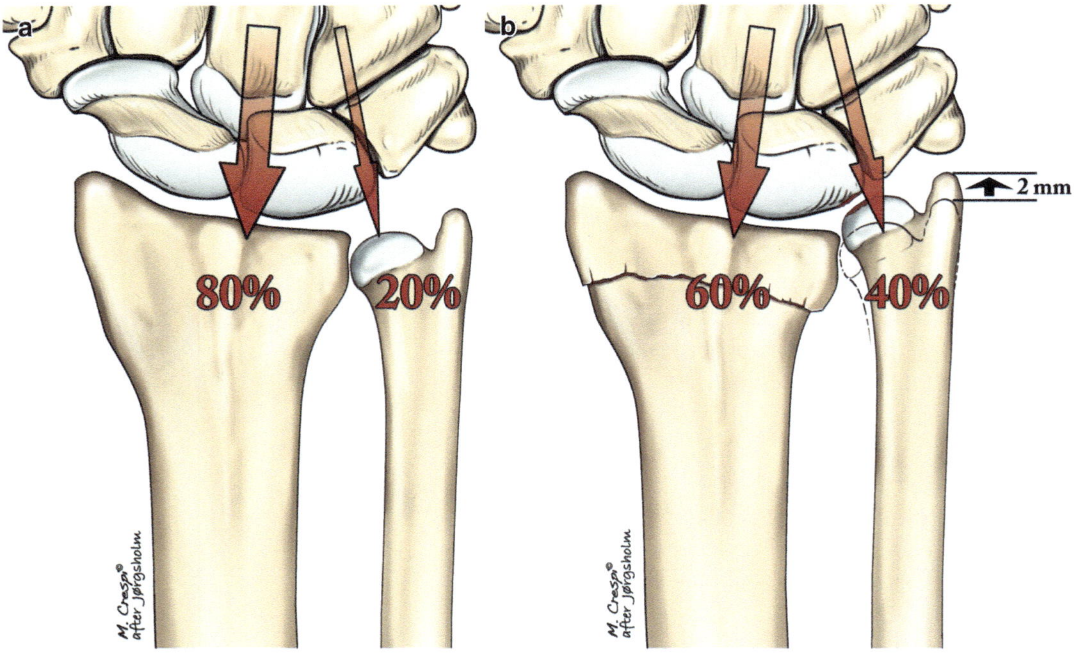

Fig. 38.3 Axial load distribution. (**a**) In a normal wrist. (**b**) In a wrist after a distal radius fracture healed with 2-mm radial shortening

38.4 Clinical Findings

The manifestation in any stage of ulnocarpal impaction can be ulnar-sided wrist pain, swelling on the dorsoulnar aspect of the wrist, impairment of forearm rotation, extension and ulnar deviation and decreased grip strength. The symptoms may show in any combination. Ulnar-sided wrist pain is one of the most common complaints after distal radius fracture.

- Ulnar-sided wrist pain: Often pain during rest referred toward the elbow.
- Aggravation during pronation/extension: Bicycling, typewriting and car driving.
- Prominent ulnar head: The patient will point out the symptomatic area around the dorsal aspect of the ulnar head.
- Swollen and tender around ulnar head: Compare to the other side.
- Limited forearm rotation and wrist extension: Especially decreased supination.
- Plus/minus DRUJ instability: Compare to the other side. Ulnar styloid non-union?
- Pronation/extension test positive: Full pronation, dorsal extension, ulnar deviation and axial load provoke pain (Nakamura 1997).
- Ulnocarpal stress test positive: With 90° flexed elbow forced ulnar deviation and axial load in the wrist during full pronation/supination reproduces the pain (Fig. 38.5).
- The ulnar impaction test positive: Pain when the ulna is held down and the wrist deviated ulnar wards and the forearm supinated (Tolat et al. 1992).

38.5 Imaging

Radiographs give a good initial screening.

- AP view:
  Ulnar positive variance (Fig. 38.1)
  Type of inclination in sigmoid notch (Fig. 38.4)
  Cystic changes ulnar/proximal in the lunate (Fig. 38.2)
  Arthritic changes in DRUJ
  Ulnar styloid non-union

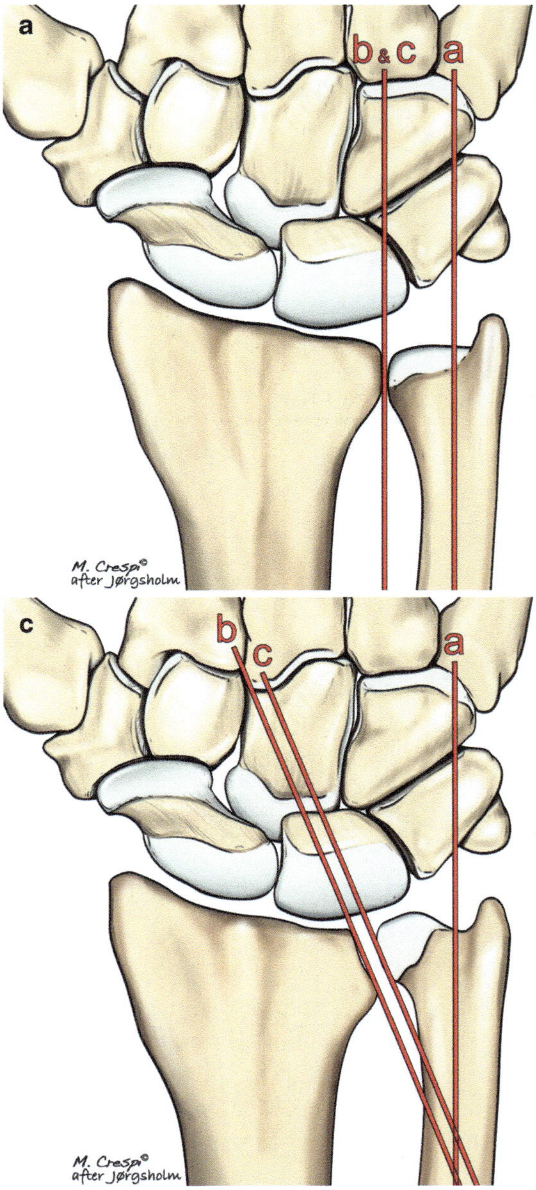

Fig. 38.4 Types of the distal radioulnar joint (DRUJ) according to Baek et al. 2011: (**a**) Type I: The apposing joint surfaces (b, c) are parallel to the long axis of the ulna (a). (**b**) Type II: The apposing joint surfaces (b, c) are oblique to the long axis of the ulna (a). The sigmoid notch and the ulnar seat angles are positive. (**c**) Type III: The apposing joint surfaces (b, c) are reversely oblique to the long axis of the ulna (a). The sigmoid notch and the ulnar seat angles are negative

- Lateral view:
  Dorsal tilt
  Dorsal subluxation of ulnar head
- Stress view:
  Forced grip and full pronation

MRI is indicated if clinical suspicion of ulnocarpal impaction or ligament tear exists.

- STIR and T1-weighted projections: Bone marrow oedema corresponding to ulnoproximal lunate and radioproximal triquetrum

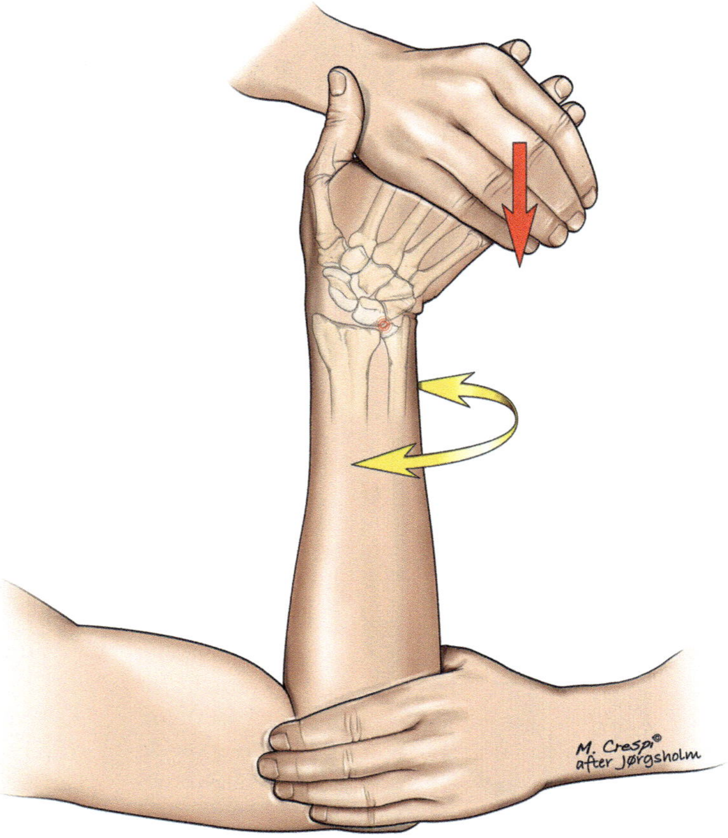

Fig. 38.5 Ulnocarpal stress test

eventually corresponding part of ulnar head ("kissing lesion") (Fig. 38.6). TFCC lesions? LT lesions? Proximal hamate oedema?

Bone scan is sensitive but has a low specificity and will show a hot spot around the lunotriquetral area.

- Early phase IV technetium injection: Hot spot in the lunotriquetral area.

SPECT/CT is promising in diagnosing impaction syndrome and probably is the most accurate investigation available but further studies are needed to support this (Krüger et al. 2011; Ito 2013).

- Late phase IV technetium injection and CT scan: A combination of bone scan and CT scan gives highly accurate placement of hot spots (Fig. 38.7).

All investigations could be negative. The diagnoses will ultimately be arthroscopic confirmation of a "kissing lesion" sometimes only chondromalacia in the ulnar dorsal corner of the proximal lunate (Fig. 38.8).

38.6 Treatment

- Radiocarpal arthroscopic evaluation of TFCC, lunate, triquetrum, lunotriquetral ligament and ulnar head and DRUJ if possible. Synovectomy and debridement of injured TFCC, chondral and ligamentous lesions.

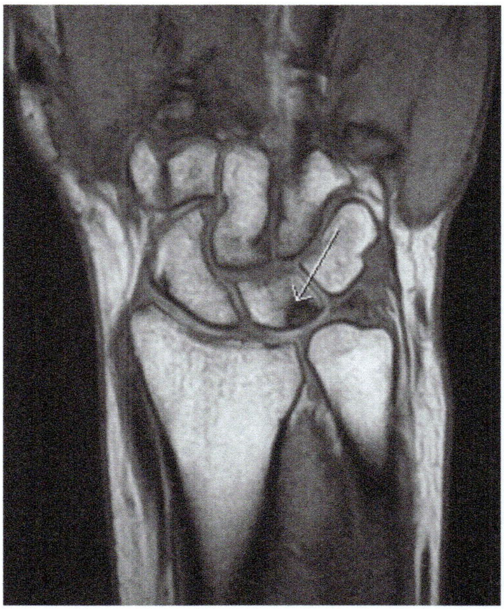

Fig. 38.6 MRI showing typical oedema in the proximal dorsal part of the lunate as seen on the T1 weighted sequences. (marked by *arrow*)

- Midcarpal arthroscopic evaluation of luno-triquetral ligament and joint and proximal hamate. Synovectomy and eventually resection of head of hamate if localized osteoarthritis.
- Ulnar shortening procedure if ulnocarpal impaction is evident (Fig. 38.9).
- Arthroscopic wafer procedure of ulnar head could be indicated if ulnar shortening osteotomy is considered troublesome (heavy smoker, pronounced osteoporosis or earlier insufficient ulnar shortening).

38.7 Operative Technique

- Arthroscopic TFCC resection and wafer procedure.
- Reinsertion of TFCC or ulnar styloid if necessary: Arthroscopic or open reinsertion of TFCC with bone anchoring or transosseous technique and high strength suturing. Open cleaning, bone grafting and fixation of non-union of ulnar styloid with tension band wiring or cannulated screw.
- Open shortening osteotomy: Preferable with oblique technique using a sawing jig for precise osteotomy and control of rotation (Fig. 38.10). Most of the available systems have a maximum of 5–10 mm shortening (Table 38.1). Step-cut osteotomy can be used if major shortening is planned or a cutting device is not available but it is technical demanding and needs special attention and technique (Fig. 38.11).

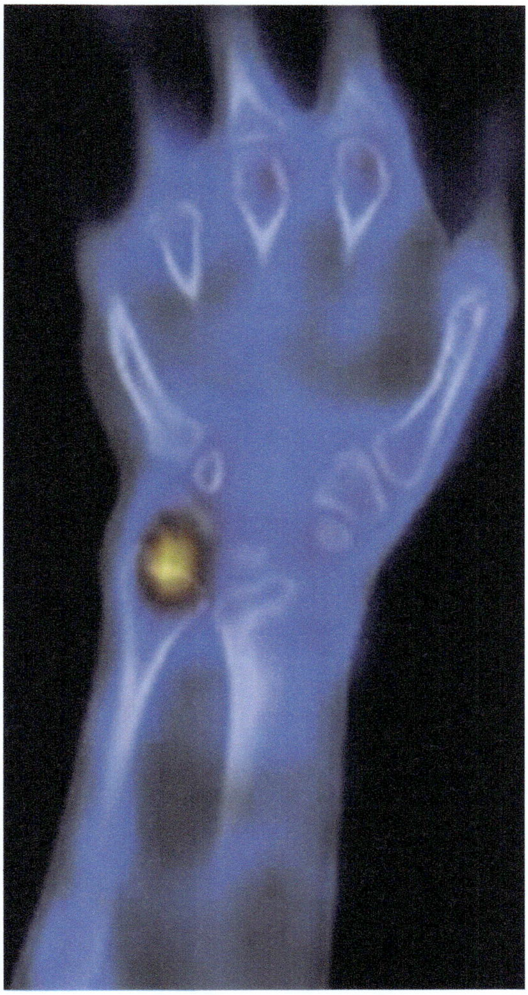

Fig. 38.7 SPECT/CT showing increased uptake in the area of the ulnar head, lunate and triqietrum. Picture by courtesy of Dr Bo Povlsen, Guy's Hospital, London.

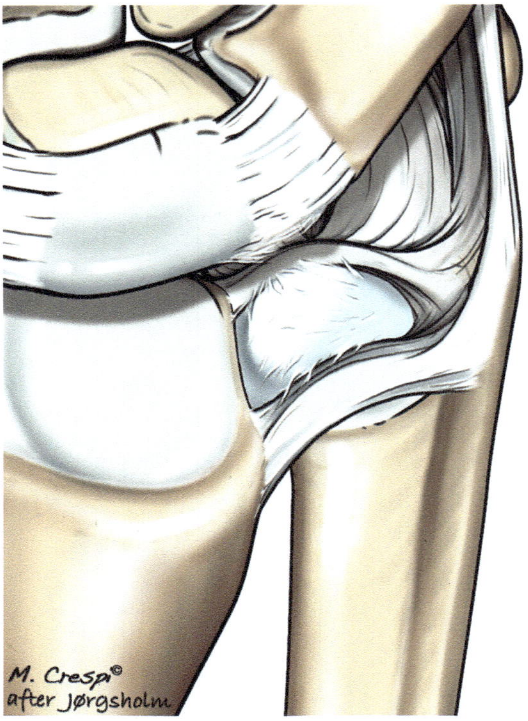

Fig. 38.8 Arthroscopic appearance of a "kissing lesion"

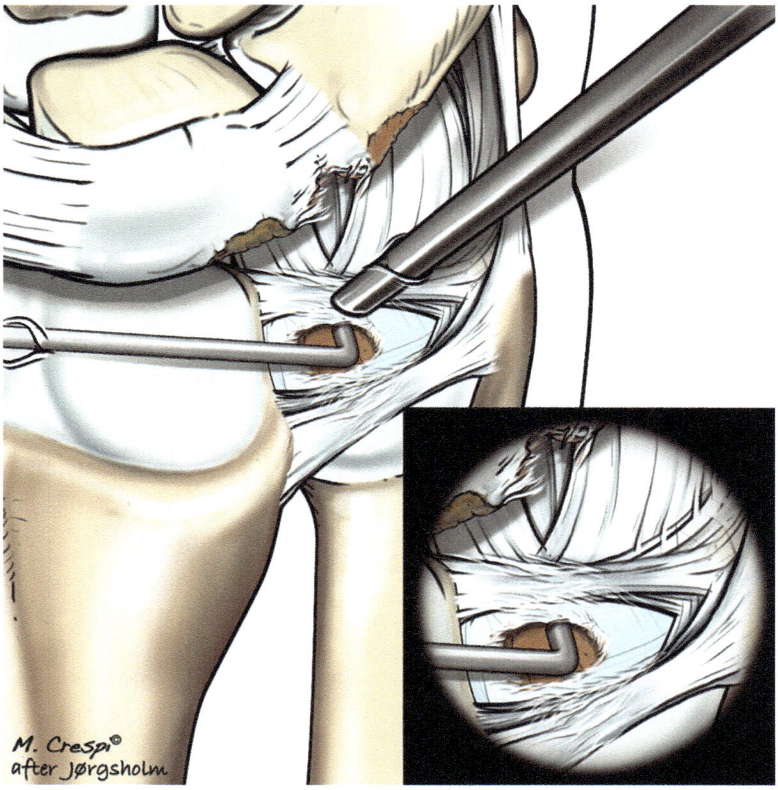

Fig. 38.9 Arthroscopic appearance of ulnocarpal impaction with discus and cartilage degeneration

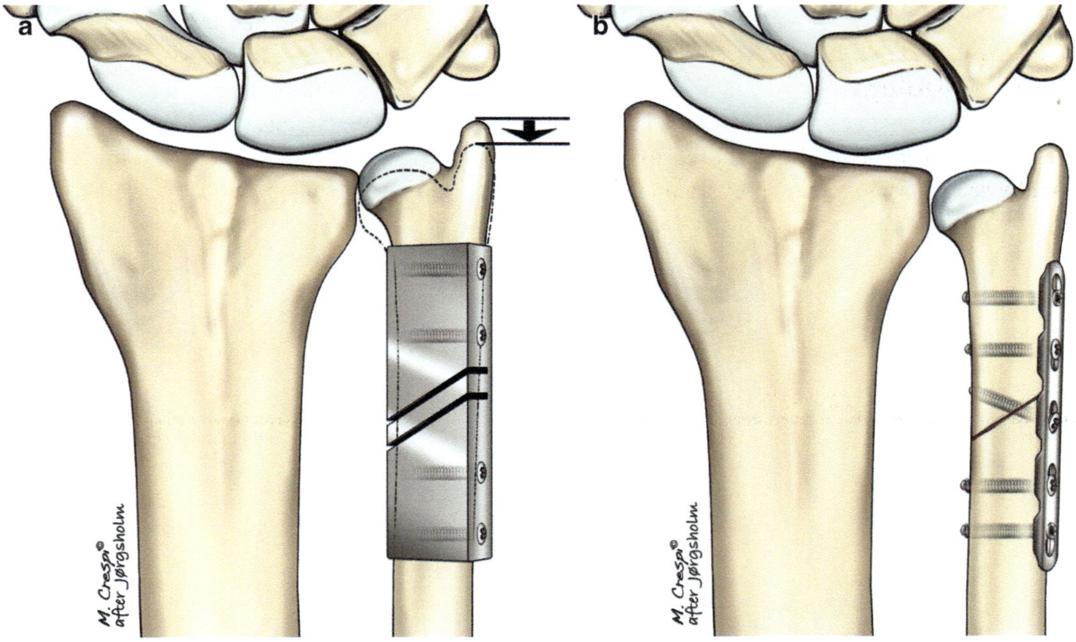

Fig. 38.10 (**a**, **b**) Oblique ulnar shortening with saw-guide

Table 38.1 Ulnar shortening osteotomy systems

System	Manufacturers	Min. size (mm)	Holes No.	Screw size (mm) Locking +/–	Shortening (mm)
Acumed	Acumed, Hillsboro, USA	85×9×3	7	3.5 +	1–10
I.T.S.	I.T.S. GmbH, Lassnitzhöhe, Austria	92	8	2.7/3.0 +	1–13
Martin	KLS Martin GmbH, Umkirch, Germany	80×10×3.2	7	2.5 +	3–10
Newclip	NewclipTecnichs, Haute Gouliane, France	77×11×2.5	6	2.8/3.5 +	0–12
Osteotec	Osteotec, Dorset, UK	72×11×3.3	5	3.5 –/+	2.5–5.5
Rayhack	Wright Medical Technique, Arlington, USA		7	2.7 –/+	3.5–18.1
Trimed	Trimed Inc., Santa Clarita, USA	75×9×4.1	5 & 7	3.2 +	2–10
Synthes	DepuySynthes, Solothurn, Switzerland	62×9×3.5	6 & 9	2.8 +	2.5–5
Ulnafix	Osteotec, Dorset, UK		5 & 7	3.5 +	2–5

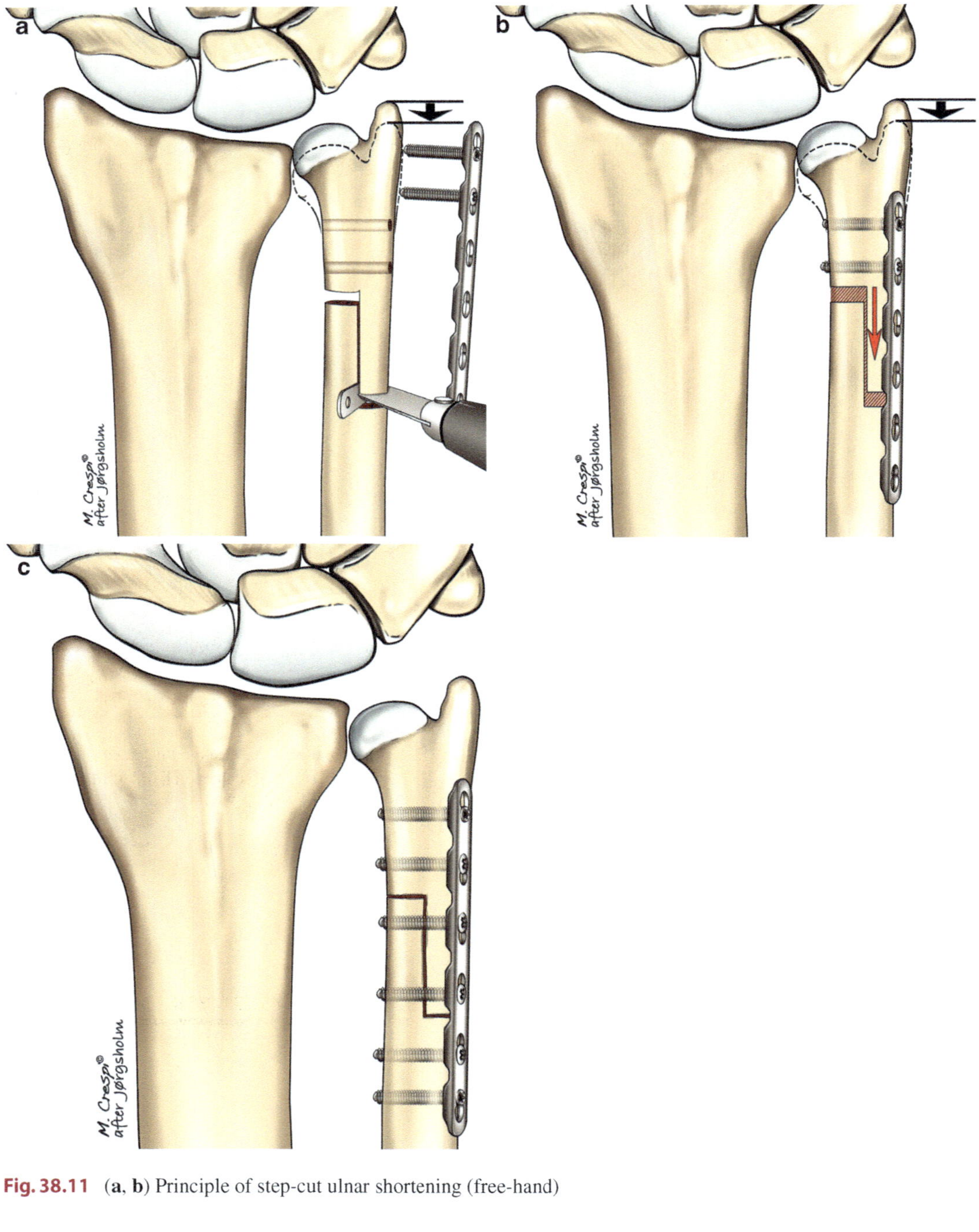

Fig. 38.11 (**a**, **b**) Principle of step-cut ulnar shortening (free-hand)

Tricks and Tips for Diagnosing and Treating Ulnocarpal Impaction Syndrome

- Think of impaction syndrome in patients with ulnar-sided wrist pain after a distal radius fracture.
- Compare the wrist joint and DRUJ on injured side to the normal opposite side.
- When measuring ulnar variance use normal side as reference.
- Imaging should always include a stress view (power grip in full pronation) compared to the contralateral side.
- Ulnocarpal impaction is often an arthroscopic diagnosis and all imaging (radiographs, CT, MRI, bone scan, SPECT/CT) could be normal.
- TFCC could be intact in ulnocarpal impaction syndrome.
- Early DRUJ osteoarthritis is not a contraindication to ulnar shortening.
- Use preferable oblique osteotomy with a sawing jig.
- Smoking and NSAID increase the risk of non-union.

References

Baek GH, Lee HJ, Gong HS, Rhee SH, Kim J, Kim KW, Kong BY, Oh WS. Long-term outcomes of ulnar shortening osteotomy for idiopathic ulnar impaction syndrome: at least 5-years follow-up. Clin Orthop Surg. 2011;3:4.

Chun S, Palmer AK. The ulnar impaction syndrome: follow-up of ulna shortening osteotomy. Hand Surg. 1993;18A:46–53.

Darrach W. Partial excision of lower shaft of ulna for deformity following Colles's fracture. 1913. Clin Orthop. 1992;275:3–4.

Field J, Majkowski RJ, Leslie IJ. Poor results of Darrach's procedure after wrist injuries. J Bone Joint Surg. 1993;75B:53–7.

Hove LM, Molster AO. Surgery for posttraumatic wrist deformity. Radial osteotomy and/or ulnar shortening in 16 Colles' fractures. Acta Orthop Scand. 1994; 65:434–8.

Imaeda T, Nakamura R, Shionoya K, Makino N. Ulnar impaction syndrome: MR imaging findings. Radiology. 1996;201(2):495–500.

Ito S, Yamamoto Y, Tanii T, Aga F, Nishiyama Y. SPECT/CT imaging in ulnocarpal impaction syndrome. Clin Nucl Med. 2013;38(10):841–2.

Köppel M, Hargreaves IC, Herbert TJ. Ulnar shortening osteotomy for ulnar carpal instability and ulnar carpal impaction. J Hand Surg. 1997;22B:451–6.

Krüger T, Hug U, Hüllner M, Schleich F, Veit-Haibach P, von Wartburg U, Strobel U. SPECT/CT arthrography of the wrist in ulnocarpal impaction syndrome. Eur J Nucl Med Mol Imaging. 2011;38:792.

Milch H. Cuff resection of the ulna for malunited Colles' fracture. J Bone Joint Surg Am. 1941;23(2):311–3.

Nakamura R, Horii E, Imaeda T, Nakao E, Kato H, Watanabe K. The ulnocarpal stress test in the diagnosis of ulnar-sided wrist pain. J Hand Surg Br. 1997;22(6):719–23.

Petersen K, Breddam M, Jørgsholm P, Schrøder H. Ulnar shortening osteotomy after Colles fracture. Scand J Plast Reconstr Surg Hand Surg. 2005;39(3):170–7.

Tatebe M, Nakamura R, Horii E, Nakao E. Results of ulnar shortening osteotomy for ulnocarpal impaction syndrome in wrists with neutral or negative ulnar variance. J Hand Surg Br. 2005;30(2):129–32.

Tolat AR, Sanderson PL, De Smet L, Stanley JK. The gymnast's wrist: acquired positive ulnar variance following chronic epiphyseal injury. J Hand Surg Br. 1992;17(6):678–81.

Uschiyama S, Terayama L. Radiographic changes in wrist with ulnar plus variance observed over a 10-year period. J Hand Surg Am. 1991;16:45–8.

Intra-articular Malunion

39

Francisco del Piñal

Contents

F. del Piñal, MD, Dr Med
Instituto de Cirugia Plastica y de la Mano,
Santander, Spain

Unit of Hand-Wrist and Plastic Surgery,
Hospital Mutua Montañesa,
Paseo de Pereda 20-1, E-39004, Santander, Spain
e-mail: drpinal@drpinal.com, pacopinal@gmail.com

39.1 Summary

Intra-articular malunion should be considered as a surgical emergency in order to avoid irreversible damage of the cartilage surfaces. In this chapter, the decision-making process and the algorithm used by the author on the management of this complex pathology are discussed. If there is a step-off but the cartilage is preserved, an intra-articular (arthroscopically assisted) osteotomy is the procedure of choice. If only a major osteochondral defect of the radius is present, then the transfer of a vascularized piece of the base of the third metatarsal is chosen. If mirror damage occurs and is less than 50 % of the radius surface, smoothing the joint surface with arthroscopic technique (arthroscopic resection arthroplasty) is selected. If massive chondral defects are present, then a partial arthrodesis is the choice (preferably arthroscopic). The techniques and results of each are described in detail. A malunion is a major derangement of the wrist as a whole: attention to the radius and any distal radioulnar joint pathology should be addressed if a good result is to be obtained.

39.2 Introduction

- Malunion is the most common complication of distal radius fractures and can cause considerable disability (Amadio and Botte 1987).
- The malunion can affect the metaphysis (extra-articular malunion), the joint itself (intra-articular malunion) or both. Any of

L.M. Hove et al. (eds.), *Distal Radius Fractures*,
DOI 10.1007/978-3-642-54604-4_39, © Springer-Verlag Berlin Heidelberg 2014

them may cause pain, restricted range of motion and osteoarthritis.
- Step-offs at the radiocarpal joint cause abnormal concentration at the edges of the step-offs (up to 8 times the base value) and abnormal motion of the corresponding carpal bone (Wagner et al. 1996). Loss of cartilage will occur early in this setting and osteoarthritis will be the end result (Knirk and Jupiter 1986).
- The surgeon should be warned that although restoration of the joint surface is important, understanding and managing ALL associated problems is paramount: a malunion implies a major derangement of the wrist as a whole and all areas should be dealt with.
- In particular, most, if not all, patients will complain of decreased range of pronation-supination and/or ulnar-sided pain. Many areas may need to be cared for and of which some may no longer have a good solution.
- Besides this, the patient in pain, handicapped and having had a negative experience many of them having being diagnosed with/treated for complex regional pain syndrome (CRPS or Reflex Sympathetic Dystrophy, RSD) needs particular care.
- Hence, before embarking on its management, a clear understanding of the aetiology of the patient's pain, limitations and the solutions planned need to be honestly discussed.
- Multiple problems (radiocarpal, ulnocarpal and distal radioulnar) may need to be addressed in the same operation.

39.3 General Management and Decision-Making Process of the Radius Component

- My approach to manage any intra-articular malunion depends on the quality of the cartilage (Fig. 39.1).
- If the cartilage is intact in the radius and the carpal bones, I prefer an arthroscopically guided intra-articular osteotomy.
- Corrective intra-articular osteotomy is not indicated if the radius articular surface is shattered or the cartilage is gone.
- If this damage is localized only to the radius joint surface, I consider the use of a vascularized osteochondral graft.
- Finally, if there is damage to the cartilage of the radius and the carpal bones ("mirror image lesions"), I opt for an arthroscopically assisted resection arthroplasty, while an arthroscopically assisted radio-scapho-lunate (RSL) arthrodesis would be my choice when the damage is generalized.
- The decision making is not simple, and to complicate things further, the decision many times has to be taken intraoperatively. Indeed, despite the fact that radiological workup (radiograms and CT) is invaluable, a difficult diagnostic arthroscopy, in the setting of a scarred arthro-fibrotic joint, is often needed before the final decision regarding the best surgical procedure can be taken.
- All in all, this is a complex group of patients: the surgeon cannot offer a single surgical option preoperatively, and the postoperative aftercare varies depending on the decision taken intraoperatively.
- Added to this uncertainty, they have many times had an incorrect diagnosis of suffering CRPS 1. It takes a lot of time and effort to convince them that they need a complex operation, which rarely will restore function back to normal. Besides this, most of the medication they may have been taken is addictive, so withdrawal may prolong this process with several weeks or months.
- Furthermore, ulnar conditions and extra-articular malunion can coexist with the intra-articular problem.
- All doubts and uncertainties should be explained fairly to the patient, as once they understand them all; it is my experience that they become extremely cooperative and keen to escape from their assumed destiny.

39.4 Arthroscopic-Assisted Osteotomies

- Any fracture with a step-off of 2 mm or more is an absolute indication for a corrective intra-articular osteotomy, whether symptomatic or

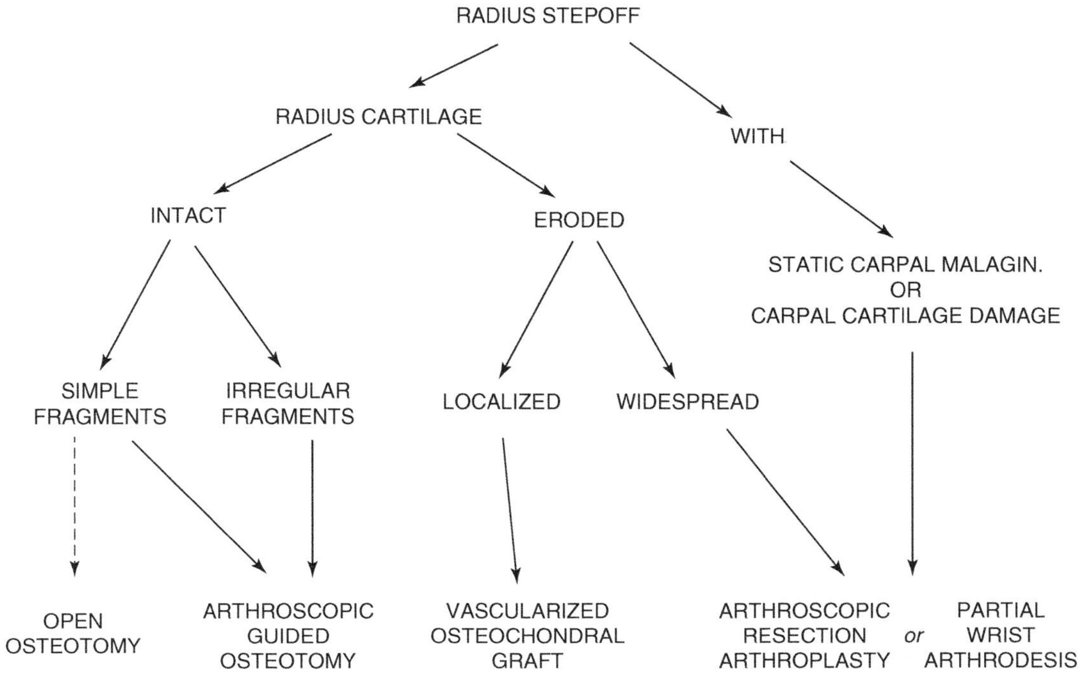

Fig. 39.1 Flow chart used by the author in the decision-making process (© Piñal in del Piñal et al. 2012)

not, as ostheoarthritis will develop (Knirk and Jupiter 1986).

- In fact, step-offs of just a millimetre (Trumble et al. 1994) may also be symptomatic, and it seems reasonable in young patients with a step-off involving the scaphoid or lunate facet (i.e. intrafacet as a horizontal step-off) to proceed as soon as possible with the osteotomy. Overloads at the intrafacet step-off are much more than at the sagittal crest (interfacet as a sagittal step-off) (Wagner et al. 1996).
- Wearing of the cartilage on the opposing carpal bone is a contraindication for an osteotomy, as restoration of the joint congruency will not prevent osteoarthritis.
- Time should not be taken as an absolute measure, but is depending upon the location in the joint, the amount of load and use of the wrist by the patient. It is my experience that a good outcome can be obtained up to 12 months or more after the fracture.
- The operation has been successfully carried out by volar, dorsal or combined approaches.
- The arthroscopic approach offers the advantages of precise cutting the fragments through the malunited cartilage with magnification and good illumination.
- Furthermore, it does not rely on fluoroscopy, which has proven unreliable (Edwards et al. 2001).

39.4.1 Technique

- The arm is exsanguinated and stabilized to the table with an arm strap.
- In early malunions (4–12 weeks from injury), the procedure is started by preparing the proposed site of plate fixation with the arm lying on the hand table.
- In order to facilitate the separation of the fragments when later doing the intra-articular osteotomy, the extra-articular callus is removed in the area exposed by at the time of plate fixation. At this stage, no attempt should be made to go all the way to the joint or use any forceful bending of the fragment nor

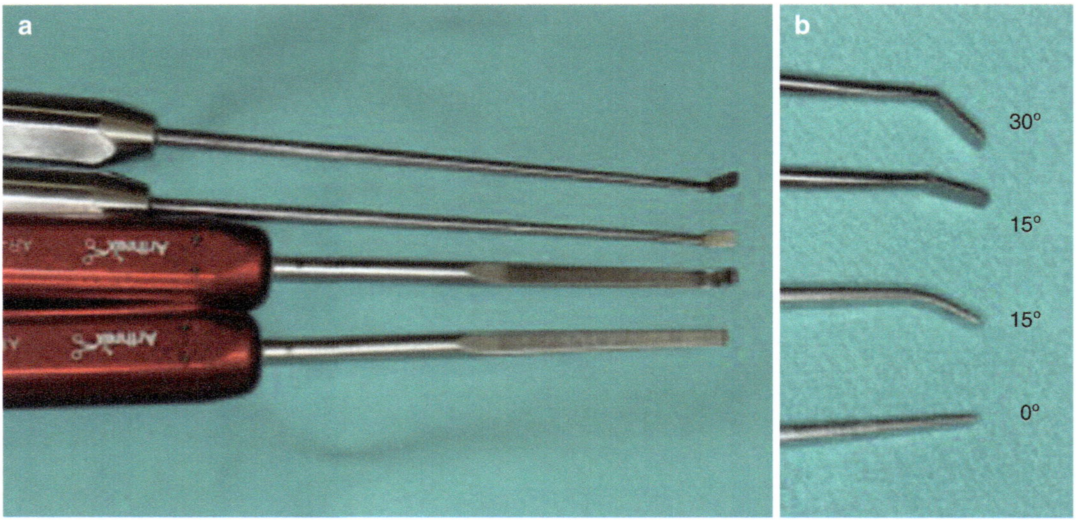

Fig. 39.2 (**a**) Two shoulder periosteal elevators and 2 sturdier osteotomes are used for cutting the bone. (**b**) Notice, on the lateral view, the different angulations of their ends, which are essential for carrying out the osteotomies (© Piñal in del Piñal et al. 2010)

attempt to force the fragment with the osteotome, as this may split the cartilage at an incorrect place.

- A plate, when needed, is provisionally placed at this stage and held in position with a single screw through its stem as recommended for an acute fracture (del Piñal 2008).
- The hand is then placed in traction with the fingers pointing upwards, with a customized traction system (del Piñal et al. 2006). In most cases we use 7–10 kg of traction applied to all fingers, but the counterweight can be increased if the joint space is still very tight.
- It is paramount to carry out the arthroscopy following the dry technique (del Piñal 2008) as otherwise the saline will escape through the portals.
- The standard dorsal 3–4 and 6R portals are made larger than usual, approximately 0.5–1 cm transverse incision, and widened with a hemostat to permit a smooth entrance of the osteotomes.
- It is crucial to remove scar and debris inside the joint and around the capsule in order to get a clear view. "Aggressive" shavers (2.9 mm gator micro bladeTM; ref: C9961. ConMed Linvatec. Largo, Fl, USA) are used to accomplish debridement in an effective manner. The quality of the articular cartilage of the radius and of the adjacent scaphoid and lunate is confirmed.
- For cutting the bone we use a shoulder periosteal elevator (of 15 and 30° angle) (Arthrex® AR-1342-30° and AR-1342-15°, Arthrex, Naples, FL, USA) and also straight and curved osteotomes (Arthrex® AR-1770 and AR-1771) (Fig. 39.2). Instruments with different angles are required as the limited joint space is not enough for manoeuvering the osteotome to get access to the malunited fracture lines.
- Straight cuts with the straight osteotome are the easiest from a technical standpoint, but only possible when the fracture line is straight and in line with one of the portals (Fig. 39.3).
- Most malunions, however, are not amenable to this "simple" osteotomy, and in those instances the fracture line is recreated by making multiple perforations or cuts with the angled osteotome. This creates a sort of "tear line" in the cartilage and subchondral bone for easy breakage when levering the fragment with the osteotomes.
- In general, the osteotomes will have to be introduced from a dorsal portal to cut a volar

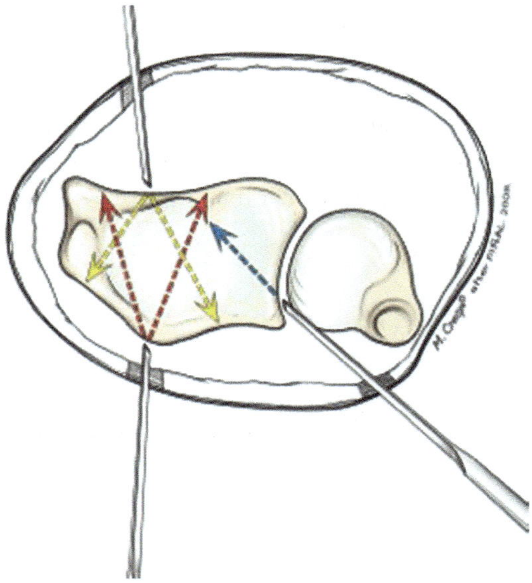

Fig. 39.3 Straight line osteotomies are only possible when the portal is lined up with the malunited fracture line (© Piñal in del Piñal et al. 2010)

fragment and vice versa. Given the space limitations and the fact that quite commonly the malunions are irregular, one has to be prepared to use any portal, any osteotome and combinations of linear and "tear line" osteotomies in order to manage a given malunion (Fig. 39.4).

- Gentle manoeuvering is necessary when hammering from dorsal to volar, as there is a risk of cutting flexor tendons if plunging through volarly or extensor tendons when doing the reverse manoeuver.
- The displaced fragments are fully mobilized by carefully moving them apart with the osteotome.
- Often, scar and new bone formation between the fragments impede perfect reduction. This early granulation tissue should be resected with the help of small curettes, shaver or burrs introduced through the portals, allowing the size of the gaps to be minimized.
- Once the reduction is acceptable, the operation proceeds with stepwise fixation exactly in the same manner as for a fracture (del Piñal et al. 2005, del Piñal 2008).
- No bone graft is used to support the fragments, as fixation is sufficiently rigid with the available volar locking plates as to allow to mobilize early (Fig. 39.5).

39.4.2 Clinical Experience

- Our initial experience consisted of 11 cases operated 1 to 5 months after the traumatic event under arthroscopic assistance (del Piñal et al. 2010).
- In 5 cases a single antero-ulnar or radial styloid fragment was osteotomized, whereas in the rest, up to 3 fragments were osteotomized. In the final patient, osteotomy of a malunited radius fragment was combined with an ulnar shortening osteotomy.
- Results have been uniformly good (del Piñal et al. 2010).

39.5 Arthroscopic Resection Arthroplasty

- Damage to the cartilage, either on the opposing carpal bone or on both the radius and the carpus (i.e. mirror lesions) (Fig. 39.6), historically forced the surgeon to select a salvage procedure: wrist denervation, partial or total wrist arthrodesis or arthroplasty.
- We have had a favourable experience with the so-called arthroscopic resection arthroplasty (del Piñal et al. 2012).
- This procedure consists of removing the articular portion of the radius fragment at the site of the arthritis (the step-off), while preserving the remaining radiocarpal joint and intact articular cartilage (Fig. 39.7).
- Conceptually, the operation we propose may be considered destructive for the wrist because we remove a part of the radius articular surface and the remaining surface may be overloaded. The rationale, however, is exactly the same as other motion preserving operations such as four-corner fusion or

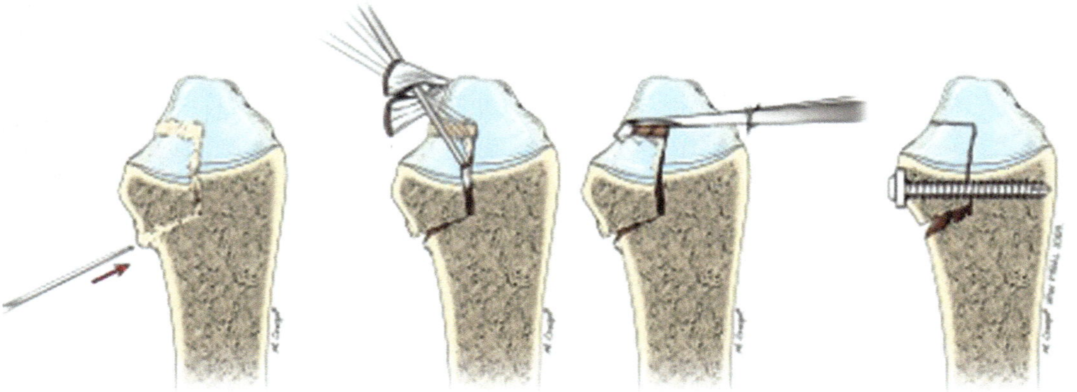

Fig. 39.4 Most malunions require multiple portals and combinations of osteotomies. Notice that the osteotome is introduced into the cleft between the radio-scapho-capitate and long radiolunate ligaments when using the volar-radial portal (© Piñal in del Piñal et al. 2010)

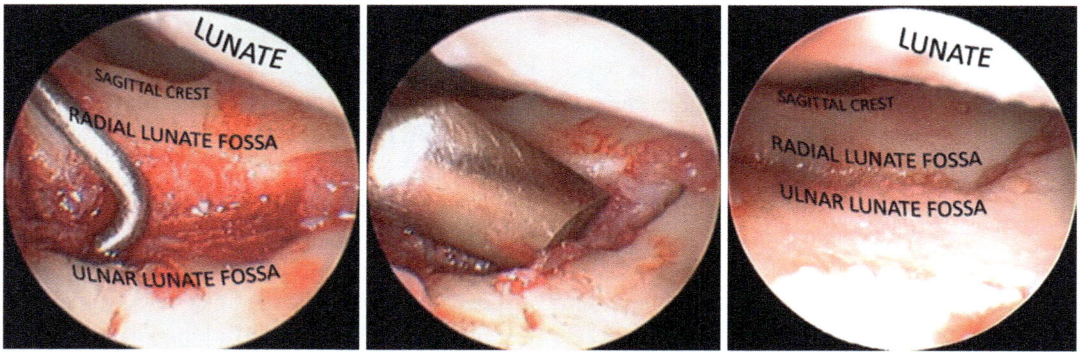

Fig. 39.5 (**a**) Correction of a 4 mm step-off on the lunate fossa (right wrist – scope in 6R). (**b**) The osteotome (entering the joint through a dorsal portal) is separating the malunited fragments. (**c**) Corresponding view after reduction (© Piñal in del Piñal et al. 2010)

proximal row carpectomy, where we remove the arthritic area and allow healthy areas to bear the load.

39.5.1 Operative Technique

- The arthroscopy was carried out using the dry technique.
- Once other pathology at the midcarpal joint was excluded, the camera was usually introduced through the 3–4 portals and the shaver through the 6R portal.
- The radiocarpal joint was debrided of loose synovium and intra-articular adherences with a 2.9-mm shaver until a working space was obtained.
- Typical findings of a stiff wrist joint were seen: widespread scarring and thickening of the capsule and ligaments with concomitant loss of their compliance. Restrictive adhesions and synechiae at the site of mal-

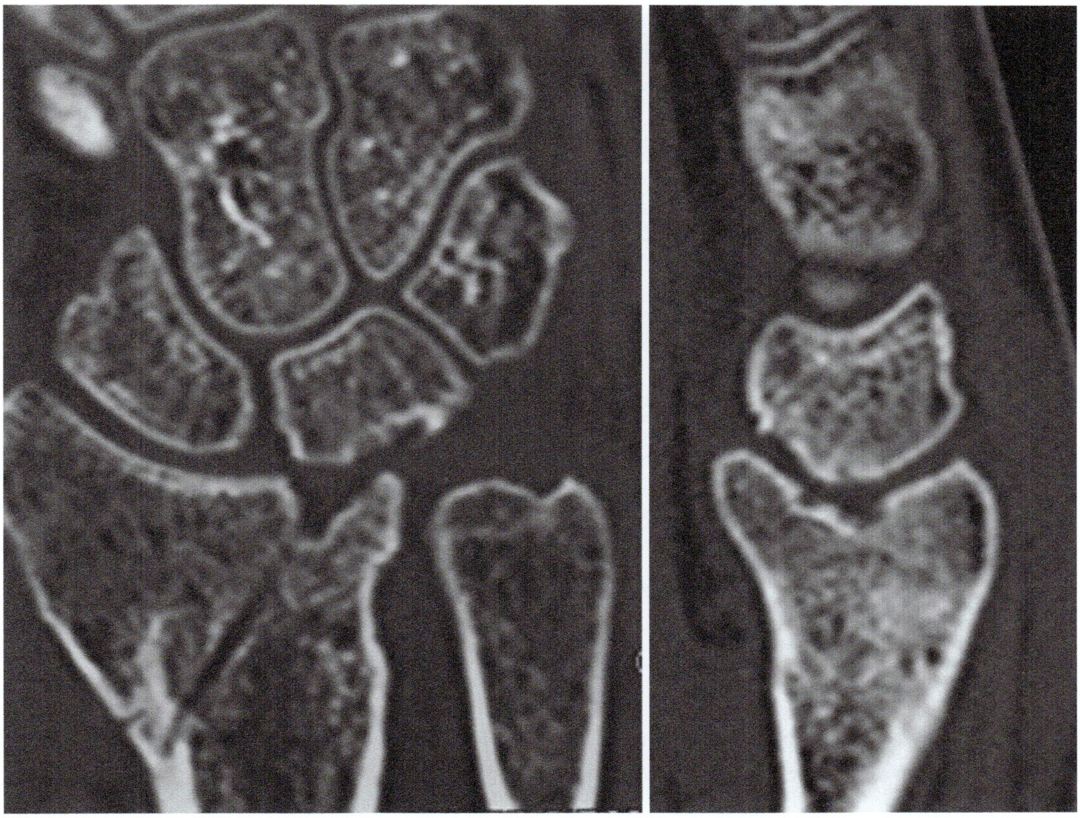

Fig. 39.6 Preoperative CT scan of a patient with severe damage on the lunate articular surface by the bony spur on the radius (© Piñal in del Piñal et al. 2012)

union and the corresponding denuded carpal bone were present in all cases in varying degrees.

- A primary goal, in order to introduce instruments, was to create a working space by removing restricting adherences and recreating the natural dorsal sulcus between the capsule and the proximal carpal row.
- Once the working space was created, the degree of step-off and chondral loss of the carpal bones was noted.
- With the camera in the most favourable portal, a 2.9-mm burr was used to resect the portion of the radius fragment causing the intra-articular step-off (Fig. 39.8).
- The aim was to produce a smooth cancellous surface that was slightly more depressed (0.5 mm) than the healthy cartilaginous surface. During the resection, great care was taken to preserve the volar rim of the radius in order not to detach the origin of the important volar ligaments.
- The margin of the opposing arthritic carpal bone was debrided with the shaver.
- At the end of the arthroscopy, the joint was extensively irrigated to remove debris.
- Postoperatively, the patients were encouraged to begin range of motion exercises immediately except when other procedures were done.

39.5.2 Clinical Experience

- Our initial experience consisted of 10 patients with step-off from 2 mm to 6 mm evenly distributed between the scaphoid fossa and the lunate fossa. The results, at an average of 28

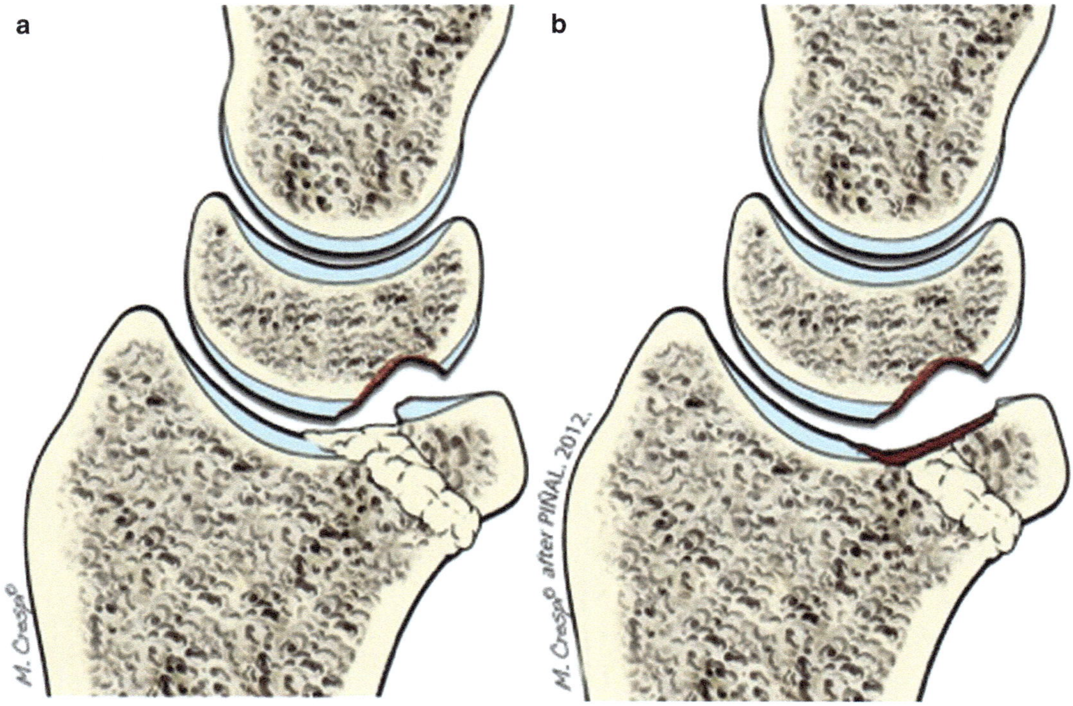

Fig. 39.7 Schematic representation of the operative principle: (**a**) The protruded fragment, which has eroded the carpal bone, is burred down to below the level of the normal cartilaginous surface. (**b**) A contoured articular surface, slightly depressed in the denuded area, is the goal of the operation (© Piñal in del Piñal et al. 2012)

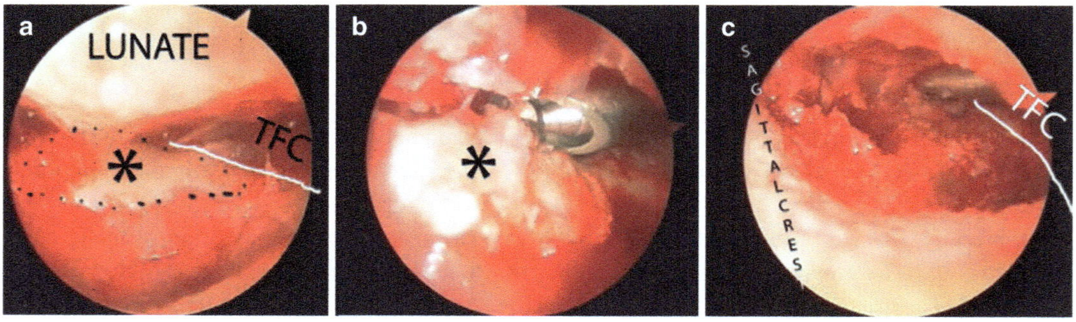

Fig. 39.8 (**a**) A protruding volar-ulnar fragment (*asterisk*) has caused a major cartilage defect on the lunate. (**b**) A 2.9 mm burr is contouring the fragment. (**c**) At the end of the operation, about 50 % of the anterior lunate fossa has been removed (the 2.9 mm shaver on the far volar-ulnar corner of the radius helps to approximate the size of the defect) (© Piñal in del Piñal et al. 2012)

months, were very satisfactory (del Piñal et al. 2012).

- Remodelling of the resected area was evident on radiograms, and there was neither cyst formation nor narrowing of the joint (Fig. 39.9).
- Admittedly, with the small number of patients and relatively short follow-up period, no definitive conclusions can be made regarding the long-term efficacy of this procedure.
- However, it may provide either a temporary alternative to partial wrist arthrodesis with minimal morbidity for active patients or perhaps a definitive operation for less demanding patients.
- This procedure has the advantage of minimal morbidity, keeping multiple future treatment

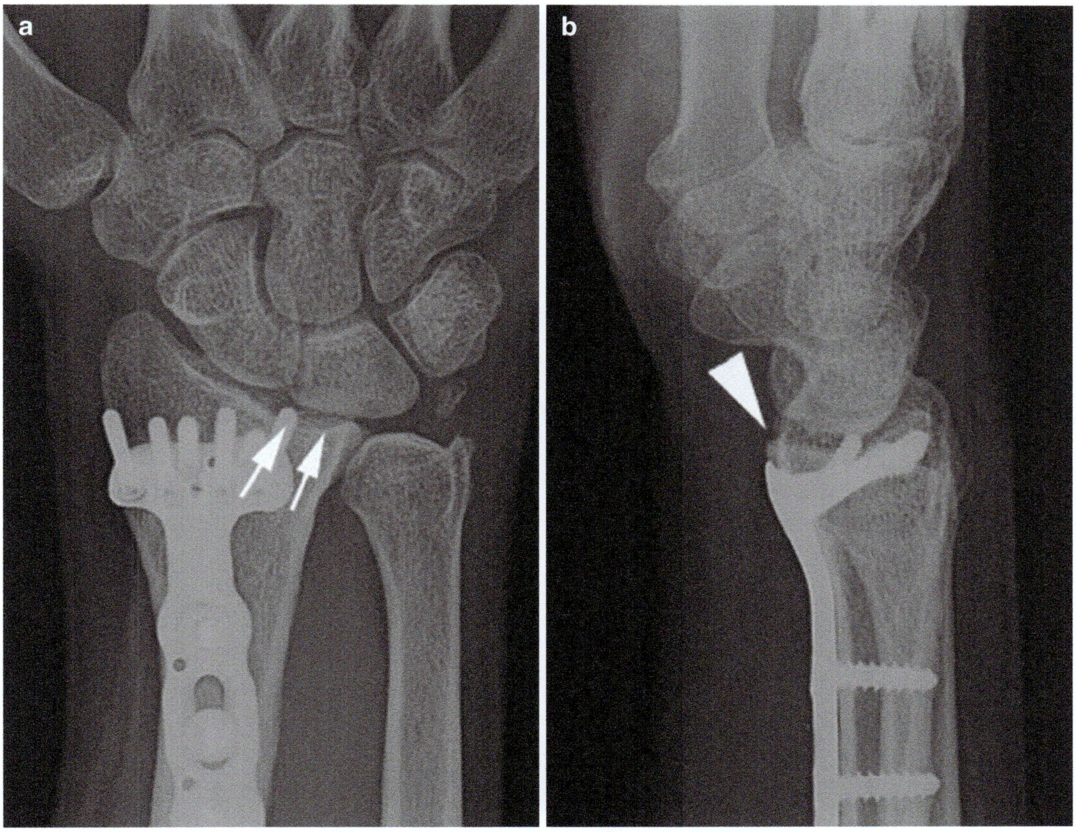

Fig. 39.9 (**a**, **b**) Radiograms at 3.5 years after the arthroplasty operation. Remodelling of the lunate fossa is evident and marked with *arrows*. Notice removal of the radius spur on the lateral view (*arrow head*) (same patient as Figs. 39.6, 39.8 and 39.9) (© Piñal in del Piñal et al. 2012)

options open, allowing immediate range of motion and providing pain relief at least in the short term.

- Although speculative, the operation is probably not indicated when more than 50 % of the radius surface is involved even if the rest of the joint surface is completely intact, as the risk of overloading the healthy part of the joint will be high.

39.6 Vascularized Osteochondral Graft

- If a large segment of the cartilage of the scaphoid or lunate fossae is irreversibly damaged, the only option is to perform some form of radiocarpal fusion: radiolunate (RL) or radio-scapho-lunate (RSL) fusion. Partial fusions, however, limit the range of motion at the wrist and overload the adjacent mobile joints.
- The blood supply of the deep layers of the subchondral bone is important in cartilage metabolism as vascularized joints maintain the articular space in the long term (Tsubokawa et al 2003), while nonvascularized joints collapse (Entin et al 1962).
- We have for several years been using the base of the third metatarsal as a vascularized osteochondral graft to reconstruct major articular defects on the radius articular surface (del Piñal et al. 2005, 2013).
- The base of the third metatarsal has a principal facet that we use for reconstructing the radius articular surface, and an accessory facet to the fourth metatarsal, which is invaluable to reconstruct the sigmoid notch (Fig. 39.10).

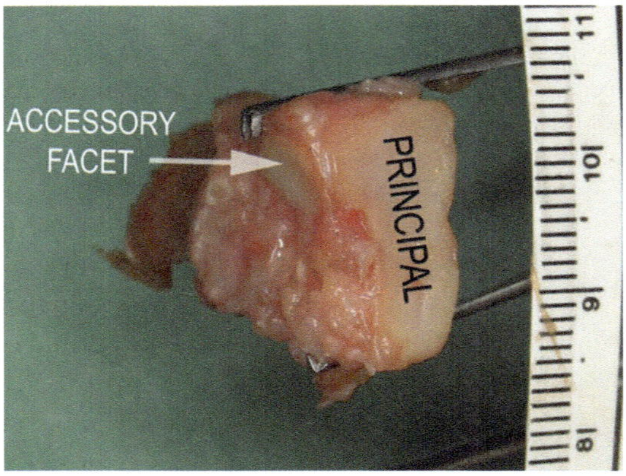

Fig. 39.10 Left third metatarsal base seen with proximal aspect in the foreground. Notice that there is accessory facet located in the most dorsal portion of the lateral side which as very useful when reconstructing the sigmoid notch (© Piñal in del Piñal et al. 2013)

- The operation requires microsurgical expertise but allows patients to maintain pain free range of motion.
- The main indication is when both the lunate facet and sigmoid notch are involved: with a single flap, the radiocarpal and distal radioulnar relationships and function are restored (Fig. 39.11).
- Due to size limitations, a flap cannot replace both the scaphoid and lunate facet at the same time. The operation cannot be done if the whole radius surface is involved.

39.6.1 Surgical Technique

- Planning is paramount and if the sigmoid notch also needs to be reconstructed only the contralateral donor side will match (Fig. 39.12). The recipient site should be assessed first as to know the donor site requirements.
- The wrist was approached through a longitudinal dorsal midline incision. The extensor pollicis longus was released from the 3rd extensor compartment, and the 2nd and 4th extensor compartments were dissected subperiosteally from the radius. The posterior interosseous nerve was identified and divided. The affected area of the distal radius was removed with an osteotome, sagittal saw or rongeur as needed. This excision included the metaphyseal bone in order to create a 3-dimensional defect to allow for placement of the flap. At this point, corrective osteotomies were performed for any salvageable malpositioned fragment (usually the volar fragments).
- To raise the flap, the foot is approached though a zigzag incision in the cleft between the extensor hallucis longus and the extensor digitorum longus (del Piñal et al. 2005). The extensor hallucis brevis is cut and retracted laterally together with the extensor digitorum longus, which will expose the blood supply to the dorsum of the foot (Fig. 39.13a). Once the anatomy is clear the base of the metatarsal is cut and a pedicle is based on the dorsalis pedis artery. A skin monitor is elevated in every case to control the transplant (Fig. 39.13b). The osteochondral graft is tailored to fit into the defect and rigidly fixed. Revascularization is done end to side to the radial artery and to local veins (Figs. 39.14 and 39.15).
- The donor site is simply closed under an aspirative drainage.
- Partial weight bearing on a rigid shoe is allowed after 3–5 days. On follow-up radiograms the metatarsal recedes slightly which seems to be the key of not having had any case of metatarsalgia to date.

39.6.2 Clinical Experience

- Our experience is limited to 7 patients (range 26–55 years).
- The majority had the lunate facet and sigmoid notch reconstructed.
- All flaps survived without complications. Good results have been obtained in the long term in this limited cohort (del Piñal et al. 2013).

39.7 Partial Arthrodeses

- When a major part of the radius articular surface and/or the opposing carpal bones are destroyed, few alternatives are left apart from some form of partial arthrodesis, i.e. RL or RSL arthrodesis.

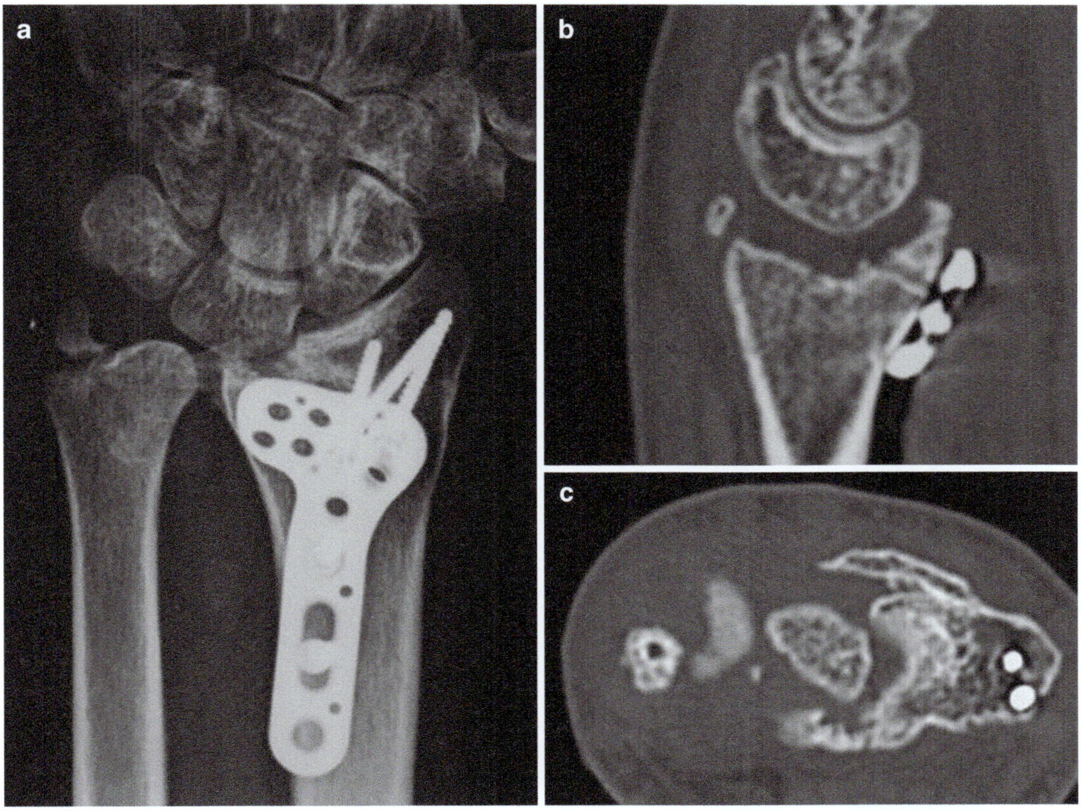

Fig. 39.11 The ideal candidate for the index operation: (**a**) A massive osteochondral defect of one of the facets of the radius. The scaphoid fossa was not damaged. (**b**) and (**c**) The sigmoid notch and lunate facet had cartilage damage, but the lunate and ulnar head cartilage were well preserved (© Piñal in del Piñal et al. 2013)

- Other types of motion preserved operations might be denervation or wrist replacement.
- The description of these techniques is beyond this chapter, but both RL and RSL arthrodeses can be done with arthroscopic assistance (Ho 2008) (Fig. 39.16).
- However, a high failure rate approaching 40 % in the short term has been reported (Mühldorfer-Fodor et al. 2012) so currently this form of salvage should be offered cautiously. It is however encouraging those complex fixations can be done through minimally invasive surgery.

39.8 Ulnar Side Procedures

Ulnar-sided pathology always accompanies the more obvious radius deformity and is a major cause of persistent pain and secondary surgery. Impaction, incongruity, instability and stiffness can all be present together, or separately, and be responsible, in differing degrees, for the patient's symptoms. The specific treatment of each one of these conditions is covered in other chapters.

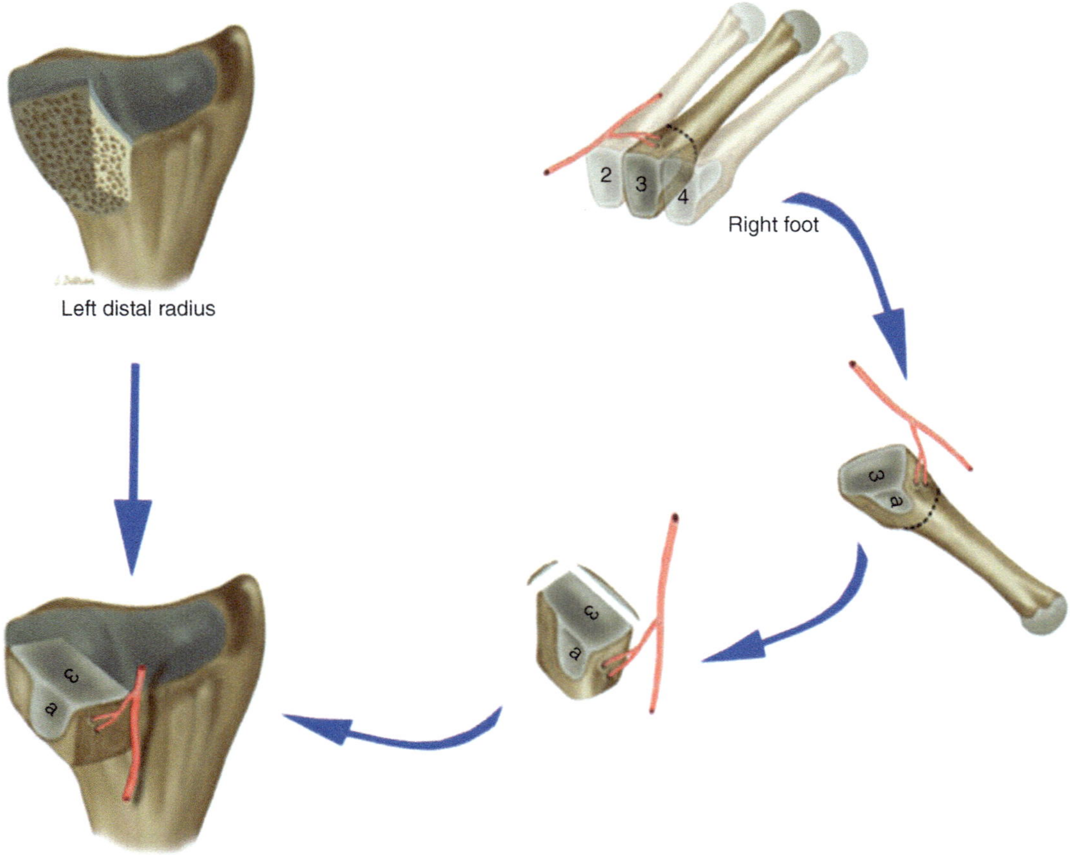

Fig. 39.12 In order to reconstruct the typical dorsoulnar radius malunited scenario, where the defect involves not only the lunate facet but also the dorsal aspect of the sigmoid notch, the contralateral metatarsal needs to be harvested (© Piñal in del Piñal et al. 2013)

Conclusions

- Intra-articular malunion should be looked upon as a surgical urgency in order to prevent irreversible damage of the cartilage surfaces.
- It is important to have a clear decision-making process and use an algorithm based upon the degree of cartilage damage (Fig 39.1).
- Good results can be achieved if the appropriate choice is made.
- Clear indications in operative planning, both preoperatively and during the procedure, is paramount for success. However, these patients are often difficult to handle due to previous experience, pain, etc.

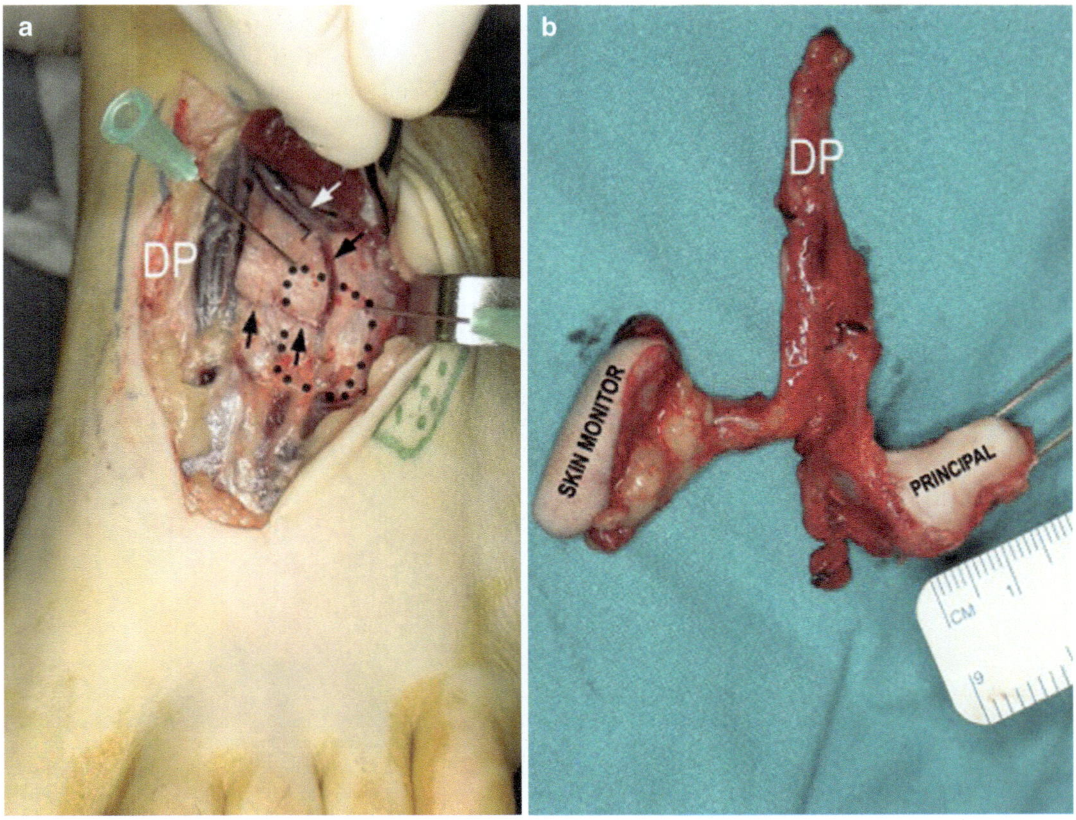

Fig. 39.13 Intraoperative view during flap harvesting. (**a**) The vessels going to the base of the third metatarsal (limited by *dots*) are highlighted by *arrows*. (**b**) The harvested flap which includes a skin monitor and the base of the third metatarsal (*DP* dorsalis pedis) (© Piñal in del Piñal et al. 2010)

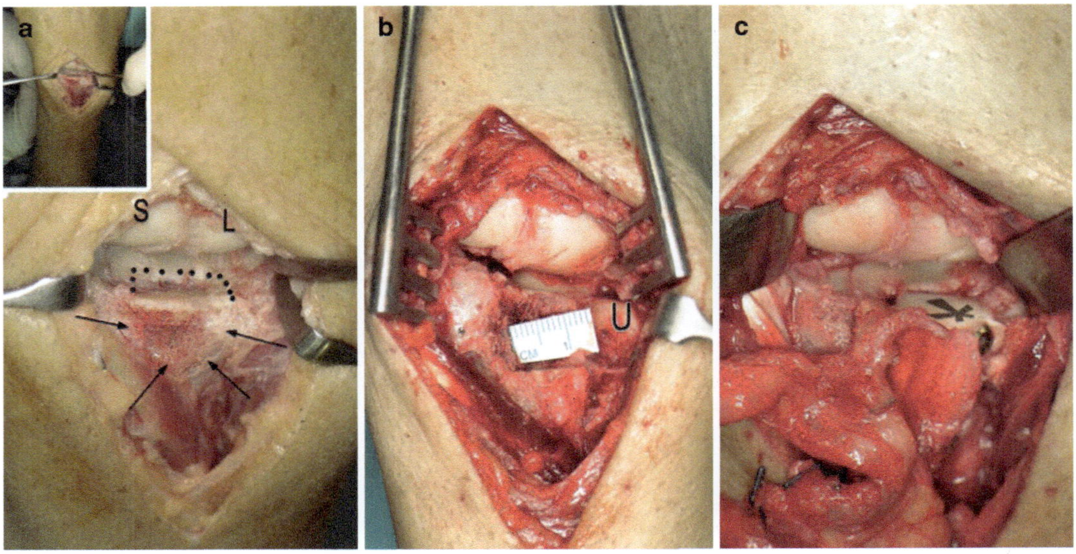

Fig. 39.14 Intraoperative view (*Inset* panoramic view). (**a**) Area of scarring and irregularities on the dorsoulnar aspect of the radius can be seen only after the hypertrophic dorsal rim was removed (*arrows*). (**b**) A three-dimensional defect has been created exposing the ulnar head (*U*). (**c**) The graft has been fixed with two screws (© Piñal in del Piñal et al. 2010)

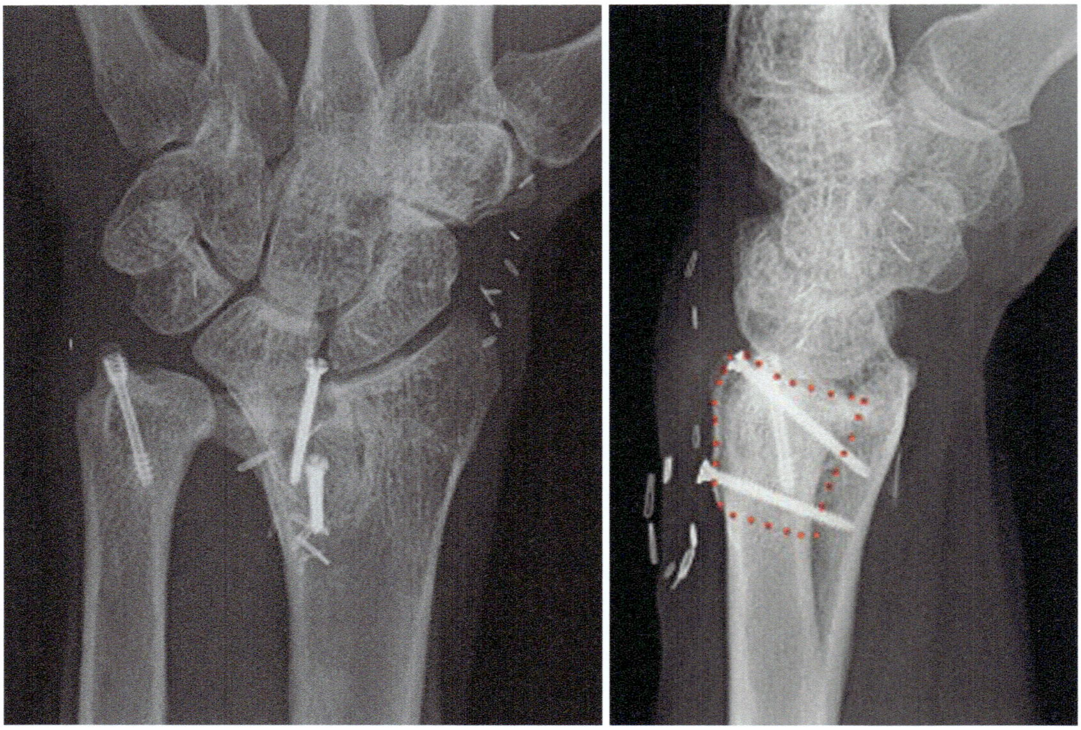

Fig. 39.15 PA and lateral X-rays at 2 years, in the same patient as Fig. 39.12 with the graft in position (marked with *red dots*). Notice that the nonunited ulnar styloid was also fixed in the same operation (© Piñal in del Piñal et al. 2013)

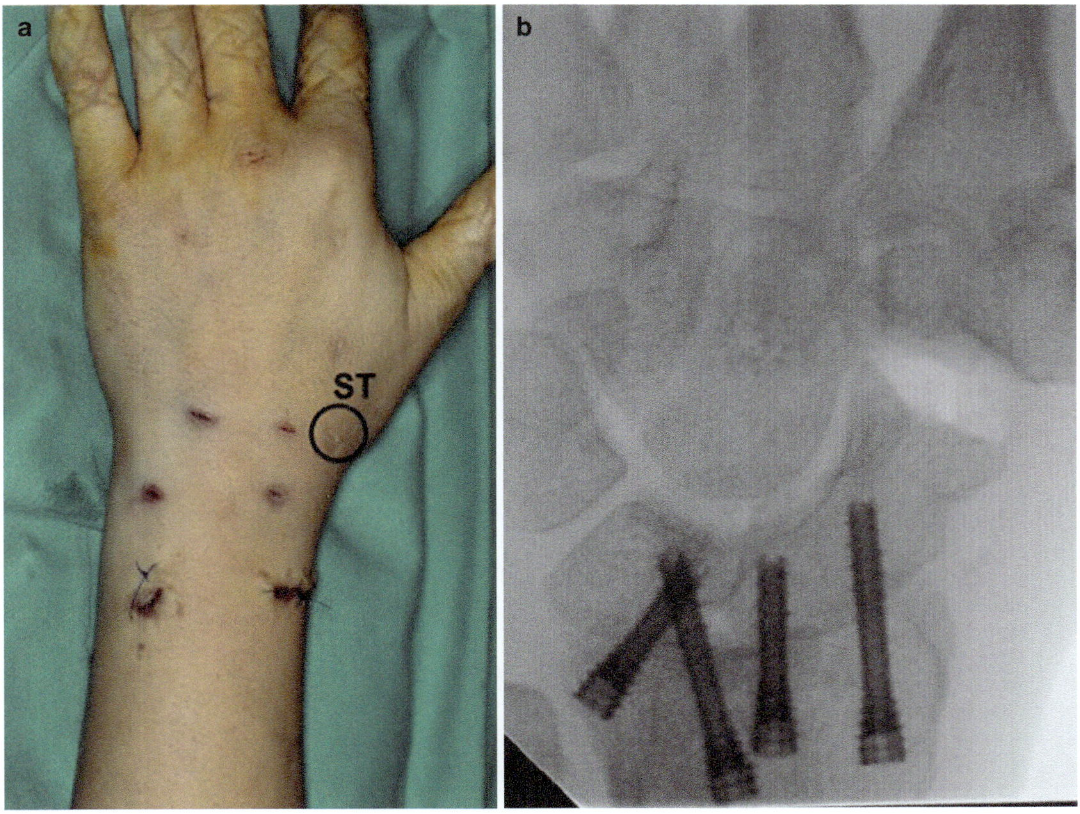

Fig. 39.16 (**a**) Notice minimal swelling at the end of the arthroscopically assisted radio-scapho-lunate arthrodesis, with resection of the distal pole of the scaphoid carried out through the ST portal. Cannulated screws were inserted through the proximal incisions (sutured most prox incisions). (**b**) Fluoroscopic view of the fixation (© Dr. Piñal, 2013)

References

Amadio PC, Botte MJ. Treatment of malunion of the distal radius. Hand Clin. 1987;3(4):541–61.

del Piñal F. Dry arthroscopy of the wrist: its role in the management of articular distal radius fractures. Scand J Surg. 2008;97:298–304.

del Piñal F, García-Bernal FJ, Delgado J, Sanmartín M, Regalado J. Reconstruction of the distal radius facet by a free vascularized osteochondral autograft: anatomic study and report of a patient. J Hand Surg Am. 2005;30(6):1200–10.

del Piñal F, García-Bernal FJ, Delgado J, Sanmartín M, Regalado J, Cerezal L. Correction of malunited intra-articular distal radius fractures with an inside-out osteotomy technique. J Hand Surg Am. 2006;31:1029–34.

del Piñal F, Cagigal L, García-Bernal FJ, Studer A, Regalado J, Thams C. Arthroscopically guided osteotomy for management of intra-articular distal radius malunions. J Hand Surg Am. 2010;35(3):392–7.

del Piñal F, Klausmeyer M, Thams C, Moraleda E, Galindo C. Arthroscopic resection arthroplasty for malunited intra-articular distal radius fractures. J Hand Surg Am. 2012;37(12):2447–55.

del Piñal F, Klausmeyer M, Thams C, Moraleda E, Galindo C, Studer A, Cerezal L. Vascularized graft from the metatarsal base for reconstructing major osteochondral distal radius defects. J Hand Surg Am. 2013:38A(10):1883–95.

Edwards III CC, Harasztic J, McGillivary GR, Gutow AP. Intra-articular distal radius fractures: arthroscopic assessment of radiographically assisted reduction. J Hand Surg. 2001;26A:1036–41.

Entin MA, Alger JR, Baird RM. Experimental and clinical transplantation of autogenous whole joints. J Bone Joint Surg. 1962;44A:1518–36.

Ho PC. Arthroscopic partial wrist fusion. Tech Hand Up Extrem Surg. 2008;12:242–65.

Knirk JL, Jupiter JB. Intra-articular fractures of the distal end of the radius in young adults. J Bone Joint Surg Am. 1986;68(5):647–59.

Mühldorfer-Fodor M, Ha HP, Hohendorff B, Löw S, Prommersberger KJ, van Schoonhoven J. Results after radioscapholunate arthrodesis with or without resection of the distal scaphoid pole. J Hand Surg Am. 2012;37(11):2233–39.

Trumble TE, Schmitt SR, Vedder NB. Factors affecting functional outcome of displaced intra-articular distal radius fractures. J Hand Surg Am. 1994;19(2): 325–40.

Tsubokawa N, Yoshizu T, Maki Y. Long-term results of free vascularized second toe joint transfers to finger proximal interphalangeal joints. J Hand Surg Am. 2003;28:443–7.

Wagner Jr WF, Tencer AF, Kiser P, Trumble TE. Effects of intra-articular distal radius depression on wrist joint contact characteristics. J Hand Surg Am. 1996;21(4): 554–60.

Distal Radius Fractures and Secondary Carpal Dysfunction

40

Marc Garcia-Elias and Guillem Salva-Coll

Contents

M. Garcia-Elias, MD, PhD
Consultant in Hand and Upper Extremity Surgery, Institut Kaplan, Passeig de la Bonanova, 9, 2°2ª, 08022 Barcelona, Spain
e-mail: garciaelias@institut-kaplan.com

G. Salva-Coll, MD, PhD
Department of Orthopaedics, Consultant in Hand and Wrist Surgery, Institut Balear de Cirurgia de Mà and Hospital Universitari Son Espases, Palma de Mallorca, Spain

40.1 Summary

The goal of treatment of a distal radial fracture is to promote bone healing and prevent complications. If these goals are not achieved, the joint may become either stiff or unstable. Instability and stiffness are at the two ends of a spectrum of dysfunctions that may appear after a distal radial fracture. Instability would be characterized by excessive passive mobility (kinematic instability) and/or inability of sustaining physiologic loads without yielding (kinetic instability). Stiffness may allow resisting loads, but may prevent normal movement. After a distal radius fracture, most carpal instabilities are secondary to radius malunion plus a variable degree of muscle imbalance and ligament insufficiency. Malunion and muscle imbalance may be prevented by proper fracture stabilization and muscle reeducation. Detecting ligament tears when the radius is fractured is not easy. When missed at presentation, chronic instability may appear. Certainly, it is difficult to discern which injuries are harmless and which are potential wrist destabilizers. This chapter will review how to diagnose and manage chronic carpal instabilities secondary to a distal radius fracture.

40.2 Introduction

- It has often been said that a fracture is a soft tissue injury complicated by a broken bone. Paraphrasing that statement, we could say

L.M. Hove et al. (eds.), *Distal Radius Fractures*, DOI 10.1007/978-3-642-54604-4_40, © Springer-Verlag Berlin Heidelberg 2014 that a distal radius fracture is an intracarpal derangement complicated by a broken distal radius. From minor elongations to complete tears of various carpal ligaments, a spectrum of soft tissue injuries may accompany a distal radius fracture.

- In the last two decades, several investigations have used wrist arthroscopy to determine the incidence of associated intracarpal ligament ruptures in patients with a distal radius fracture (Table 40.1) (Geissler et al. 1996; Lindau et al. 1997; Richards et al. 1997; Mehta et al. 2000; Shih et al. 2001; Kordasiewicz et al. 2006; Forward et al. 2007). Before those studies, such injuries were believed to be unusual and harmless. Now we know that they are not infrequent and probably less benign than previously assumed.
- Posttraumatic carpal instability may appear under different clinical forms:
  1. Adaptive malalignment secondary to fracture malunion
  2. Non-dissociative radiocarpal dysfunction with intact scapholunate (SL) and lunotriquetral (LT) joints
  3. Non-dissociative midcarpal dysfunction
  4. SL dissociative problem with the lunate adopting a "dorsal intercalated segment instability" (DISI) pattern of malalignment
  5. LT dissociative problem with "volar intercalated segment instability" (VISI) pattern of malalignment (Garcia-Elias 2011).

Table 40.1 Incidence of scapholunate (SL) and lunotriquetral (LT) injury associated to a distal radial fracture, according to different authors

Authors	*N*	SL (%)	LTq (%)
Geissler et al. (1996)	60[a]	32	15
Lindau et al. (1997)	50[c]	54	65
Richards et al. (1997)	64[a]	21	7
Richards et al. (1997)	73[b]	7	13
Mehta et al. (2000)	31[a]	85	61
Mathoulin et al. (2001)	27[a]	37	15
Shih et al. (2001)	33[a]	18	12
Kordasiewicz et al. (2006)	21[a]	33	5
Forward et al. (2007)	51[c]	86	29
Varitimidis et al. (2008)	20[a]	45	20
Total	430	41	22

[a]Intra-articular fractures
[b]Extraarticular fractures
[c]Intra- and extraarticular fractures

40.3 Adaptive Carpal Malalignment

- Once fractured, the distal radius fragment may displace and consolidate in a variety of ways: it may rotate along the sagittal, the axial, and/or the coronal planes, but also it may translate palmarly, dorsally, radially, or proximally. Combining all possible displacements, there are at least 120 different forms of distal radius malunion. Of all, the most frequent deformity is one in which the distal radius fragment has healed abnormally extended, proximally migrated, and slightly supinated relative to the radius shaft.
- Patients with an abnormal tilt of their distal articular surface of the radius do not keep the hand inclined along the malunited distal fragment; usually, they realign it along the longitudinal axis of the forearm. For instance, if the distal fragment is extended and supinated, the patient will position the metacarpals in flexion and pronation to compensate for the distal radius deformity. This implies that some ligaments are permanently taut while others are relaxed. The consequence is an abnormal carpal kinematics. Despite the misalignment, however, there is not an intrinsic carpal pathology needing repair; it is an adaptive phenomenon which will disappear when the deformity is corrected (Fig. 40.1). This particular type of malalignment has been called "carpal instability adaptive" (Garcia-Elias 2011; Wolfe et al. 2012) and should not be confused with the malalignment induced by intracarpal pathology (Box 40.1). With time, such an abnormal alignment may cause permanent damage to the ligaments resisting more strain, and the case may evolve into a true dissociative pattern of instability.
- Instability and pain at the midcarpal joint secondary to distal radius malunions should therefore be treated by a distal radius osteotomy and

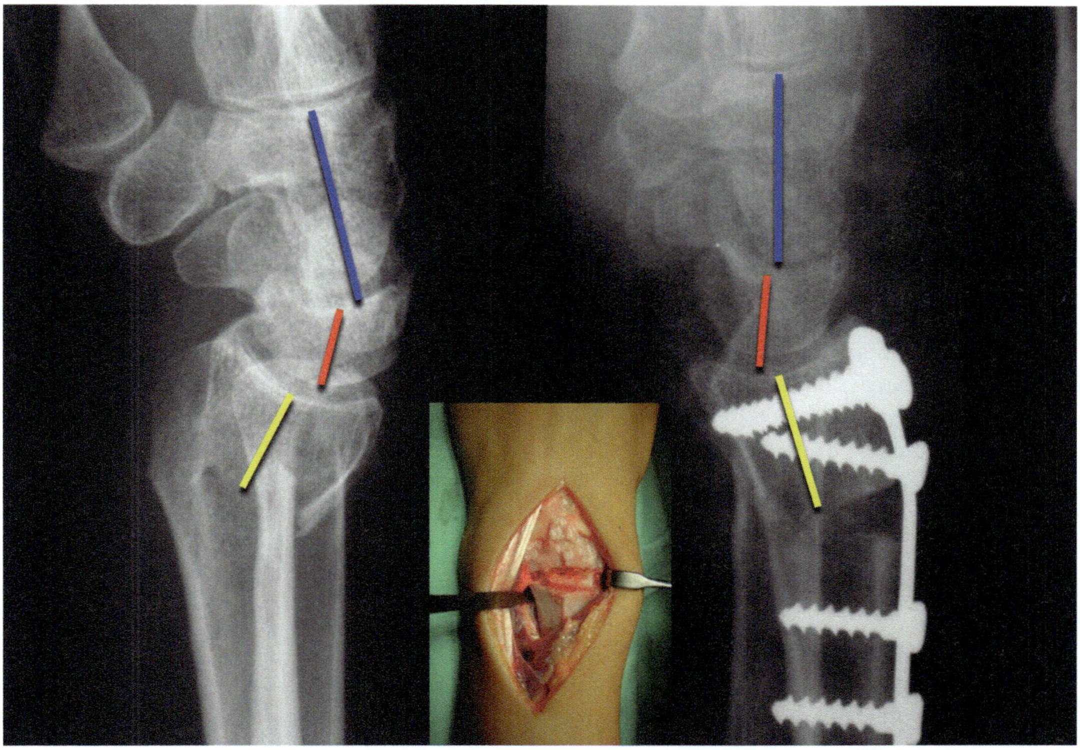

Fig. 40.1 Adaptive carpal malalignment. The distal fragment is tilted dorsally, the lunate is in DISI, and the distal row is in flexion. An open wedge osteotomy, stabilized with a dorsal plate, brought the carpal alignment to normal (*color lines*)

not with a midcarpal soft tissue stabilization (Taleisnik and Watson 1984). This condition should not be categorized as a true midcarpal instability, as the cause of the instability is not a ligament derangement but a repetitive overload of the midcarpal joint capsule and ligaments. This view would be supported by the fact that the instability often manifests months after the injury.

Box 40.1: Adaptive Carpal Malalignment: Pearls and Pitfalls

- Radius deformity is the primary cause of the midcarpal dysfunction. Because the underlying pathology is not in the carpus, this type of instability has been called "extrinsic" or "adaptive."
- When there is malalignment, the lunate often appears rotated into extension adopting a dorsal intercalated segment instability type deformity (DISI).
- In this type of dorsal CIND (carpal instability non-dissociative), the capitate is reduced in neutral or radial deviation and subluxates dorsally in ulnar deviation.
- Treatment should address the bone deformity, usually restored by a corrective osteotomy.

40.3.1 Pathomechanics

- In the presence of a malunited distal radius, the primary cause of midcarpal dysfunction is the radius deformity. In some cases, there may also be a secondary insufficiency of the extrinsic ligaments. When these ligaments are inadequate to resist dorsolaterally

directed forces, the lunate tends to rotate into extension, adopting a DISI type of deformity, while the capitate adopts a flexed position to realign the hand along the forearm axis (Wolfe et al. 2012).
- Patients with distal radius malunion may present with clunking and pain in the dorsoradial corner of the wrist. That pain may be explained as the consequence of the capitate subluxing over the dorsal rim of the midcarpal socket in ulnar deviation. Postural adaptation of the carpal bones to the abnormal radial slope, inducing distension of the dorsal intercarpal ligament, explains such an extrinsic carpal clunking.

40.3.2 Treatment

- It is important to emphasize that, in these cases, the underlying pathology is not in the carpus and that carpal dysfunction disappears when the radius deformity is corrected by an osteotomy (Taleisnik and Watson 1984; Wolfe et al. 2012).
- Sometimes the distal radius deformity is not in the sagittal but in the coronal plane, often in the form of an increased inclination of the radius articular surface and an ulna minus variance. In such instances, a radioulnar leveling procedure plus normalization of the distal radial slope by a closing wedge osteotomy has been used (Garcia-Elias 2011; Wolfe et al. 2012). This appears to inhibit the rotational clunking of the proximal row by pushing the triangular fibrocartilage complex (TFCC) against the ulnar corner of the lunate.
- Additional intracarpal soft tissue procedures are only occasionally necessary.

40.4 Radiocarpal Instability

- The palmar extrinsic radio- and ulnocarpal ligaments have been portrayed as two inverted V-shaped ligamentous bands arising from the radius and the ulna; the proximal V converges onto the palmar aspect of the lunate and the distal V onto the palmar aspect of the neck of the capitate. These ligaments are disposed in superficial and deep layers. The only dorsal extrinsic radiocarpal ligament is the dorsal radiotriquetral ligament.
- It is known that, under load, the normal carpus has an inherent tendency to slide down ulnarly and palmarly due to the inclined distal articular surface of the radius. This tendency is resisted by the palmar and dorsal radiocarpal ligaments, which oblique disposition is ideal to resist such subluxing forces.
- If the ligaments fail, the carpus, or rather the carpal condyle, may sublux or even dislocate in a palmar and ulnar direction. In normal circumstances, the extrinsic radiocarpal ligaments do not disrupt completely in the course of a distal radius fracture. However, if the fracture has displaced dorsoradially, the carpal condyle will be forced to sublux in a direction that the extrinsic radiocarpal ligaments cannot constrain. In such cases, the only ligaments that could hold the carpus in place would be the ulnocarpal, but those are often avulsed off the fovea together with the rest of the TFCC. The radiocarpal dysfunction so created should be categorized as a carpal instability non-dissociative (CIND) (Box 40.2) (Wolfe et al. 2012).
- The contact area and peak pressure change significantly when the distal radius is dorsally angulated (Pogue et al. 1990). As the dorsal tilt increases, the centroids of load across the radioscaphoid and radiolunate joints shift dorsally with a final point where the scaphoid stands the dorsoradial edge of the joint, where there is no cartilage. It is assumed that the loss of volar tilt may cause extension to the lunate and a compensatory flexion of the capitate or a dorsal subluxation of the radiocarpal joint, which in turn may lead to degenerative osteoarthritis.
- Surgical management of a radiocarpal dysfunction secondary to malunited distal radius fracture is based on the correction of the radius deformity (Fig. 40.2a–g). The osteotomy needs to be carefully planned and

executed to restore the normal length, volar tilt, radial inclination, and axial rotation of the distal radius. By restoring the radius anatomy, tension of the undisrupted ligaments and surrounding tendons is rebalanced.

- Only exceptionally the torn ligaments need to be repaired to stabilize the carpus. For this to be necessary, the tears must be massive, in which case a partial radiocarpal fusion may be more effective than an unpredictable ligament repair.
- Because the clinical result depends on the status of the articular surfaces, the corrective osteotomy should be performed before the development of osteoarthritic changes. If left untreated, these wrists develop early osteoarthritis either at the radiocarpal joint, at the midcarpal joint, or both (Fig. 40.3).

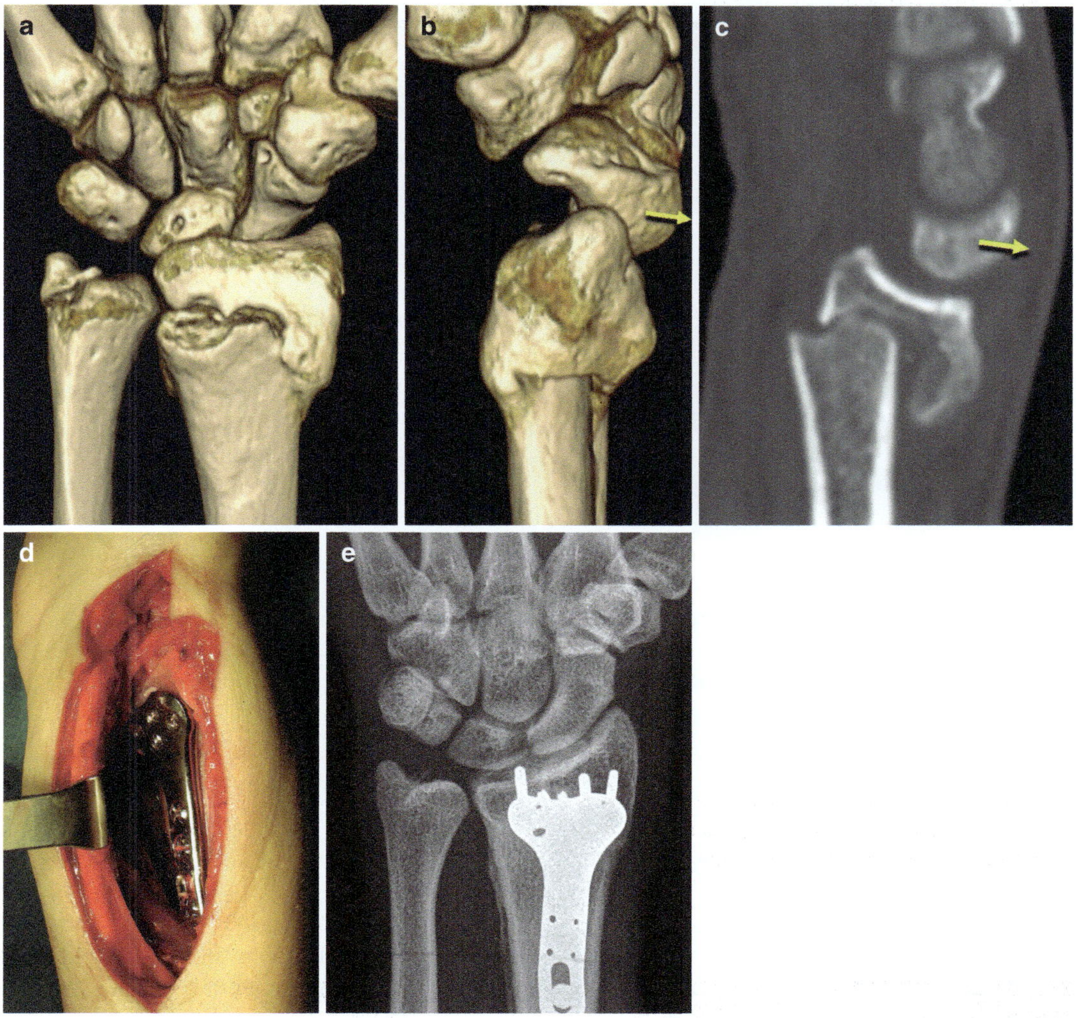

Fig. 40.2 (**a**–**c**) An 18-year-old man, university student, sustained a dorsoradially displaced extraarticular distal radius fracture while practicing motocross. The injury was treated by closed reduction and cast immobilization. The fracture healed into a dysfunctional malunion: the malrotated distal fragment had healed in pronation, extension, and slight radial deviation and both scaphoid and lunate exhibited a dorsoradial subluxation over the dorsoradial rim of the radius as seen in the 3D reconstruction and sagittal CT scan image (*yellow arrow*). (**d**, **e**) A corrective osteotomy, stabilized with a fixed-angle volar plate, was done. (**f**, **g**) Clinical result at final follow-up

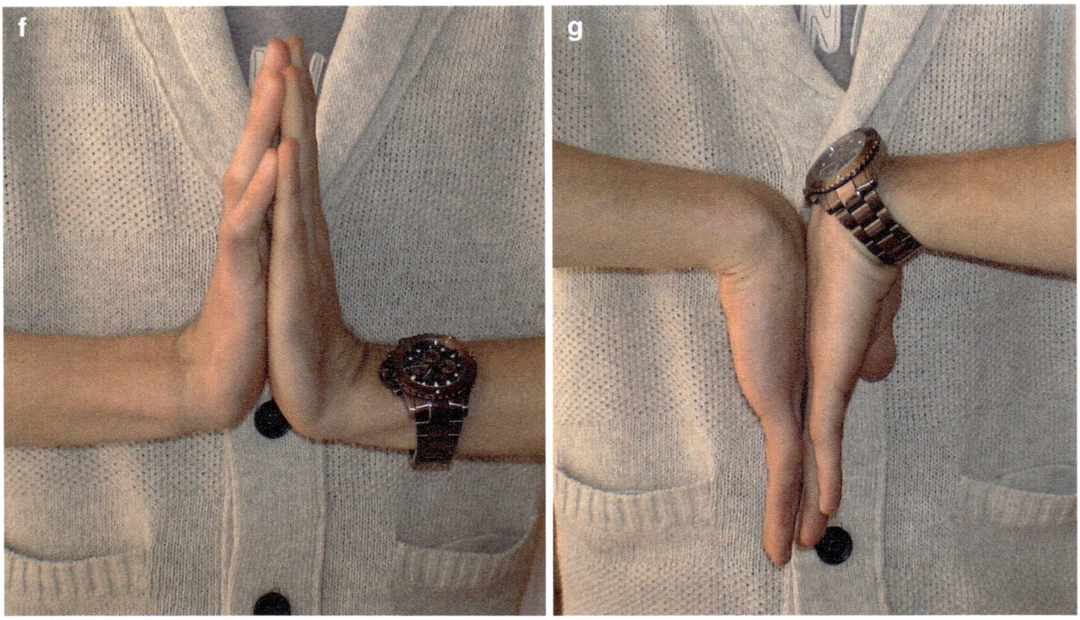

Fig. 40.2 (continued)

Box 40.2: Radiocarpal Instability: Pearls and Pitfalls

- The tendency of the radiocarpal joint to slide down ulnarly and palmarly due to the inclined distal articular surface of the radius is resisted by both palmar and dorsal radiocarpal ligaments.
- Subluxation of the radiocarpal joint may occur acutely, indicating complete radiocarpal ligament ruptures or as radiocarpal fracture dislocations, or in the chronic phase, as a result of ligament failure due to chronic overload.
- Most cases respond well by restoring the normal length and inclination of the distal radius surface with a corrective osteotomy.

40.5 Midcarpal Dysfunction

- A variety of conditions (fractures, ligament injuries, congenital defects, bone deformities, etc.) may result in midcarpal dysfunction. The combination of a true palmar midcarpal instability and a distal radius fracture is very rare.
- Midcarpal instability is one of the most challenging forms of carpal instability.
- It induces sudden positional changes of the distal row relative to the proximal row in a variety of ways (dorsal, palmar, combined). Abnormal kinematics of the radiocarpal joint may also be part of the problem.
- Each form of midcarpal instability has its own pathophysiology, each deserving specific treatment (Garcia-Elias 2011; Wolfe et al. 2012).

40.6 Scapholunate Dissociation

- In general, it is admitted that one segment never presents with two injuries occurring at the same time. In the wrist, the disrupting energy is usually spent either disrupting the distal radius metaphysis or producing an intracarpal derangement.
- Most commonly, a hyperextension injury to the wrist results in a distal radius fracture, while a hyperextension-ulnar deviation-supination injury results in an intracarpal ligament rupture.

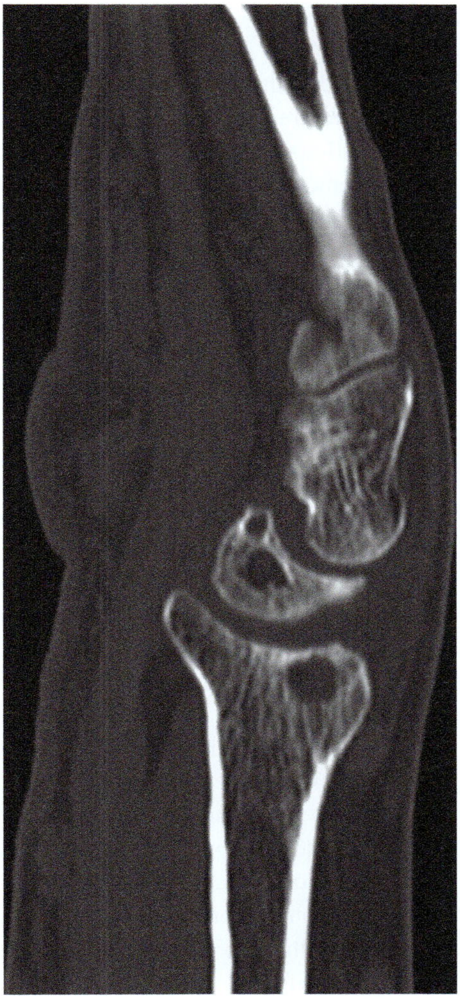

Fig. 40.3 CT sagittal image of a dorsal malunion of the distal radius that developed a chronic dorsal midcarpal instability, with early midcarpal degeneration characterized by joint narrowing and subchondral cysts

- In the first case, the unstable distal fragment may displace in different ways. If there is a predominant proximal impaction, the fracture may become stable again. In that case, the traumatizing energy may keep on twisting the wrist, inducing a progressive interosseous perilunate derangement, usually starting at the SL joint, and progressing ulnarly to cause a perilunate dislocation. Indeed, in those cases, the SL tear would be the first stage of a more extended perilunate destabilization pattern (Box 40.3) (Garcia-Elias 2011).
- About one third of all fractures of the distal radius have an associated SL ligament injury (Table 40.1). Intra-articular fractures are more prone to have concomitant ligament injury. Most often, the SL injury consists of a partial tear of the anterior and proximal components of the SL interosseous complex, stages 1 to 3 according to Geissler et al.'s classification (1996). Complete ruptures are much less frequent.
- If those ligaments do not heal spontaneously, an overall carpal dysfunction may appear progressively as a result of failure of the secondary scaphoid stabilizers, namely, the scaphotrapezial-trapezoidal (STT), scaphocapitate (SC), and radioscaphocapitate (RSC) ligaments.
- Multiple treatment options have been proposed to salvage these forms of carpal instability when symptomatic. From capsule tenodesis to bone-ligament-bone transfers and from partial fusions to proximal row carpectomies, there are multiple treatment alternatives all aiming to recover acceptable function with minimum morbidity (Garcia-Elias et al. 2006).
- Restoring function in such cases involves not only regaining adequate range of motion but also recovering the ability of carrying physiologic loads without yielding.

Box 40.3: Scapholunate Instability: Pearls and Pitfalls

- About 40 % of all distal radial fractures have a concomitant SL ligament injury.
- Intra-articular fractures are more prone to have these ligament injuries in line with the progressive greater arch mechanism seen in perilunate dislocations.
- The more common pattern of SL injury consists of a partial tear of the SL interosseous complex.
- Arthroscopy is the best way to diagnose not only SL tears but also all associated injuries and to evaluate the cartilage, key point to determine the best method of treatment.

- The rigidity of the carpal collapse and the degree of secondary degenerative changes must be determined, since they will influence treatment alternatives.
- Each stage of progressive instability deserves a different strategy depending on individual needs, injury characteristics, and chronicity of the dysfunction.

40.6.1 Diagnosis

- Certain fracture patterns are more prone to be associated with ligament injuries than others. Particular attention needs to be paid to all intra-articular fractures involving the inter-facet prominence between the scaphoid and lunate fossae and the so-called "die-punch" fractures. In addition, horizontal shear fractures of the radial styloid are also associated with SL ligament damage, in line with the greater arch mechanism of the perilunate dislocation.
- Patients with SL instability present with a history of pain and weakness. As the scaphoid malalignment increases, the adjacent joints become dysfunctional, making for a global carpal destabilization characterized by pain and decreased grip strength. A typical snap may appear during radial inclination as a result of the proximal scaphoid subluxing over the dorsolateral rim of the radius.
- In distal radius malunion it could be difficult to assess carpal angles. Indirect radiographic signs of SL tears may be seen, such as an increased gap at the SL joint or a subluxation of the scaphoid over the dorsal edge of the malunited radius. CT or MRI arthrogram is the next option to diagnose such ligament injuries.
- Arthroscopy is the final and best way to diagnose not only SL tears but all associated injuries and to evaluate the cartilage of the radiocarpal and midcarpal joints, key point to determine the best method of treatment.
- The rigidity of the carpal collapse and the degree of secondary degenerative changes must be determined, since they will influence treatment alternatives.

40.6.2 Treatment

- None of the therapeutic options reported in the literature have been shown to be efficient in all stages of instability nor is there full agreement on when each technique is eligible. Each stage of progressive instability deserves a different strategy depending on a number of factors including individual needs, injury characteristics, and chronicity of the dysfunction.
- If distal radius malunion is present, it should be taken in consideration when planning the SL ligament reconstruction, regardless of the treatment that will be performed, as a distal radius osteotomy could be mandatory when planning the definitive treatment.
- Chronic SL tears without wrist arthritis have been reconstructed by a variety of procedures including limited carpal arthrodesis, capsulodesis, and tenodesis. Carpal-based capsulodesis and tenodesis have been advocated to ameliorate the tethering effect of dorsal distal radius-based capsulodeses and tenodeses. These procedures alone may improve or restore the adaptive midcarpal collapse, but they do not reestablish SL continuity and kinematic integration. Consequently, outcomes after these procedures are relatively similar and often only palliative. Recently, interest has been revived in dynamic tendon transfers as an alternative to capsulodesis or tenodesis (Peterson and Freeland 2010) (Fig. 40.4a, b).
- In late presented cases after fracture union, the SL joint may remain unstable clinically and dissociated radiographically. In such instances, not only the ligaments have to be repaired or reconstructed, but the secondary capsular contractures have to be released, in order to both facilitate reduction of the SL joint and recover an acceptable and durable hand function generally. It is particularly important to excise the fibrosis that obliterates the space of Poirier palmarly and the capsule of the scaphotrapezoid joint dorsally. Unless all this is done correctly, the ligamentoplasty is not going to be successful. Occasionally, in combined problems with

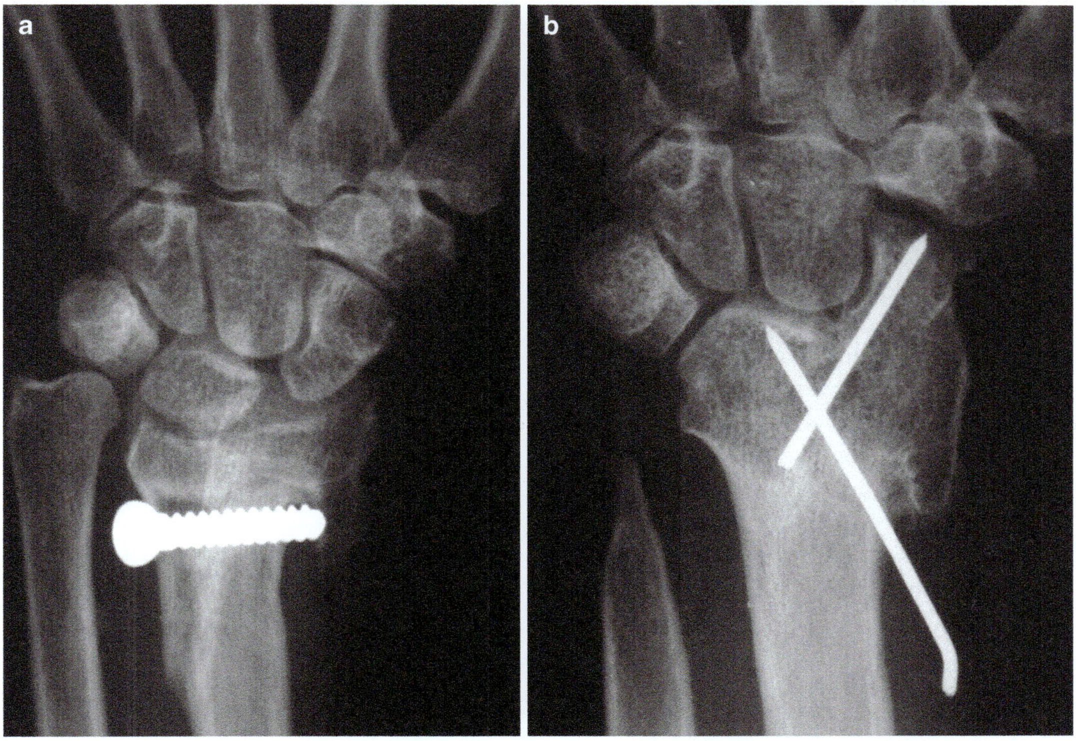

Fig. 40.4 (**a**) Late presentation of a distal radius malunion with chronic SL dissociation. Note the distal radial deformity, shortening of the radius with an ulna plus, and an increased SL gap. (**b**) This patient was treated by a radio-scapho-lunate arthrodesis with a matched ulna procedure to address the distal radioulnar and ulnocarpal conflict

malunion and SL dissociation, a corrective osteotomy in addition to the ligamentoplasty has to be considered, or alternatively, salvage procedures such as a radio-scapho-lunate (RSL) arthrodesis.

40.7 Lunotriquetral Dissociation

- About one fifth of all distal radius fractures have an associated lunotriquetral (LT) ligament injury (Table 40.1). The ligament injury is produced by shear forces exerted on the LT joint, as a result of the pisiform pushing the triquetrum dorsally, while the lunate is blocked by the distal radius.
- Rupture of the LT ligaments induces a carpal instability, which is different from the SL instability. If the dorsal radiotriquetral ligament is also insufficient, in addition to a torn LT ligament, the lunate is no longer connected to the triquetrum and is therefore moved into flexion, the so-called VISI pattern of malalignment. When this happens, the triquetrum also becomes unstable and migrates proximally. The consequence of all of this is a midcarpal joint incongruity and LT dysfunction, characterized by painful crepitation in ulnar deviation (Osterman and Seidman 1995; Garcia-Elias 2011).

40.7.1 Diagnosis

- The spectrum of LT ligament injury ranges from partial tears with variable pain and weakness to complete dissociation with static collapse, causing a forklike deformity of the wrist and prominence of the distal ulna. Symptoms are usually intermittent and are especially prominent with wrist deviation or pronation/supination. They include diminished motion, weakness, a sensation of instability or giving way, and ulnar nerve paresthesias. A painful wrist clunk with deviation is often present (Shin et al. 2000).

- A careful history followed by a systematic physical examination can often identify an injury to the LT ligament.
- Confirmation of the diagnosis by means of radiography, arthrography, or arthroscopy is essential before initiating treatment.
- LT ligament rupture is commonly diagnosed by arthroscopy. As for SL dissociations, the degree of instability is determined by attempting to insert a curved probe in the joint space. If the probe can be entered and rotated in the joint space, the joint is dynamically unstable. If aside from that, the two articulating bones can be easily displaced from each other, the instability is severe, indicating an injury of both the intrinsic and extrinsic ligaments.

40.7.2 Treatment

- A number of factors have to be considered when deciding a treatment for a LT dissociation: degree of instability, healing potential of the ruptured ligaments, reducibility, status of cartilage, presence of other injuries, etc. (Garcia-Elias 2011). Based on this, one of the following treatments is decided:
  - Percutaneous LT joint fixation with K-wires (indicated in the acute injury)
  - LT fusion (indicated in the chronic instability without carpal collapse)
  - Tendon reconstruction of the LT ligaments (indicated in chronic instability with partial LT tears)
  - Salvage procedures (proximal row carpectomy, radiocarpal or midcarpal fusion) for the chronic carpal collapse into VISI

References

Forward DP, Lindau TR, Melsom DS. Intercarpal ligament injuries associated with fractures of the distal part of the radius. J Bone Joint Surg Am. 2007;89A:2334–40.

Garcia-Elias M. Carpal instability. In: Wolfe S, Hotchkiss R, Pederson W, Kozin S, editors. Green's operative hand surgery. 6th ed. Philadelphia: Churchill Livingstone Elsevier; 2011. p. 465–521.

Garcia-Elias M, Lluch AL, Stanley JK. Three-ligament tenodesis for the treatment of scapholunate dissociation: indications and surgical technique. J Hand Surg Am. 2006;31:125–34.

Geissler WB, Freeland AE, Savoie FH, et al. Intracarpal soft-tissue lesions associated with a intra-articular fracture of the distal end of the radius. J Bone Joint Surg Am. 1996;78A:357–65.

Kordasiewicz B, Pomianowski S, Orłowski J, Rapała K. Interosseous ligaments and TFCC lesions in intraarticular distal radius fractures – radiographic versus arthroscopic evaluation. Ortop Traumatol Rehabil. 2006;8:263–7.

Lindau T, Arner M, Hagberg L. Intraarticular lesions in distal fractures of the radius in young patients. J Hand Surg Br. 1997;22B:638–43.

Mathoulin C, Sbihi A, Panciera P. Interest in wrist arthroscopy for treatment of articular fractures of the distal radius: report of 27 cases. Chir Main. 2001;20(5):342–50.

Mehta JA, Bain GI, Heptinstall RJ. Anatomical reduction versus fluoroscopic reduction in the management of intra-articular distal radius fractures. An arthroscopically assisted approach. J Bone Joint Surg Br. 2000;82B:79–86.

Osterman AL, Seidman GD. The role of arthroscopy in the treatment of lunatotriquetral ligament injuries. Hand Clin. 1995;11:41–50.

Peterson SL, Freeland AE. Scapholunate stabilization with dynamic extensor carpi radialis longus tendon transfer. J Hand Surg Am. 2010;35A:2093–100.

Pogue DJ, Viegas SF, Patterson RM, et al. Effects of distal radius fracture malunion on wrist joint mechanics. J Hand Surg Am. 1990;15A:721–7.

Richards RS, Bennett JD, Roth JH, et al. Arthroscopic diagnosis of intra-articular soft tissue injuries associated with distal radial fractures. J Hand Surg Am. 1997;22A:772–6.

Shih JT, Lee HM, Hou YT, Tan CM. Arthroscopically-assisted reduction of intra-articular fractures and soft tissue management of distal radius. Hand Surg. 2001;6:127–35.

Shin AY, Battaglia MJ, Bishop AT. Lunotriquetral instability: diagnosis and treatment. J Am Acad Orthop Surg. 2000;8:170–9.

Taleisnik J, Watson HK. Midcarpal instability caused by malunited fractures of the distal radius. J Hand Surg Am. 1984;9A:350–7.

Varitimidis SE, Basdekis GK, Dailiana ZH, et al. Treatment of intra-articular fractures of the distal radius: fluoroscopic or arthroscopic reduction? J Bone Joint Surg Br. 2008;90(6):778–85.

Wolfe SW, Garcia-Elias M, Kitay A. Carpal instability nondissociative. J Am Acad Orthop Surg. 2012; 20:575–85.

Secondary Osteoarthrosis: Partial or Total Arthrodesis Versus Wrist Arthroplasty

41

Michel E.H. Boeckstyns

Contents

M.E.H. Boeckstyns, MD
Clinic for Hand Surgery,
Gentofte Hospital – University of Copenhagen,
Copenhagen, Denmark
e-mail: michel.boeckstyns@regionh.dk

41.1 Summary

Secondary osteoarthrosis of the wrist typically develops after intra-articular distal radius fractures with articular incongruity (step-off) of 1–2 mm or more or with an associated rupture of the scapholunate ligament. If the condition is painful and conservative measures fail, surgical treatment may be necessary. Total wrist fusion is the standard procedure but total- or hemi-wrist arthroplasty may also be used. Other motion preserving solutions are feasible, if the midcarpal joint is normal: total or partial radiocarpal fusion or a modified proximal row carpectomy, depending on the condition of the cartilage in the radioscaphoid fossa.

41.2 Treatment Options

Secondary osteoarthrosis (OA) of the wrist may result after a distal radius fracture (DRF) in which there are cartilage changes due to the intra-articular nature of the fracture (Fig. 41.1). Accurate reduction of the articular surface is a critical factor in avoiding this complication: articular incongruity of 1–2 mm or more carries a high risk of developing OA (Knirk and Jupiter 1986; Catalano et al. 1997; Fernandez et al. 1997). Associated scapholunate ligament disruption may lead to wrist instability and scapholunate advanced collapse (SLAC wrist), increasing the risk of OA. The radiographic presence of OA does not necessarily correlate with

L.M. Hove et al. (eds.), *Distal Radius Fractures*,
DOI 10.1007/978-3-642-54604-4_41, © Springer-Verlag Berlin Heidelberg 2014

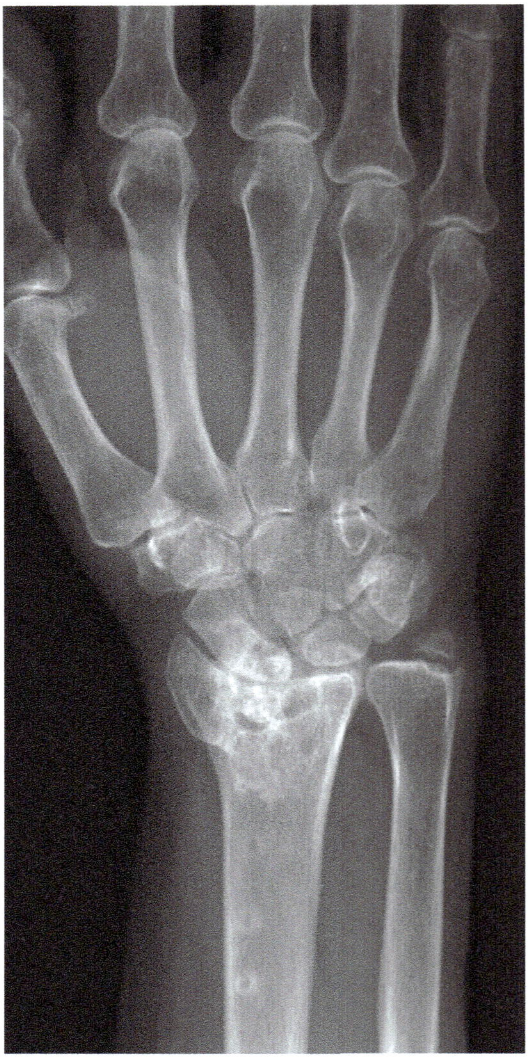

Fig. 41.1 Secondary OA after intra-articular distal radius fracture

the functional outcome, but painful and disabling OA requires treatment. If the condition does not respond adequately to conservative treatment (anti-inflammatory medication, splinting and steroid injections), it may have to be treated surgically. Before making a decision of performing surgery on the radiocarpal joint, it is important to make sure that the pain is related to the radiocarpal joint and does not originate from the distal radioulnar joint, a TFCC lesion or ulnocarpal abutment.

- Total wrist fusion (TWF) is the standard procedure for OA of the wrist from whatever cause, including posttraumatic conditions, and patients may accommodate well for the loss of motion (Murphy et al. 2003). With the use of special wrist fusion plates (Fig. 41.2), the number of carpal or carpometacarpal nonunions is low (2–7 %) (Meads et al. 2003; Houshian and Schroder 2001). Nevertheless, TWF may have an important negative impact on the health status of patients with posttraumatic OA (Adey et al. 2005), and with increasing interest in functional outcome after surgery, the importance of preserving some range of wrist movement to allow activities of daily living such as writing, personal care, dressing and combing hair has become apparent. This has encouraged developing techniques with preservation of motion: total wrist arthroplasty or limited intracarpal fusions.
- Radio-scapholunate fusion (RSL-fusion) may be an option in patients with radiocarpal OA, where both the radiolunate and radioscaphoid joints are involved, provided the midcarpal joint is normal. This procedure blocks the natural rotation of the scaphoid, limiting radial deviation and flexion of the distal row relative to the fused proximal row. Nonunion is frequent and symptomatic secondary OA in the midcarpal joint may develop in as much as 22–33 % at an early stage (Muhldorfer et al. 2009; Nagy and Buchler 1997). Thus RSL-fusion may only be a step towards TWF. ROM is rather limited but can be improved with excision of the distal scaphoid, resulting in approximately 50 % of the normal range of movement of the wrist (Garcia-Elias et al. 2005). This supplementary procedure may even diminish the risk of early midcarpal OA. Motion can be further improved if the triquetrum is excised (McGuire and Bain 2012) (Fig. 41.3).
- In case of a die-punch lesion, in which the lunate has crushed the lunate fossa of the distal radius, a radiolunate fusion may also be an option. This is only feasible, if the radioscaphoid as well as the midcarpal joints are intact. Fixation of these partial fusions can be provided by using K-wires, powered staples or a Spider plate. Another solution may be to

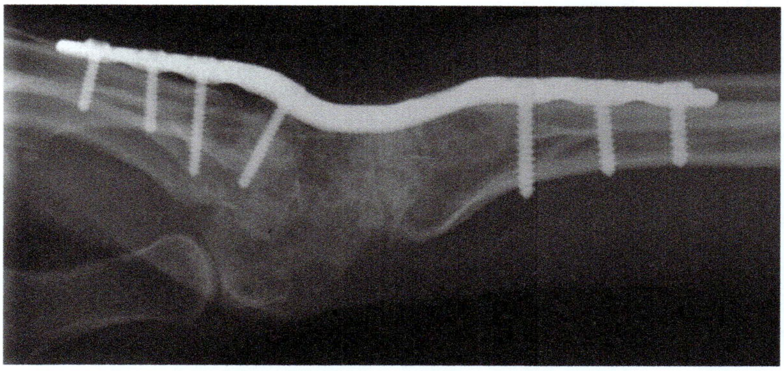

Fig. 41.2 Total wrist fusion with wrist fusion plate

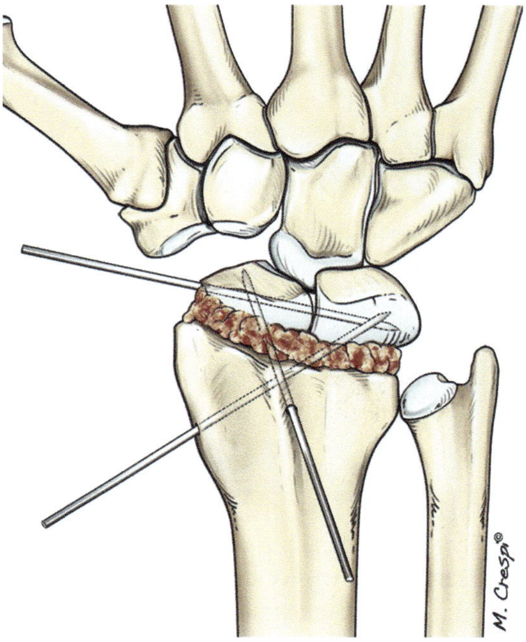

Fig. 41.3 Radio-scapholunate fusion with excision of the distal scaphoid pole and the triquetrum

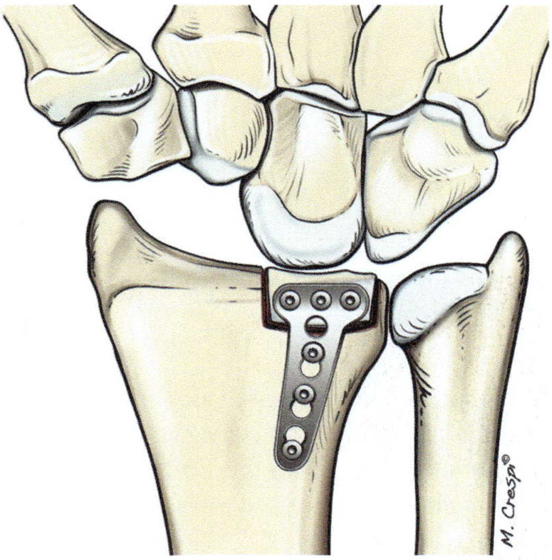

Fig. 41.4 OA after die-punch lesion. The lunate is used to replace the lunate fossa of the radius. The scaphoid and triquetrum are excised (Modified proximal row carpectomy)

excise the scaphoid and triquetrum while the lunate is incorporated in the radius at the lunate fossa, thus replacing the damaged cartilage with the lunate cartilage towards the capitate (Fig. 41.4, modified proximal row carpectomy).

- TWA can be used as a motion preserving procedure in posttraumatic situations (Herzberg et al. 2012), mostly reported for the salvage of SLAC and SNAC wrists (scaphoid non-union advanced collapse), more rarely for OA after DRF. According to the European Re-motion TWA registry (April 2013), 58 of 258 TWA were done on posttraumatic indications and of these only 13 after DRF (Fig. 41.5). Wrist motion is depended on that before operation and in average 35° in extension, 35° in flexion, 22° in ulnar deviation and 9° in radial deviation can be expected. Grip strength improves moderately (25 %).

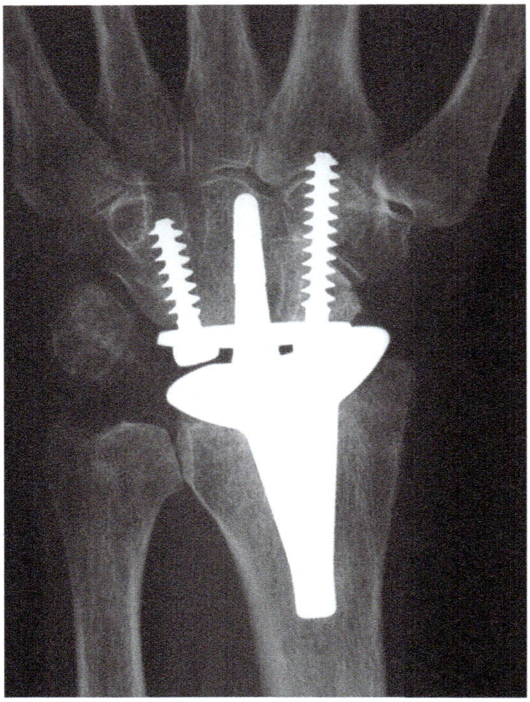

Fig. 41.5 Total wrist arthroplasty with the Re-motion prosthesis

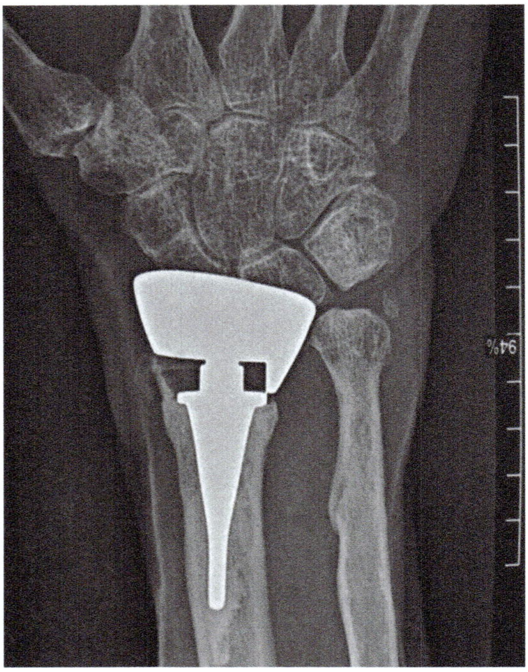

Fig. 41.6 The Roux hemi-wrist arthroplasty (Courtesy Jean-Luc Roux)

Cumulated implant survival is approximately 90 % at 9 years. The Universal 2 TWA has a similar design. Both the Re-motion and the Universal 2 can be used (off label) as a hemi-wrist arthroplasty (HWA), using the radial component only. The Roux prosthesis is a specially designed HWA, so far reported in a small series of six patients, of whom one had OA after a DRF (Roux 2009). These implants can also be used in acute comminuted DRF, where restoration of a congruent joint surface is impossible (Fig. 41.6).

- A different concept is the recently introduced Amandys pyrocarbon interposition arthroplasty (Fig. 41.7). In a series of 25 cases, the mean extension of operated wrists was 36° and flexion 32°, and efficient pain reduction was obtained in most patients (Bellemere et al. 2012).

Conclusion

There are several possibilities for the surgical treatment of radiocarpal OA after a DRF (Fig. 41.8). Limited fusions can be used if the midcarpal joint is preserved. TWA and HWA are also feasible as motion preserving solutions and must certainly be tried in selected patients, especially with panarthritic wrists. It is important to remember that both limited fusions and arthroplasties may eventually lead to TWF and the patients should have this information.

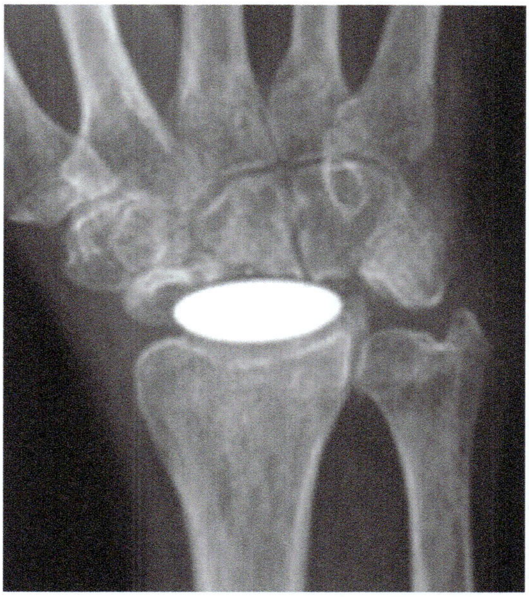

Fig. 41.7 The Amandys pyrocarbon interposition implant (Courtesy Philippe Bellemère)

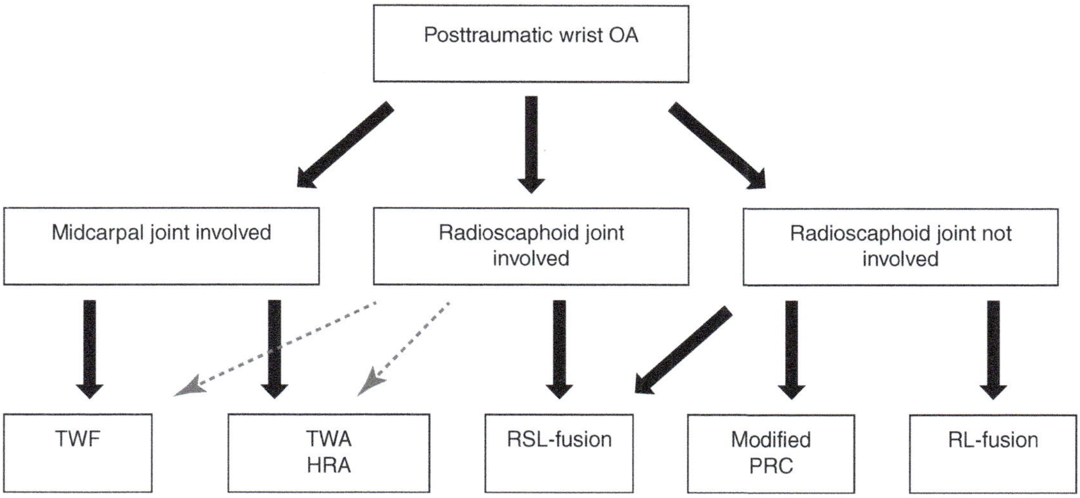

Fig. 41.8 Treatment options. *TWF* total wrist fusion, *TWA* total wrist arthroplasty, *HRA* hemi-wrist arthroplasty, *RSL-fusion* radio-scapholunate fusion, *Modified PRC* modified proximal row carpectomy, *RL-fusion* radiolunate fusion

References

Adey L, Ring D, Jupiter JB. Health status after total wrist arthrodesis for posttraumatic arthritis. J Hand Surg Am. 2005;30(5):932–6.

Bellemere P, Maes-Clavier C, Loubersac T, Gaisne E, Kerjean Y. Amandys((R)) implant: novel pyrocarbon arthroplasty for the wrist. Chir Main. 2012; 31(4):176–87.

Catalano 3rd LW, Cole RJ, Gelberman RH, Evanoff BA, Gilula LA, Borrelli Jr J. Displaced intra-articular fractures of the distal aspect of the radius. Long-term results in young adults after open reduction and internal fixation. J Bone Joint Surg Am. 1997; 79(9):1290–302.

Fernandez JJ, Gruen GS, Herndon JH. Outcome of distal radius fractures using the short form 36 health survey. Clin Orthop Relat Res. 1997;341:36–41.

Garcia-Elias M, Lluch A, Ferreres A, Papini-Zorli I, Rahimtoola ZO. Treatment of radiocarpal degenerative osteoarthritis by radioscapholunate arthrodesis and distal scaphoidectomy. J Hand Surg Am. 2005; 30(1):8–15.

Herzberg G, Boeckstyns M, Ibsen Sørensen A, Axelsson P, Kroener K, Liverneaux P, Obert L, Merser S. "Remotion" total wrist arthroplasty: preliminary results of a prospective international multicenter study of 215 cases. J Wrist Surg. 2012;01(01):17–22.

Houshian S, Schroder HA. Wrist arthrodesis with the AO titanium wrist fusion plate: a consecutive series of 42 cases. J Hand Surg Br. 2001;26(4):355–9.

Knirk JL, Jupiter JB. Intra-articular fractures of the distal end of the radius in young adults. J Bone Joint Surg Am. 1986;68(5):647–59.

McGuire DT, Bain GI. Radioscapholunate fusions. J Wrist Surg. 2012;1(2):135–40.

Meads BM, Scougall PJ, Hargreaves IC. Wrist arthrodesis using a Synthes wrist fusion plate. J Hand Surg Br. 2003;28(6):571–4.

Muhldorfer M, Hohendorff B, Prommersberger KJ, van Schoonhoven J. Medium-term results after radioscapholunate fusion for post-traumatic osteoarthritis of the wrist]. Handchir Mikrochir Plast Chir. 2009; 4(3): 148–55.

Murphy DM, Khoury JG, Imbriglia JE, Adams BD. Comparison of arthroplasty and arthrodesis for the rheumatoid wrist. J Hand Surg Am. 2003; 28(4):570–6.

Nagy L, Buchler U. Long-term results of radioscapholunate fusion following fractures of the distal radius. J Hand Surg Br. 1997;22(6):705–10.

Roux JL. [Replacement and resurfacing prosthesis of the distal radius: a new therapeutic concept]. Chir Main. 2009;28(1):10–7.

Secondary DRU Joint Problems Instability, Nonunion Styloid, and Ulnocarpal Abutment

42

Jan-Ragnar Haugstvedt

Contents

J.-R. Haugstvedt, MD, PhD
Department of Orthopedics,
Østfold Hospital Trust, Moss, Norway
e-mail: jrhaugstvedt@gmail.com

42.1 Summary

Following a fracture of the distal radius, poor or improper treatment may result in later ulnar-sided wrist pain and instability. A TFCC rupture could involve the distal component, capsular detachment, or the proximal component, avulsion from the foveal attachment, the latter giving major instability. After arthroscopic evaluation, these injuries could be treated open or with an arthroscopic-assisted procedure. When there is no healing potential of the ligaments, a ligament reconstruction using a free tendon graft should be performed. If instability is combined with osteoarthritis of the DRUJ, a semi-constrained prosthesis is advised.

A fracture of the ulnar styloid seldom gives late pain or discomfort; however, sometimes the tip of the nonunion styloid impinges with the carpus and should be removed. If the nonunion styloid presents with DRUJ instability, a fracture involving the foveal DRU ligament attachment should be suspected, and the ulnar styloid, or the ligaments, should be reattached.

L.M. Hove et al. (eds.), *Distal Radius Fractures*,
DOI 10.1007/978-3-642-54604-4_42, © Springer-Verlag Berlin Heidelberg 2014

Ulnocarpal abutment as a result of shortening of the radius gives ulnar-sided wrist pain, especially when radial deviating the wrist with a pronated forearm. A partial arthroscopic resection of the ulnar head or an ulnar shortening osteotomy should be performed.

42.2 Introduction

- Following a trauma to the hand, wrist, or forearm, a patient may suffer from a soft tissue injury, a fracture of the distal radius, a forearm fracture, or a dislocation fracture of the forearm bones.
- When diagnosed and properly treated at the time of injury, most injuries will heal without any (major) sequelae.
- Some injuries are overlooked or not diagnosed at the time of injury. This may be due to lack of attention from the doctor to listen to the patient and examine the wrist and hand for the extent of the injury or not using available tools for diagnosing, such as X-ray, CT, MRI, or arthroscopy.
- Conservative treatment of a distal radius fracture may result in malalignment, shortening of one bone, or instability of the carpus, wrist, or forearm.
- With the increasing use of osteosynthesis, especially plates and screws for stabilization of a fracture of the distal radius, patients are allowed to mobilize before soft tissue or ligament injuries are allowed to heal.
- Many patients with primarily overlooked injuries or not adequate postoperative treatment will later complain from symptoms and signs from the ulnar side of the wrist.

42.3 Anatomy

- The distal radioulnar joint (DRUJ) is the connection between the lower ends of the radius and ulna. The joint is stabilized by the following structures: (1) triangular fibrocartilage complex (TFCC), (2) the ulnocarpal (UC) ligament complex (the ulno-lunate (UL) and the ulno-triquetral (UT) ligaments with a superficial layer of fibers connecting the distal ulna to the distal carpal row, the ulno-capitate ligament), (3) the extensor carpi ulnaris (ECU) tendon and subsheath, (4) the pronator quadratus (PQ) muscle, (5) the radioulnar interosseous membrane (IOM) and interosseous ligament (IOL), (6) the bony structures of the radius and ulna itself, and (7) the joint capsule.
- The "seat," the part of the distal ulna articulating with radius, is conical with an articular cartilage about an arc of approximately 110°. The radius of the curvature is approximately 8 mm.
- The sigmoid notch of the radius is a shallow concave articular surface for the ulnar head, the arc being approximately 70° and the radius of the curvature about 15 mm.
- In neutral forearm rotation, approximately 60 % of the articular surface of the sigmoid notch is in contact with the ulnar head. This percentage is reduced in both extremes of forearm rotation to about 10°. The deeper the sigmoid notch, the greater the osseous stability (Fig. 42.1).

42.4 Biomechanics

- Approximately 20 % of load transmitted across the wrist is transmitted through the ulnocarpal joint. This load will increase with ulnar deviation, pronation, and radial shortening.
- The TFCC functions as a cushion for the ulnar carpus and is the major stabilizer of the DRUJ (Palmer and Werner 1981).
- When tested for dynamic stability under loaded conditions, the foveal ligament insertion has a greater effect on stability than the styloid insertion (Haugstvedt et al. 2006).
- The PQ and ECU are both important dynamic stabilizers of DRUJ.
- The axis of forearm rotation runs through the radial head to the foveal region of the ulnar head.
- Due to the differences of the radii of the seat and the sigmoid notch, a rotation as well as a

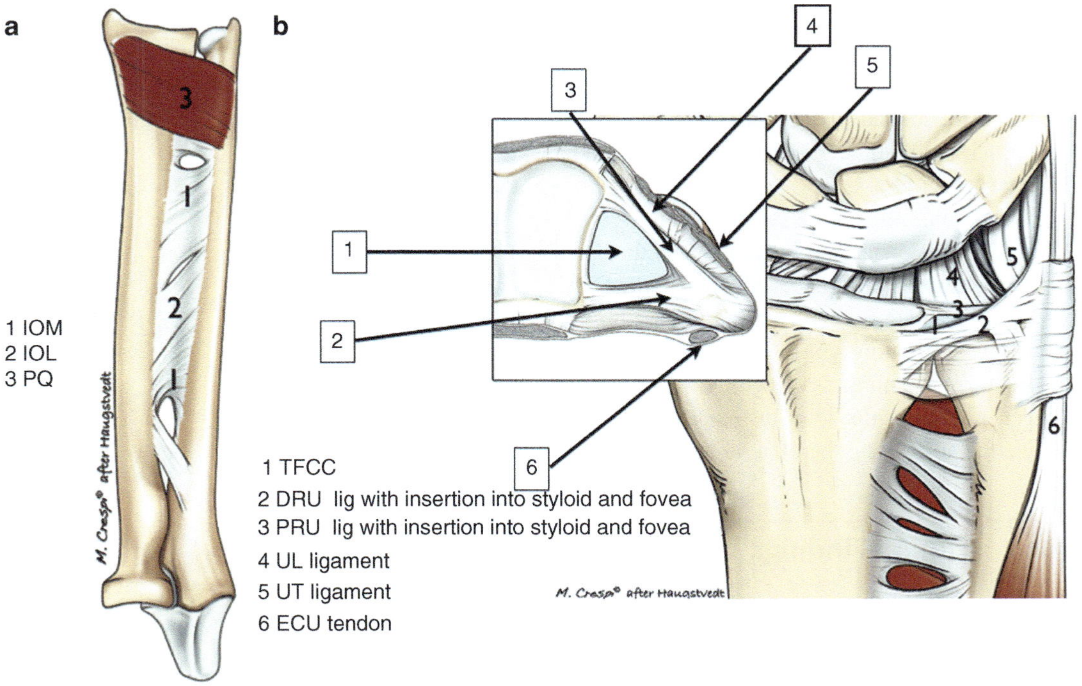

Fig. 42.1 (**a**) This figure displays the forearm bones, the radius, and the ulna. The IOM and IOL run from radius to ulna to transform load from the radius distally to the ulna proximally. Along with the PQ muscle, these structures also stabilize the DRUJ. (**b**) Other structures stabilizing the DRUJ are the TFCC with the meniscus and the distal radioulnar ligaments, the UC ligaments, the ECU tendon and tendon sheath, as well as the bone itself and the capsule. See text

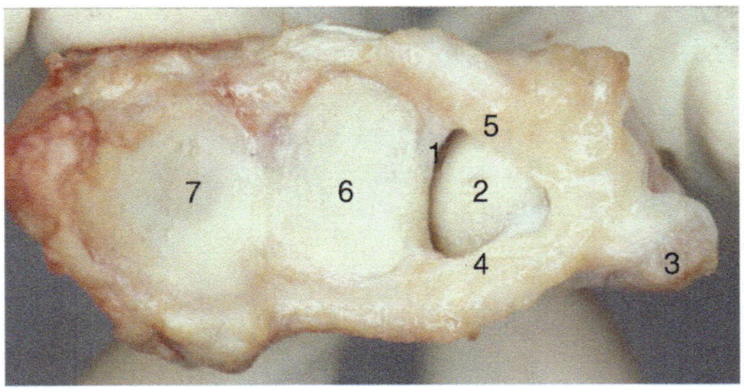

Fig. 42.2 This picture shows a dissected distal end of the forearm from a distal view. The meniscus has been removed; the DRU ligaments are intact. The sigmoid notch of the radius and the seat of the ulna are shown to illustrate the different size and radii of the two structures. Upon supination or pronation of the forearm, a rotation as well as a translation will occur (in addition to a proximo-distal migration). *1* The sigmoid notch, *2* the ulnar head (the meniscus removed), *3* the ulnar styloid, *4* DRU ligament, *5* PRU ligament, *6* the lunate fossa, distal radius, *7* the scaphoid fossa, distal radius

translation (and a proximal or distal migration) will take place in the DRUJ when the forearm is being rotated (Fig. 42.2).

42.5 Pathomechanics

- When falling on an outstretched hand, a person may sustain an injury of the bone and/or the soft tissue.
- A fracture of the distal radius with a dorsal displacement of more than 34° from the normal anatomic position will give an injury of the ulnar-sided soft tissues (Scheer and Adolfsson 2011).
- In young patients with a fracture of the distal radius, more than 90 % were found to have concomitant ligamentous injuries in the wrist (Lindau et al. 1997).
- TFCC injuries are classified according to Palmer (1989). Atzei described injuries of the proximal component (foveal detachment of DRU ligaments) and of the distal component (capsular detachment of the TFCC) (Atzei 2009).
- Disruption of the ulnar attachment of the ligament complex through the fovea and/or the

styloid attachment will affect both the palmar and dorsal radioulnar ligaments, which may lead to more destabilization of the DRUJ compared to isolated disruption of either dorsal or palmar radioulnar ligament at their radial attachment.
- If the sigmoid notch cavity is shallow or the palmar or dorsal margins have been displaced by a fracture, the chances of an unstable DRUJ in full pronation or full supination are high.
- Upon shortening of the radius following a fracture, the ulna may become relatively longer, changing the load distribution across as well as impacting the ulnar side of the wrist.

42.6 Clinical Findings

- Patients suffering from ulnar-sided wrist pain due to DRU instability, pseudarthrosis of an ulnar styloid fracture, or ulnar abutment syndrome may suffer from symptoms such as pain, clicking, locking, instability, reduced range of movement, tenderness especially upon deviation or rotation, subluxation of the ulnar head, or difficulties opening a door, turning a door knob, lifting a pan, etc. (Haugstvedt and Husby 1999).
- Clinical testing for DRUJ instability should be performed with the forearm in neutral rotation as well as in supinated and pronated positions.
- All testing should include the noninjured side for comparison (Fig. 42.3).
- Patients with a suspect ulnar abutment syndrome should be tested with the arm in pronated position, using an active grip and deviating the wrist in a radial-ulnar direction. This will give pain and discomfort. (Again, compare to the noninjured side.)

42.7 Imaging

- Posterior-anterior (PA) images of the wrist should be performed with the shoulder of the examined hand 90° abducted from the trunk and the elbow flexed at 90° with the ulna perpendicular to the humerus and the forearm in pronated position. The wrist should be in neutral flexion-extension and radial-ulnar deviation. The palm of the hand should face down on the cassette with the fingers extended. In this view, the radial and ulnar styloid should be far apart.
- In a lateral view, the elbow is flexed to 90° and adducted to the trunk, the wrist should be midprone, and wrist in a neutral position. A "true" lateral view (within 10°) is obtained if the palmar margin of the pisiform is projected midway between the palmar margins of the distal pole of the scaphoid and the capitate head.
- In a nonunion of the ulnar styloid, the distal fragment could be displaced and could be seen

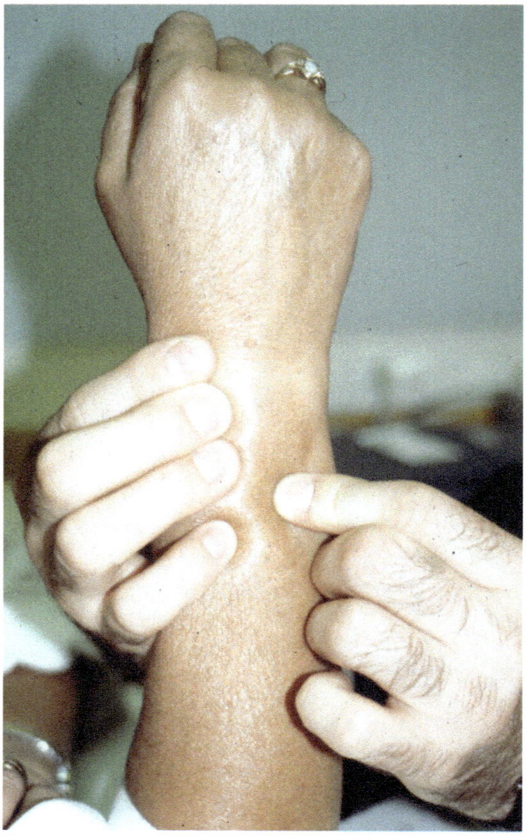

Fig. 42.3 When testing for DRUJ instability, one forearm bone should be stabilized while the other should be moved in dorsal followed by volar direction. The test should be carried out in neutral forearm rotation as well as in maximum supinated, respectively, pronated position. The noninjured side should always be tested for comparison

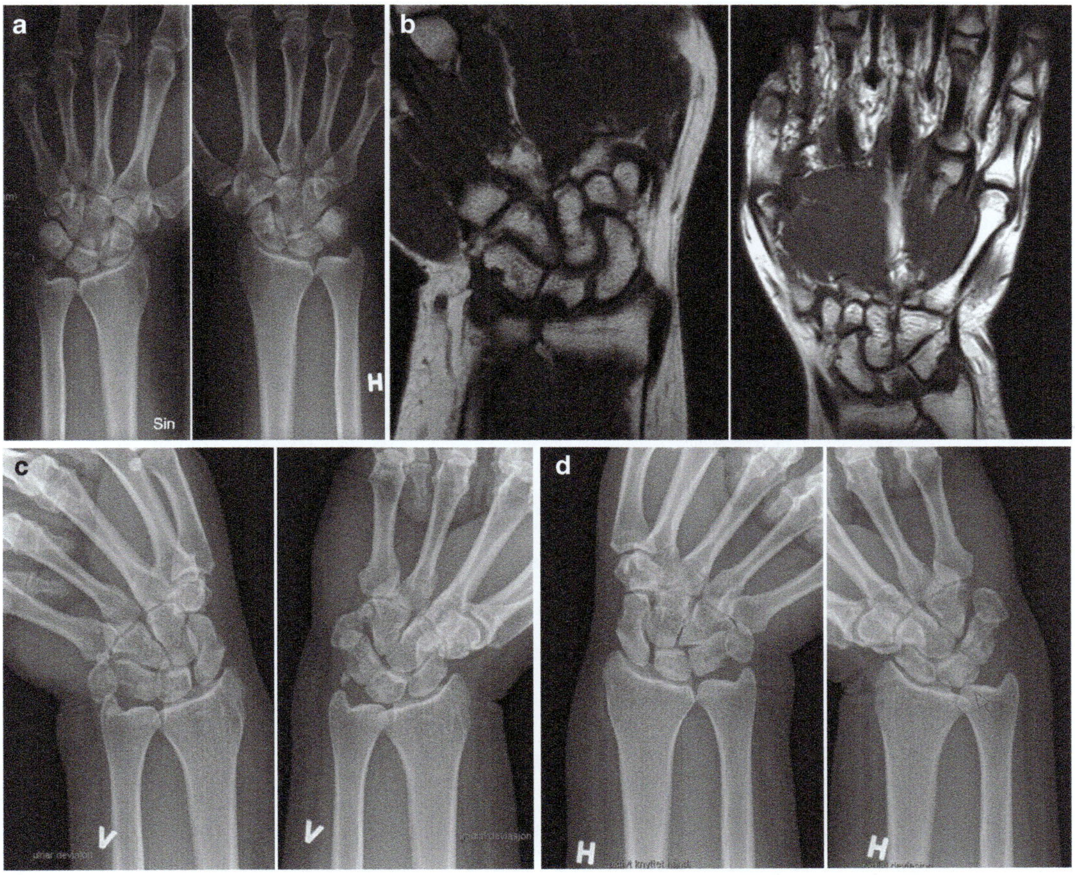

Fig. 42.4 (**a**) PA view of both wrists in a patient suspect of ulnar abutment syndrome. The left wrist to the left, the right wrist to the right. (**b**) MRIs of the same patient. Notice the changes in the lunate on both sides. (**c**) The patient is making a fist (observe the flexed fingers) as he is placing the left hand in an ulnar- and radial-deviated position, respectively. (**d**) The same as for (**c**), however displaying the right hand. In (**c**) and (**d**), notice the conflict between the ulnar head and the lunate in the radial deviated positions

conflicting with the ulnar carpus in a PA view of an ulnar-deviated wrist.

- If ulnar abutment syndrome is suspected, a PA view should be taken with the patient's arm in pronation and having the patient making a fist. (This will provoke proximal migration of the radius.) Images should be taken with the wrist in neutral as well as with the wrist in radial and ulnar deviation, respectively (Fig. 42.4).
- CT could be of great value to verify displacement of the DRUJ, nonunions of the styloid, as well as changes of the carpal bones in ulnar abutment syndrome.
- When DRUJ instability is suspected, CT should be performed with the forearm in neutral as well as in supinated and pronated forearm rotation. The instability might however be dynamic; thus, the instability will not be revealed unless the patient exerts variable rotational torque against resistance while the testing/imaging is performed (Tay et al. 2007).
- MRIs could be of great help in revealing changes in the carpus when ulnar impaction is suspected, but, however, is of less help (in the author's practice) for other wrist disorders. (MRI is highly dependent on the equipment being used as well as the radiologist interpreting the images.) Plain X-rays and CT scans are usual of better help than MRIs.
- *All imaging should be performed on both sides to compare the injured to the noninjured side.*

42.8 Treatment of DRU Instability, Nonunion of the Ulnar Styloid, and Ulnocarpal Abutment

42.8.1 Treatment of DRU Instability

- If the patient's history, clinical findings, and testing for instability arise suspicion of DRU instability, an arthroscopy should be performed to verify the diagnosis.
- For Palmer type I A and type I D (Palmer 1989), repair is (usually) not performed. For Palmer type I C, please see Chap. 28 where injuries around the distal ulna are discussed. For Palmer type I B, the author will suggest to use Atzei's approach to the problem (Atzei 2009).
- In order for the best treatment to be given, the status of the distal TFCC component (dc-TFCC; the TFCC proper, the hammock structure (Nakamura et al. 1996); and the UCL as well as the capsular attachment of the TFCC) should be examined. Furthermore, assessments of the proximal TFCC component (pc-TFCC; the foveal attachment of the distal radioulnar ligaments) as well as the healing potential of the TFCC tear and the DRUJ cartilage should be done.

42.8.2 Repair of dc-TFCC

- Patients with capsular detachment of TFCC following a distal radius fracture usually suffer from clicking, tenderness, and pain upon rotating the forearm more than major instability. The treatment is reattachment of the TFCC to the capsule where a variety of techniques have been performed such as "outside-in," "inside-out," or "all-inside." The "outside-in" technique is shown in Fig. 42.5. Postoperative immobilization should include a long arm cast for at least 4 weeks; return to activities allowing resisted forearm rotation should be awaited for at least 8 weeks. The results of these repairs, even a long time after the primary injury, are good in 60–80 % (Haugstvedt and Husby 1999) (Fig. 42.5).

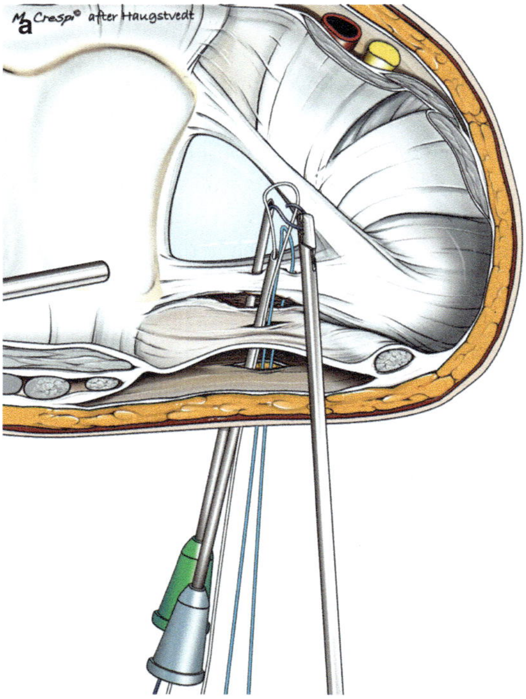

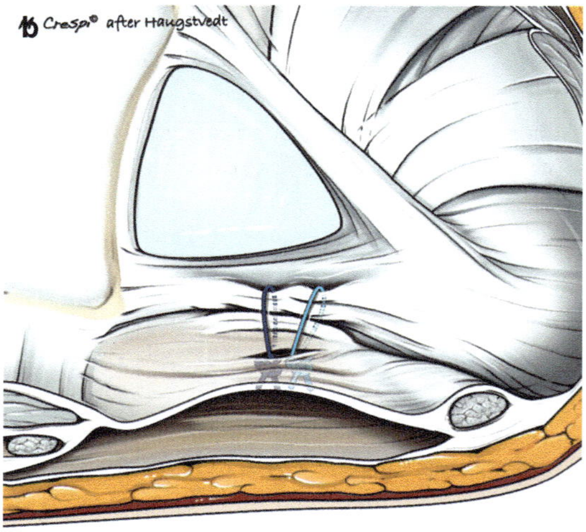

Fig. 42.5 This shows an "outside-in" technique for capsular reattachment of TFCC. (**a**) A suture is inserted into a needle; the needle is then passed in a proximal to distal direction through the TFCC, central to the rupture, and into the radiocarpal joint. With a "mosquito" or a grasper, the suture is withdrawn to outside the capsule. Another one or two sutures are placed in a similar manner. Before tightening the sutures, the subcutaneous space should be inspected for the dorsal sensible branch of the ulnar nerve to avoid having the nerve in the suture. (**b**) When the sutures have been tightened, the TFCC is reattached to the capsule

42.8.3 Repair of pc-TFCC

- If severe instability of the DRU is found upon testing, foveal detachment of the DRU ligament insertion should be suspected. The testing should be performed in neutral as well as in supinated and pronated forearm rotation, and the noninjured side should be tested for comparison.
- When wrist arthroscopy is performed, a positive trampoline as well as a positive hook test is found (Atzei 2009). The DRUJ should be evaluated using arthroscopy to inspect the status of the foveal attachment as well as the DRUJ cartilage.
- Repair of the foveal detachment could be done through an open or an arthroscopic-assisted approach. Postoperative immobilization is the same as for repair of dc-TFCC (Fig. 42.6).

42.8.4 Reconstruction of DRU Ligaments

- When the integrity of the ligaments is questionable, when there are degenerative changes and the ligaments could be approximated only under tension, a repair as described above is not possible. For these cases, a ligament reconstruction should be performed.
- There are several techniques for DRU ligament reconstruction, the author having good experience with the technique described by Adams and Berger (2002) (Fig. 42.7).
- The results after DRU ligament reconstruction are good (Adams and Berger 2002). Patients may suffer from a new injury with rupture of the reconstructed ligament; it is then possible to perform another similar reconstruction with a new graft. Today, it is becoming more and more popular to perform this procedure as an arthroscopic-assisted procedure.

42.8.5 Salvage Procedure or Joint Replacement

- When there is DRU instability without potential for ligament repair and/or the status of the DRUJ joint (cartilage) is poor, then a salvage procedure should be planned for.
- A variety of prosthesis has been made for the DRUJ; however, when there is instability in combination with a destroyed joint, the author has good experiences with a semi-constrained prosthesis (Aptis®).
- Long-time results show good results for this prosthesis (Laurentin-Pérez et al. 2008) (Fig. 42.8).

42.8.6 Treatment of Nonunion of the Ulnar Styloid

- Treatment of fractures of the ulnar styloid is discussed in Chap.28. Three types of styloid fractures are described: Type I is distal to the base of the styloid and involves in part or total of the superficial horizontal fibers of the TFCC. Type II runs through the base of the styloid into the proximal foveal area, but does not involve the articular surface of the ulnar head. Type III extends proximal to the foveal insertion (Fig. 42.9).
- When a patient with a nonunion of an ulnar styloid fracture is seen, the DRUJ should be examined for instability (Scheer et al. 2010). A wrist arthroscopy is the gold standard for evaluating intra-articular pathology.

42.8.7 Excision/Resection of the Tip of the Ulnar Styloid

- If the DRUJ is stable and the patient suffers from ulnar-sided wrist pain, this could arise from a non-united ulnar styloid. When performing arthroscopy, synovitis could be visualized in the dorsal recess, and sometimes

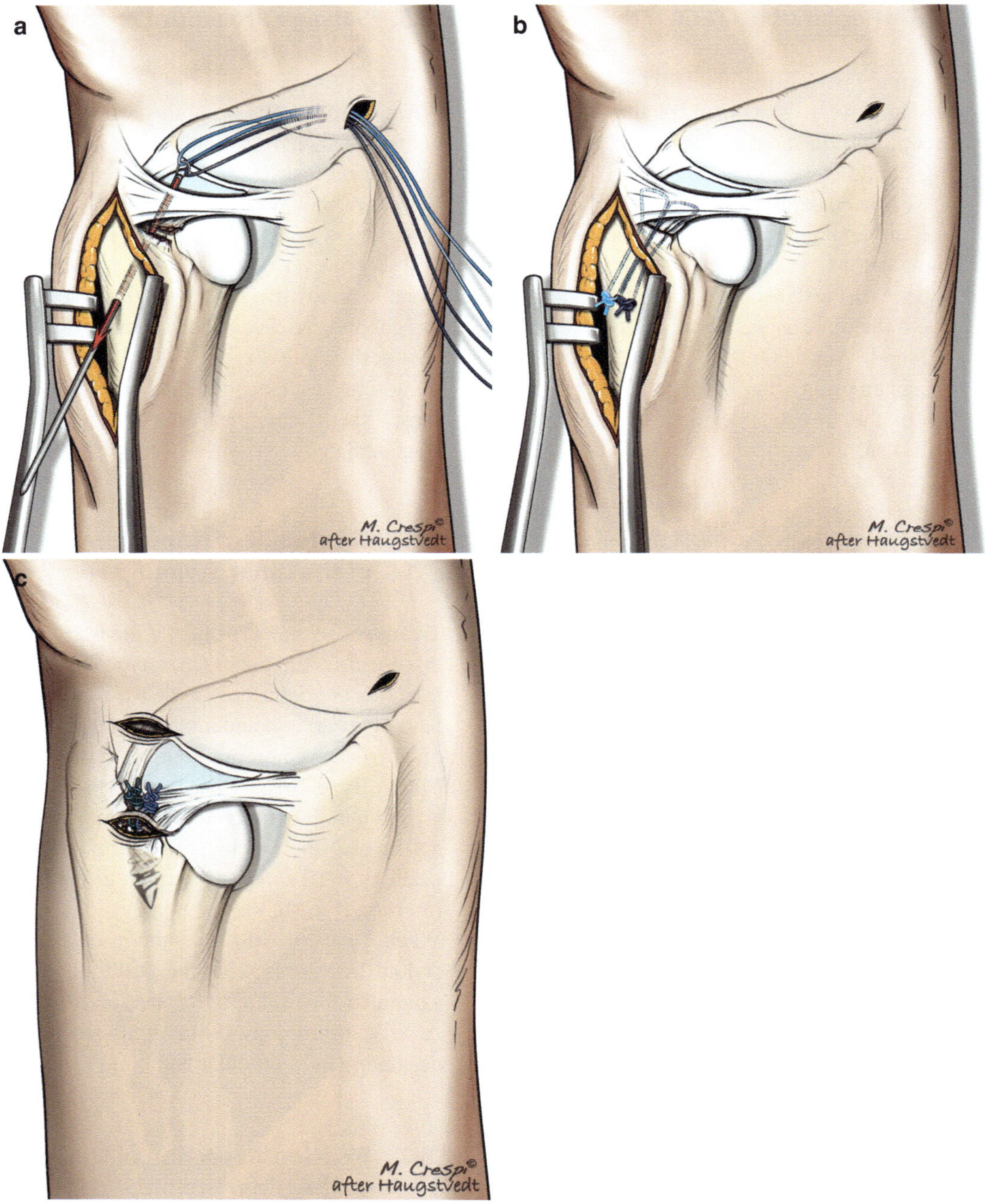

Fig. 42.6 For foveal repair, an arthroscopic-assisted or open repair could be performed. (**a**) After having debrided the foveal region using a direct foveal portal, it is possible to use a special guide and a flexible K-wire to drill through the TFCC into the foveal region and through the ulna. An incision is made where the K-wire exits. Two sutures could be pulled through the drill hole: one end should be left behind on the radial side of the wrist and the other end pulled through to the ulnar side. (**b**) Using the same guide and K-wire, two additional holes can be drilled: one in the volar component of the DRU ligaments and the other in the dorsal component. The remaining end of the sutures is entered into the K-wires, one at the time, and is then pulled through the two new drill holes. The two sutures are tightened over the bone giving a very solid repair. (**c**) If an open repair is preferred, exposure is done through the EDM compartment. An alternative to drill holes through ulna is using a bone anchor to fix the TFCC down to the foveal region

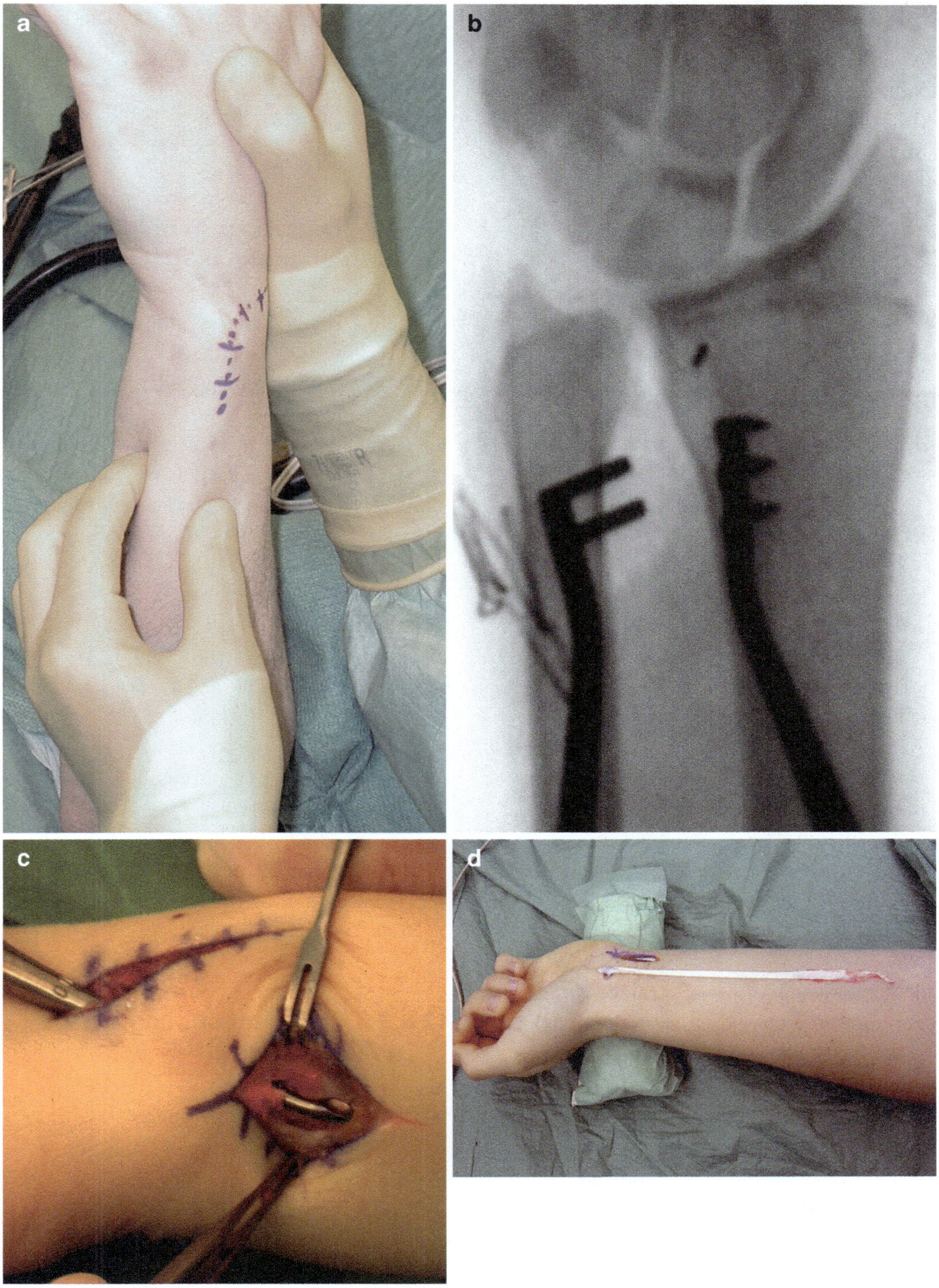

Fig. 42.7 DRU ligament reconstruction. (**a**) Preoperatively testing of DRU instability. (**b**) Using a fluoroscope, drill a K-wire through radius at a point close to the distal ulnar corner of the radius without conflicting the articular surface of the distal radius or the sigmoid notch. (**c**) Make another hole through the ulna from the foveal region to exit through the ulnar cortex between the FCU and ECU. (**d**) Harvest the PL tendon; however, other grafts may also be used such as a strip of the FCU tendon. (**e**) The tendon graft is then passed through the holes in the radius and ulna and is fixed by passing the ends of the graft in opposite directions around the ulnar neck and then sutured to each other or by using an interference screw in the ulna. (**f**) Schematic drawing of the tendon reconstruction

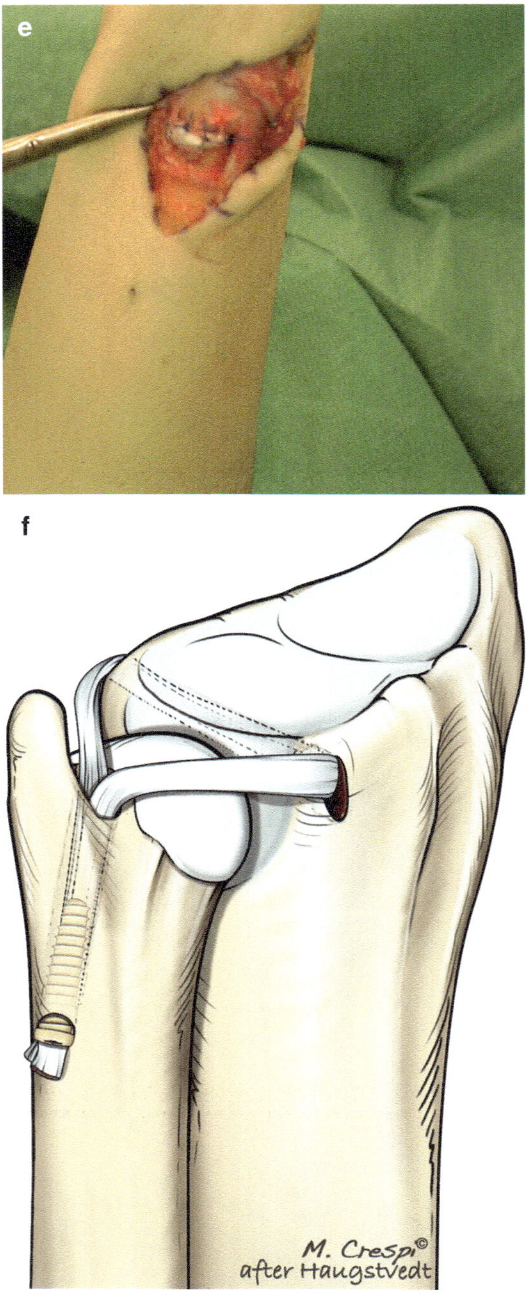

Fig. 42.7 (continued)

even injury on the cartilage of the triquetrum can be found due to impingement between the non-united ulnar styloid and the triquetrum. In this situation, resection of the non-united ulnar styloid should be performed. This could be done through an open or preferably arthroscopically assisted procedure. (If open procedure is chosen, be careful not to injure the ECU tendon and tendon sheath.)

42.8.8 Reattachment of the Non-united Ulnar Styloid

- If the DRU is unstable, this could imply that the non-united ulnar styloid fragment involves the foveal attachment of the DRU ligaments.
- A patient might also present with an old tip fracture that has caused no problems for many years; however, following a new trauma, the patient now suffers from ulnar-sided wrist pain and instability. While the first tip fracture caused neither pain nor instability, the new trauma has caused a TFCC injury. Only wrist arthroscopy can reveal the status.
- If there is instability and the foveal attachment is involved, reattachment of the non-united styloid should be performed. This could be done using K-wires and cerclage or a screw(s). (See Chap. 28.)
- If arthroscopy shows that reinsertion of TFC is possible, then excision of the non-united styloid could be performed even in these cases.

42.8.9 Treatment of Ulnocarpal Abutment

- While clinical findings combined with X-rays, CT scans, or MRI arise suspicion on ulnocarpal abutment (see above), wrist arthroscopy will reveal the diagnosis.
- Typically, a degeneration of the central part of TFC is seen; there are chondral changes of the ulnar head as well as of the proximal row bones (lunate and triquetrum). In long-standing cases, instability of the LT interval is often found in midcarpal arthroscopy.

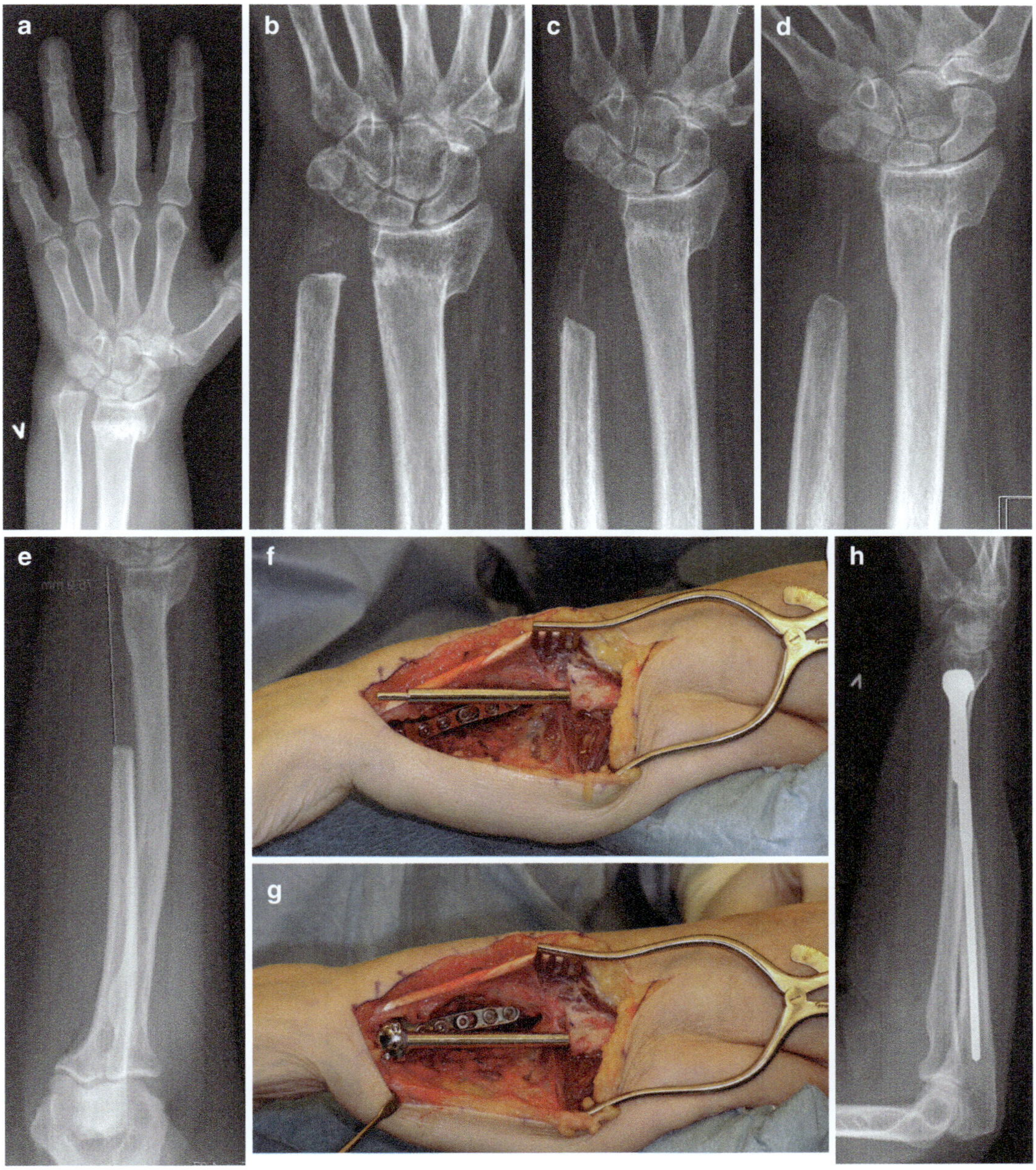

Fig. 42.8 (**a**) The result after treatment of a distal radius fracture in an elderly lady. She complained of ulnar-sided wrist pain and a Darrach procedure was performed; the result is shown in (**b**). She was pain-free for a short period of time and returned with new ulnar-sided wrist pain, and a wider resection of the ulna was done (**c**). She returned again; X-rays showed an impingement between the stump of the ulna and the radius (**d**); however, this problem was not addressed. Instead, a wider resection of the ulna was performed (**e**). When she later returned with new ulnar-sided wrist pain she was offered a semi-constrained, custom-made prosthesis (Aptis®). (**f**) This shows the plate fixed on the radius while the custom-made ulnar part is in place within the ulnar stem. (**g**) The head of the ulna has been placed. (**h**) Postoperative X-rays

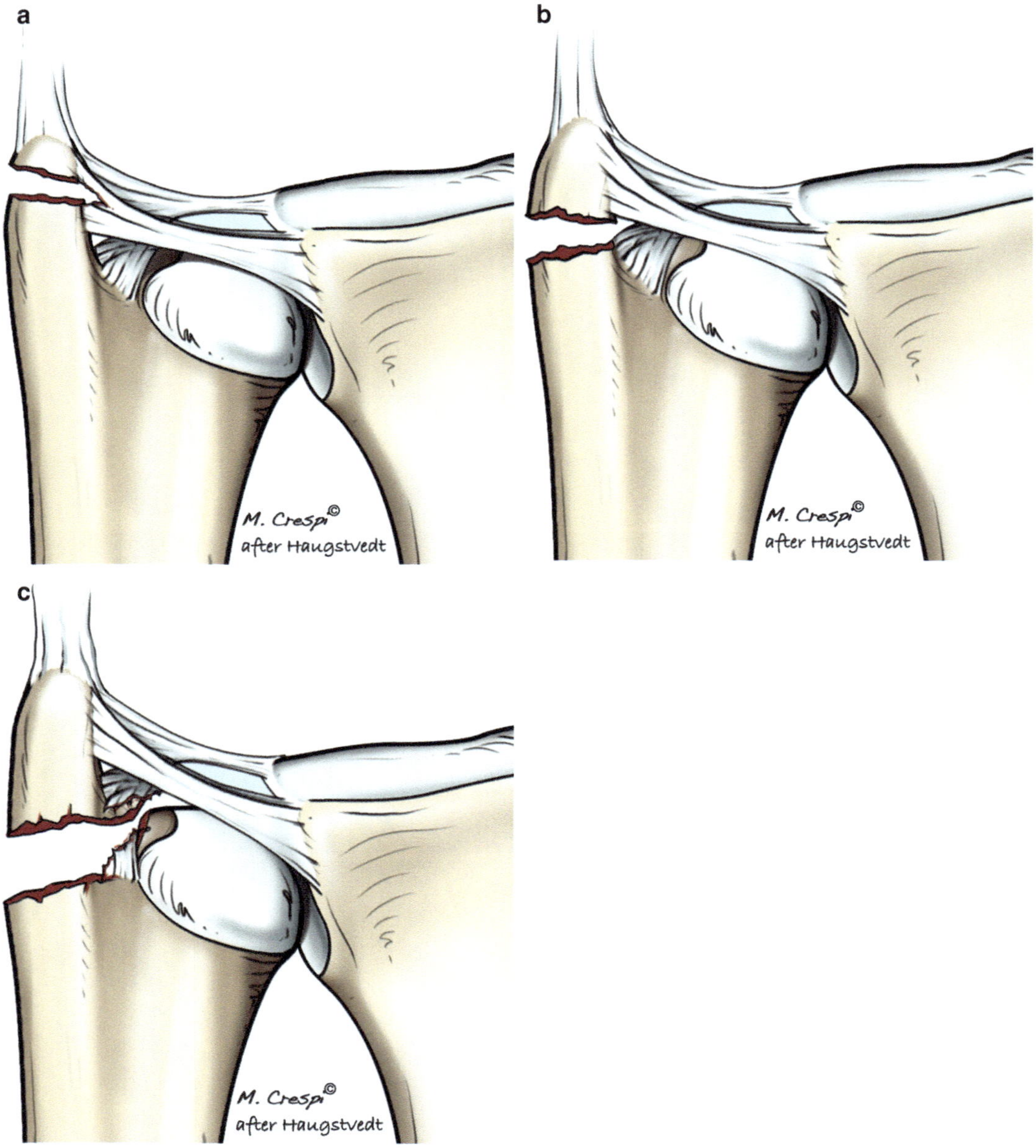

Fig. 42.9 Fractures through the ulnar styloid could run (**a**) through the tip of the styloid, (**b**) through the base of the styloid involving the foveal attachment of the DRU ligaments, or (**c**) extend proximalt to the foveal region. Whenever a styloid fracture is seen, clinical testing is carried out for testing of DRU stability. See text

42.8.10 Arthroscopic Partial Resection of Distal Ulna

- If arthroscopy is performed and ulnocarpal abutment is verified, it is possible to go on with an arthroscopic-assisted partial resection of the distal ulna. The TFC is resected for wide exposure of the ulnar head; a synovectomy is then performed to resect soft tissue. While the forearm is rotated into supination and pronation, a burr is used to resect the bone of the distal ulna in an oblique and helicoidally manner without getting into the articular surface of the DRUJ.
- To unload the ulnocarpal abutment, resection of 2–4 mm is often necessary. It may take

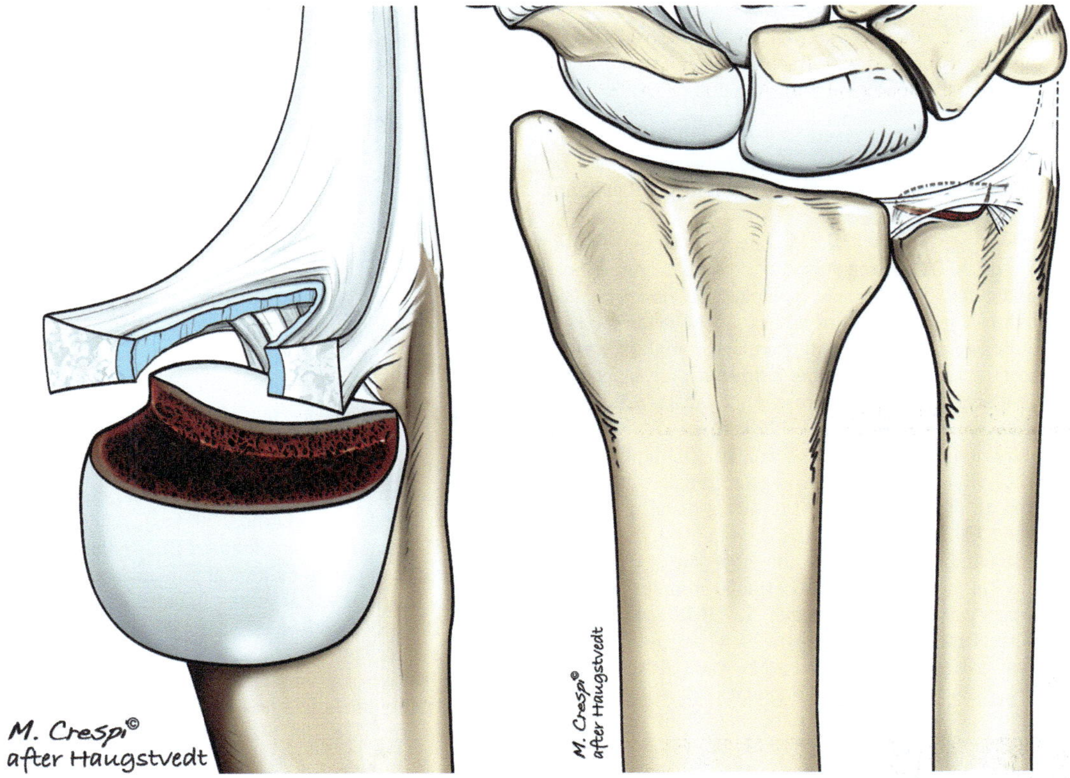

Fig. 42.10 In an arthroscopic wafer procedure, the forearm should be rotated while the resection of bone is performed. It is imperative not to resect the DRUJ joint, however only the part of the ulnar head impinging on the carpal bones

some months before the patients are fully recovered and pain-free (Fig. 42.10).

42.8.11 Ulnar Shortening Osteotomy

- Ulnar shortening osteotomy may seem to be the most logical way of treating ulnocarpal abutment following a radial fracture. If minor instability is found, ulnar shortening has been found to stabilize the DRUJ if the radioulnar ligaments are attached to the fovea (Nishiwaki et al. 2005).
- There are several designed plates for rigid fixation after ulnar shortening osteotomy. Usually, 3–7 mm is resected; however more than 10 mm have also been reported (Fig. 42.11).
- The results after arthroscopic debridement of TFCC followed by partial resection of ulnar head or ulnar shortening osteotomy are reported to be 70–80 % good or excellent (Bernstein et al. 2004).

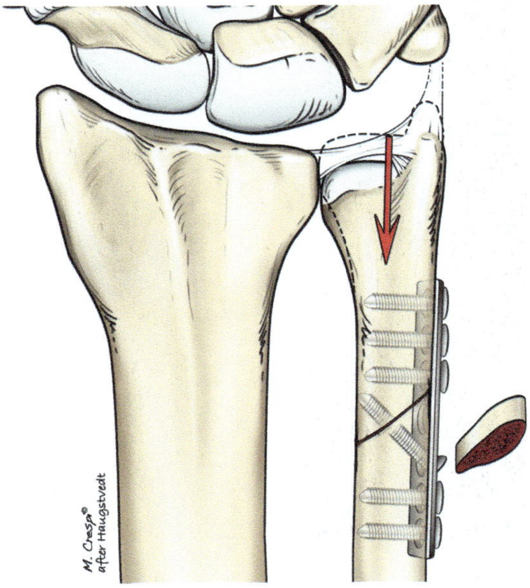

Fig. 42.11 There are many plates designed for ulnar shortening osteotomy. If an oblique parallel resection is made, a screw perpendicular to the cut will give good compression and the plate provides good stability for early mobilization

References

Adams BD, Berger RA. An anatomic reconstruction of the distal radio ulnar ligaments for posttraumatic DRUJ instability. J Hand Surg Am. 2002;27:243–51.

Atzei A. New trends in arthroscopic management of type 1-B TFCC injuries with DRUJ instability. J Hand Surg Eng. 2009;34(5):582–91.

Bernstein MA, Nagle DJ, Martinez A, Stogin Jr JM, Wiedrich TA. A comparison of combined arthroscopic triangular fibrocartilage complex debridement and arthroscopic wafer distal ulna resection versus arthroscopic triangular fibrocartilage complex debridement and ulnar shortening osteotomy for ulnocarpal abutment syndrome. Arthroscopy. 2004;20(4):392–401.

Haugstvedt JR, Berger RA, Nakamura T, Neale P, Berglund L, An KN. Relative contributions of the ulnar attachments of the triangular fibrocartilage complex to the dynamic stability of the distal radioulnar joint. J Hand Surg Am. 2006;31:445–51.

Haugstvedt JR, Husby T. Results of repair of peripheral tears in the triangular fibrocartilage complex using an arthroscopic suture technique. Scand J Plast Reconstr Surg Hand Surg. 1999;33(4):439–47.

Laurentin-Pérez LA, Goodwin AN, Babb BA, Scheker LR. A study of functional outcomes following implantation of a total distal radioulnar joint prosthesis. J Hand Surg Eng. 2008;33(1):18–28.

Lindau T, Arner M, Hagberg L. Intraarticular lesions in distal fractures of the radius in young adults. A descriptive arthroscopic study in 50 patients. J Hand Surg Br. 1997;22(5):638–43.

Nakamura T, Yabe Y, Horiuchi Y. Functional anatomy of the triangular fibrocartilage complex. Hand Surg. 1996;21:581–6.

Nishiwaki M, Nakamura T, Nakao Y, Nagura T, Toyama Y. Ulnar shortening effect on distal radioulnar joint stability: a biomechanical study. J Hand Surg Am. 2005;30(4):719–26.

Palmer AK, Werner FW. The triangular fibrocartilage complex of the wrist—anatomy and function. J Hand Surg Am. 1981;6(2):153–62.

Palmer AK. Triangular fibrocartilage complex lesions: a classification. J Hand Surg Am. 1989;14(4): 594–606.

Scheer JH, Adolfsson LE. Pathomechanisms of ulnar ligament lesions of the wrist in a cadaveric distal radius fracture model. Acta Orthop. 2011;82(3):360–4.

Scheer JH, Hammerby S, Adolfsson LE. Radioulnar ratio in detection of distal radioulnar joint instability associated with acute distal radius fractures. J Hand Surg Eur. 2010;35(9):730–4.

Tay SC, Berger RA, Tomita K, Tan ET, Amrami KK, An KN. In vivo three-dimensional displacement of the distal radioulnar joint during resisted forearm rotation. J Hand Surg Am. 2007;32(4):450–8.

Salvage Procedures to the DRU Joint

43

Dorte Engelund and Camilla Ryge

Contents

D. Engelund, MD (✉)
Hand Surgery Clinic, Department of Orthopedics,
Hillerød Hospital, University of Copenhagen,
DK 3400 Hilleroed, Denmark
e-mail: dorte.engelund@regionh.dk

C. Ryge, MD, PhD
Section of Hand Surgery, Department of Orthopedics,
Hillerød Hospital, University of Copenhagen,
DK 3400 Hilleroed, Denmark

43.1 Summary

When the distal radioulnar joint (DRUJ) is destroyed after a distal radius fracture with or without additional laxity, the remaining surgical option is to salvage function and try to remove pain. Historically the option was to remove the ulnar head. This has turned out to produce new problems such as ulnar stump impingement and severe instability. The Sauvé-Kapandji procedure gives more stability to the wrist, but the stump impingement is still a problem in some cases. Ulnar head implants of different shapes have been developed. An ulnar head replacement can restore the biomechanical properties of the joint. The choice of method is depending on the patient's specific needs. None of the methods are ideal and none can restore normal function, strength, durability and absence of pain. Nevertheless until now, most reports are promising.

43.2 Introduction

The distal radioulnar joint is affected in most distal radius fractures. The initial energy that causes the fracture inevitably also affects the DRUJ. This results in cartilage lesions of the ulnar head and/or the sigmoid notch and damage to the soft tissue that stabilises the joint – these are the TFCC, the ECU subsheath and the joint capsule. Both lesions deteriorate with time, leading to arthritis, instability or both. Some lesions are

L.M. Hove et al. (eds.), *Distal Radius Fractures*,
DOI 10.1007/978-3-642-54604-4_43, © Springer-Verlag Berlin Heidelberg 2014

recognised and dealt with acutely, most, however, in the months or even years thereafter.

The authors of the previous chapters describe interventions to restore well-functioning DRUJ: TFCC reinsertion, TFCC reconstruction and corrective osteotomies of the distal radius and/or ulnar shortening. The topic of this chapter is the salvage procedures. They become relevant when all methods to restore the joint are exhausted, the laxity is irreparable and joint surfaces are destroyed.

Salvage procedures are not ideal solutions for anybody, but offer the best results we can obtain with the methods at our disposal.

It is therefore of the outmost importance that the patient is informed about the possibilities regarding his or her particular situation and is involved in the decision making between the different surgical options or even the possibility of doing nothing surgically.

Salvage procedures for the DRUJ can be divided into two categories: arthroplasties with autologous material or procedures with prosthetic implants.

43.3 The Role of the Ulnar Head

Until the beginning of the 1990s, autologous methods were the only possible methods (except for the Swanson silicone ulnar head, which failed unacceptably early). For that reason, we have long-term experience with these methods and have knowledge of the drawbacks.

In the 1980s, anatomic and biomechanical studies disclosed that the DRUJ is a complex structure of outmost importance providing stability, strength and mobility in the connection between the forearm and the wrist (Hagert 1979; Palmer and Werner 1981; Ekenstam and Hagert 1985).

The DRUJ comprises the ligamentous apparatus, TFCC, ulnocarpal ligaments, ECU sheath, and the bony elements, the sigmoid notch of the radius and the ulnar head itself. The recognition of the importance of the DRUJ is the basis for the development of the different prosthetic implants on the market today.

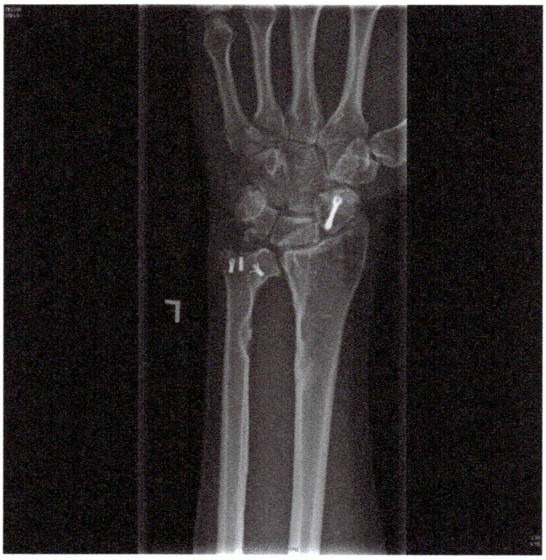

Fig. 43.1 A typical candidate for salvage procedures. Evidence of several prior surgeries – not all successful. Scaphoid fracture, distal radius fracture, TFCC reinsertion and DRU ligament reconstruction a.m. Scheker

The relevant patients have often had one or more previous surgeries to their wrist. They complain with pain, instability, diminished force and sometimes restricted movement. Figure 43.1 shows an X-ray of the wrist of a candidate for salvage procedures. The situation now is a painful arthritic instable DRUJ with restricted rotation and ulnocarpal abutment.

43.4 Autologous Methods

43.4.1 Ulnar Head Excision

- The first method to address pain in the distal forearm after a Colles fracture was the Darrach method, which dates back to 1912. It is a total resection of the ulnar head. It is supposed to relieve pain and to restore forearm rotation.
- Several authors have invented modifications of the simple ulnar head resection. In short, Bowers performs a hemiresection of the head with preservation of the ulnocarpal ligaments and creates an interposition with tendon material between the ulnar stump and the radius. Watson and Wolf have described other

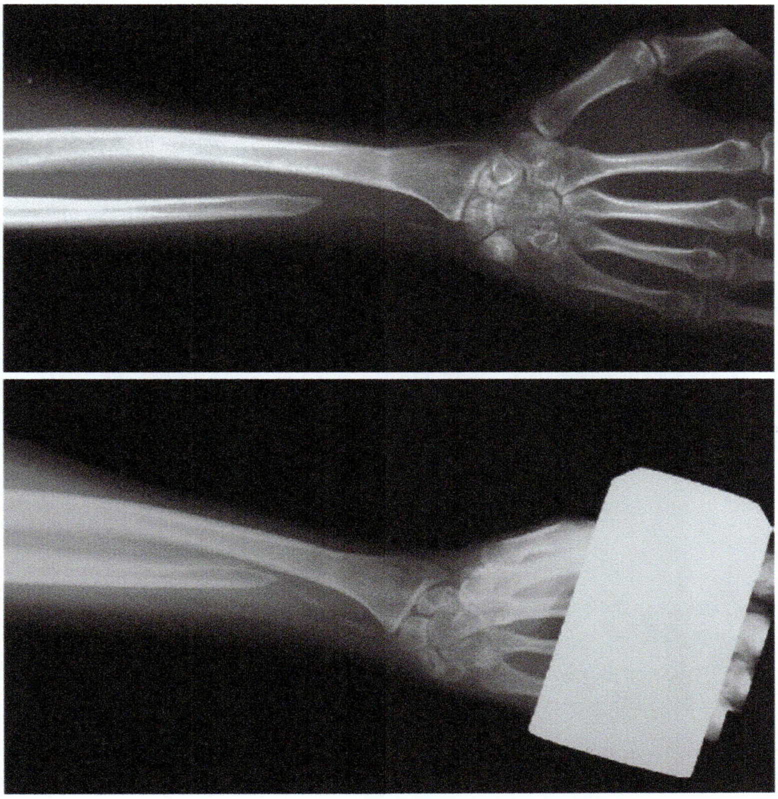

Fig. 43.2 The impingement occurs with load and is not seen on a normal AP view, but requires a load in the lifting hand, neutral rotation and the X-ray taken with horizontal beams. Luis Scheker with permission

modifications, but the problems are not solved. The patients can rotate their DRUJ, but cannot lift any weight without pain (Scheker 2012).

- The Darrach procedure and the above modifications have been widely used. There are two main problems. The carpus is unsupported and drifts ulnarly and the radius impinges on the proximal stump of the ulna. The impingement mechanism is described in Fig. 43.2 (Lees and Scheker 1997).

43.4.2 Sauvé-Kapandji

- In 1936, Sauvé and Kapandji described another approach. They perform a fusion of the DRUJ, so that the aching surfaces are locked. In order to re-establish rotation, they create a pseudarthrosis proximal to the ulnar head, by taking out a small wafer of the ulnar neck and thus creating the possibility of a new rotation centre (Fig. 43.3).

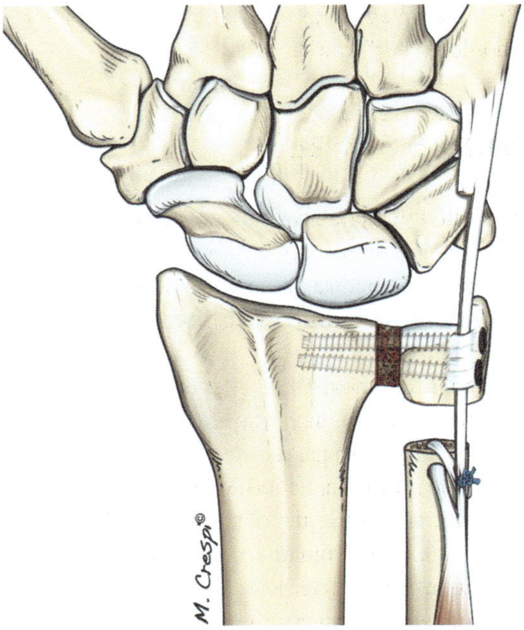

Fig. 43.3 Sauvé-Kapandji procedure with recommended details. See text

- The advantages are that it stops the arthritic pain from moving the DRUJ. It gives better support to the carpus and less ulnar translation. But the problem with instability and impingement of the proximal ulnar stump is not eradicated. In addition, non-union of the fusion is not rare.

"Sauvé-Kapandji Tips and Tricks"
Rotate the head correctly.
- Place in supination, and predrill with a K-wire guide volarly to the styloid into the radius. This places the ulnar styloid, as well as the ECU sheath and tendon, in continuity with the dorsal radius.

In order to prevent non-union, we propose these cautions:
- Decorticate the joint surfaces.
- Put bone graft in between (from the resected bone).
- Fix with two screws or pins to avoid movement in the fusion site. Two headless cannulated compression screws are easy and effective (Fig. 43.3).

To avoid ulnocarpal abutment:
- In any way, place the ulnar head stump in an ulna minus position.

To obtain the best possible stability of the proximal ulnar stump:
- Always perform one of the recommended soft tissue stabilisations, e.g. ECU tenodesis.

43.4.3 Soft Tissue Stabilisation

The efforts to stabilise the ulnar stump have yielded different techniques. Although none is ideal, it seems rational to recommend a dynamic ECU tenodesis for Sauvé-Kapandji. The ECU is an important stabiliser of the ulnar head as it is constrained within the six compartments. After resection of the ulnar head or resection of a distal part of the ulnar shaft, the tendon's constraining effect on the distal ulna is lost. The ECU tenodesis (Fig. 43.3) has been proven to last in a follow-up study, of 95 months (Akio Minami et al. 2006).

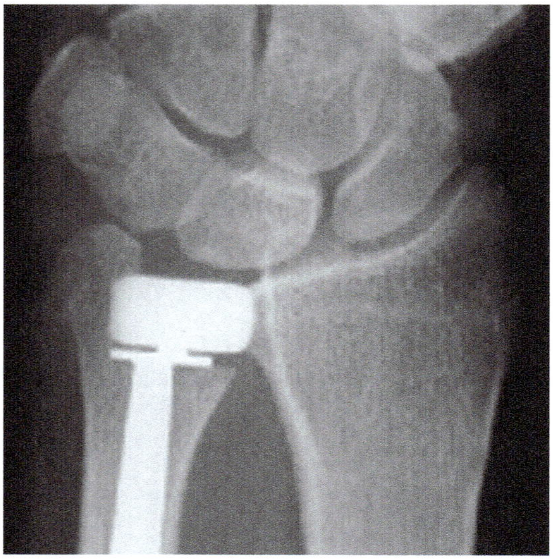

Fig. 43.4 Partial head implant. A pyrocarbon spacer on a titanium stem

43.5 Methods with Prosthetic Implants

There are different prosthetic devices to address different levels of mismatch problems of the DRUJ.

43.5.1 Partial Ulnar Head Implants

- The ulnar head implant (hemiarthroplasty or ulnar head spacer) solves problems of isolated ulnar head damage with preserved TFCC.
- In order to replace the joint surface alone and to save the ligamentous apparatus and its insertion on the healthy part of the ulna, the partial ulnar head prosthesis has been developed. The current prosthetic types on the market require resection of the joint-bearing part of the ulnar head, while the TFCC and its attachments to the fovea and to the styloid are left untouched. Figure 43.4 shows a partial head implant in place.

43.5.2 Total Ulnar Head Implants

- These are the implants that were manufactured first. The total ulnar head is resected and replaced. Most are modular with either a metal

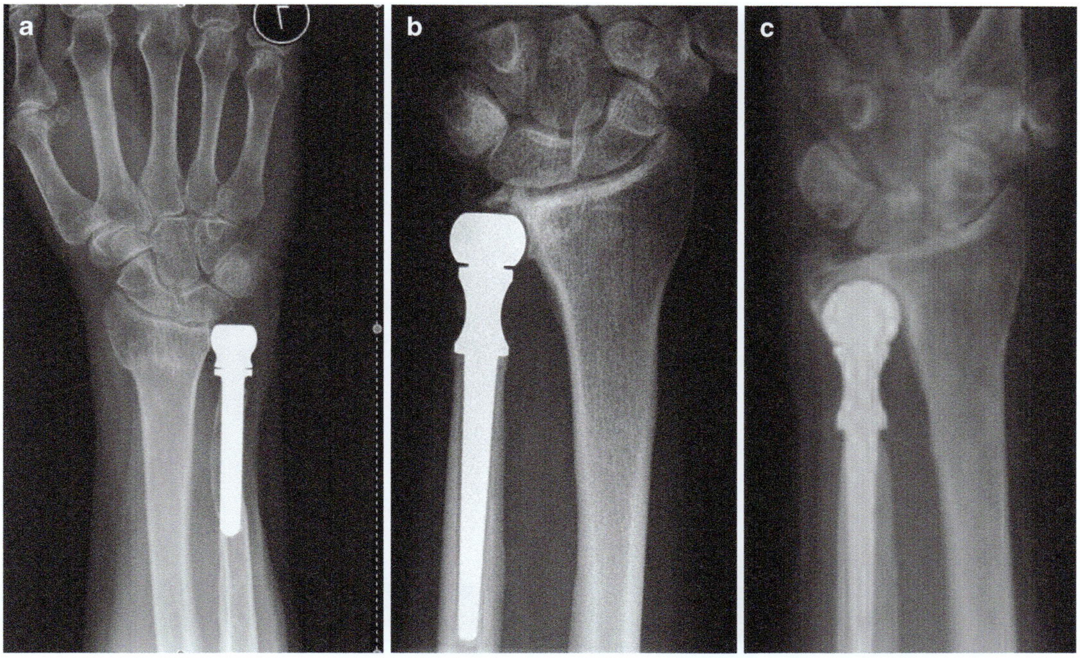

Fig. 43.5 Examples of total ulnar head implants. (**a**) uHead from SBI. (**b**) ulnar head from Martin (Herbert). (**c**) spherical ulnar head from Martin (Herbert) especially for Sauvé-Kapandji revision

or ceramic head. With all of them, some reattachment of the TFCC remnants and accessible soft tissue is recommended.

- The first series reported 23 patients with failed Darrach procedures who had an ulnar head replacement (Herbert prosthesis). At 2 years, all participants had a significant improvement of symptoms (Van Schonhooven et al. 2000).

The same group of patients was reviewed in a long-term follow-up study 11 years on Van Schonhooven et al. 2012. Only 16 patients were reachable, but the results were impressive. There was no deterioration in any of the results.

- Recently, a follow-up study of 30 months, encompassing 25 patients that had ulnar head replacement, as the first treatment for arthritic DRUJ, showed even better results than as a second procedure after ulnar head resection (Sauerbier et al. 2013).
- There are several designs for total ulnar head replacement (Fig. 43.5), even some are designed as salvage for previously performed Sauvé-Kapandji.
- Over the last 10–15 years, increasing numbers of studies reflect successful ulnar head replacements. Restoration of stability, rotation and pain-free strength is the rule. Even arthritic sigmoid joint surfaces seem to tolerate and adapt. Some have reported visible wear of the sigmoid on X-ray, but with surprisingly little clinical importance (Willis et al. 2007; Herzberg 2010).

43.5.3 Total DRUJ Replacement

- The ulnar head prostheses only address the problems on the ulnar part of the joint.
- The next step in the evolution of distal ulnar joint prostheses addresses the radial part as well. Two different concepts are available at the time being.
- One is an unconstrained system where a sigmoid notch implant of metal-backed polyethylene is developed to match the existing ulnar head implant (Fig. 43.6). Movement is possible in rotation, in the axial plane and a little in the AP plane – as in the physiologic joint. The stability depends on soft tissue remnants and optional additional stabilising procedures. The

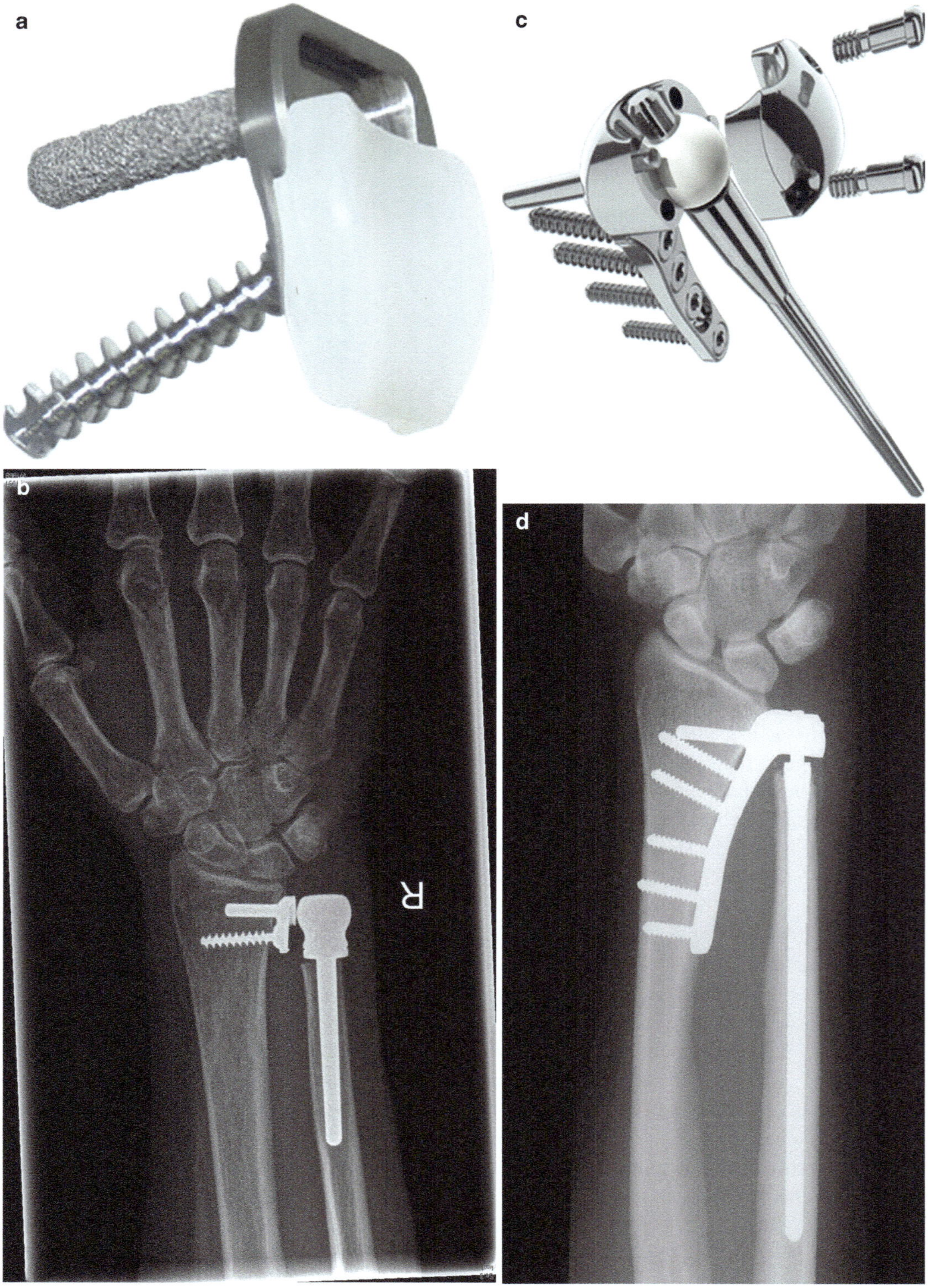

Fig. 43.6 (**a**) sigmoid component (Stability) from SBI to match the uHead. (**b**) the components of the Aptis prosthesis. (**c**) X-ray of DRUJ replacement with Stability and uHead unconstrained system. (**d**) X-ray of DRUJ replacement with Aptis semi-constrained system

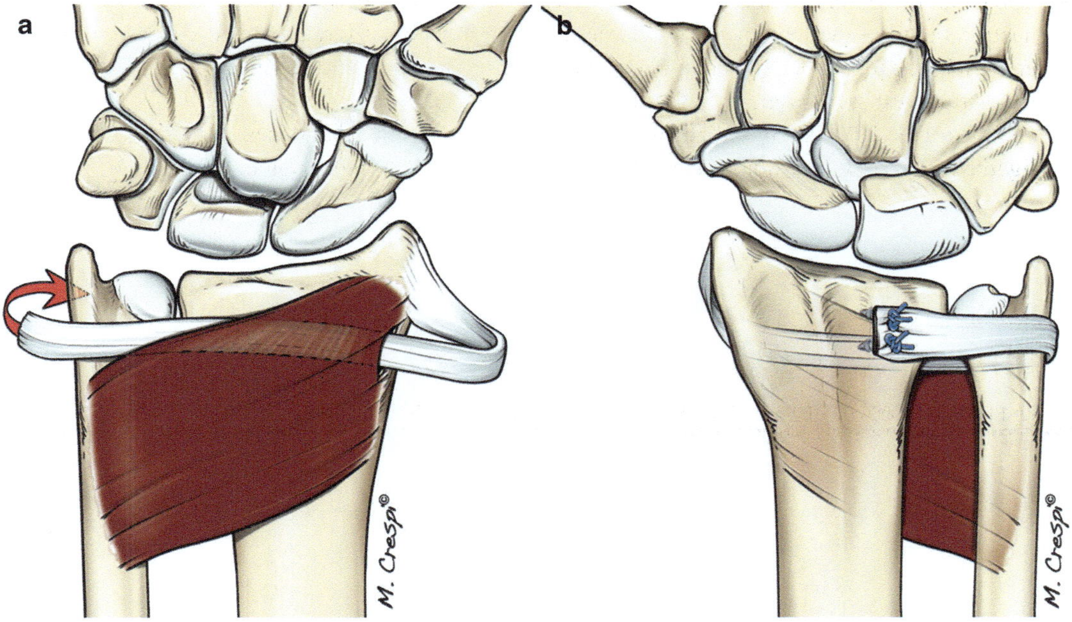

Fig. 43.7 Brachioradialis wrap technique (**a**) the tendon is passed deep to the pronator quadratus from radial to ulnar. (**b**) then around the ulnar head (implant) and dorsally anchored to the rim of the sigmoid notch

system is relatively new and there are no follow-up studies yet. Though, the ulnar head part has been tested over time (Willis et al. 2007).

- The other concept is a so-called semi-constrained implant, where the prosthetic joint is a metal on metal joint with a ball core of polyethylene. With this device, movement is possible in the axial plane and in rotation (Fig. 43.6).

The semi-constrained implant is naturally very stable and meets the expectation of a pain-free, stable and moveable joint. No additional soft tissue stabilisation is necessary. The future will show if the rigidity of the system will cause loosening. The latest studies with 6-year follow-ups report lasting improvement in ROM and weight-bearing capacity. No loosening was reported (Laurentin-Pérez et al. 2008; Savvidou et al. 2013).

43.6 Stabilisation of Unconstrained Prosthesis

43.6.1 The Brachioradialis Wrap

When dealing with unconstrained implants, local soft tissue remnants are not always strong enough to stabilise the DRUJ. This challenge is met in an elegant way with the brachioradialis wrap (Amit Gupta 2013) (Fig. 43.7).

Identify the musculous border of the brachioradialis tendon proximally radially on the forearm. Harvest and cut as proximal as possible, getting a good long tendon. Take care not to damage the branch of the radial nerve. Draw the graft down to the radial styloid, were it remains attached. Pass it underneath the pronator quadratus. Hereafter, take it round the head/collar of the implant and lastly insert it on the dorsal rim of the sigmoid notch of the radius, usually with two anchors in the radius.

We use it for stabilising an ulnar head implant with or without a sigmoid notch component.

43.6.2 The Need of a Sigmoid Notch Component

In hip surgery, hemiarthroplasties are given to elderly people with a short life expectancy. In all other femoral head replacements, an acetabular component is mandatory in order to avoid the wear of the prosthetic head against the cartilage of the acetabulum.

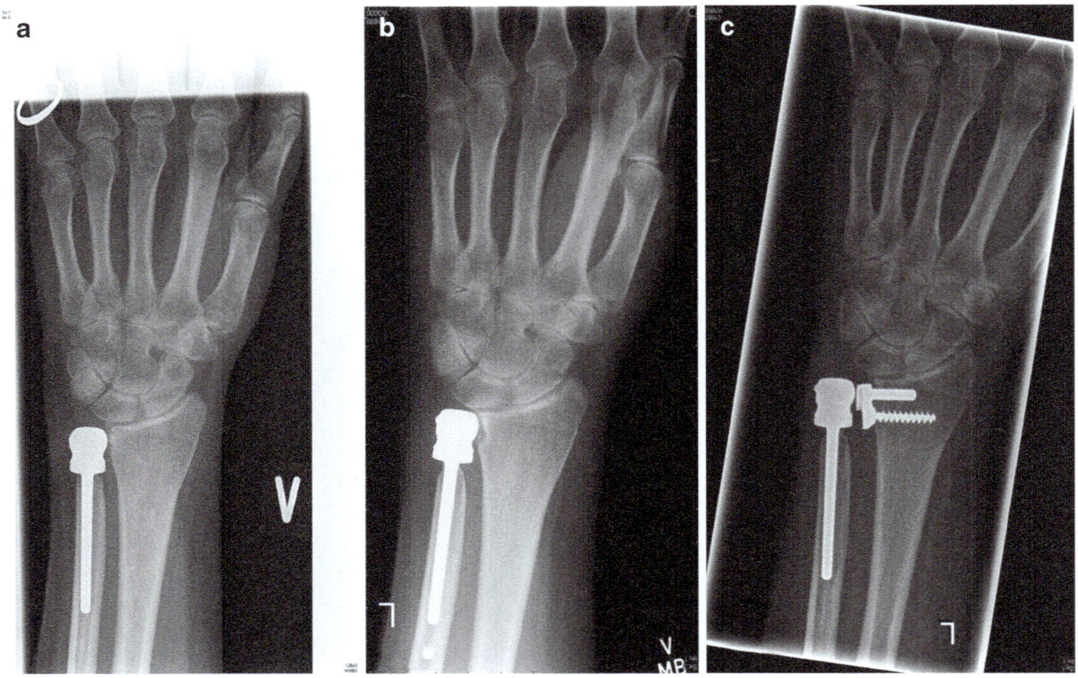

Fig. 43.8 Symptomatic sigmoid wear after 5 years. Pain free after addition of a sigmoid component. (**a**) Primary ulnar head replacement. (**b**) 5 years down the line sigmoid wear. (**c**) addition of sigmoid component

The patients we have met with an ulnar head replacement alone have come back in pain. We know that literature tells not to worry (Willis et al. 2007; Herzberg 2010), but despite this, we suspect that the subchondral bone of a worn sigmoid could yield pain when loaded on a metal head. The work of Herzberg (2010) is prospective and will presumably give a valid answer with time.

We often prefer to do a total DRUJ replacement at once with a modular ulnar head implant and a sigmoid notch implant combined with the BR wrap.

In some instances, the osteoarthritis has deformed the original shape of the sigmoid notch, and it is necessary to plan preoperatively on the basis of a 3D CT scan where to resect bone and where to place a sigmoid notch implant for good congruency of the DRUJ.

43.6.3 Cases with Sigmoid Wear

One patient had had an ulnar head implant 5 years earlier. It had functioned perfectly for the first 3 years. Hereafter, the wrist became increasingly painful. X-ray showed slight wearing of the sigmoid notch corresponding to the clinical findings. She had a revision with a sigmoid notch implant and replacement of the ulnar head implant. In addition, we performed a BR wrap for stability. The pain promptly disappeared and has lasted for 3 years now (no further follow-up) (Figs. 43.8 and 43.9).

Another patient had had an Eclypse pyrocarbon spacer. Although the material should be less harmful to the cartilage than metal, she did not experience any pain relief after the operation.

Clinically the most probable reason was the arthritic sigmoid shown on CT (Figs. 43.10 and 43.11). The final solution for this patient was a modification to the Bowers procedure. The implant was removed and a fascia lata soft tissue graft was used for interposition (Fig. 43.12).

43.7 Discussion

Many of the prosthetic devices described above have given promising results in the short term. But surgeons and patients must remember that

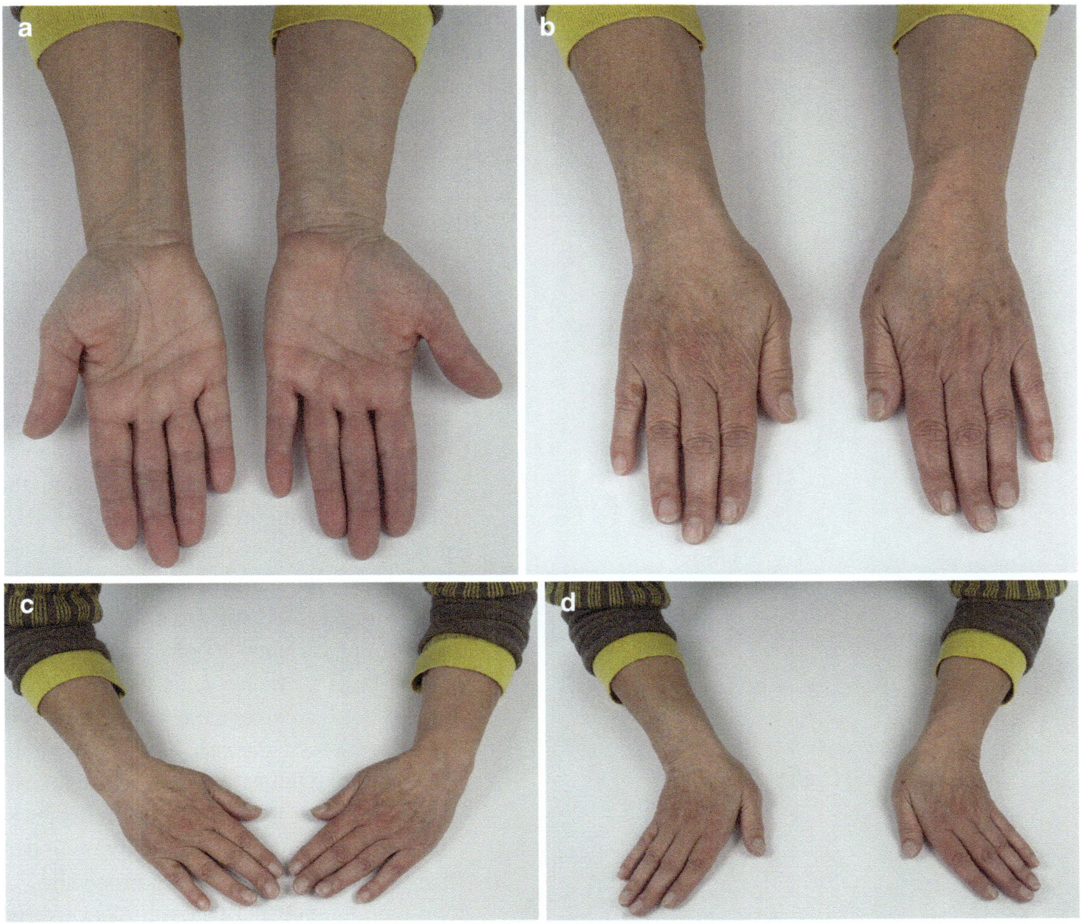

Fig. 43.9 Range of motion 3 month after total DRUJ replacement in the right wrist. (**a**) supination. (**b**) pronation. (**c**) radial deviation. (**d**) ulnar deviation

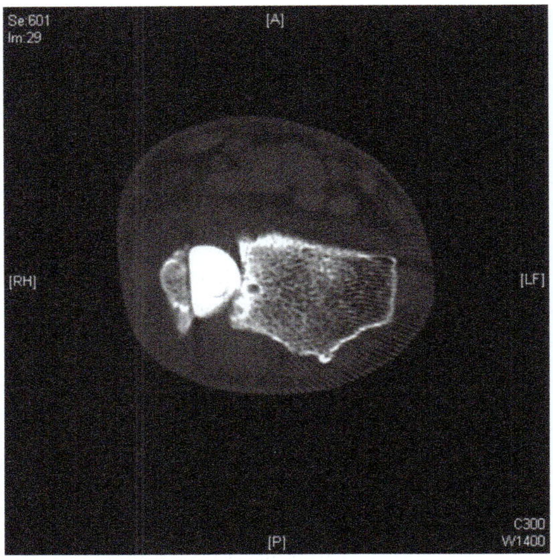

Fig. 43.10 Arthritic sigmoid shown on CT

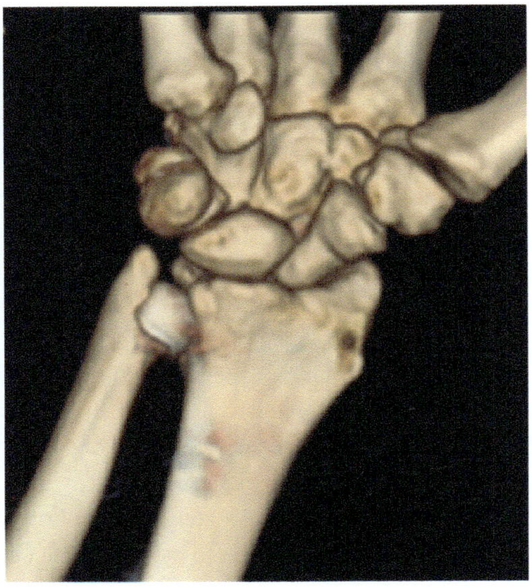

Fig. 43.11 The implant in place before removal. Apparently well placed

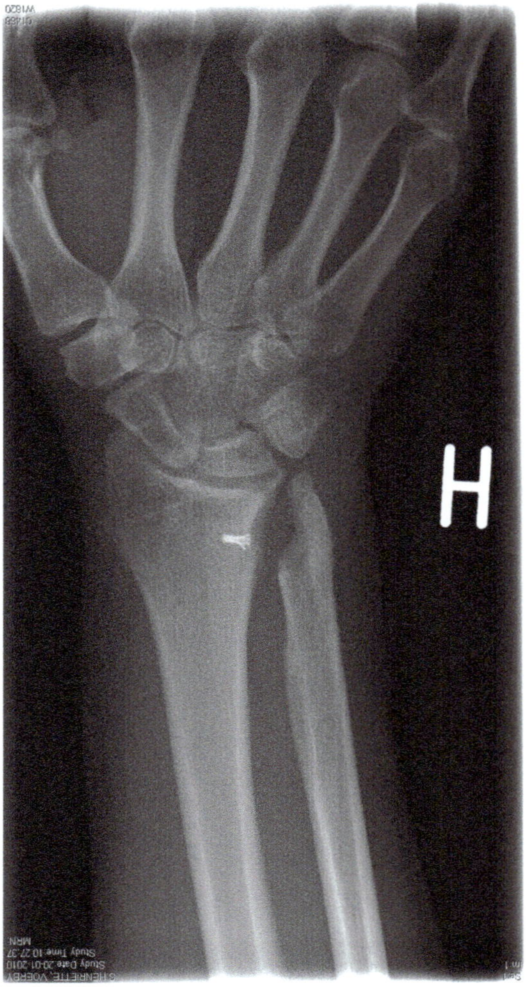

Fig. 43.12 Modified Bowers procedure with fascia lata soft tissue interposition

we still lack a solid, long- term follow-up of these relatively new items. We must bear in mind the lessons learned by our colleagues and their patients concerning prosthetic implants in other joints.

Although the manufacturers of the prosthetic devices can benefit from others' experiences with orthopaedic implants, special problems will probably show up related to this joint. The classic risks are loosening, periprosthetic fractures and material wear.

The first studies with a long-term follow-up (up to 11 years) give reason to be optimistic (Van Schonhooven et al. 2012).

Still we have only seen publications of series from the clinics involved in developing the implants. Economic interests might bias the results. It will be interesting to see the results when the operations become widely spread.

Conclusion

- Excision arthroplasty can only restore forearm rotation at the expense of stability; the ulnar head is an important part of the joint and has to be replaced in case of malfunction.
- The first encouraging reports, from more than 10 years follow-up after ulnar head replacement, have been published. It seems rational to replace the ulnar head in the majority of patients with desolate DRUJ problems. It is increasingly safe to do DRUJ replacement surgery.
- Unfortunately, we still have to be cautious with young patients. People under 40 have a life span of so many years ahead of them that it seems naïve to expect the implants to last. Because of the risk of complications, loosening and future need for replacement(s) of prosthesis, it is probably still most feasible to treat a painful DRUJ in a young person with the Sauvé-Kapandji procedure.
- We recommend that Darrach, Bowers and other excision procedures should be used solely as a last solution in patients with failed prosthesis or in elderly patients with low functional demands.
- As for the distribution of distal radius fractures, the pattern of patients with posttraumatic DRUJ problems ranges from young to old and high to low demands to strength and mobility.
- It is essential for a successful outcome that the patient and the surgeon make decisions on an informed basis. The decision should be based on the operative options, the risks, postoperative immobilisation, physiotherapy and the expected functional result and its limitations. Nonoperative treatment should even be considered.
- Detailed operative techniques of the procedures described in this chapter are beyond the scope of this book.

References

Ekenstam F, Hagert CG. Anatomical studies on the geometry and stability of the distal radio ulnar joint. Scand J Plast Reconstr Surg Hand Surg. 1985;19:17–25.

Gupta A. Brachioradialis wrap: a new method of stabilizing the distal radioulnar joint. In: Slutsky DJ, editor. Principles and practice of wrist surgery. Philadelphia: Saunders; 2013; chapter 32.

Hagert CG. Functional aspects of the distal radioulnar joint. J Hand Surg Am. 1979;4:585.

Herzberg G. Periprosthetic bone resorption and sigmoid notch erosion around ulnar head implants: a concern. Hand Clin. 2010;26(4):573–7.

Laurentin-Pérez LA, et al. A study of functional outcomes following implantation of a total distal radioulnar joint prosthesis. J Hand Surg Eur. 2008;33(1): 18–28.

Lees VC, Scheker LR. The radiological demonstration of dynamic ulnar impingement. J Hand Surg Br. 1997; 22B(4):448–50.

Minami A, Norimasa I, Ishikawa J, Suenaga N, Kato H. Stabilization of the proximal ulnar stump in the Sauvé-Kapandji procedure by using the extensor carpi ulnaris tendon: long-term follow-Up studies. J Hand Surg Am. 2006;31A(3):440–4.

Palmer AK, Werner FW. The triangular fibrocartilage complex of the wrist: anatomy and function. J Hand Surg Am. 1981;6:153–62.

Sauerbier M, et al. Ulnar head replacement and related biomechanics. J Wrist Surg. 2013;2:27–329.

Savvidou C, et al. Semiconstrained distal radioulnar joint prosthesis. J Wrist Surg. 2013;2(1):41–8.

Scheker LR. Is there a place for Salvage Procedures of the Distal Radio Ulnar Joint in the 21th century. ASSH meeting 2012, Chicago, Symposium 09.

van Schoonhoven J, Fernandez DL, Bowers WH, Herbert TJ. Salvage of failed resection arthroplasties of the distal radioulnar joint using a new ulnar head prosthesis. J Hand Surg Am. 2000;25:438–46.

van Schonhooven J, et al. Salvage of failed resection arthroplasties of the distal radioulnar joint using an ulnar head prosthesis: long-term results. J Hand Surg Am. 2012;37(7):1372–80.

Willis AA, Berger RA, Cooney WP. Arthroplasty of the distal radio ulnar joint using a new ulnar head endoprosthesis: preliminary report. J Hand Surg Am. 2007; 32A:177–89.

Wrist Denervation

44

Carlos Heras-Palou

Contents

C. Heras-Palou, MD
Consultant Hand and Wrist Surgery,
Pulvertaft Hand Centre, Royal Derby Hospital,
Derby, UK
e-mail: carlos.heraspalou2@gmail.com

L.M. Hove et al. (eds.), *Distal Radius Fractures*,
DOI 10.1007/978-3-642-54604-4_44, © Springer-Verlag Berlin Heidelberg 2014

44.1 Summary

The purpose of wrist denervation is to decrease pain by surgically dividing the nerves that transmit the afferent pain signal from the wrist. Osteoarthritis following distal radius fractures is a rare problem, which can be treated by denervation. Patient selection using local anaesthetic blocks and functional assessment help to identify patients that are good candidates for this procedure. Wrist denervation can be complete or partial. Results seem to be good in the long term in two-thirds of cases.

44.2 Indications

- The purpose of wrist denervation is to decrease pain by surgically dividing the nerves that transmit the afferent pain signal from the wrist.
- It is indicated in cases of wrist osteoarthritis (OA) that present with significant pain, but have functional movement and no carpal or distal radioulnar (DRU) joint instability. Denervation is a surgical alternative to arthrodesis, either partial or total.
- The main indications for wrist denervation are in cases of scapholunate advanced collapse (SLAC), scaphoid nonunion advanced collapse (SNAC), Kienbock's disease, degeneration secondary to crystalline arthropathy and inflammatory arthritis. Its use after distal radius fractures is uncommon.

- A particular indication for isolated denervation of the posterior interosseous nerve (PIN) is relatively unknown.
  - In the weeks following a distal radius fracture, some patients develop intense pain in the wrist with tenderness over the dorsum of the distal forearm, where the posterior interosseous nerve (PIN) is.
  - This is due to injury of this nerve at the time of the fracture, pressure on the nerve due to swelling and tight cast or encasement of the nerve in scar tissue. If left untreated, persistent pain, swelling and stiffness will follow.
  - The diagnosis of PIN-mediated pain is easily confirmed by injecting 1 ml of local anaesthetic around the nerve, just proximal to the fracture. Clinical examination of the patient 20 min later will demonstrate significantly decrease in pain and increased movement. The pain usually returns when the effect of the local anaesthetic wears off.
  - In this case, surgical excision of a segment of the nerve will stop the pain and allow comfortable mobilisation.
- When the radial nerve has been damaged at the time of injury or treatment, due to a tight cast or the introduction of external fixator pins, pain and allodynia may become a significant problem. In these cases, excision of the PIN resolves the allodynia and the wrist pain (Lluch and Beasley 1989). If a radial nerve laceration, compression or neuroma is present, it should be treated as required by the individual situation.

44.3 Patient Selection for Denervation

- Patients with wrist OA, being after radius fractures or other causes, present with wrist pain, weakness of the grip, swelling and stiffness. Often there is a sensation of grating during wrist movement.
- It is important to rule out a neurogenic cause for the pain, in particular carpal tunnel syndrome.

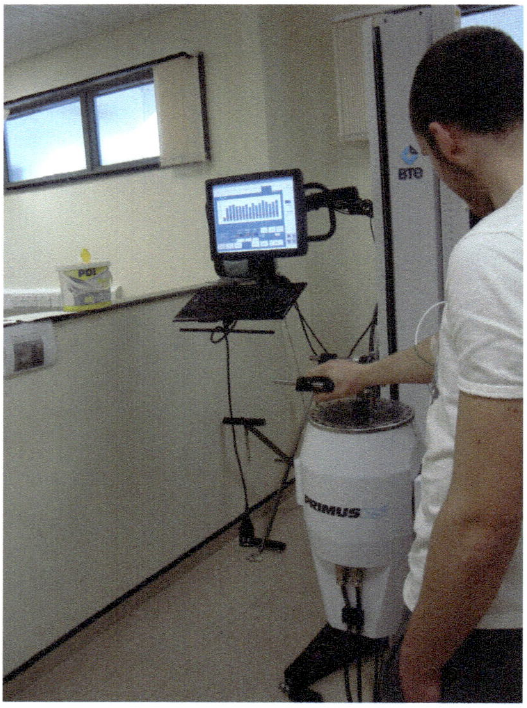

Fig. 44.1 Denervation test is done by assessing wrist function, pain and work output, which is measured before and after a local anaesthetic block. Decrease in pain by 75–90 % and a doubled increase in work output predict a good outcome after denervation

- Patient selection for wrist denervation is controversial. In our experience, a denervation test comprising of local anaesthetic blocks and functional assessment are useful in determining which patients will benefit from the procedure (Storey et al. 2011).
  - We test the patients on a BTE work simulator (Fig. 44.1), before and after injections of 1 ml of marcaine 0.5 % around each of the nerves involved: PIN, anterior interosseous nerve (AIN), under the superficial branches of the radial nerve (SBRN), under the dorsal cutaneous branch of the ulnar nerve, under the palmar branch of the median nerve and around the recurrent intermetacarpal branches.
  - In order to recommend the patient to have a denervation, we would expect the pain to reduce by 75–90 %, the work output to double and no feeling of instability during testing.

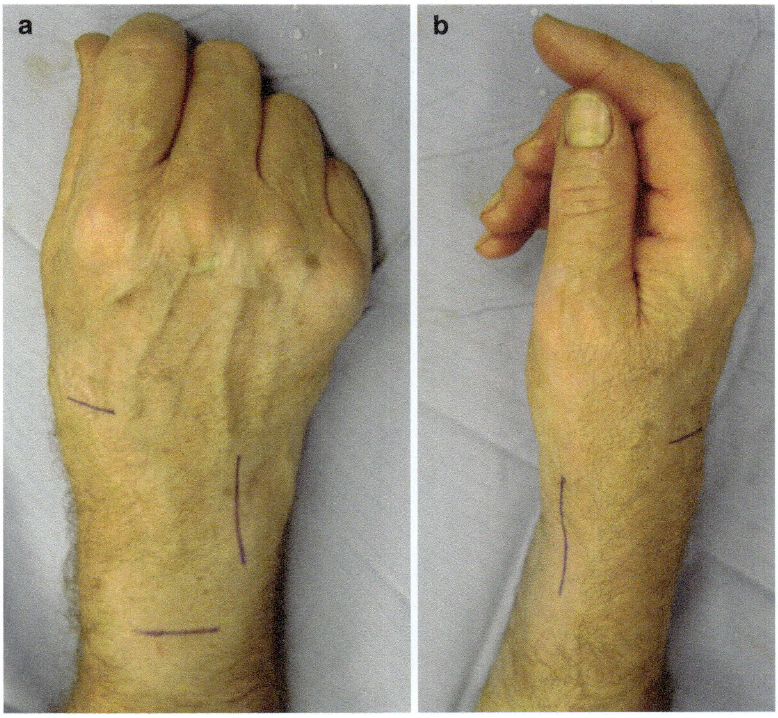

Fig. 44.2 (**a**, **b**) The classical approach to wrist denervation involves four incisions

- Alternatively, the assessment can be done by just examining the patient, with or without grip strength measurements, before and after blocks, or by using a pain diary, but the functional testing gives a more accurate prediction of success, and the patient has a better idea of what to expect after surgery.

44.4 Technique for Wrist Denervation

- Wrist denervation can be done in isolation or combined with other procedures, such as excision of osteophytes, radial styloidectomy, removal of metalwork or arthroscopic debridement of the wrist.
- The objective of a wrist denervation is to divide the afferent nerves that transmit the pain signal from the wrist (Ferreres et al. 1995). The most important nerve involved is the PIN. Other nerves involved are branches of the AIN and of the SBRN, the dorsal branch of the ulnar nerve, the palmar branch of the median nerve and recurrent intermetacarpal nerve branches.
- A full wrist denervation aims to divide all the wrist branches from these nerves. It is not possible to completely denervate a wrist with surgery. A partial denervation involves less surgery, typically involving division of the PIN with or without division of the AIN.
- The classical technique (Buck-Gramcko 1977) for a wrist denervation involves four incisions (Fig. 44.2):
  1. Transverse incision 5 cm proximal to the wrist in the dorsal forearm. The fourth extensor compartment incised and extensor tendons to the fingers retracted towards the ulnar side
  2. Dorso-ulnar incision, down to extensor retinaculum and then raising flap of skin containing the dorsal branch of the ulnar nerve
  3. Volar-radial incision, allowing to develop a plane under the radial vessels, under the palmar branch of the median nerve and under the radial nerve
  4. Transverse incision over the base of the second and third metacarpals, though the fascia, to expose recurrent intermetacarpal branch

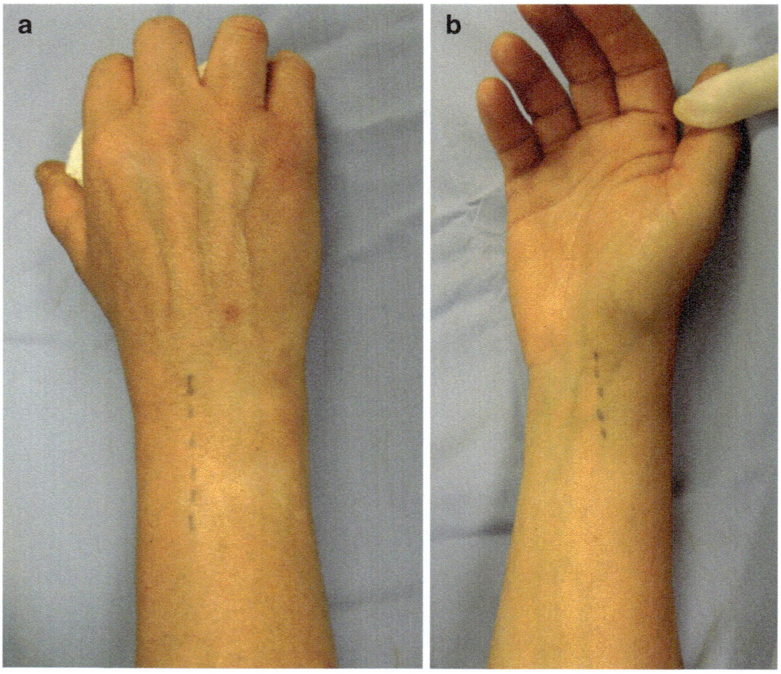

Fig. 44.3 (**a**, **b**) A modified approach using two incisions is simpler and effective

44.5 Our Preferred Technique for Wrist Denervation

- Our preferred method is a modified approach with two incisions, one longitudinal dorsal incision and a second one volar-radial (Fig. 44.3). This makes the operation simpler and provides good access to the areas required. Care must be taken not to damage the radial nerve, the dorsal branch of the ulnar nerve or the palmar branch of the median nerve.
  - Through the dorsal approach, the skin and subcutaneous tissue are raised in a "degloving" fashion from the extensor retinaculum, keeping the SBRN (Fig. 44.4a) and the dorsal branch of the ulnar nerve (Fig. 44.4b) within the flap raised. Communicating branches of the nerves, most often in conjunction with a perforator vein, going into the wrist are diathermised and divided (Fig. 44.4b). A longitudinal incision in the fourth extensor compartment, and retraction of the extensor tendons, will expose the dorsal interosseous pedicle (Fig. 44.4c). The PIN is identified and a 1 cm segment excised.
  - Deep to the PIN, through a longitudinal incision in the distal ulnar part of the interosseous membrane, the anterior interosseous pedicle is exposed, the nerve is identified and a 1cm segment is excised (Fig. 44.4d).
  - Through the volar-radial incision, a plane is developed deep to the radial vessels and to the palmar branch of the median nerve. It is thought that concomitant sympathetic nerve fibres travel with the radial artery and are involved in the transmission of the pain signal.
  - After washout, the skin is sutured. A soft bandage is applied for 10 days, till the sutures are removed and then free movement is allowed. Patients usually return to work between 2 and 4 weeks, mainly depending on their occupation.

44.6 Outcomes of Denervation

- Denervation seems to provide a significant decrease in pain in most patients, particularly if a denervation test with nerve block has come out successfully.
- Full denervation provides good long-term results in 2/3 of patients, while 1/3 may have recurrent

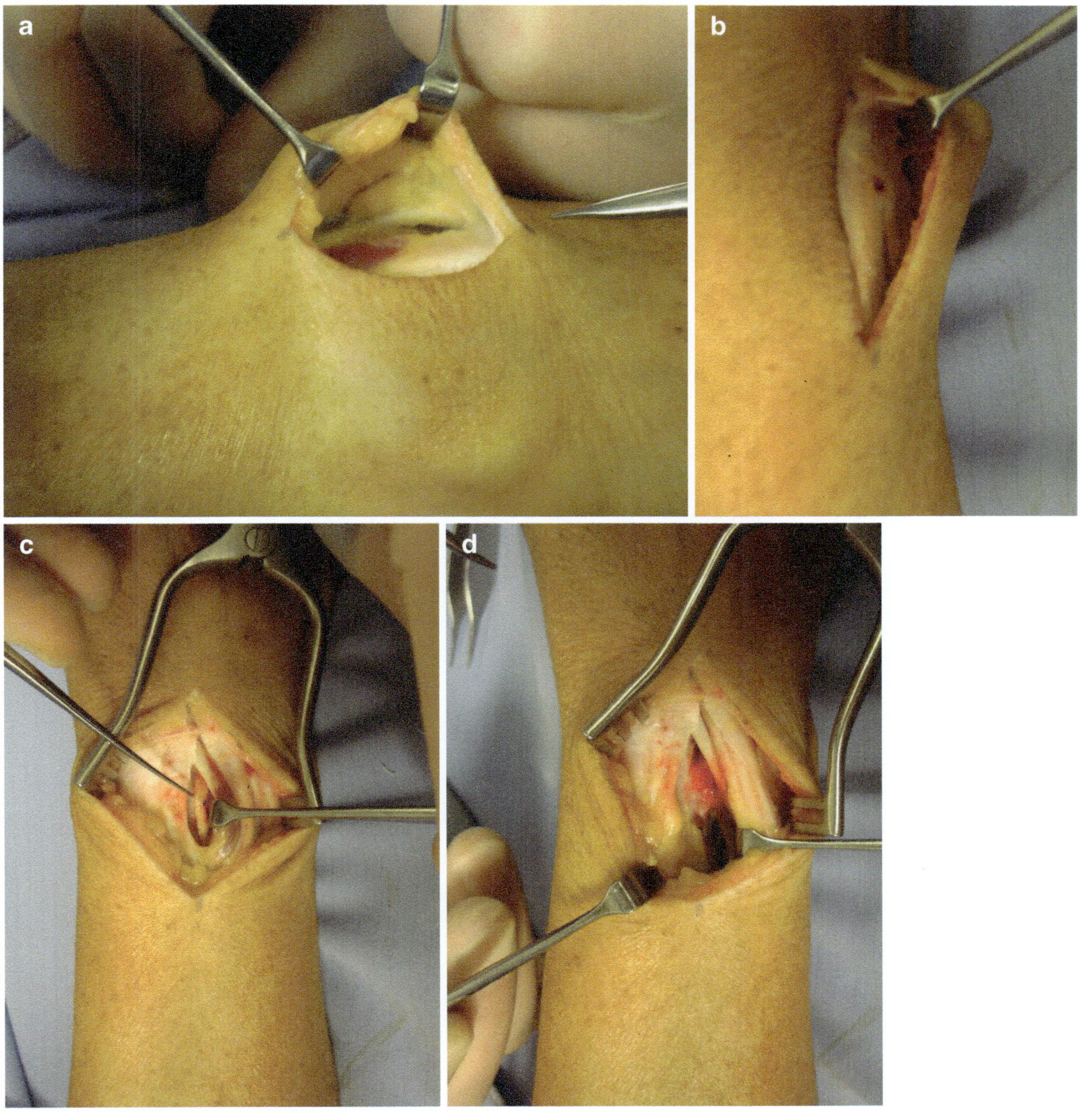

Fig. 44.4 (**a–d**) Through a dorsal approach, the skin and subcutaneous tissues are raised from the fascia in a "degloving" fashion, dividing the branches going into the wrist. (**a**) On the radial side, it is important to include the superficial branch of the radial nerve (SBRN) and all its superficial branches with the flap. (**b**) On the ulnar side, the dorsal branch of the ulnar nerve is protected and the deep branches divided. (**c**) Through a dorsal incision in the fourth extensor compartment, after retraction of the tendons, the posterior interosseous nerve (PIN) is identified and a segment 1cm long is excised. (**d**) Through an incision in the interosseous membrane, the anterior interosseous pedicle is identified and a 1cm segment of the nerve is excised

pain within 10 years of the procedure (Storey et al. 2011). Partial denervation seems to provide good results initially (Weinstein and Berger 2002), but there is often deterioration after 12 months.

- Although there is a theoretical risk of causing a neuropathic Charcot joint, it has never been reported. This probably means that complete denervation of the joint is never achieved.
- Distal numbness is a very rare complication and neuroma formation has been reported in 2 % of patients.

References

Buck-Gramcko D. Denervation of the wrist joint. J Hand Surg Am. 1977;2(1):54–61.

Ferreres A, Suso S, Foucher G. Wrist denervation. Surgical considerations. J Hand Surg Br. 1995;20:769–72.

Lluch AL, Beasley RW. Treatment of dysesthesia of the sensory branch of the radial nerve by distal posterior interosseous neurectomy. J Hans Surg Am. 1989;14(1): 121–4.

Storey PA, Lindau T, Jansen V, Woodbridge S, Bainbridge LC, Burke FD. Wrist denervation in isolation: a prospective outcome study with patient selection by wrist blockade. Hand Surg. 2011;16(3):251–7.

Weinstein LP, Berger RA. Analgesic benefit, functional outcome, and patient satisfaction after partial wrist denervation. J Hand Surg Am. 2002;27A(5):833–9.

Part V

Miscellaneous

Associated Fractures of the Distal Ulna

45

Hebe Désirée Kvernmo

Contents

H.D. Kvernmo, MD, PhD, MHA
Department of Orthopedic, Plastic and Hand Surgery, University Hospital of North Norway, 9038, Tromsø, Norway

Department of Clinical Medicine, University of North Norway – Arctic University of Norway, 9038, Tromsø, Norway
e-mail: hebe.desiree.kvernmo@unn.no

45.1 Summary

Whereas operative treatment of the distal radius fracture in adults has gained much attention, there are only a few reports on the associated fracture of the distal ulna head or neck. Little guidance on how to manage these fractures exists. This can result in inadequate treatment and contribute to less favorable results. Understanding the effect of the two-bone fracture on the stability of the forearm complex is important in proper management of these fractures. The length, alignment, and rotation have to be reestablished and maintained. By providing stable fixation of these fractures, function may be preserved and late complications minimized. During the last decade, an improved management of these challenging distal forearm fractures has followed with the introduction of locking plate technology.

45.2 Introduction

- One-third of distal radius fractures in adults are accompanied with a distal ulna fracture. Most of these occur through the ulnar styloid, but some occur through the ulna head and/or neck.
- The first report on the latter fractures came in 1995 (Biyani et al. 1995). Both the distal radius and the concomitant ulna head or neck fractures were treated conservatively. Excellent and good results were observed in

L.M. Hove et al. (eds.), *Distal Radius Fractures*,
DOI 10.1007/978-3-642-54604-4_45, © Springer-Verlag Berlin Heidelberg 2014

only 60 % of the patients. At the same time, an association between a concomitant distal ulna fracture and the rare distal radius nonunion was reported (McKee et al. 1997; Fernandez et al. 2001; Ring 2005), leading to the knowledge that these associated fractures can affect stability of the forearm.

- Later, a few reports on operative fixation have followed (Ring et al. 2004; Walz et al. 2006; Dennison 2007; Lee et al. 2012), demonstrating greatly improved results.
- This chapter gives an overview of the different aspects in management of associated ulna head and neck fractures. A tailored approach for treatment based on current literature is outlined.

45.3 Epidemiology

- Only one study has given the national incidence on forearm fractures (Wigg et al. 2003). However, the study included all fractures of the distal forearm. The true incidence of a distal radius fracture with an associated distal ulna fracture is therefore unknown.
- Reports on operated distal radius fractures with concomitant ulna head or neck fractures in adult patients (>18 years of age) indicate that these fractures are rare:
  - In a study of associated distal ulna fractures in elderly patients (mean age 70 years) operated for a distal radius fracture, an ulna head fracture was seen in 6 % (Biyani et al. 1995). All were high-energy injuries.
  - In a study of both ulna head and neck fractures, 12.4 % sustained the injury (Walz et al. 2006).
  - In a study of younger adults, even less patients were identified (Gschwentner et al. 2008).
- Widely displaced distal radius fractures are most likely to be accompanied by a distal ulna fracture and most with a comminuted neck fracture (Ring et al. 2004).
- Thirteen percent of the fractures were open fractures, and most of them Grade 1, according to the Gustilo and Anderson classification.

45.4 The Forearm Complex

- To evaluate and treat concomitant distal radius and ulna fractures, a thorough understanding of normal forearm anatomy and biomechanics is crucial. It is important to recognize that this two-bone fracture acts as a forearm fracture rather than a wrist fracture, affecting the stability of the forearm complex.
- The forearm complex is comprised of the proximal radioulnar joint (PRUJ), the interosseous membrane (IOM), and the distal radioulnar joint (DRUJ). These three areas function in a coordinated manner to rotate the hand in space and allow performance of functional tasks (LaStayo and Lee 2006). If one structure of the forearm complex is disrupted, this can adversely affect the function at any of the other areas of the forearm complex.
- The radioulnar joints are considered as a single bicondylar articulation or one functional forearm joint.
- According to the concept of Hagert (1994), the center of forearm rotation is the radial head at the elbow and the fovea at the DRUJ. The distal radius swings around the ulnar head, which is the isometric point for rotational forces (Fig. 45.1). For this movement, the radius is dependent on stability and alignment of the distal ulna. For stability, the radius is attached to the fixed ulna head by the dorsal and volar radioulnar ligaments. These ligaments are parts of the triangular fibrocartilaginous complex (TFCC), stabilizing the DRUJ.
- Histological analysis reveals two predominant attachments to the distal ulna (Nakamura et al. 2001). The deep portion of the ligaments inserts into the fovea, whereas the superficial part inserts into the styloid. When no load is

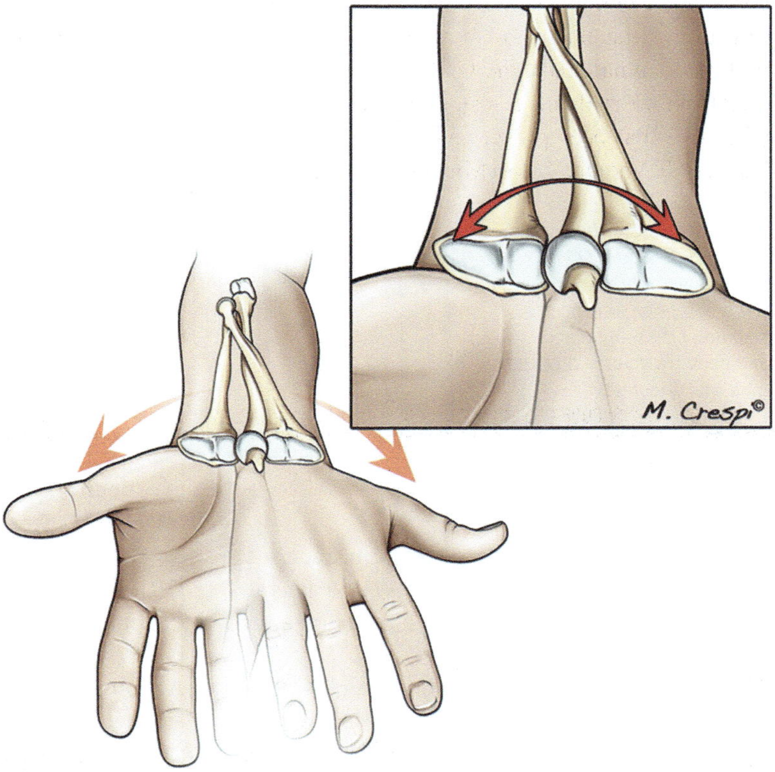

Fig. 45.1 Under rotation, radius swing around the fixed ulna. For distal ulna fractures associated with fractures of the radius, radius is dependent on stability and alignment of the distal ulna

applied across the wrist, each part plays an equal role in stability (Haugstvedt et al. 2006). However, when load is applied of this weight-bearing joint, the deep fibers are found to contribute to significantly greater stability of the DRUJ than the superficial fibers.

- Fractures of the distal ulna may result in incongruency and instability of DRUJ, leading to chronic pain and limited forearm rotation.

45.5 Clinical Examination

- In order to give primary definitive fracture care, pitfalls in diagnosis and treatment should be avoided. The key to diagnosis is a high index of suspicion and a careful clinical examination.
- Early assessment should focus on identifying an open fracture, neurovascular compromise, and/or associated injuries. Check the entire forearm, including the joints above and below the fracture site with every injury, since the frame-anatomy of the forearm makes a double injury likely.

Key Points Clinical Examination

- *Open fracture?* In contrast to an abrasion or puncture from the outside, a small puncture resulting from an open fracture tends to ooze blood.
- *Neurovascular compromise?* Check pulses and the median, ulnar, and radial nerves for motor and sensory disturbances.
- *Associated injuries?* Check the entire arm, including the joint above and below the fracture site.

- Differential diagnosis is multiple fracture patterns including combined fracture dislocations as Monteggia, Galeazzi, and Essex-Lopresti.

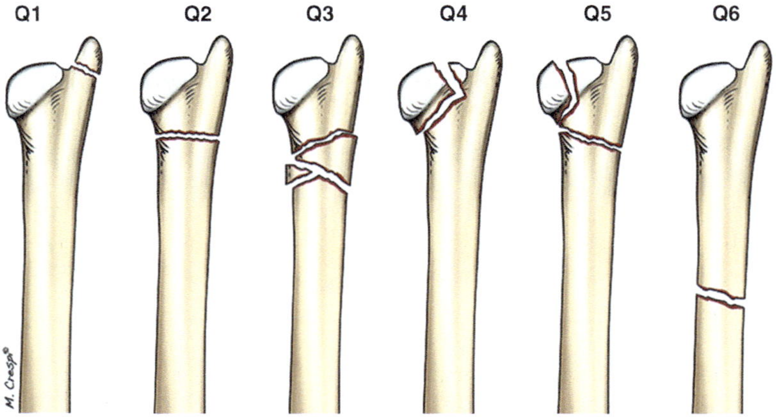

Fig. 45.2 The distal ulna fractures associated with fractures of the distal radius are according to the comprehensive classification of fractures classified according to a Q-modifier. *Q1* designates a simple ulna styloid fracture, *Q2* a simple ulna neck fracture, *Q3* a comminuted ulna neck fracture, *Q4* an ulna head fracture, *Q5* an ulna head and neck fracture, and *Q6* an ulna shaft fracture

45.6 Imaging

- All patients with suspected forearm fractures need a true posteroanterior (PA) and lateral view of the injured forearm, including the wrist and distal humerus.
- For proper wrist evaluation, it is mandatory to perform a standardized radiograph with an elbow position that is 90° of flexion, as the relative position of the two bones can change as much as 2 mm with forearm rotation.
- Comparative views of the opposite wrist can be helpful.
- In articular, partial articular, or displaced fractures, an additional CT scan is recommended.

45.7 Classification

- Both fractures are classified according to the comprehensive classification of fractures (AO/ASIF), where a Q-modifier is used for classification of the associated distal ulna fracture (Fig. 45.2).
- The angulation and malrotation of the distal ulna fracture are noted.
- For open fracture, the grading according to the Gustilo and Anderson classification is noted.

45.8 Conservative Treatment, an Option?

- In conservative treatment of the distal radius and the associated distal ulna fracture, abnormality of the DRUJ is seen in 46 % and excellent and good results are seen in only 60 % at 2 years follow-up (Biyani et al. 1995). As a result, the authors recommended ORIF of the radius as the keystone in the treatment of concomitant injuries of the two bones.
- Although many associated distal ulna head and neck fractures are reported realigned and stable once the radius is realigned and secured (Ring et al. 2004; Dennison 2007), these fractures must be watched carefully for signs of failure of closed treatment due to dislocating forces in the frontal and sagittal plane (McKee et al. 1997).
- As many as 75 % of associated ulna head or neck fractures may be unstable or malaligned after reduction and stabilization of the distal radius fracture (Walz et al. 2006).
- Unless the radius is realigned and stabilized, the DRUJ function and distal forearm stability diminishes due to disruption of the distal radioulnar ligament or loss of structural support for the TFCC (Solan et al. 2003; Seitz and Raikin 2007; Carlsen et al. 2010).
- This may be the cause of distal radius nonunion and callus encroachment of the DRUJ seen with concomitant fractures of the distal radius and ulna (McKee et al. 1997; Fernandez et al 2001; Ring et al. 2004; Ring 2005).
- Proper management of the distal ulna head and neck fracture is therefore an important determinant of the final outcome in order to avoid chronic pain, instability, and diminished pronation and supination.

Key Points Conservative Treatment

- ORIF of the distal radius fracture is mandatory.
- Conservative treatment of the associated distal ulna fracture is an option only if the ulna is realigned and stable after ORIF of the distal radius fracture.
- Plaster cast is then advocated for 6 weeks, with close follow-ups.
- Operative intervention is warranted if reduction is lost or delayed union develops.

45.9 Indication for Surgery

- The key to a successful treatment is near anatomical reduction of the fractures:
  - A study of artificially created forearm fractures in fresh cadaver specimens with intact soft tissue, and thereby intact soft tissue tension, demonstrated clinical important decrease in forearm rotation at *fracture angulation* of more than 10° in the forearm (Tarr et al. 1984).
    - The decrease in pronation and supination is less than 18 % for deformities of 10° or less, but increases to 27 % when the angulation is increased to 15°.
    - The loss of supination is, however, less for fractures in the distal third compared to fractures in the middle third.
  - For *rotatory deformity*, losses of pronation and supination equal the degree of the rotatory deformity.
  - More than 1/2 translation and articular displacement is considered unacceptable for proper forearm stability and DRUJ function (Tarr et al. 1984; Yasutomi et al. 2002) and warrants operative treatment.
- Instability of the distal ulna tested after fixation of the distal radius fracture.
- The same criterion applies to the rare isolated distal ulna fractures.
- The indication for operative treatment is summarized below:

Indication for Operative Treatment

Malalignment

- Angular deformity of the distal ulna fracture >10° in any direction
- Translation >1/2 of ulna head relative to radius
- Articular displacement

Instability of the distal ulna fracture after stabilization of the distal radius fracture

45.10 Operative Treatment and Outcome

- In the past, the distal ulna fracture was likely to have poor outcomes, due to difficulties in achievement of a stable fixation of the often small and metaphyseal fragments of the ulna, which are covered with articular surface over a 270° arc (Ring et al. 2004; Gschwentner et al. 2008).
- The improvements in operative results came with the introduction of the locking plate technology, which allows patients of all ages to be considered for internal fixation (Fig. 45.3), regardless of the bone quality.
- Although operative treatment of the isolated distal ulna fracture was described early (Buterbaugh and Palmer 1988; Jakab et al. 1993), reports of the concomitant distal ulna fracture followed in the recent decade.
- Using the condylar blade plate (Ring et al. 2004), the 2.0-mm Y-, T-, or L-shaped locked plate from the fragment plating system (Dennison 2007), and the ulna hook plate (Lee et al. 2012), a good and excellent functional score was achieved in more than 92 % of the patients, and range of motion were 102–141° in the sagittal plane and 139–159° for rotation at 1-year follow-up.

45.11 Surgical Technique for Locking Plating

- All open fractures are debrided and irrigated.
- The distal radius fracture is then approached depending on fracture type and degree of

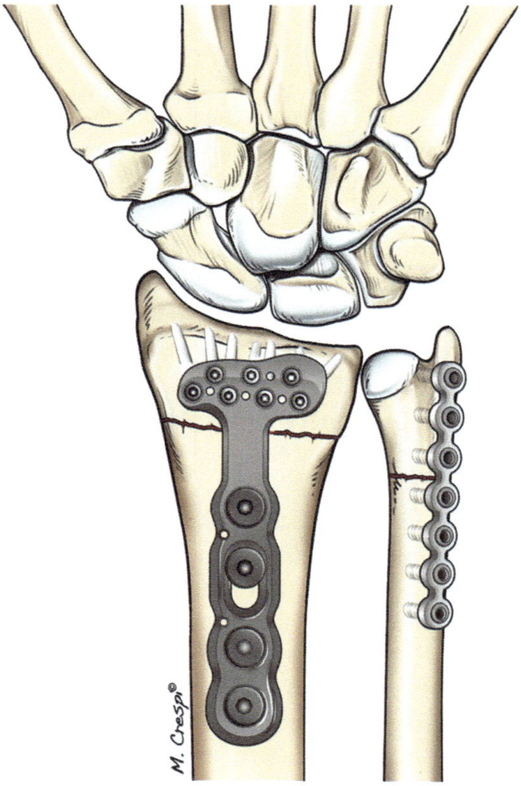

Fig. 45.3 Locking plate of concomitant radius and ulna fracture

instability. Most often, a volar locking plate is used, through a flexor carpi radialis approach.

- After fixation of the distal radius, stability of the distal ulna fracture is determined clinically and radiologically.
- Unstable distal ulna fractures are operated.

Operative Technique of Concomitant Unstable Distal Ulna Fracture (Dennison 2007)

- After fixation of the distal radius fracture, the distal ulna fracture is exposed through a longitudinal incision ulnarly to the sixth extensor compartment, in the extensor carpi ulnaris-flexor carpi ulnaris interval.
- The dorsal sensory branch of the ulnar nerve is identified and protected.
- The fracture is reduced and temporarily held with K-wires.
- A distal K-wire is placed in an ulnar to radial direction, underneath the TFCC complex to identify the distal end of the ulna.
- A 2.0-mm locking plate is the best size for most patients. The plate is bent slightly, forming a concavity toward the bone surface, and contoured to fit along the diaphysis of the ulna. The distal end of the plate is positioned adjacent to the ulna. Alternatively, depending on the fracture plane, the plate is positioned more volarly, carefully avoiding impingement upon radius in full pronation.
- Locked pegs are inserted into the head and plate. Avoid bicortical placement of the distal locking screws to prevent penetration into the DRUJ.
- The plate is then secured to the proximal ulna extraperiosteally.
- When a fracture of the ulna styloid process is present as well, the styloid is reduced and secured with a figure-of-eight suture.
- The extensor retinaculum is repaired.
- The patients are immobilized in a sugar-tong splint for 7–10 days.
- Flexion, extension, and rotational exercises are started after 7–10 days, as tolerated.

- Alternatively, if the fracture extends intra-articular, these locking plates may be insufficient in fixation of the articular surface (Lee et al. 2012). In these cases, the distal ulna hook plate may be favorable. It is precontoured. It is best placed on the ulnar border, directly in line with the ulnar styloid, and acts as a buttress for the fracture fragment of the ulnar styloid.
- The instability criteria and operative technique yield also for the rare isolated distal ulna fractures, which are sustained when the forearm is raised to shield against a blow.

45.12 Postoperative Complications

- From the studies of Ring et al. (2004), Dennison (2007), and Lee et al. (2012), three of the 54 patients had transient paresthesias in the dorsal sensory branch of the ulnar nerve and one in the median nerve distribution area. All nerves recovered completely. Two patients with increased ulnar angulation developed DRUJ arthritis and pain. There were two non-union of the radius and one of the distal ulna. Plate removal had to be performed in 11 of the patients due to plate prominence.

Key Learning Points of this Chapter

- Associated fractures of distal ulna occur in 6–12 % of all operated distal radius fractures (Biyani et al. 1995; Walz et al. 2006).
- For this two-bone fracture, ORIF of the distal radius is indicated.
- After ORIF of the distal radius, intraoperative evaluation of stability of the ulna is performed.
- If the concomitant ulna fracture is reduced and tested stable during passive rotation, cast immobilization may provide sufficient stability for the ulna fracture to heal. It is mandatory to watch the fracture carefully for signs of failure during the healing period.
- If the concomitant ulna fracture is unstable or malaligned, open reduction and internal fixation is advocated also for the distal ulna fracture.
- Different operative methods have been advocated; however, locking plate technology seems to offer the best outcome with acceptable complications.

References

Biyani A, Simison AJM, Klenerman L. Fractures of the distal radius and ulna. J Hand Surg Eur. 1995;20(3):357–64.

Buterbaugh GA, Palmer AK. Fractures and dislocations of the distal radioulnar joint. Hand Clin. 1988;4:361–75.

Carlsen BT, Dennison DG, Moran SL. Acute dislocations of the distal radioulnar joint and distal ulna fractures. Hand Clin. 2010;26(4):503–16.

Dennison DG. Open reduction and internal locked fixation of unstable distal ulna fractures with concomitant distal radius fracture. J Hand Surg Am. 2007;32(6):801–5.

Fernandez DL, Ring D, Jupiter J. Surgical management of delayed union and nonunion of distal radius fractures. J Hand Surg Am. 2001;26:201–9.

Geschwentner M, Arora R, Wambacher M, et al. Distal forearm fracture in the adult: is ORIF of the radius and closed reduction of the ulna a treatment option in distal forearm fracture? Arch Orthop Trauma Surg. 2008;128(8):847–55.

Hagert CG. Distal radius fracture and the distal radioulnar joint: anatomical considerations. Handchir Mikrochir Plast Chir. 1994;26:22–6.

Haugstvedt JR, Berger RA, Nakamura T, et al. Relative contributions of the ulnar attachments of the triangular fibrocartilage complex to the dynamic stability of the distal radioulnar joint. J Hand Surg Am. 2006;31:445–51.

Jakab E, Ganos DL, Ganon S. Isloated intra-articular fracture of the ulnar head. Case report. J Orthop Trauma 1993;7:290–2.

LaStayo PC, Lee MJ. The forearm complex: anatomy, biomechanics and clinical considerations. J Hand Ther. 2006;19(2):137–44.

Lee SK, Kim KJ, Park JS, et al. Distal ulna hook plate fixation for unstable distal ulna fracture associated with distal radius fracture. Orthopedics. 2012;25(9):e1358–63.

McKee MD, Waddel JP, Yoo D, et al. Nonunion of distal radius fractures associated with distal ulnar shaft fractures: a report of four cases. J Orthop Trauma. 1997;11:49–53.

Nakamura T, Takayama S, Horiuchi Y, et al. Origins and insertions of the triangular fibrocartilage complex: a histological study. J Hand Surg Br. 2001;26:446–54.

Ring D, McCarty P, Campbell D, et al. Condylar blade plate fixation of unstable fractures of the distal ulna associated with fracture of the distal radius. J Hand Surg Am. 2004;29(1):103–9.

Ring D. Nonunion of the distal radius. Hand Clin. 2005;21:443–7.

Seitz Jr WH, Raikin SM. Resection of comminuted ulna head fragments with soft tissue reconstruction when associated with distal radius fractures. Tech Hand Up Extrem Surg. 2007;11(4):224–30.

Solan MC, Rees R, Molloy S, et al. Internal fixation after intra-articular fracture of the distal ulna. J Bone Joint Surg Br. 2003;85(2):279–80.

Tarr RR, Garfinkel AI, Sarmiento A. The effects of angular and rotational deformities of both bones of the forearm. An in vitro study. J Bone Joint Surg Am. 1984;66(1):65–70.

Walz M, Kolbow B, Möllenhoff G. Fracture of the distal ulna accompanying fracture of the distal radius. Minimally invasive treatment with elastic stable intramedullary nailing (ESIN). Unfallchirurg. 2006;109(12):1058–63.

Wigg AE, Hearn TC, McCaul KA, et al. Number, incidence, and projections of distal forearm fractures admitted to hospital in Australia. J Trauma. 2003; 55(1):87–93.

Yasutomi T, Nakatsuchi Y, Koike H, et al. Mechanism of limitation of pronation/supination of the forearm in geometric models of deformities of the forearm bones. Biomechanics. 2002;17:456–63.

Galeazzi's Fracture and Essex-Lopresti Injuries: Dislocation Fractures of the Forearm

46

Jan-Ragnar Haugstvedt

Contents

46.1 Summary

The PRUJ and DRUJ should be looked upon as one functional unit: "the forearm joint." If one joint is injured, the function of the entire forearm could suffer. There are many structures of great importance for stabilizing these joints. When a person falls on an outstretched hand or wrist, the person falling could sustain a variety of lesions depending on the position of the wrist and elbow, the direction and action of the muscles, as well as the age of the person at the time of the impact. Correct diagnosis is of outermost importance for the best treatment and outcome. X-ray examination should include the entire forearm as well as the elbow and wrist of the injured and noninjured side. Clinical examination for tenderness and instability should be carried out. A Galeazzi's fracture is a fracture of the shaft of the radius with an associated dislocation of the DRUJ. An Essex-Lopresti injury is a fracture through the radial head with dislocation of the DRUJ. The integrity of a well-functioning forearm is dependent on intact structures of the bones, ligaments, muscles, tendons, and joint capsules, as

J.-R. Haugstvedt, MD, PhD
Department of Orthopedics, Østfold Hospital Trust, Olav Aukrusts vei 58 c, N-0785, Oslo, Moss, Norway
e-mail: jrhaugstvedt@gmail.com

L.M. Hove et al. (eds.), *Distal Radius Fractures*,
DOI 10.1007/978-3-642-54604-4_46, © Springer-Verlag Berlin Heidelberg 2014

well as the TFCC and the IOM. Early recognition and treatment are critical for the best outcome. For a Galeazzi's fracture and an Essex-Lopresti injury, open surgery with stable fixation and postoperative immobilization for the ligaments to heal should be the treatment of choice.

46.2 Introduction

- Forearm rotation is necessary to use spears, axes, and knives, all activities that allowed hominids to evolve from a food gatherer to a food producer. "In primate evolution, the size of the brain and the opposable thumb have perhaps received the most attention in the literature, yet the significance of the distal radioulnar joint is possibly of equal, if not greater, significance in aspects differentiating the most highly developed hominids" (Almquist 1992).
- When falling on an outstretched hand/arm, the person falling could sustain a variety of different (soft tissue or bony) injuries of the hand and forearm.
- Any untreated injury of the forearm could leave a person with a painful and restricted movement of the forearm giving a reduction in quality of life.
- Early recognition and treatment are critical for successful treatment and the best result.

46.3 Anatomy

- The proximal part of the radius, the head, articulates with the capitulum humeri and the ulnar notch of the proximal part of the ulna. The annular ligament surrounds the radial head. These structures form the proximal radioulnar joint (PRUJ).
- The lower, wide part of the radius ends in the radial styloid on the lateral side, while the medial side has a concave sigmoid notch for articulation with the distal ulna (ulnar head). Together with the triangular fibrocartilage complex (TFCC), these structures basically form the distal radioulnar joint (DRUJ).
- The extensor carpi ulnaris tendon (ECU) and tendon sheath and the pronator quadratus (PQ) muscle are both dynamic stabilizers of the DRUJ. Other structures stabilizing the DRUJ are the TFCC, the bone, the ulnocarpal (UC) ligaments, the interosseous membrane and ligament (IOM and IOL), and the capsule.
- The IOM has oblique running fibers running from the radius in an ulnar and distal direction. The central part of the IOM, the IOL, has a width of 4–5 cm; the fibers fan out, the origin being approximately 8 cm distal of the PRUJ, the insertion 14 cm distal to the tip of the olecranon (Skahen et al. 1997).
- The rotation of the forearm takes place in the proximal radioulnar joint (PRUJ) and the distal radioulnar joint (DRUJ). These two joints should be looked upon as one joint, the "forearm joint" (Hagert 1994).

46.4 Biomechanics

- Approximately 80 % of the load that is transmitted across the wrist is transmitted across the radiocarpal joint.
- The IOM transmits load from the radius distally to the ulna proximally, the amount depending on the position of the elbow as well as the relative length of the forearm bones due to injuries, fractures, surgical procedures, or individual variance of the bones.
- The IOL behaves biomechanically like a ligament, has material properties like the patellar tendon and stiffness comparable to the ACL, and will fail at a load of 250–1,000 N.
- Without the IOM there is no load transfer between the radius and the ulna.
- Normally, the radial head serves as the primary restraint to proximal migration of the radius.
- After radial excision, the IOL (71 %) and the TFCC (8 %) resist axial shear and prevent proximal migration.

46.5 Pathomechanics

- When a person falls on an extended wrist, the hand will be fixed against the ground. Increasing axial and rotational load is applied to the wrist,

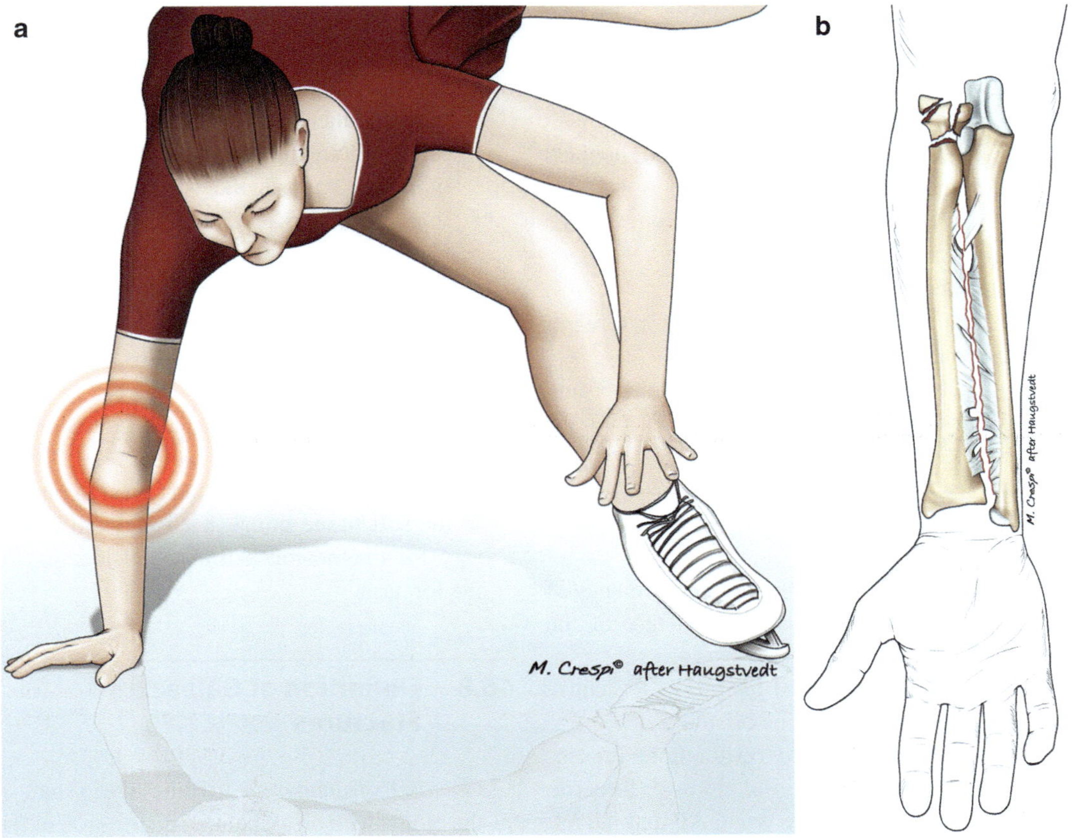

Fig. 46.1 Pathomechanics of a dislocation fracture of the forearm. (**a**) The hand is fixed to the ground, the force is transmitted over the wrist to the radius, and with an intact interosseous membrane, the force is transferred to the ulna. (**b**) With increasing force, the distal ulna will displace in a distal direction and the interosseous membrane will rupture from proximally on the radial side to distally on the ulnar side. A fracture-dislocation of the forearm may occur (see text)

forearm, and elbow. The load is transferred to the radius being stabilized between the elbow and the ground. With an intact IOM, this leads to a higher force to the proximal ulna that will not displace in a proximal direction; however, the ulnar column will displace toward the ground causing tension in the IOM, leading to an ulnar shaft fracture of joint disruption.

- The IOM is torn from the proximal radius to the distal ulna following the orientation of the fibers of the IOM.
- The pattern shows the lesion on the radial side of the forearm being more proximal to the lesion on the ulnar side.
- The proximal displacement of the radius depends on the force of injury and the position of the arm at the time of the impact (Hotchkiss 1994).
- There is probably a continuum of injury from an isolated fracture of the radial head to the more advanced fracture-dislocations that involve the PRUJ, DRUJ, as well as the IOM (Edwards and Jupiter 1988).
- Different people sustain different injuries due to the position of the wrist and elbow, the direction and action of the muscles, as well as the age of the person at the time of the impact.
- It should be noted that it has not been possible to reproduce a Galeazzi's fracture-dislocation in the laboratory by applying axial loading in a pronated forearm. Thus the true mechanism of injury remains uncertain.
- A direct blow to the forearm could cause a dislocation fracture of the forearm bones (Fig. 46.1).

46.6 Clinical Findings

- Swelling at the elbow, forearm, and/or the wrist
- Angular deformity of the forearm and dislocation of the ulnar head
- Open wound due to fractured forearm bones or dislocated joints
- Tenderness upon palpation
- Discomfort or pain when testing for forearm rotation and stability of the DRUJ
- Reduced range of motion of the elbow and wrist or forearm rotation

46.7 Imaging

- Anterior-posterior (AP) and lateral images of the elbow usually reveal the fracture of the radial head.
- Images (at least AP and lateral) of the entire forearm should always be obtained.
- The wrist may be asymptomatic upon presentation due to a more painful elbow or forearm. However, images of the wrist, AP and lateral, are mandatory.
- Any shortening of one forearm bone necessitates a fracture of the other bone or a dislocation at the proximal radioulnar joint (PRUJ) or the distal radioulnar joint (DRUJ).
- Images of the contralateral, noninjured arm and wrist should always be taken for comparison. (Due to pain true 90–90 images of the wrist may be difficult to obtain. Be sure to have identical images of the noninjured side.)
- Always perform a CT scan when in doubt. This is important for verifying the extent and position of the fragments of a radial head fracture as well as verifying any dislocation of the DRUJ.
- Ultrasound and/or MRI could reveal the extent of the soft tissue injury, but is seldom necessary for diagnosing a fracture-dislocation of the forearm.

Tricks and Tips

Tricks and tips for diagnosing a fracture-dislocation of the forearm:

- Whenever seeing a patient with a forearm fracture, be suspicious of a possible dislocation of the PRUJ or DRUJ.
- Although the wrist is asymptomatic upon presentation, always examine for tenderness and instability.
- Always compare the injured side to the uninjured opposite side.
- Imaging of a forearm fracture should always include the wrist and the elbow. Images of the uninjured opposite side should always be obtained for comparison.

46.8 Definition of Galeazzi's Fractures

- *Galeazzi's fracture* is a fracture of the shaft of the radius with an associated dislocation of the DRUJ (Mikic 1975).
- There are several classification systems based on the distance from the fracture site to the styloid process of the radius or to the mid-articular surface of the distal radius. The fracture has also been referred to as "simple" or "complex" related to the stability of the DRUJ after fixation of the associated fracture.
- In children the DRUJ could be intact; however, a dislocation through the ulnar epiphysis could occur. This is sometimes referred to as a Galeazzi's equivalent lesion (Fig. 46.2).

46.9 Natural History of Galeazzi's Fractures

- If left untreated, or with insufficient reduction and stabilization, a deformity of the distal radius and the DRUJ will occur. This could give a shortening of the radius with angulation of the bone, prominence of the ulnar head with swelling, and tenderness of the wrist.

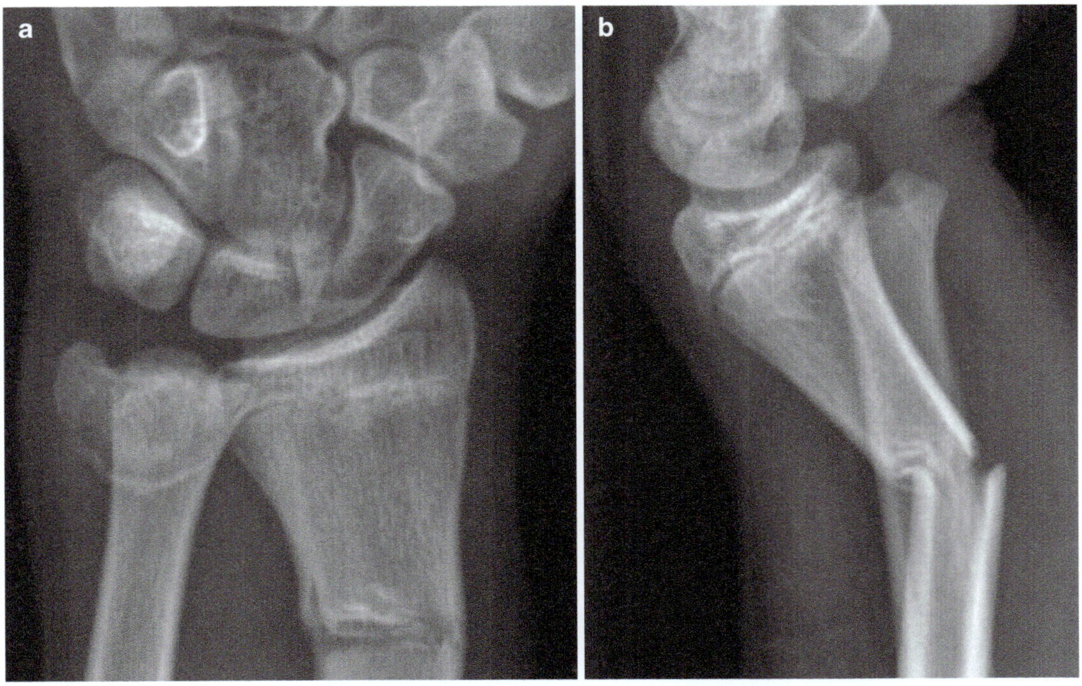

Fig. 46.2 In a child an equivalent to a Galeazzi's fracture lesion is a fracture of the radial shaft with separation of the distal ulnar epiphysis. (**a**) AP view. (**b**) Lateral view

46.10 Treatment of Galeazzi's Fractures

- In any fracture-dislocation of the forearm, open surgery should be the treatment of choice (Atesok et al. 2011).
- The exception to open surgery is Galeazzi's fracture-dislocations in children where treatment with closed reduction and a long arm cast is possible. (If interposed soft tissue prevents relocation, open reduction is necessary, however not necessarily requiring internal fixation.)
- In adults internal fixation with plate and screws should be the treatment of choice. In special cases such as open fracture-dislocations, external fixation and/or percutaneous pinning has been used.
- A volar approach to the radius is preferred for performing the osteosynthesis. Fluoroscopic guidance is necessary. When the internal fixation has been performed, intraoperative examination of the stability of the DRUJ should be done.
- When relocation of the DRUJ is not possible, exploration should be performed to remove interposed tissue (usually extensor tendons).
- If the DRUJ is unstable after fixation of the radial fracture, especially if the ulnar head can be translated dorsally out of the sigmoid notch with the forearm in supination, the DRUJ should be explored and the TFCC repaired.
- If found unstable, the DRUJ may be treated by transfixation of the ulna to the radius with a K-wire.
- If stability of the DRUJ is not achieved during surgery, postoperative treatment should include a long arm cast for 6–8 weeks with the forearm in a neutral or slight supinated forearm rotation (Fig. 46.3).

46.11 Results of Treatment of Galeazzi's Fractures

- Closed reduction and a long arm cast for 6 weeks give usually excellent results in children.

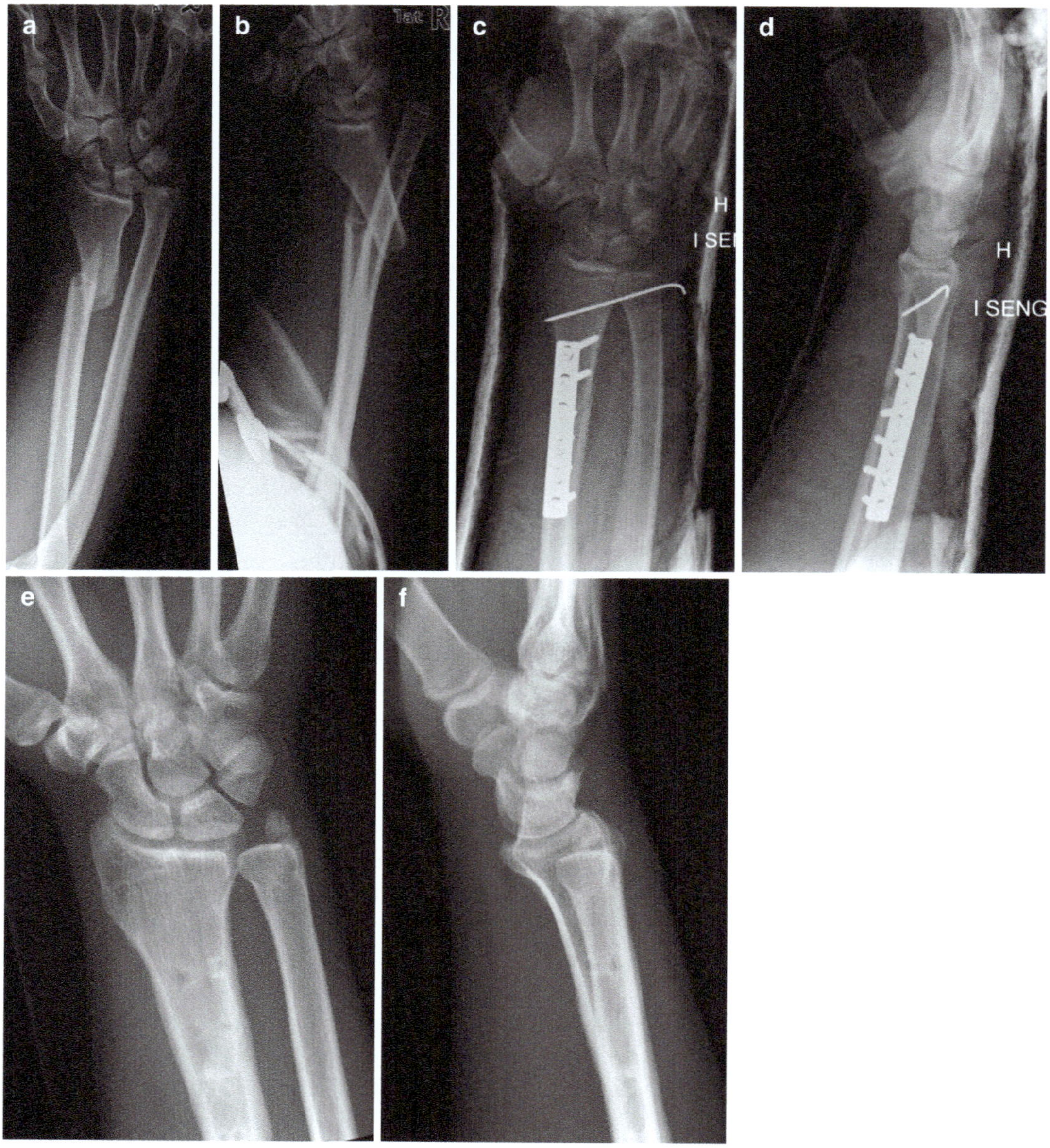

Fig. 46.3 A Galeazzi's fracture in a 23-year-old man. (**a**) AP view of the fracture. (**b**) Lateral view of the fracture. (**c**, **d**) Immediate postoperative views. (**e**, **f**) AP and lateral views after hardware removal 3 years after surgery

- Conservative treatment gives inferior results in adults.
- Open surgery with stabilization of the fracture, reduction of the dislocated DRUJ, and immobilization gives good results in adults (Reckling 1982).

46.12 Complications of Treatment of Galeazzi's Fractures

- Timing of surgery is of importance with inferior results for late treatment (more than 10 days) after injury.

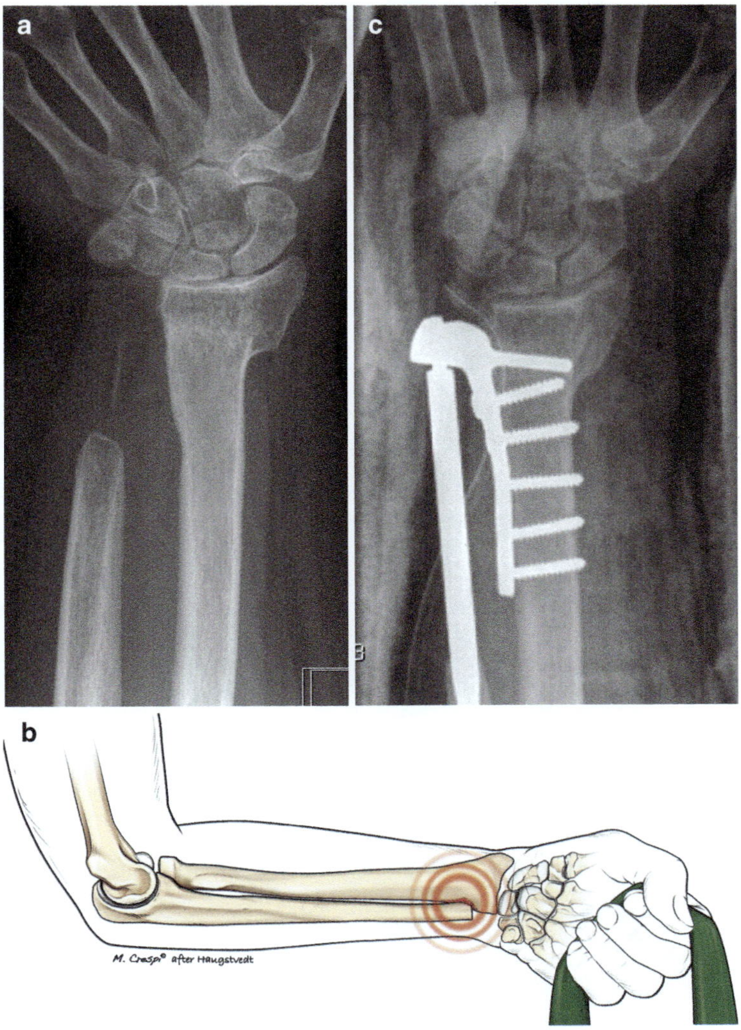

Fig. 46.4 (**a**) An old lady has had two Darrach's procedures before this picture was taken. She had temporarily relief of surgery; however, as the X-ray shows there is an impression on the radius at the level of the ulnar stump indicating impingement when she lifts her arm with a flexed elbow. (**b**) In a flexed elbow position, like the one in the figure, the radius is resting on the ulna. When the ulnar head has been removed, the radius will impinge with the stump of the ulna resulting in pain and discomfort. (**c**) The patient (in a) was finally relieved by stabilizing ulna using a semi-constrained custom made DRUJ prosthesis (see Chap. 42)

- Nonunion of the ulnar styloid has been reported, however shown to be of less importance for the final outcome.
- If anatomic reduction and rigid fixation of the radial fracture gives stability of the DRUJ, then the literature does not conclude that postoperative immobilization influences the result of treatment. However, if TFCC repair has been performed, if the DRUJ is unstable after fixation, or if a K-wire has been used for transfixation, postoperative immobilization with a long arm cast should be carried out.
- Instability, or a subluxation or dislocation of the DRUJ, could be the final result after a Galeazzi's fracture.

46.13 Treatment of Complications of Galeazzi's Fractures

- If the symptoms from the DRUJ are mild, a brace to support the wrist is helpful.
- If DRUJ symptoms persist reducing the patience's quality of life, an arthroscopic examination and treatment should be performed. This should include debridement of any synovitis and evaluation of TFCC and the distal radioulnar ligaments, followed by treatment/repair of any TFCC rupture or ligament reconstruction of any instability.
- Long-standing symptoms from permanent dislocation of the DRUJ are difficult to treat. Avoid

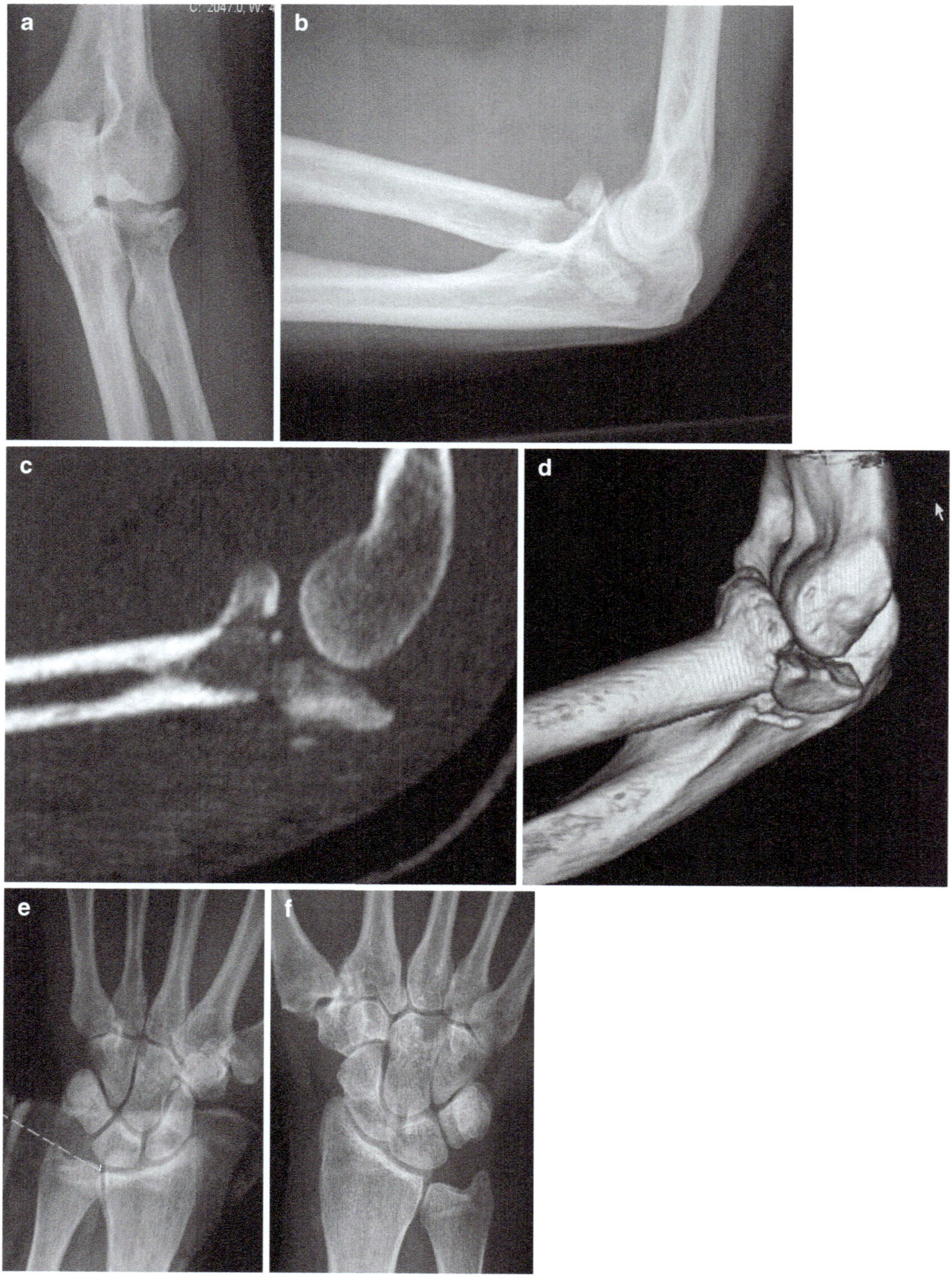

Fig. 46.5 A patient suffering from an Essex-Lopresti injury. The pictures display (**a**) AP view of the elbow and (**b**) a side view of the fracture of the radial head. (**c**, **d**) Demonstrate how a CT scan of the radial head fracture gives more information about the fracture fragments. (**e**, **f**) Show the wrist from the injured and noninjured arm. Observe the discrete ulnar plus variance found in (**e**) the injured side. This finding, combined with examination of both wrists, gives us information about the extent of the injury

any form of resection arthroplasty, Darrach or Sauve-Kapandji procedures, as these techniques will often give problems from an unstable distal end of the ulna impinging on the radius.

- If open surgical intervention is necessary, consider a DRUJ joint replacement (Fig. 46.4).

46.14 Definition of Essex-Lopresti Injuries

- Essex-Lopresti injury is a fracture through the radial head with dislocation of the DRUJ. There is a rupture of the IOM with instability of the forearm and the DRUJ (Essex-Lopresti 1951) (Fig. 46.5).

46.15 Natural History of Essex-Lopresti Injuries

- If left untreated gradual proximal migration of the radius will occur resulting in a positive ulnar variance, changes in the DRUJ, and possible changes in the elbow as well.
- The patient will suffer from swelling and tenderness of the wrist and the elbow, reduced forearm rotation, and ulnar deviation.

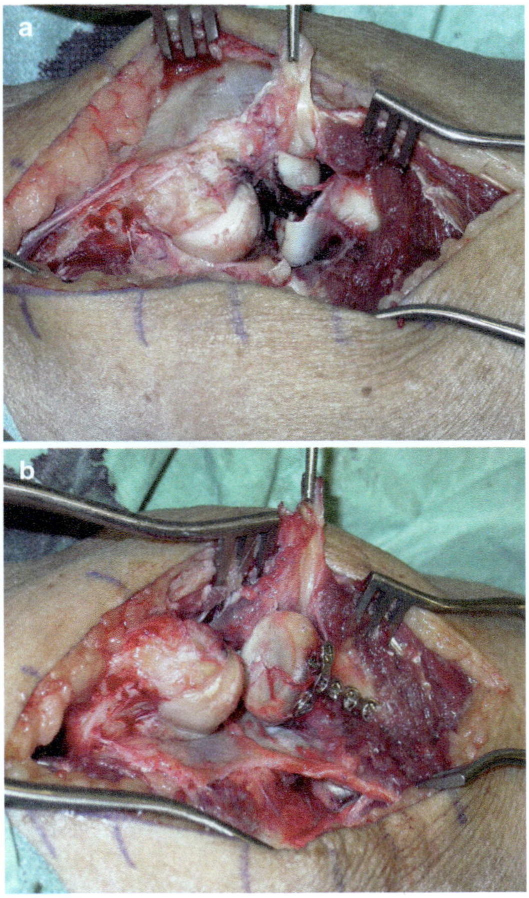

Fig. 46.6 Intraoperative pictures showing the fracture of the radial head before (**a**) and after (**b**) the osteosynthesis

46.16 Treatment of Essex-Lopresti Injuries

- In any fracture-dislocation of the forearm, open surgery should be the treatment of choice.
- When the extent of the injury is realized, one should address both the PRUJ and the DRUJ.
- The radial head should be repaired or, if not possible, replaced by radial head prosthesis to preserve the length of the radius to prevent proximal migration of the radius. The choice of prosthesis is less important than the fact that a spacer is inserted to restore radial length and possibly allowing the soft tissue to heal and become stabilized (Figs. 46.6 and 46.7).
- Acute repair of the IOM and IOL is usually not performed, as it may not be possible to approximate the edges of the membrane to allow for healing. If acute repair is thought of, a strong tendon (such as FCR) or a bone-tendon-bone graft harvested from the patellar tendon should be used (Hotchkiss 1994).
- The DRUJ is usually reduced when the PRUJ is stabilized. If relocation of a displaced DRUJ is not possible, open surgery should be performed to remove interposed soft tissue or bony fragments. When open surgery is performed, TFCC repair should be done.
- Transfixation of the ulna to the radius should be considered, especially if there are difficulties in keeping DRUJ in position. Immobilization in a long arm cast for 6–8 weeks is recommended to allow the extensive soft tissue and ligament injuries to heal.
- Forearm rotation should be permitted after 8 weeks when rehabilitation is started guided by a hand therapist.

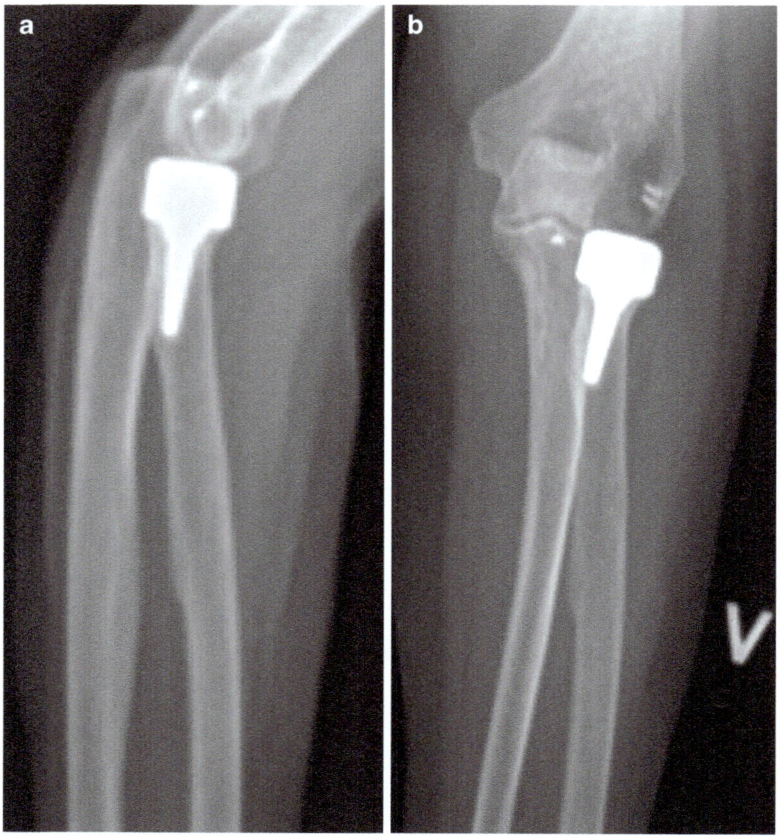

Fig. 46.7 If osteosynthesis of the radial head fracture is not possible, a radial head prosthesis should be inserted in order to keep intact the length of the radius while the soft tissue heals (**a**, **b**)

46.17 Results of Treatment of Essex-Lopresti Injuries

- The extent of the injury involving the PRUJ, DRUJ, and IOM leaves the surgeon with a challenge. There are no studies in the literature including a larger number of patients showing the results of different treatment options. Good results are reported when the radial head is preserved or replaced, steps are taken to prevent proximal migration of the radius, the DRUJ is relocated and stabilized, and the arm is immobilized for weeks.
- If osteosynthesis of the radial head is performed, pain and decreased range of forearm rotation could necessitate hardware removal.
- When a radial head implant has been inserted, silicone prostheses could fragment or break. A metal prosthesis has also possibilities for complications necessitating removal of the prosthesis. If the prosthesis has functioned as a “spacer” long enough for the soft tissue to heal or to stabilize, the prosthesis could simply be removed. The alternative, and probably a better option, is to replace it with a new prosthesis.

46.18 Complications of Treatment of Essex-Lopresti Injuries

- The best results are achieved if the surgery is performed early after the injury. Late surgery, delayed more than 4–6 weeks, gives worse results.

46.19 Treatment of Complications of Essex-Lopresti Injuries

- Upon removal of the radial head (or prosthesis), a gradual stretching of the IOM may occur with proximal migration of radius. This will lead to a positive ulnar variance

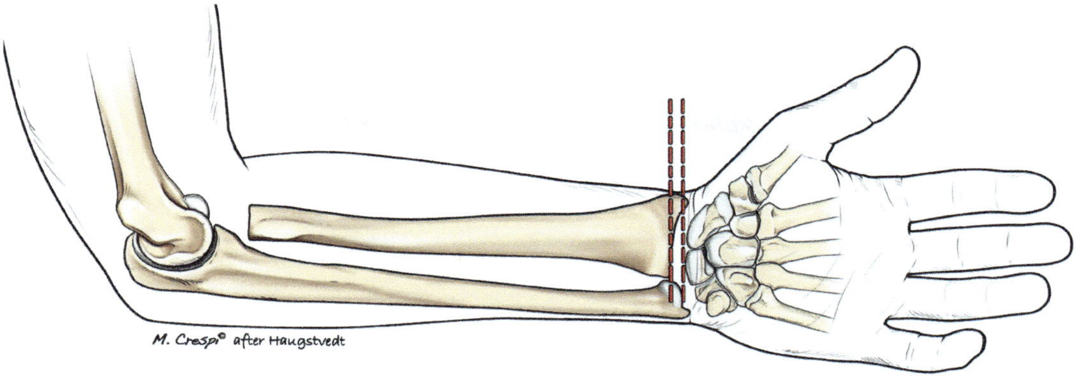

Fig. 46.8 Resection of the radial head will in most cases eventually lead to proximal migration of the radius resulting in a positive ulnar variance at the wrist. An ulnar shortening osteotomy will not solve the problem as the radius will again start migrating in the proximal direction unless a radial head replacement is performed (*dotted lines*). A resection of either the ulnar head (see Fig. 46.4b) or the radial should be performed with great caution

with symptoms from the ulnar side of the carpus. There is no simple solution to this problem. Ulnar shortening may sound tempting and will often relieve the patient's symptoms in the beginning; however, if there is no proximal stability between the proximal radius and capitulum humeri and the IOM is incompetent, the radius may shorten further starting a vicious cycle of proximal radius migration, distal ulnar shortening, etc. (Fig. 46.8).

- For chronic radioulnar longitudinal dissociation reconstruction, using a bone-patellar tendon-bone graft has been useful (Adams et al. 2010).
- Any symptoms from the DRUJ should be addressed in the same manner as described previously, in the Galeazzi part.

The best treatment for complications of fracture-dislocations is preventive.

References

Adams JE, Culp RW, Osterman AL. Interosseous membrane reconstruction for the Essex Lopresti injury. J Hand Surg Am. 2010;35(1):129–36.

Almquist EE. Evolution of the distal radioulnar joint. Clin Orthop Relat Res. 1992;275:5–13.

Atesok KI, Jupiter JB, Weiss AP. Galeazzi fracture. J Am Acad Orthop Surg. 2011;19(10):623–33.

Edwards Jr GS, Jupiter JB. Radial head fractures with acute distal radioulnar dislocation. Essex-Lopresti revisited. Clin Orthop Relat Res. 1988;234:61–9.

Essex-Lopresti P. Fractures of the radial head with distal radio-ulnar dislocation. Report of two cases. J Bone Joint Surg. 1951;33:244–7.

Hagert CG. Distal radius fracture and the distal radioulnar joint-anatomical considerations. Handchir Mikrochir Plast Chir. 1994;26(1):22–6.

Hotchkiss RN. Injuries to the interosseous ligament of the forearm. Hand Clin. 1994;10(3):391–8.

Mikic ZD. Galeazzi fracture-dislocations. J Bone Joint Surg. 1975;57:1071–80.

Reckling FW. Unstable fracture-dislocations of the forearm (Monteggia and Galeazzi lesions). J Bone Joint Surg. 1982;64:857–63.

Skahen 3rd JR, Palmer AK, Werner FW, Fortino MD. The interosseous membrane of the forearm: anatomy and function. J Hand Surg Am. 1997;22(6):981–5.

Distal Radius Fractures in Children

47

Per-Henrik Randsborg

Contents

P.-H. Randsborg, MD, PhD
Health Services Research Unit,
Akershus University Hospital, Oslo, Norway
e-mail: pran@ahus.no

47.1 Summary

Fractures of the distal radius are the most common fractures in children. Most fractures are buckle-type factures which are inherently stable and are treated with a removable splint for 3 weeks. Greenstick fractures are unstable and continue to displace also after the first week. To maintain reduction, a three-point molded plaster should be applied. Complete fractures are unstable, and percutaneous pinning is often necessary.

Because of the remodeling potential of the distal radius, displacement will often correct itself fully. Displacement of 25° in boys younger than 8 years and 20° in boys younger than 12 years is acceptable. The potential for remodeling is slightly less for girls since they reach puberty earlier.

Fractures of the physis are categorized according to the Salter-Harris or Peterson classifications. Type 2 fractures are the most common. Remodeling potential is great, and complications are rare. The risk of growth arrest increases if the fracture is reduced more than 3 days after injury or if reduction is repeated. Intra-articular physeal injuries should be anatomically reduced and secured with smooth pins. If possible the pins should avoid the physis to avoid risk of growth arrest.

Soft tissue is sometimes interposed in the fracture preventing reduction. To permit safe extraction of the interposed tissue, a volar approach is advised. Open fractures need formal debridement in the theater and stabilization with smooth pins. Prophylactic antibiotics and delayed suture

L.M. Hove et al. (eds.), *Distal Radius Fractures*,
DOI 10.1007/978-3-642-54604-4_47, © Springer-Verlag Berlin Heidelberg 2014

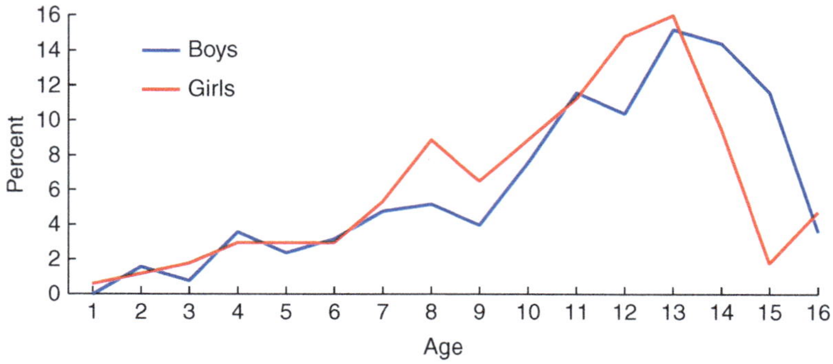

Fig. 47.1 The distribution of 419 distal radius fractures in children by age and gender (From Akershus University Hospital Fracture Register 2011)

should be considered according to the degree of the open fracture.

47.2 Epidemiology

Distal radius fractures are the most common fracture in childhood, representing 23–36 % of all childhood fractures (Brudvik and Hove 2003; Randsborg et al. 2013).

- These fractures are more common in boys.
- The nondominant arm is affected in about 60 % of cases.
- They occur at any age but are most common during the adolescent growth spurt (Fig. 47.1).
- The mean age for metaphyseal fractures are 10 years and 12 years for fractures involving the physis.
- The most common mechanism of injury is a fall on an outstretched hand.
- In Scandinavia the most common activities involved are football and ski (about 15 % each). 80 % of injuries happen outdoors.
- During the last half century, children in the Western world have enjoyed increasing prosperity, leisure time, and access to recreational and organized sport. During this increase in welfare, the number of fractures in children has increased enormously.
- In his classic study of 8,682 pediatric fractures, Lennart Landin reported a twofold increase in fracture rate between 1950 and 1979 (Landin 1983).
- The largest increase is seen in the incidence of fractures of the distal radius.

47.3 Diagnosis and Classification

47.3.1 Clinical Presentation

The patient presents a painful and often swollen distal radius. In cases with dislocation a classical dinner fork deformity such as seen in adults is often present. There is reduced range of movement in the wrist.

- Neurovascular deficits are rare (<1 %).
- Open fractures are also rare in childhood, but occasionally the proximal fragment can penetrate the thin volar skin.
- Smith's type (volar displacement of the distal fragment) is rare in childhood, but because of the high incidence, it is seen occasionally in busy fracture clinics.

47.3.2 Diagnosis

Anteroposterior and lateral radiographs are sufficient for diagnosis in the vast majority of cases.

- Only rarely, for intra-articular physeal fractures, are CT scans necessary to evaluate the articular surface, assisting preoperative planning.
- The articular surface is difficult to identify on plain radiographs, especially in younger children where the distal epiphysis has not yet ossified.
- To measure the degree of displacement caused by the fracture, the angle of the physis on the radial axis on the lateral radiograph is measured (Fig. 47.2). This angle is normally 90°

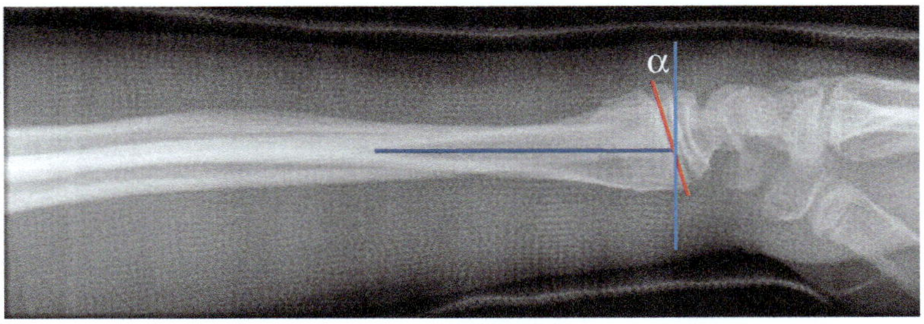

Fig. 47.2 Measuring the sagittal displacement of distal radius fractures in children by the method described by Lautman et al. The physis is normally 90° on the axis of the radius. *α* represents the degree of displacement caused by the fracture

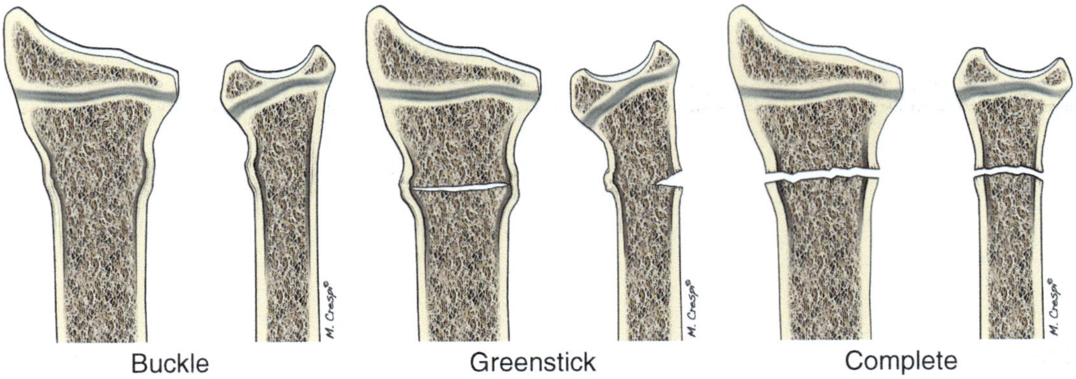

Fig. 47.3 Classification of metaphyseal fractures of the distal radius in children. Buckle, greenstick, and complete fractures. Buckle (torus) fractures are characterized by a compression failure of the bone without disruption of the cortex on the tension side of the bone. The greenstick fractures differ from the buckle fracture as the cortex is disrupted on the tension side but intact on the compression side of the fracture. Complete fractures (adult type) have disruption of both cortices in one plane

(Lautman et al. 2002), and any deviation from this is the displacement caused by the fracture.

47.3.3 Classification

The distal metaphysis of the radius is defined as the part of the bone that lays within a square, with the sides the length from the ulnar most point of the ulna to the radial styloid. Although this definition includes the physis, injuries to the growth plate are classified separately. Fractures of the distal metaphysis of the radius in children are commonly grouped into three categories (Fig. 47.3): buckle (or torus) fractures, greenstick fractures, and complete fractures.

- Buckle (torus) fractures are characterized by a compression failure of the bone without disruption of the cortex on the tension side of the bone.
- The greenstick fractures differ from the buckle fracture as the cortex is disrupted on the tension side, but intact on the compression side of the fracture.
- Complete fractures (adult type) have disruption of both cortices in one plane.

The follow-up algorithm of these different categories varies; thus the classification will provide guidelines for management and prognosis. The distribution of fracture types is demonstrated in Table 47.1 and examples are presented in Fig. 47.4.

Injuries to the physis have traditionally been classified according to the Salter-Harris classification, introduced in 1963 (Salter and Harris 1963). Hamlet Peterson challenged this system in 1994, questioning the existence of the Salter-Harris type V, while adding two other fracture patterns in his new classification of physeal injuries (Peterson 1994). The Salter-Harris classification is still the dominant system, but the Peterson system has introduced a new type I fracture which is a transmetaphyseal fracture with an extension to the physis, which has some clinical relevance and should therefore be kept in mind. Both classifications are demonstrated and compared in Fig. 47.5.

Table 47.1 Distribution of fracture types in 301 distal radius fractures in children

Fracture type	No (%)
Buckle	208 (69.1)
Greenstick	44 (14.6)
Complete	17 (4.7)
Physeal	32 (10.6)

From Akershus University Hospital, Norway (Randsborg and Sivertsen 2009)

47.4 Management of Metaphyseal Fractures

47.4.1 Buckle Fractures

Buckle (or torus) fractures are inherently stable fractures (Randsborg and Sivertsen 2009).

- Several studies have demonstrated that these fractures do not need clinical or radiological follow-up.
- The management consists of applying a splint for comfort which can be removed by the parents after 3 weeks (Plint et al. 2006).
- Most fractures of the distal radius in children are buckle fractures, and many unnecessary visits to the fracture clinic can be avoided by identifying these fractures on the first visit.

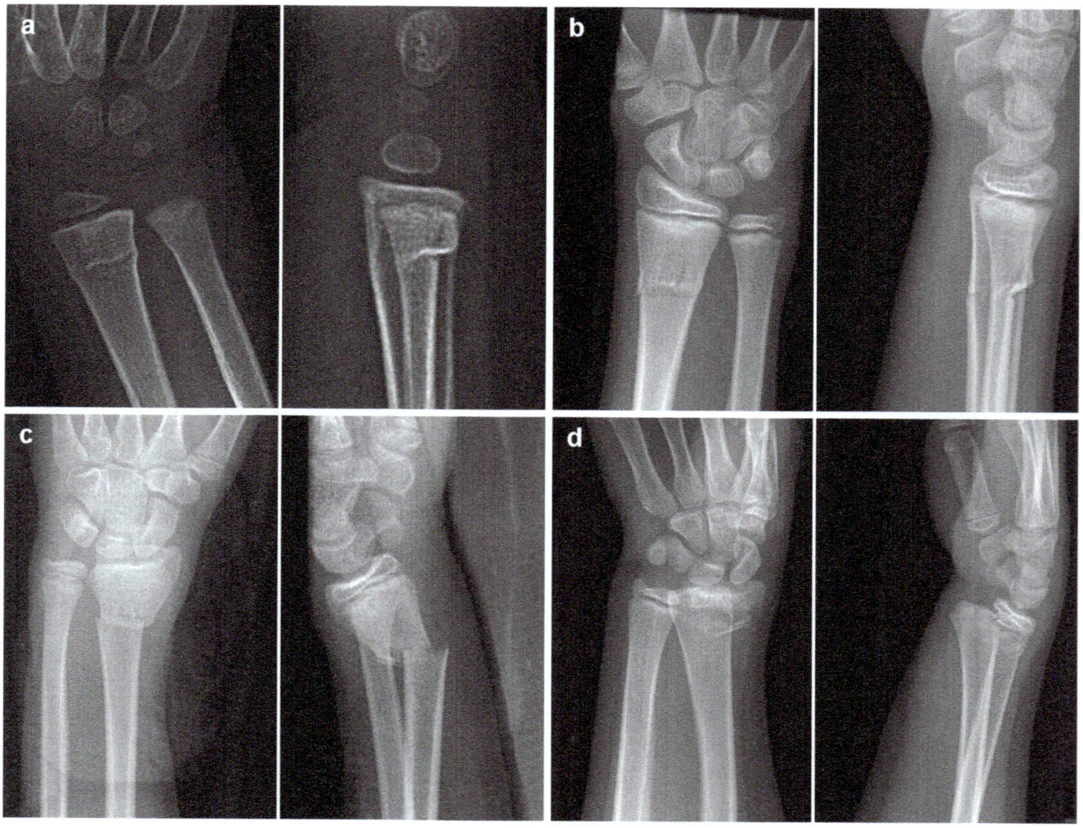

Fig. 47.4 Examples of fractures from the four categories: (**a**) buckle (torus) fracture, (**b**) greenstick fracture, (**c**) complete fracture, and (**d**) physeal fracture (From Randsborg and Sivertsen (2012), Reprinted with permission from BioMed Central Musculoskeletal Disorders)

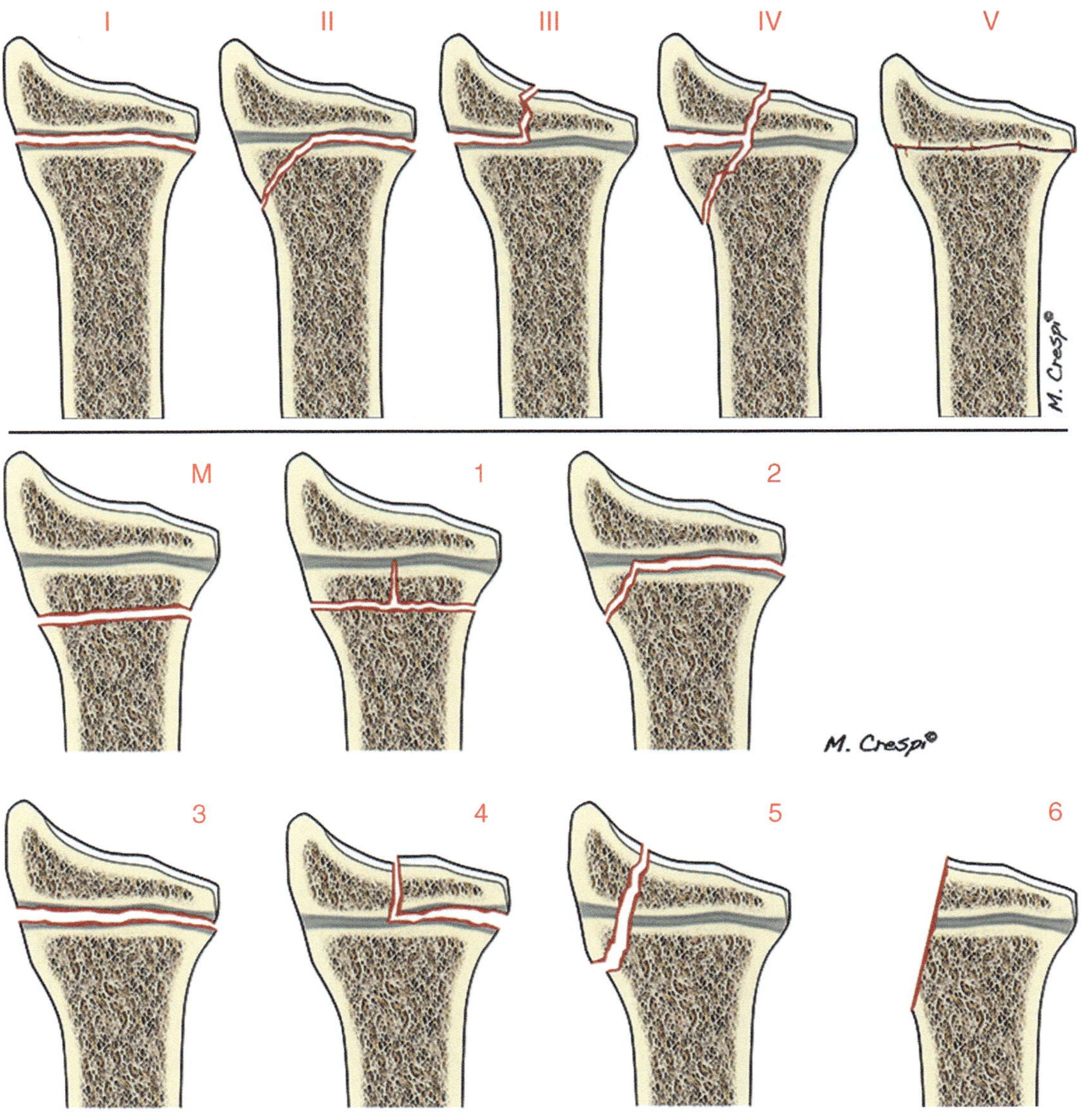

Fig. 47.5 Classification of physeal injuries according to the Salter-Harris system (*top row*) and Peterson system (*lower two rows*). Type 2 (same in both systems) is the most common type in the distal radius. Note that the category M in the Peterson classification system is not a physeal injury

47.4.2 Greenstick Fractures

Greenstick fractures are, however, unstable. Moreover, they continue to displace also after the first 2 weeks (Fig. 47.6) (Randsborg and Sivertsen 2009). Unfortunately, it is difficult to identify which fractures will displace beyond 20°.

- Fractures with acceptable angulation (Table 47.2) are managed in a short cast for 4–5 weeks (longer immobilization for older children).
- They should be reviewed after 1 week.
- Surgical management consists of closed reduction with or without percutaneous pinning.
- It is difficult to assess the stability perioperatively, and it is therefore wise to have a low threshold for pinning.
- The pins are left proud of the skin to facilitate removal without the need for a second general anesthetic.

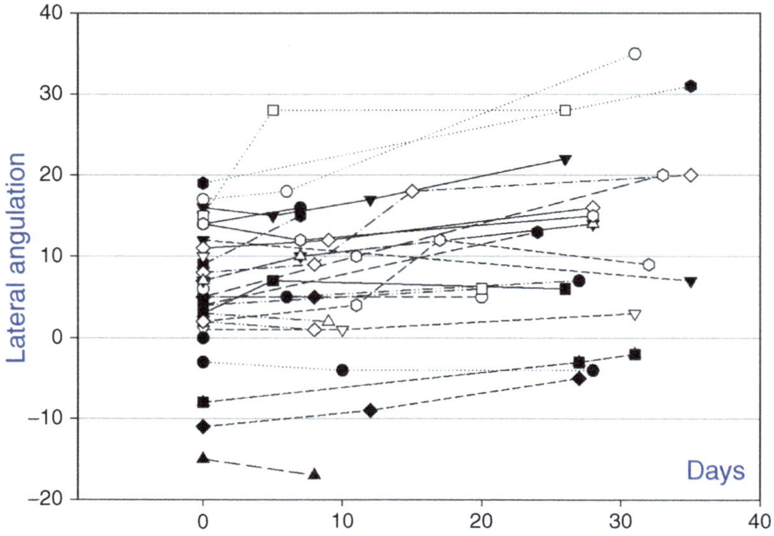

Fig. 47.6 Lateral angulation during the immobilization period in plaster of unreduced greenstick fractures. Note the tendency of the lateral angulation to increase throughout the period. The various geometric figures represent different fractures followed over time (*x-axis*) with lateral angulation measured on repeat radiographs (*y-axis*)

Table 47.2 Limits of angulation of distal radius metaphyseal fractures that will lead to anatomic remodeling

Age	Sagittal plane		Frontal plane
	Boys	Girls	
0–7	25°	20°	10°
8–12	20°	15°	5°
>13	10°	0	0

47.4.3 Complete Fractures

Complete fractures (also sometimes referred to as "adult-type" fractures) are highly unstable.

- Percutaneous pinning to stabilize the fragments should be considered also for fractures with acceptable angulation (Fig. 47.7).
- Conservative managed complete fractures of the distal radius should be reviewed at day 5 or 10 radiologically and clinically, and displacement should initiate surgical consideration.
- Complete fractures are immobilized for 5–6 weeks.

47.4.4 Conservative Management

When managing a distal radius fracture without surgical fixation, i.e., conservatively, the goals are to immobilize the fracture and maintain the reduction. When the cortex is disrupted on the distraction side of the fracture (greenstick), the fracture tends to displace to end up in its originally displaced position.

- It is therefore of paramount importance that the plaster is applied appropriately to counteract the displacing forces.
- A proper three-point molded plaster will help maintain reduction. This is the art of conservative management, which should not be forgotten (Fig. 47.8).
- Avoid the common mistake to apply the distal pressure too distally, so that the wrist joint is flexed, causing pain and discomfort.
- The cast index (CI), as proposed by Chess et al. (1994), is a useful tool to assess how well the plaster is molded.
- The CI is the ratio between the internal width of the cast in the sagittal plane and the width of the cast at the coronial plane at the fracture site.
- A CI >0.8 increases the risk of redisplacement of the fracture.

47.4.5 Operative Management

The most common method of surgical fixation is by smooth pins that are inserted percutaneously or via a mini incision to protect the dorsal tendons and sensory branch of the radial nerve.

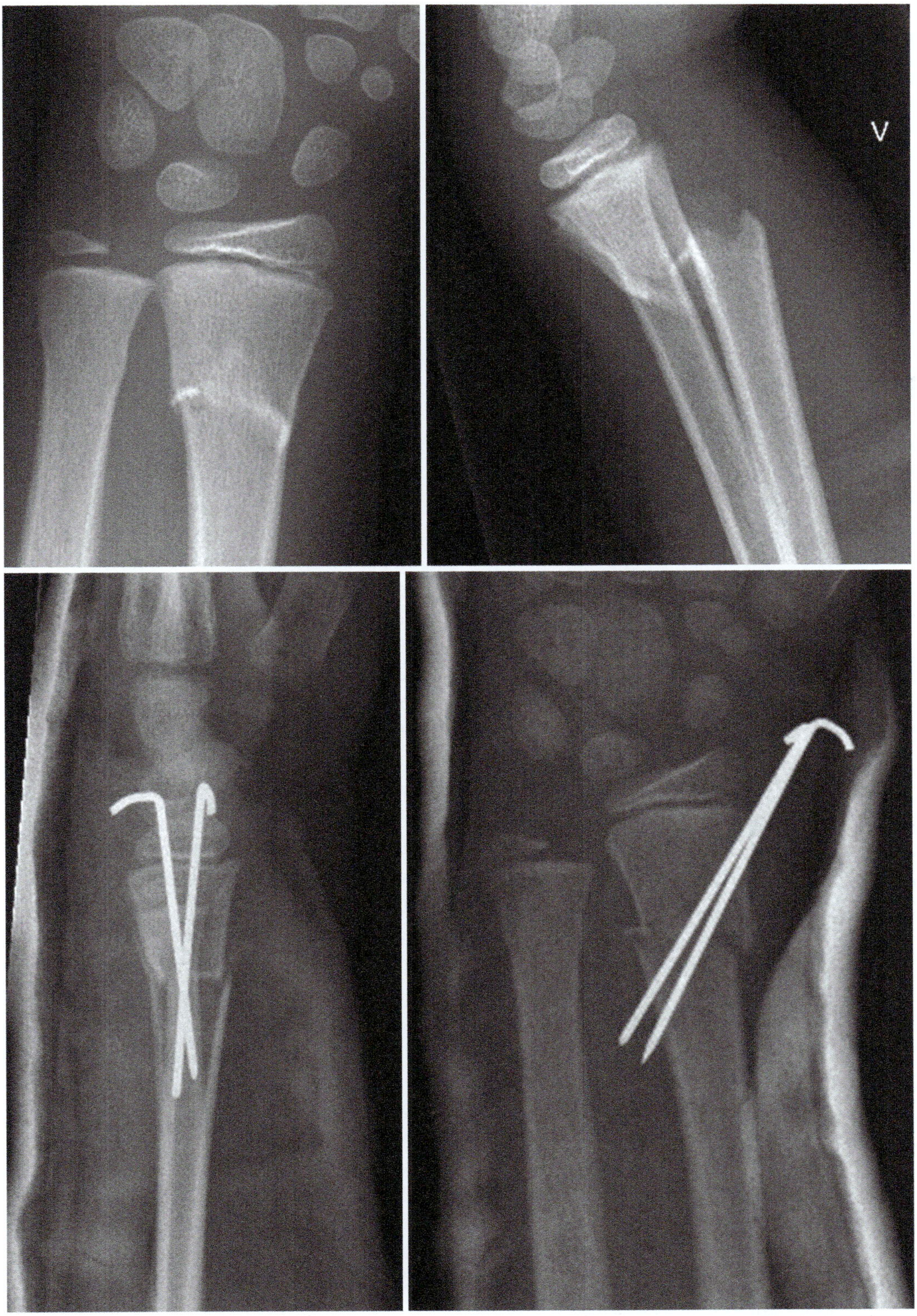

Fig. 47.7 A complete fracture in an 8-year-old boy, managed with closed reduction and percutaneous pinning. Note that the pins avoid the physis

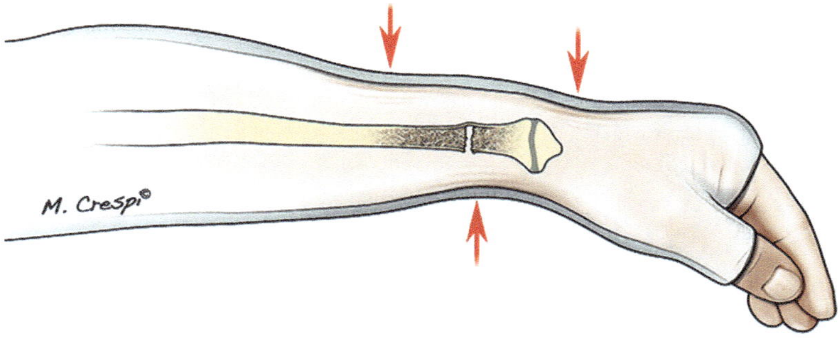

Fig. 47.8 A bent plaster makes a straight bone. Application of a three-point molded plaster counteracts the displacing forces and helps maintain reduction. In a volarly displaced fracture (Smith's type), the molding should be reversed, i.e., two pressure points volarly and one dorsally

- If at all possible it is preferable to avoid passing the pins through the growth plate.
- For some comminuted, highly unstable fractures, a plate fixation can be considered.
- External fixation is not used to the same degree as for adults, but might be an option for unstable open fractures, especially in multitrauma.
- Open reduction is indicated for all open factures.
- The wound should be extended in both directions and formally irrigated in the operation theater.
- The fracture should be reduced anatomically and stabilized, normally with two crossed pins.
- Prophylactic antibiotics and delayed primary suture should be considered according to the severity of the compound fracture.
- Open reduction is also indicated for irreducible fractures. The irreducibility might be caused by interposed soft tissue such as the muscle, periosteum, tendons, or rarely neurovascular structures. A dorsal mini incision permits the introduction of a lever to assist reduction (Fig. 47.9), but does not give appropriate overview of the interposing tissues.
- A formal volar approach is recommended for irreducible fractures to permit safe extraction of the interposed soft tissues, especially in neurovascular compromised cases.

47.4.6 Complications and Remodeling

Complications after metaphyseal fractures of the distal radius are rare and mostly transient, such as stiffness and pressure sores from the plaster.

- Since greenstick and complete fractures displace during the immobilization period, malunion at the time of removal of the plaster is not uncommon.
- However, the distal radius exhibits an amazing potential for remodeling (Fig. 47.10).
- In children under 5 years, sagittal plane angulation up to 35° can remodel completely.
- In patients younger than 10 years, up to 25° of lateral angulation is acceptable (Friberg 1979; Johari and Sinha 1999; Wilkins 2005).
- Excellent long-term functional and anatomic results have been reported (Hove and Brudvik 2008).

Because of this wonderful ability to remodel, it is difficult to agree on strict recommendations for when a displaced fracture is in need for reduction and consequently on follow-up routines. If displaced greenstick factures of the distal radius remodel over time, it can be argued that immobilization alone is sufficient. However, little is known about the consequences of a bent wrist on the physical activity of children, even if it is transient. The degree of acceptable angulation diminishes as the child approaches puberty. Since girls reach puberty before boys, the acceptable lateral displacement is greater for boys than for girls (Table 47.2).

47.5 Management of Physeal Fractures

47.5.1 Management

Most physeal fractures can be managed conservatively in a plaster for 3–5 weeks. The limits of

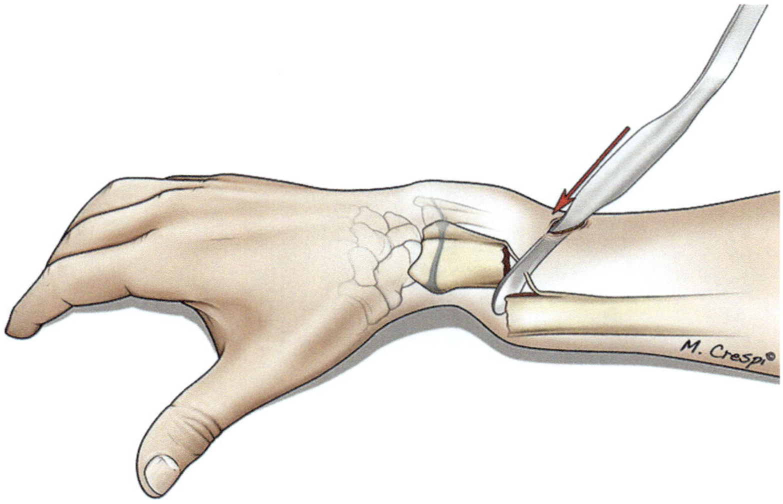

Fig. 47.9 The pin leverage technique is useful to assist a difficult reduction. A small dorsal incision permits the insertion of a lever which assists the reduction

acceptable angulation or dislocation are difficult to agree on because of the tremendous remodeling potential of the distal physis.

- Peterson recommended gentle closed reduction for Peterson type 1 and 2 fractures with more than 10° displacements in the lateral view (Fig. 47.11).
- For Peterson type 3 (corresponding to Salter-Harris type 1) reduction is recommended if the physis is displaced more than 50 % or if the tilted epiphysis is riding upon the metaphysis, causing damage to the physis which might lead to premature growth arrest.
- The intra-articular Salter-Harris type 3 and 4 fractures (Peterson type 4 and 5) often need surgery because the joint surface must always be reduced anatomically.
- A step in the joint surface indicates indirectly that the physis is displaced, and growth disturbances are common after these injuries.
- An anatomic reduction will therefore not only secure a congruent joint but also reduce the risk of premature growth arrest.
- Intra-articular fractures are difficult to maintain reduced by closed means, and pinning is often necessary.
- When a physeal fracture needs reduction, the manipulation should be done carefully without the use of excessive force to avoid iatrogenic injury to the growth plate.
- The patient must be comfortable and relaxed, and general anesthesia is often necessary.
- It is acceptable to place a smooth K-wire through the physis to stabilize the reduction, but repeat drilling through the growth plate must be avoided.
- There is some evidence to suggest that closed reduction and percutaneous pinning (CRPP) reduce the risk of growth disturbance, possibly because it stabilizes the physis and prevents harmful movement of the fragments.
- On the other hand, pinning through the physis may cause growth disturbance, so when possible the fracture should be stabilized by pins that avoid the physis (if the metaphyseal fragment is big enough). In Peterson type 4 fractures a transversely placed pin through the epiphysis is preferable, avoiding the physis.

47.5.2 Complications, Growth Arrest, and Remodeling

Complications following injuries to the distal radius physis are rare due to the great remodeling potential (Fig. 47.12). However, fractures involving the physis might lead to growth disturbances. The risk of distal radius growth arrest is esti-

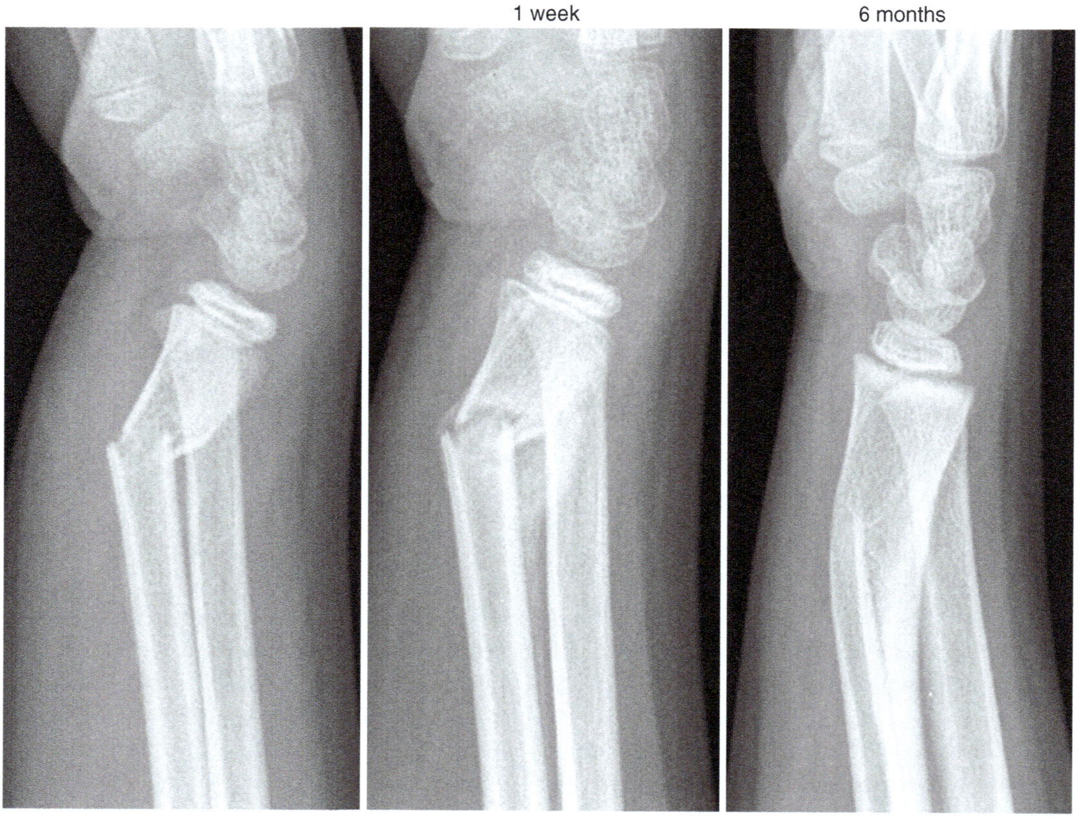

Fig. 47.10 Remodeling of a displaced, complete fracture in a 7-year-old girl

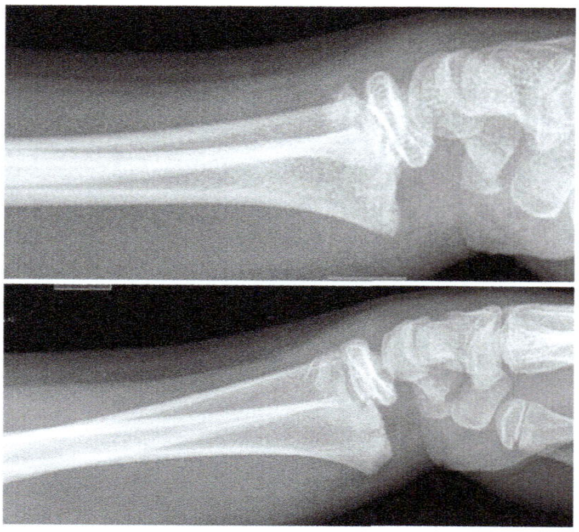

Fig. 47.11 Type 2 fractures with more than 10° of angulation or Peterson type 3 fractures with more than 50 % dislocation (or if the physis is riding on the metaphysis) should be managed by gentle closed reduction

mated to 4–5 % for displaced radial physeal fractures (Cannata et al. 2003).

- The risk of growth disturbances increases, however, if the fracture is reduced more than 3 days after the fracture or if repeat attempts of reduction are performed.
- Therefore, reduction should not be repeated if the position is lost during immobilization or if the patient presents several days after injury (Fig. 47.13).
- If the fracture is deemed unstable perioperatively during a closed reduction, percutaneous pinning is advised, even if it involves crossing the physis.

Complete growth arrest occurs when the entire radial physis closes. This leads to positive ulnar variance and radial deviation of the wrist and might contribute to degenerative changes in the

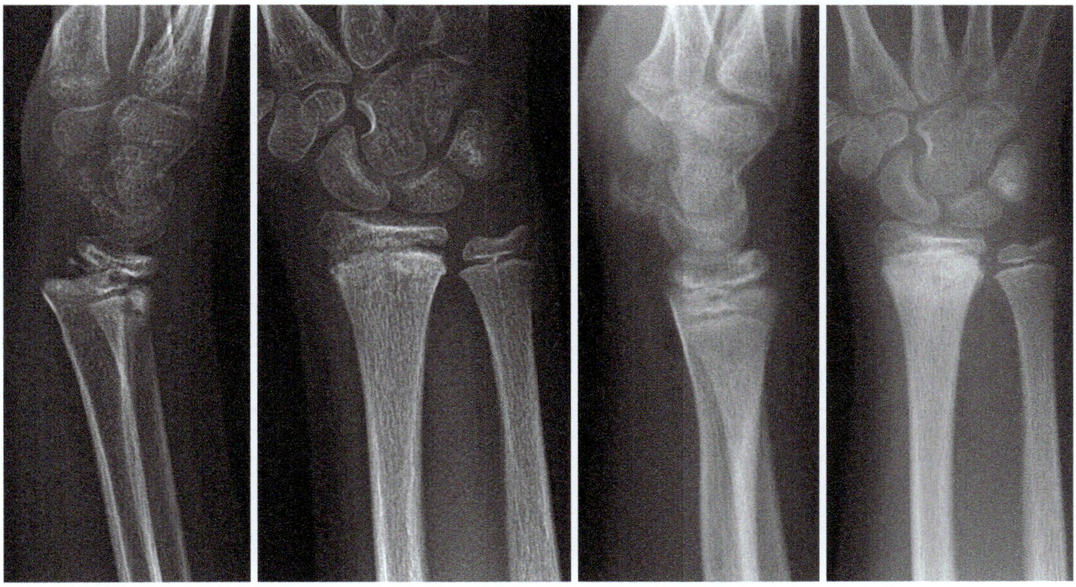

Fig. 47.12 This physeal fracture presented to the hospital over 2 weeks after the injury. It was left unreduced, and 14 months later it had completely remodeled without sign of growth disturbance

wrist later in life. The natural ulnar variance varies between individuals and between the dominant and nondominant hand. Measuring the ulnar variance in children is slightly different because of the open growth plates. In 1989 Hafner, Poznanski, and Donovan described a method which has become standard for skeletal immature patients (Fig. 47.14) (Hafner et al. 1989).

- The average ulnar variance is – 2 mm.
- Clinical deviation is not apparent before the relative radial shortening is >4 mm.
- If radial growth disturbances are discovered, early surgical closure of the distal ulna is indicated in children older than 8 years (Peterson 2007).
- In younger children, closure of the ulnar physis will lead to an unacceptable short forearm; therefore, radial lengthening should be considered, if necessary combined with ulnar arrest or shortening (Hove and Engesaeter 1997) (Fig. 47.15).

Partial growth arrest is a more complicated problem because it leads to deformity of the articular surface as well as positive ulnar variance. Partial growth arrest can be managed by bar resection if less than 40 % of the physis is affected. Resection of the affected physis will permit the physis to resume growth, but not at the same speed as the other wrist. Therefore, physiodesis of the ulna physis must also be considered to avoid positive ulnar variance. The timing for this procedure is difficult, and according to Hamlet Peterson, it is common to leave it for too long.

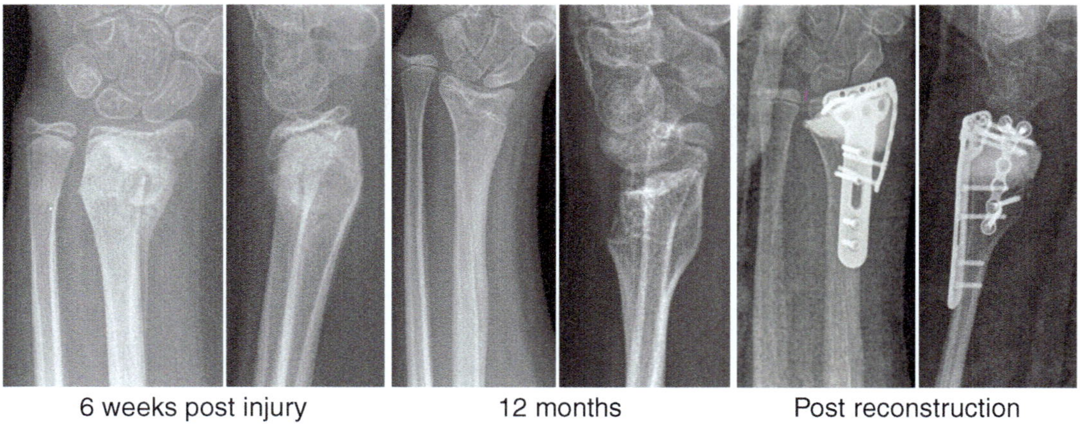

Fig. 47.13 Physeal arrest in a 12-year-old girl. The fracture was reduced on the day of injury and then re-manipulated 3 days after injury. One year later she had a cosmetic disturbing radial deviation of the wrist and positive ulnar variance. The radius was lengthened and the joint surface reconstructed

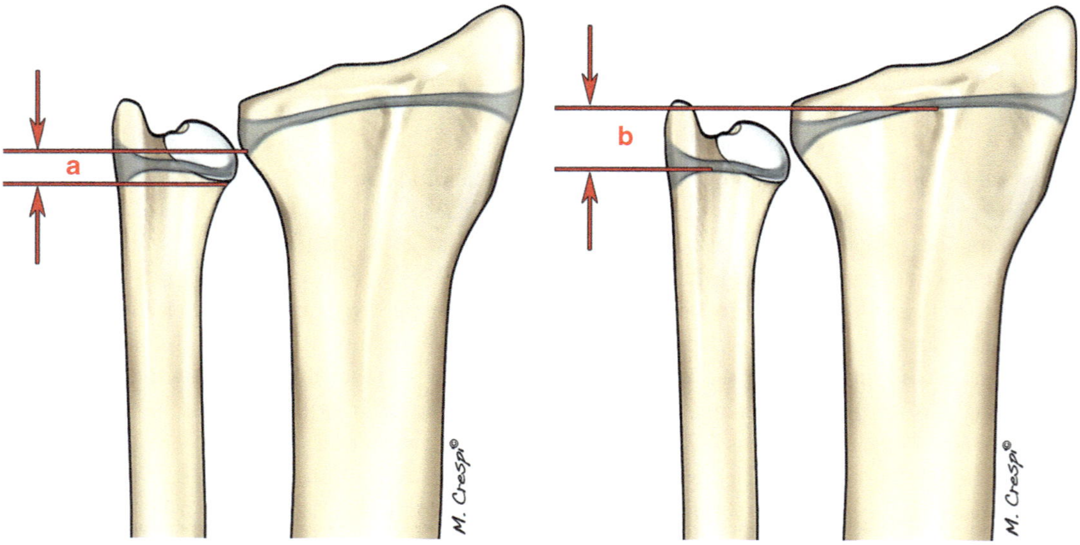

Fig. 47.14 Measuring ulnar variance. In children, the ulnar variance is measured by the Hefner method, which takes the difference between the physis of the ulna and the radius, measuring from either the most proximal (**a**) or the most distal (**b**) portion of the physis

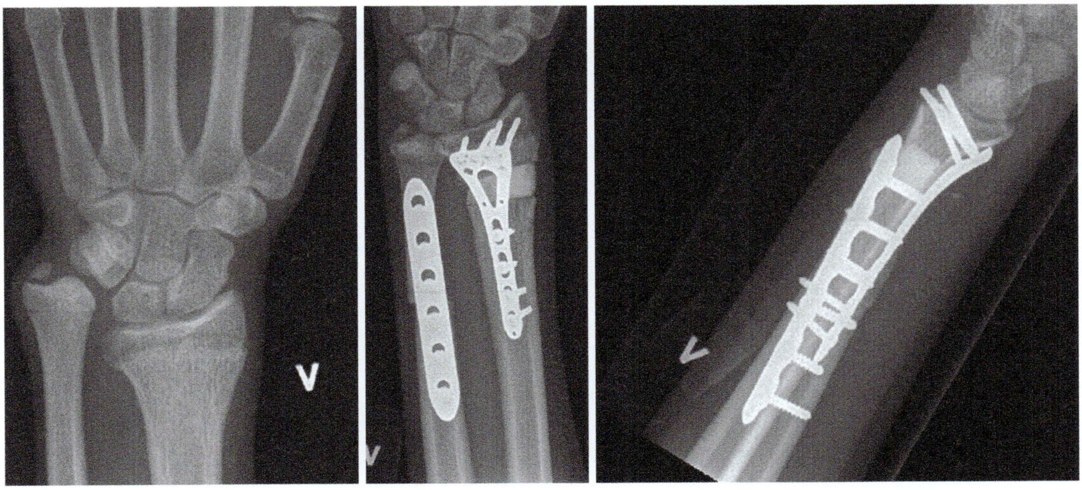

Fig. 47.15 A 16-year-old boy complained of gradual deviation of his left wrist. Radiographs demonstrated physeal arrest of the distal radius (*left*). He had several injuries to his wrist in the past, but had never seen a doctor or had a radiograph taken. The primary physeal injury was therefore not diagnosed or treated. The patient underwent radial lengthening combined with ulnar shortening when he reached skeletal maturity (Courtesy of Dr Ole Reigstad, Rikshospitalet, Oslo, Norway)

References

Brudvik C, Hove LM. Childhood fractures in Bergen, Norway: identifying high-risk groups and activities. J Pediatr Orthop. 2003;23(5):629–34.

Cannata G, De Maio F, Mancini F, Ippolito E. Physeal fractures of the distal radius and ulna: long-term prognosis. J Orthop Trauma. 2003;17(3):172–9.

Chess DG, Hyndman JC, Leahey JL, Brown DC, Sinclair AM. Short arm plaster cast for distal pediatric forearm fractures. J Pediatr Orthop. 1994;14(2):211–3.

Friberg KS. Remodelling after distal forearm fractures in children. II. The final orientation of the distal and proximal epiphyseal plates of the radius. Acta Orthop Scand. 1979;50(6 Pt 2):731–9.

Hafner R, Poznanski AK, Donovan JM. Ulnar variance in children–standard measurements for evaluation of ulnar shortening in juvenile rheumatoid arthritis, hereditary multiple exostosis and other bone or joint disorders in childhood. Skeletal Radiol. 1989;18(7):513–6.

Hove LM, Brudvik C. Displaced paediatric fractures of the distal radius. Arch Orthop Trauma Surg. 2008;128(1):55–60.

Hove LM, Engesaeter LB. Corrective osteotomies after injuries of the distal radial physis in children. J Hand Surg Br. 1997;22(6):699–704.

Johari AN, Sinha M. Remodeling of forearm fractures in children. J Pediatr Orthop B. 1999;8(2):84–7.

Landin LA. Fracture patterns in children. Analysis of 8,682 fractures with special reference to incidence, etiology and secular changes in a Swedish urban population 1950–1979. Acta Orthop Scand Suppl. 1983;202:1–109.

Lautman S, Bergerault F, Saidani N, Bonnard C. Roentgenographic measurement of angle between shaft and distal epiphyseal growth plate of radius. J Pediatr Orthop. 2002;22(6):751–3.

Peterson HA. Physeal fractures: Part 3. Classification. J Pediatr Orthop. 1994;14(4):439–48.

Peterson HA. Distal radius. In: Peterson HA, editor. Epiphyseal growth plate injuries. Berlin: Springer; 2007. p. 227–72.

Plint AC, Perry JJ, Correll R, Gaboury I, Lawton L. A randomized, controlled trial of removable splinting versus casting for wrist buckle fractures in children. Pediatrics. 2006;117(3):691–7.

Randsborg PH, Gulbrandsen P, Saltyte BJ, Sivertsen EA, Hammer OL, Fuglesang HF, Aroen A. Fractures in children: epidemiology and activity-specific fracture rates. J Bone Joint Surg Am. 2013;95(7):e421–7.

Randsborg PH, Sivertsen EA. Distal radius fractures in children: substantial difference in stability between buckle and greenstick fractures. Acta Orthop. 2009;80(5):585–9.

Salter RB, Harris WR. Injuries involving the epiphyseal plate. J Bone Joint Surg Am. 1963;45(3):587–622.

Wilkins KE. Principles of fracture remodeling in children. Injury. 2005;36 Suppl 1:A3–11.

Index

L.M. Hove et al. (eds.), *Distal Radius Fractures*,
DOI 10.1007/978-3-642-54604-4, © Springer-Verlag Berlin Heidelberg 2014

GPSR Compliance

The European Union's (EU) General Product Safety Regulation (GPSR) is a set of rules that requires consumer products to be safe and our obligations to ensure this.

If you have any concerns about our products, you can contact us on ProductSafety@springernature.com

In case Publisher is established outside the EU, the EU authorized representative is:

Springer Nature Customer Service Center GmbH
Europaplatz 3
69115 Heidelberg, Germany

Batch number: 10731332

Printed by Printforce, the Netherlands